MEDICAL RADIOLOGY
Diagnostic Imaging

Springer
Berlin
Heidelberg
New York
Hong Kong
London
Milan
Paris
Tokyo

M. Forsting (Ed.)

Intracranial Vascular Malformations and Aneurysms

From Diagnostic Work-Up to Endovascular Therapy

With Contributions by

C. Cognard · A. Dörfler · M. Forsting · W. Küker · L. Pierot · L. Spelle · I. Szikora
I. Wanke

Foreword by

K. Sartor

With 157 Figures in 587 Separate Illustrations, 16 in Color and 9 Tables

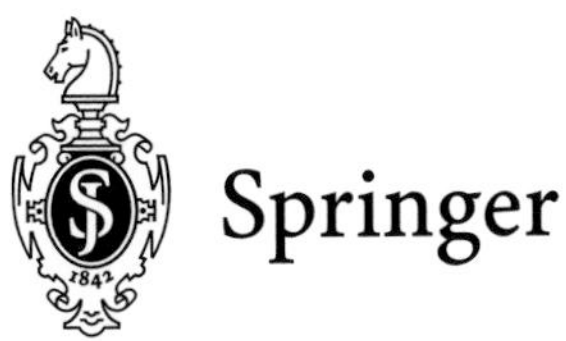

Springer

Michael Forsting, MD
Professor of Neuroradiology
Institute of Diagnostic and Interventional Radiology
Department of Neuroradiology
University of Essen
Hufelandstrasse 55
45122 Essen
Germany

Medical Radiology · Diagnostic Imaging and Radiation Oncology
Series Editors: A. L. Baert · L. W. Brady · H.-P. Heilmann · M. Molls · K. Sartor

Continuation of Handbuch der medizinischen Radiologie
Encyclopedia of Medical Radiology

ISBN 3-540-42430-X Springer-Verlag Berlin Heidelberg New York

Library of Congress Cataloging-in-Publication Data

Intracranial vascular malformations and aneurysms : from diagnostic work-up to endovascular therapy / M. Forsting (ed.) ; with contributions by C. Cognard ... [et al.] ; foreword by K. Sartor.
p. ; cm. -- (Medical radiology)
Includes bibliographical references and index.
ISBN 354042430X (hardcover : alk. paper)
1. Intracranial aneurysms. 2. Subarachnoid hemorrhage. 3. Diagnostic Imaging. I. Forsting, M. (Michael), 1960- II. Cognard, C. (Christophe) III. Series.
[DNLM: 1. Intracranial Arteriovenous Malformations--diagnosis. 2. Diagnostic Imaging. 3. Intracranial Aneurysms--diagnosis. 4. Intracranial Aneurysm--therapy. 5. Intracranial Arteriovenous Malformations--therapy. WL 355 I615 2003]
RD594.2 .I586 2003
616.1'33--dc21 2002075766

Springer-Verlag is part of Springer Science+Business Media

http//www.springeronline.com

Printed in Germany

Cover-Design and Typesetting: Verlagsservice Teichmann, 69256 Mauer

21/3150xq – 5 4 3 2 1 0 – Printed on acid-free paper

Foreword

The radiology of vascular malformations and aneurysms is intimately related to the evolution of magnetic resonance (MR) imaging, digital subtraction angiography (DSA) and catheter-based endovascular therapy. Prior to the advent of MR imaging radiologists knew little of so-called venous angiomas (today: developmental venous anomalies), cavernous hemangiomas (cavernomas) or capillary teleangiectasias, as most of these angiodysplasias could not be diagnosed reliably by computed tomography (CT) or invasive angiography, let alone the earlier encephalographic techniques with positive or negative contrast. But only after MR imaging at field strengths of 1 T or higher had become standard did it become clear how common these aberrations of vascular development actually are, in particular cavernomas and developmental venous anomalies. This surprised even the pathologists and again required the radiologists to learn more about these anomalies and abnormalities, such as their pathogenesis, histopathology, epidemiology, genetics, and natural history, including their propensity to bleed. It also required them to be able to differentiate these angiodysplastic lesions from non-vascular lesions of potentially graver significance.

Advanced knowledge regarding vascular malformations and aneurysms is now there, but the interested radiologist is still forced to gather it from multiple sources, mostly original articles in journals, treatises on specific topics, and other publications of a more or less limited scope. This is why Michael Forsting, a neuroradiological "all-rounder" with a strong bent towards and considerable experience in minimally invasive endovascular therapy of intracranial vascular abnormalities, has put great effort into producing a book that condenses the existing information in one handy volume. In doing so he has been helped by members of his department at University of Essen as well as by friends and colleagues from leading neuroradiologic institutes in several European countries.

What came out of this joint effort is a well-organized, beautifully illustrated monograph that leaves little to be desired: Whenever one is in need of concise, comprehensive clinical, diagnostic and (endovascular-) therapeutic information on intracranial vascular malformations and aneurysms – here it is. The book, rich in important facts, numbers and details, impresses perhaps most by its didactic structure and overall style. For this reason, I believe, it will quickly find a large readership among radiologists and neuroclinicians alike. Possibly quite a number of copies will end up on the desks of clinical pathologists who sometimes do envy us for the possibility to visualize and diagnose most brain lesions in vivo rather than in tabula.

Heidelberg

Klaus Sartor

Preface

Why a book about the diagnostic imaging and endovascular therapy of vascular malformations? There is a simple answer: This is a fascinating part of neuroradiology, it has many interdisciplinary aspects and it has become a large field of my and our professional life. The book should have been ready at least one year earlier, but there was always something new that had to be included. Still, I am sure, each reader will miss something he or she has just heard at a meeting or read in the current issue of a journal. On the other hand, there is already a wealth of established basic knowledge about diagnostic imaging and endovascular therapy that will not change fast and justifies writing a book instead of a review paper.

There are a lot of basics one should know about vascular malformations of the brain, and during our daily practice my colleagues and I see a lot of images and patients that do not have a proper diagnosis or have had a lengthy odyssey before finding an expert. We all hope that our book will find readers who are willing to go into this important aspect of radiology and will enable them to care for their patients in a professional way. And it is not only written for interventional neuroradiologists: it should be of interest for everybody working in "neuro-disciplines".

Although we belong to the younger generation of European neuroradiologists – we know that age is a moving target, but never mind – we chose not to write a modern book with colored "memory boxes" or other such aids, but an old-fashioned textbook. It is something to read at leisure – perhaps on a pleasant evening with a glass of red wine beside you - and memory will be supported by some redundancies and repetitions. Anyone in a hurry can run through the book just looking at the many images.

We invite all readers to help us improve the next edition. If something is good, let us know! More importantly, if something is not good or even wrong, please give us a call or send us an e-mail!

It was tough work, but finally we enjoyed it. We owe a debt of thanks to Ursula Davis of Springer-Verlag, who continuously pushed us to finalize it, always friendly and always stimulating.

Last but not least, a lot of people contributed substantially to this book without writing a chapter by themselves. They include my academic teachers Hermann Zeumer (Hamburg), Armin Thron (Aachen) and Klaus Sartor (Heidelberg), who gave the first impulse to write this book. I would like to thank them for supporting me during my whole professional career and for numerous stimulating discussions on vascular problems of the brain.

Essen MICHAEL FORSTING

Contents

1 Developmental Venous Anomalies

M. Forsting and I. Wanke

CONTENTS

In a typical neurovascular working day, developmental venous anomalies (DVAs) are causing a lot of confusion. In part, this confusion is related to the term "venous angioma", which is used in many institutions as a synonym for DVA! But, "venous angioma" is clearly a misnomer, because the term "angioma" usually suggests a severe disease with a substantial risk of bleeding. In contrast, DVAs must be considered as unusual, but nonpathological, venous drainage and an embryologically determined variant of venous drainage. On the other hand: DVAs are considered to be the most common form of cerebral vascular malformations, occurring in up to 4% of the population (Garner et al. 1991; Ostertun and Solymosi 1993; Truwit 1992). This high incidence is a good reason to familiarize oneself with these lesions and keep abreast of new findings in this area.

In my experience, another factor contributing to the DVA-related confusion is that many radiologists and clinicians just see abnormal vessels on magnetic resonance imaging (MRI) scans, immediately tell the patient something about a vascular malformation, and refer the patient for neurosurgical extirpation of the lesion.

To avoid too much irritation, specifically within the group of referring doctors, the term "venous angioma" should be avoided and DVA should be used. However, if you are reporting about a DVA, it is usually necessary to explain what this is. And this is a good reason to read the upcoming chapter.

M. Forsting, MD, PhD; I. Wanke, MD
Institute of Diagnostic and Interventional Radiology, Department of Neuroradiology, University of Essen, Hufelandstrasse 55, 45147 Essen, Germany

1.1 Pathology

The pathogenesis of a DVA is still unknown. Saito and Kobayashi et al. (1981) hypothesized that an intrauterine event during formation of the medullary veins or tributaries induces the formation of collateral venous drainage pathways. This hypothesis is supported by the absence of normal draining veins in the region of the large draining collector vein.

Another assumption is that an in-utero acquired venous occlusion maintains the intrinsic venous anastomoses within the white matter. The DVA then expresses an early collateral adaptation, but develops on a preexisting venous system that has been transformed. However, the majority of DVAs are not associated with any sort of neural tissue damage or dysfunction. Lasjaunias (1997) commented on this theory that it can hardly be imagined that a significant venous disorder (such as thrombosis) at an early stage of development would not be associated with some tissue abnormality. Furthermore, the fact that DVAs do not exist in the diencephalon, brain stem, or spinal cord and are only encountered where tectum derivates exist, excludes DVAs from the group of pathological malformations (Lasjaunias 1997).

The association of venous malformations with other vascular malformations gave further room for speculation. Mullan et al. (1996) hypothesized that true arteriovenous (AV) malformations may be fistulized venous malformations and that both vascular anomalies may be related to a developmental failure of the cortical venous system. However, these are nice theories, but do not have any impact on diagnostic work-up or patient management, nor are they supported by any study. Kilic et al. (2000) looked for expression of structural proteins and angiogenic factors in cerebrovascular anomalies. Whereas AVM and cavernomas had expression of vascular endothelial growth factor, DVAs did not express any of the studied growth factors and mainly consisted of structural proteins of angiogenically mature tissue. This finding strongly supports the idea of a simple variation of the venous drainage instead of being a true vascular malformation.

In contrast, the relationship of DVAs with cavernous hemangiomas has been well documented (Abe et al. 1990; Comey et al. 1997; Goulao et al. 1990; Rigamonti and Spetzler 1988; Wilms et al. 1994). There are also reports about de novo formation of cavernous hemangiomas in the vicinity of DVAs (Ciricillo et al. 1994). The close relationship of mixed malformations may be related to venous hypertension within the regional microenvironment with erythrocyte diapedesis and angiogenic growth factor release (Cirillo et al. 1994; Robinson et al. 1995). Another interesting finding is that in families affected with cavernomas – an autosomal dominant inheritance has been established in these families – none of the patients described to date with the combination of cavernoma and DVA has a positive familial history, nor has any genotypic classification been found. However, we have to accept the coincidence between DVAs and cavernomas, but have to admit that we do not have any substantial hypothesis what the pathogenetic origin of this coincidence is.

The histologic examination does not reveal any vessel abnormality. The vessel wall is completely normal in DVAs. The anomaly in DVAs is the course of the draining vein. There is no arterial component in this entity. Intervening brain tissue is present between the veins compromising the lesion, and this brain tissue is usually normal without evidence of hemosiderin staining or gliosis. On MRI, there is sometimes a high T2-signal visible around the draining vein. However, this should not be interpreted as gliosis, but can be explained by dilated perivascular and cerebrospinal fluid (CSF)-containing space (see Fig. 1.4).

Developmental venous anomalies represent the most common vascular variant, accounting for 63% of intracranial vascular malformations in one large autopsy study, with an overall incidence of 2%–4% (Sarwar and McCormick 1978). The lesion consists of a tuft of abnormally enlarged medullary venous channels that are radially arranged around, and drain into a central venous trunk. The common trunk drains intracerebrally into the deep or superficial venous system (Lasjaunias 1997). It is important to bear in mind that the vein's course is not normal; however, it does drain normal functioning brain tissue. This should be of particular interest when surgery has to be performed around the draining vein, e.g., if the DVA is associated with a cavernoma. In these patients, it is of the utmost importance to preserve the draining vein and to remove only the cavernoma (see Fig. 1.7).

1.2 Clinical Presentation

Hemodynamically, DVAs represent low-flow, low-resistance lesions that are less likely to bleed. Garner et al. (1991) calculated the hemorrhage rate to be 0.22% per year; McLaughlin et al. (1998) found a symptomatic hemorrhage rate of 0.34% per year. This range of hemorrhage risk is within the range we expect from cavernous hemangiomas alone. Based on these data and on hemodynamics, one might already conclude that hemorrhages in the presence of a DVA are not related to the DVA itself, but in nearly all patients related to an associated cavernous angioma! My opinion is that the risk of hemorrhage

a

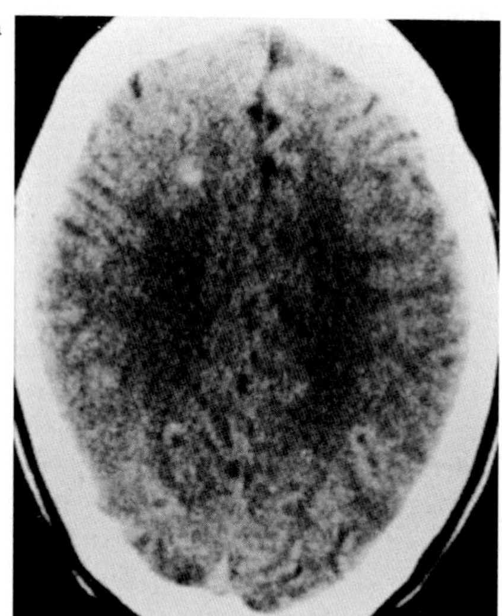

b

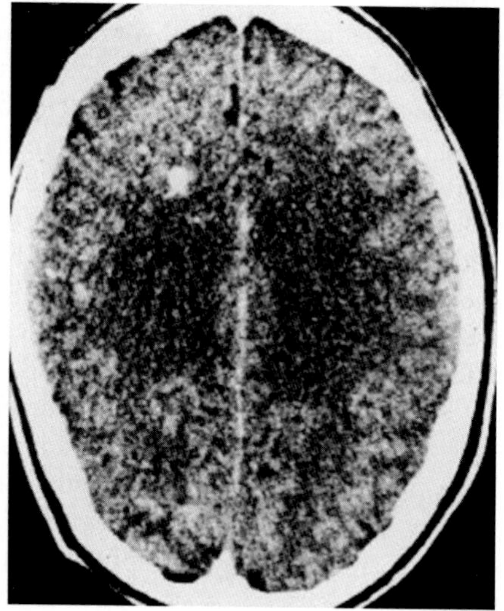

Fig. 1.1. a Axial nonenhanced computed tomography scan reveals a hyperdense dot within the right frontal lobe representing the transcerebral draining collector vein. **b** The contrast-enhanced scan with a 4-mm slice thickness [explaining the decreased signal-to-noise ratio compared to (**a**)] shows the marked enhancement of the vein and confirms the diagnosis of a developmental venous anomaly

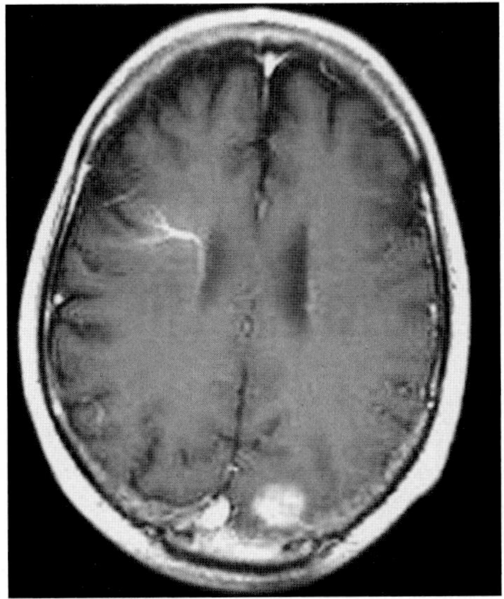

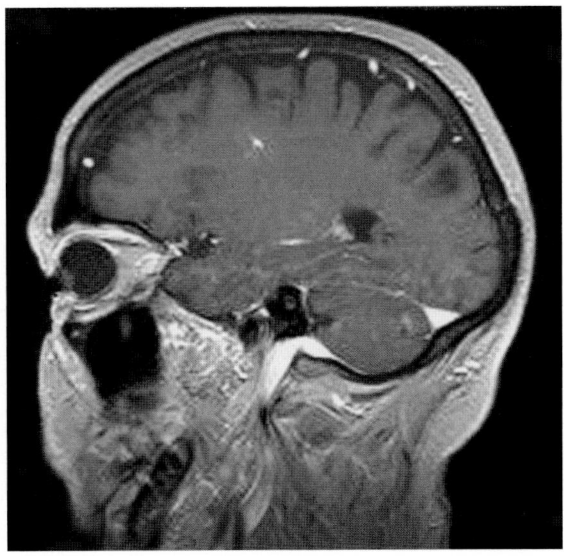

Fig. 1.2a, b. Axial (**a**) and sagittal (**b**) contrast-enhanced T1-weighted magnetic resonance imaging with a typical right frontal developmental venous anomaly. Conspicuous on both views is the transcerebral draining vein. A second look reveals the "Medusa head", small venules radially arranged around and draining into the transcerebral collector vein

in a pure DVA is around zero! I did not find a single case report with a well documented intracerebral hemorrhage (ICH) due to a pure DVA. However, this is not evidence-based, just a simple clinical impression gained over the years. In all cases mentioning a pure DVA as the cause of an ICH, imaging was not optimal and did not rule out the more common constellation with an associated cavernoma.

The coincidence of DVAs and cavernomas, however, is evidence-based and therefore has to be taken into consideration whenever facing a cavernoma or a DVA. Up to one third of DVAs are associated with cavernomas (see Figs. 6–9).

A major problem of most studies reporting hemorrhages due to a DVA is how they ruled out an associated cavernoma. It is clearly not enough just to perform T2-weighted images in patients with DVAs. All these patients need an imaging work-up with T2*-weighted MRI sequences to exclude or to visualize associated cavernomas with the highest sensitivity.

Beside the risk and discussion of hemorrhagic complications, DVAs have been associated with vague neurological symptoms, such as nonspecific headaches and dizziness, or with more specific symptoms and/or signs like seizures (McLaughlin et al. 1998). However, having in mind the association of caver-

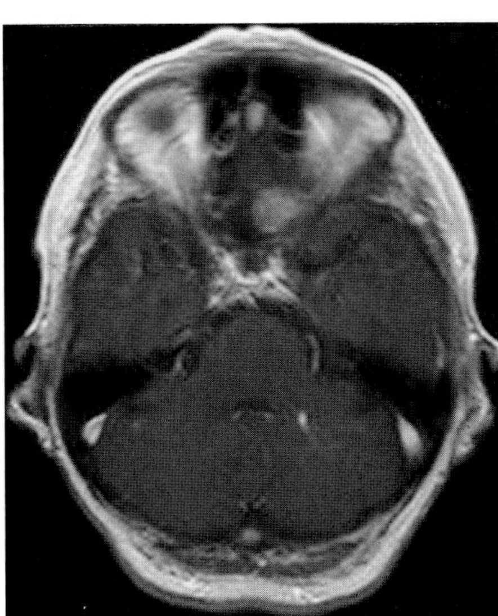

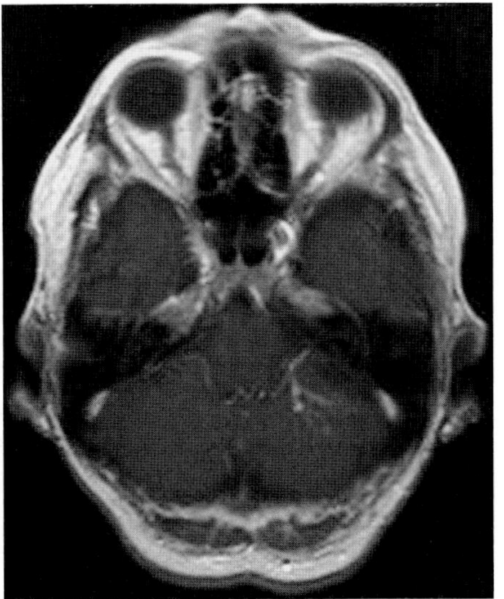

Fig. 1.3a, b. Axial contrast-enhanced T1-weighted magnetic resonance imaging with a developmental venous anomaly located in the left cerebellar hemisphere. Again, the transparenchymal draining vein is the most striking sign. On (**b**), the Medusa head is clearly visible. There is no need for an additional digital subtraction angiography

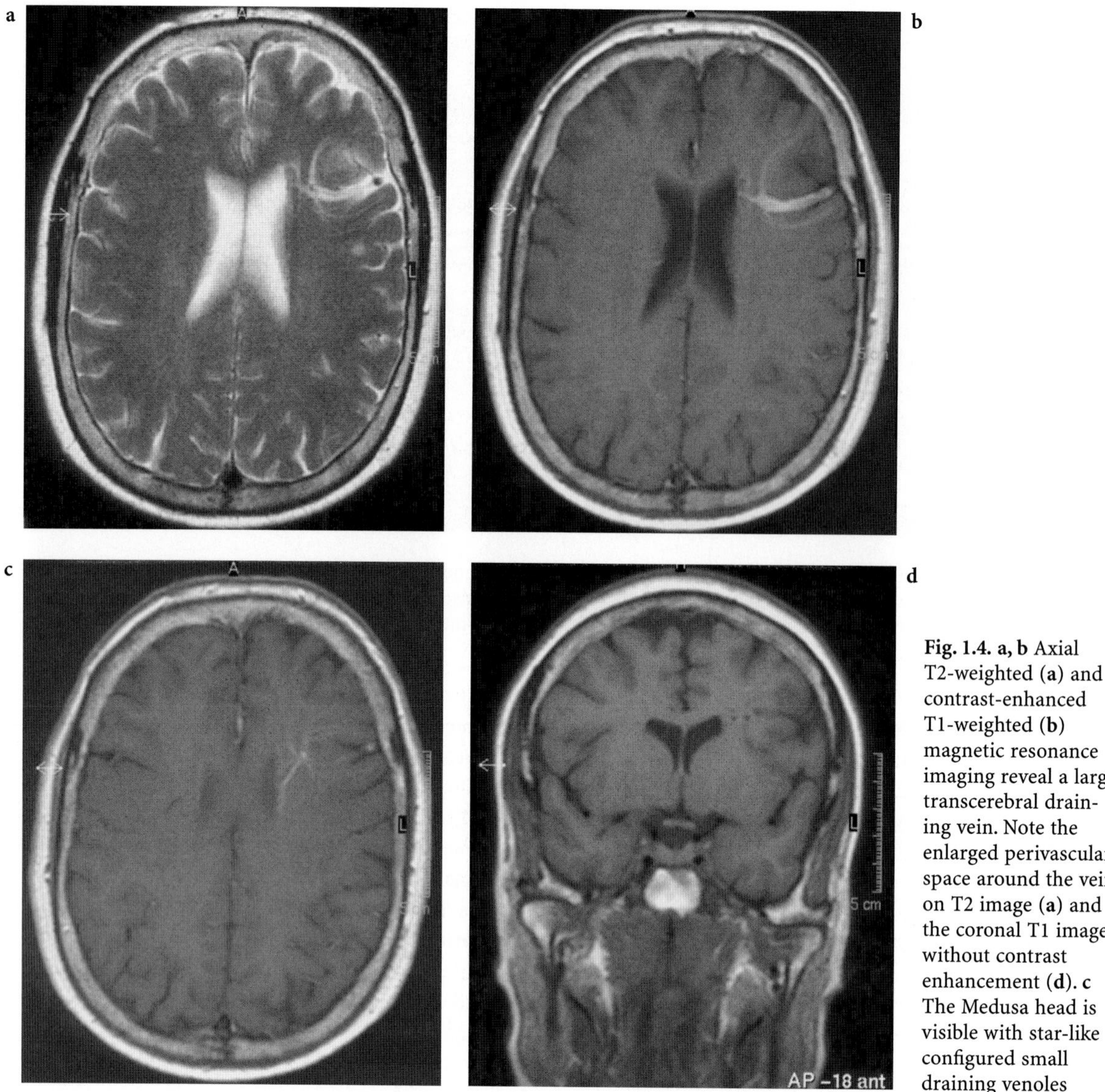

Fig. 1.4. a, b Axial T2-weighted (**a**) and contrast-enhanced T1-weighted (**b**) magnetic resonance imaging reveal a large transcerebral draining vein. Note the enlarged perivascular space around the vein on T2 image (**a**) and the coronal T1 image without contrast enhancement (**d**). **c** The Medusa head is visible with star-like configured small draining venoles

noma and DVA, all these findings have to be critically reviewed. In 1998, McLaughlin and colleagues published their series of 80 patients with DVAs focused on the prospective natural history of cerebral developmental venous malformations. According to their interpretation, 22/80 DVAs were symptomatic: nine patients had headaches related to the DVA, four presented with DVA-related seizures. Three patients had sensory symptoms, three other patients motor deficits. Two patients presented with trigeminal neuralgia and a single patient with an extrapyramidal movement disorder. Korinth et al. (2002) described another patient with trigeminal neuralgia due to a DVA in the cerebellopontine angle. After microvascular decompression, the typical symptoms of the neuralgia disappeared completely. At the time of registration, 16/80 patients in the McLaughlin series had sustained previous intracranial hemorrhage in the region of the venous malformation, two of them suffered subsequent hemorrhage during the prospective follow-up period. Most of the venous malformations were located in the posterior fossa (36/80). In three patients, there was an association of the DVA with a cavernous hemangioma. McLaughlin and colleagues did excellent work while collecting all these data and it is clearly one of the most important papers dealing with DVAs.

However, it is questionable whether the symptoms of the patients were really related to the DVA. It is not surprising that a substantial proportion of patients with these lesions reaching neurosurgical centers had some history of associated neurological events. Such selection bias is not unusual and is likely to overestimate the risk of any associated neurological manifestation. Symptoms like headache and sensory symptoms are difficult to dissociate from the lesion, but it is also often impossible to attribute the symptoms causally to the DVA. Another problem of the study is that imaging was not optimized to get maximal sensitivity for cavernomas. Symptoms like bleeding, seizures, and headache are known to be associated with cavernomas. Therefore, T2*-weighted MRI sequences should be standard for all DVA imaging protocols. However, some patients really might have local symptoms due to the large caliber of the draining vein, specifically when located within the cerebellopontine angle. ABDULRAUF and coworkers (1999) found a coincidence of cavernous malformation and DVA in 24% of patients referred for surgical removal of a cavernous malformation. They additionally deduced that, specifically in the posterior fossa, the likelihood of an association of both entities increases significant. Another interesting hypothesis of theirs is that association of a cavernoma and a DVA may increase the probability of a cavernoma-related hemorrhage. In their study population, 38% of patients with cavernoma alone presented with hemorrhage, but 62% of patients with cavernoma and DVA. Additionally, the incidence of repeated symptomatic hemorrhage was increased in the group with combined malformations (23%) compared to the pure cavernoma patients (9.5%). COMEY et al. (1997) described *similar* cases with parenchymal enhancement around the DVA, and speculated that this finding might be secondary to local venous hypertension. Other surgeons (LITTLE et al. 1990)

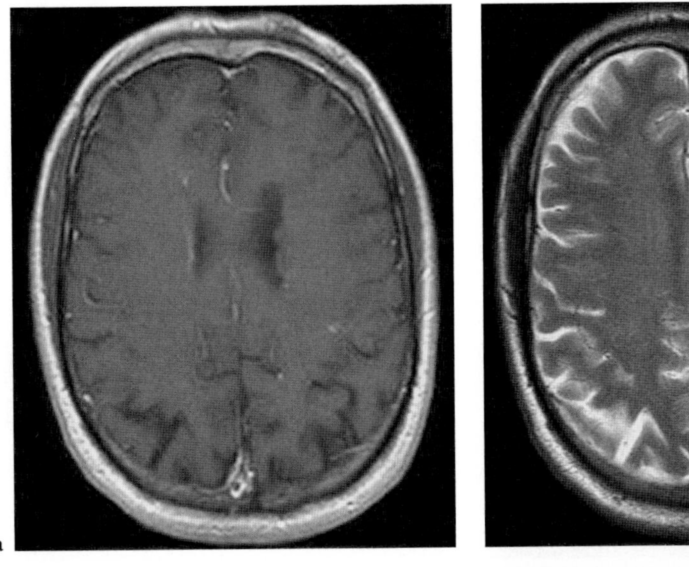

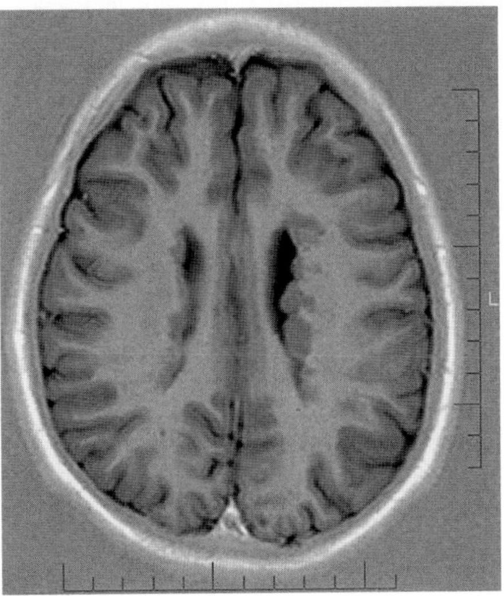

Fig. 1.5. a Axial contrast-enhanced T1-weighted image with a small developmental venous anomaly (DVA) in the left hemisphere. The typical transcerebral draining vein is diagnostic. However, the epileptic seizures of the patient are not associated with the DVA. **b, c** T2-weighted (**b**) and inversion recovery sequence (**c**) nicely reveal the nodular subependymal heterotopic gray matter in the wall of the left ventricle. This cellular migration disorder is the cause of the seizures

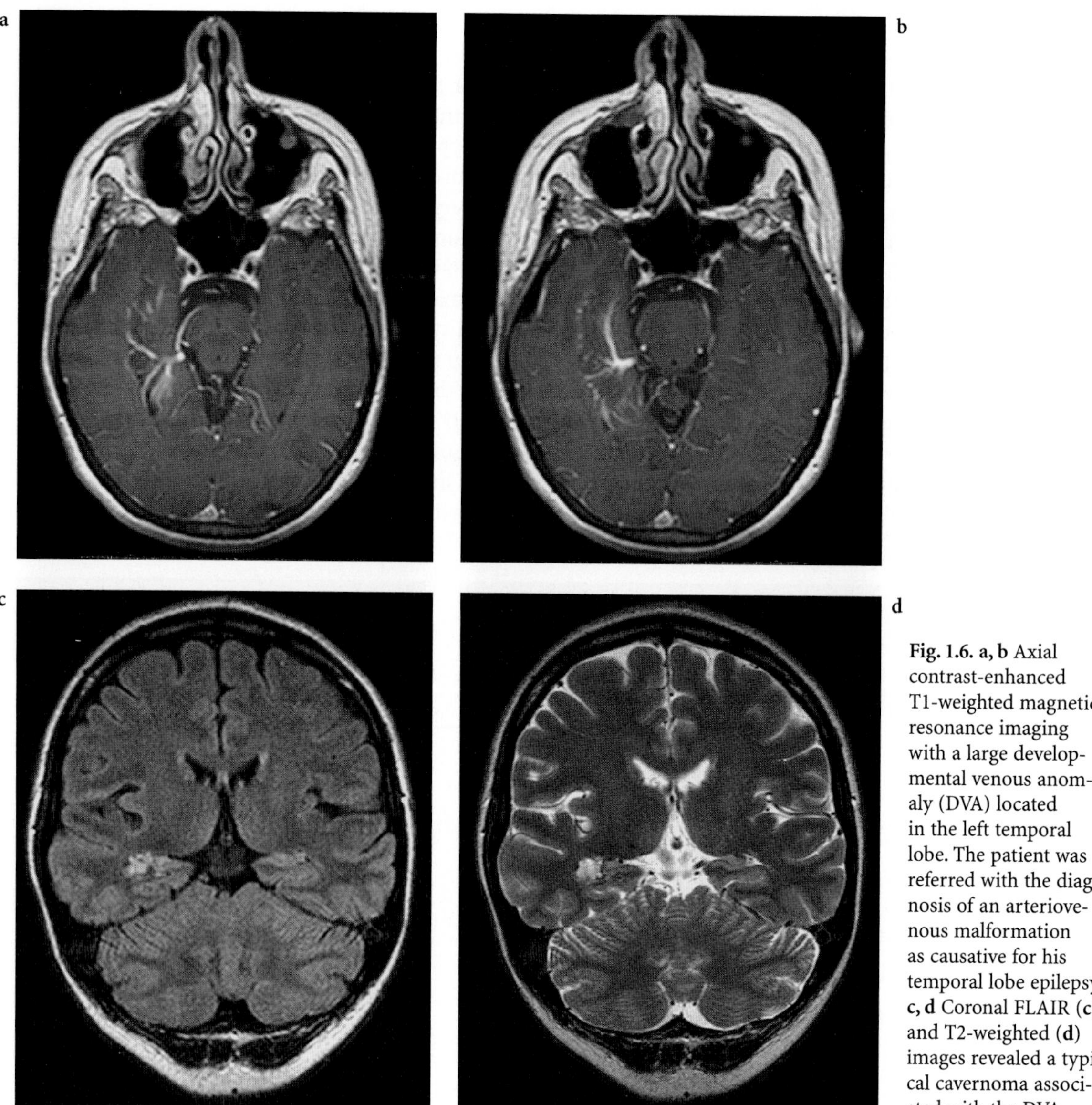

Fig. 1.6. a, b Axial contrast-enhanced T1-weighted magnetic resonance imaging with a large developmental venous anomaly (DVA) located in the left temporal lobe. The patient was referred with the diagnosis of an arteriovenous malformation as causative for his temporal lobe epilepsy. **c, d** Coronal FLAIR (**c**) and T2-weighted (**d**) images revealed a typical cavernoma associated with the DVA

found an anatomical and physiological communication between cavernomas and associated DVAs. Therefore, it might indeed be possible that venous hypertension in association with DVA can predispose a cavernoma to bleed. Another explanation for this finding may be that the majority of cavernomas were located in the supratentorial compartment, but the majority of cavernomas plus DVA were located in the infratentorial compartment. Because of their eloquent location, it is likely that smaller hemorrhages in the posterior fossa manifest overt symptoms and may hence be detected clinically.

In 1999, Töpper et al. reported 67 patients with the MRI-based diagnosis of DVA. In 12 patients, an associated cavernoma was found. And again: there was no hemorrhage in a patient with a pure DVA. All hemorrhages were due to an associated cavernoma.

The first thing to memorize in clinical presentation of DVA is: There is no, or at least an extremely low, risk of hemorrhage due to a DVA. All hemorrhages are related to an associated cavernoma. You just have to find the cavernoma or urge a radiologist to do so.

In Töpper's study, the main reasons for referring the patient to the MRI suite included seizures and headaches. In contrast to McLaughlin, these authors did not find any association between the complaints that led to MRI and the location or diagnosis of a DVA. In both groups, there were a lot of patients with headaches and epilepsy; in fact, these two groups represented the main referral reason in both groups. Whereas McLaughlin classified many DVAs as symptomatic because the patients suffered from headaches, Töpper et al. never found an association between headache and a DVA. And I agree: I don't think that there is an association between DVA and headache. Remember, DVAs do not cause any steal effect (like true AVMs), and it is more than difficult to explain how the pathomechanism for headache could be. In general, there are two explanations for the coincidence of headaches and DVAs in the same patient. First, both findings are common and there is no causal relationship at all. Second, a small subgroup of patients with DVA and headache might have an additional cavernoma located near the surface of the brain. Some of these patients suffer from headache due to subarachnoid microhemorrhages. And then again, the cavernoma is responsible for the clinical picture and not the DVA.

Another reason for patient's referral to an MRI unit are seizures. There might be an association between DVA and epilepsy, even if the EEG focus in not congruent with the location of the DVA. If this is true, one should take a careful look for an associated cavernoma, cavernomas being known to cause different types of epilepsy, mainly due to their content of hemosiderin.

And if you don't find a cavernoma as a source for the ictus: there is little evidence that the development of a DVA during embryology might be associated with some more severe developmental problems like small-scale migration deficits (Barkovich 1988; Watanabe et al. 1990). Lasjaunias (1997) pointed

Fig. 1.7. a Axial contrast-enhanced T1-weighted image reveals the typical transcerebellar draining vein. The patient had a history of transient cerebellar symptoms with ataxia. **b, c** Again, careful additional imaging [coronal T2 (**b**) and axial T2* (**c**)] clearly shows the associated cavernoma. Notice the increased visibility of the cavernoma on the T2* image (**c**) compared to the standard T2 (**b**). **d** Magnetic resonance imaging after surgical removal of the cavernoma reveals the preservation of the developmental venous anomaly not to affect the normal venous drainage of the cerebellar hemisphere

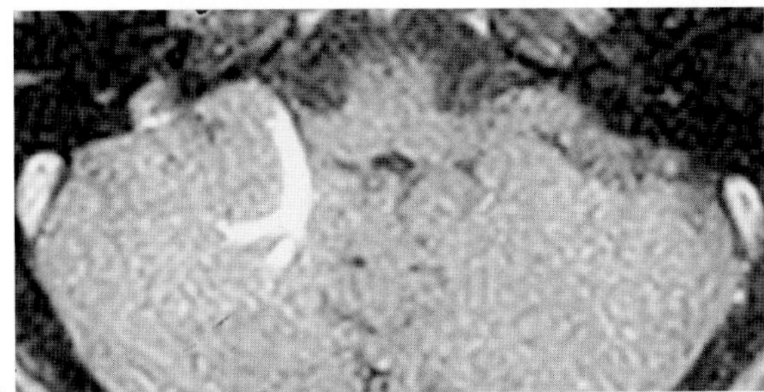
a

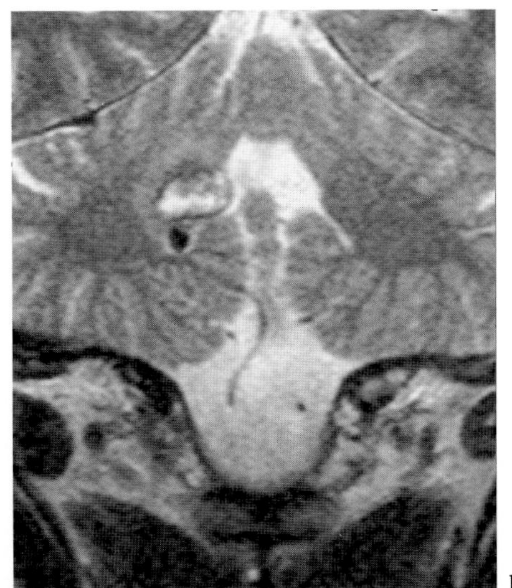
b

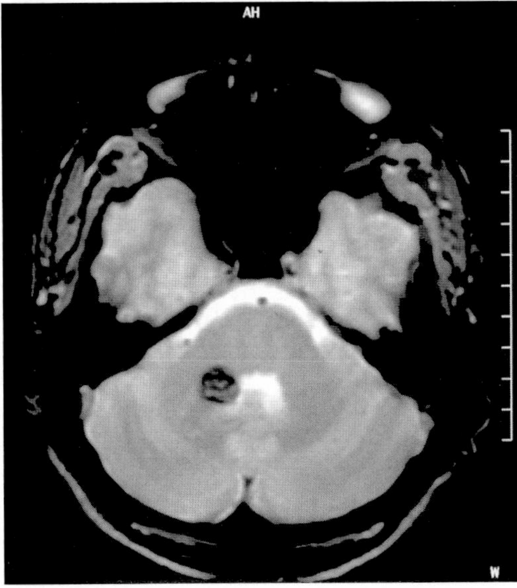

c

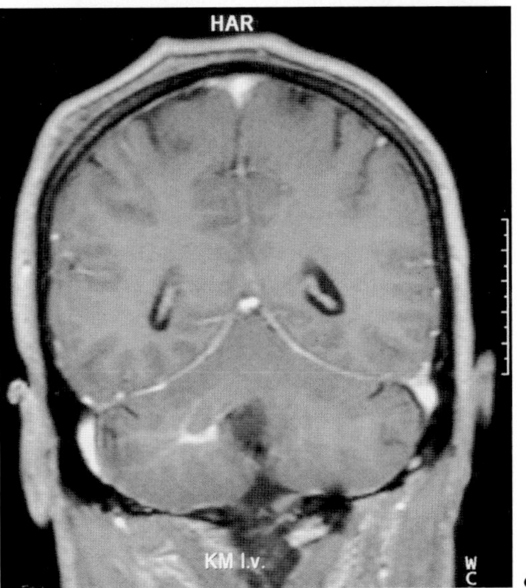

d

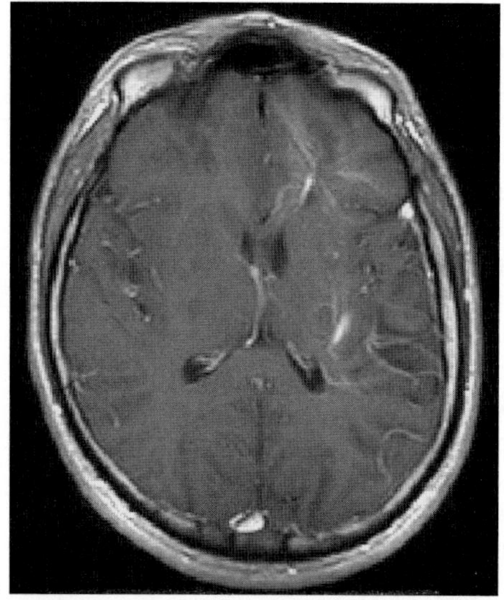

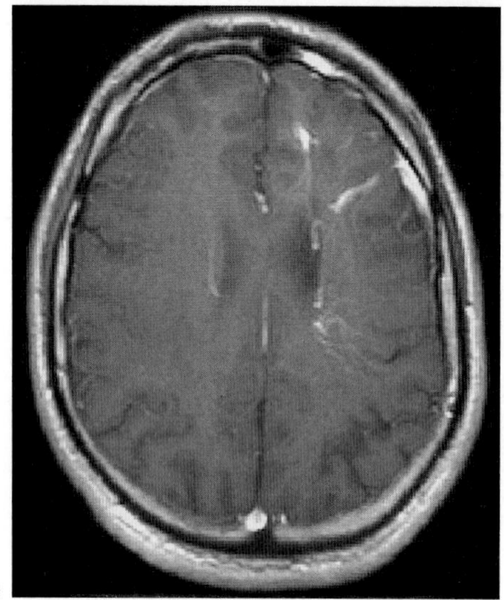

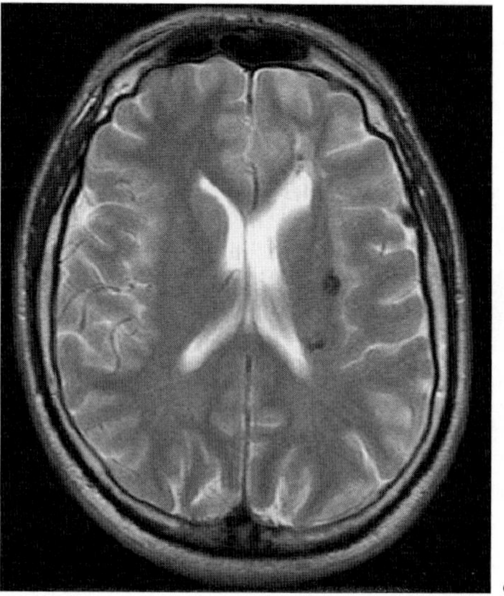

Fig. 1.8. a, b Patient with two interconnected developmental venous anomalies (DVAs) periinsular and frontal on the left side (contrast-enhanced T1-images). **c** T2-image reveals additional intracerebral cavernomas

out that the DVA is clearly not responsible for the cortical changes. However, the coincidence of both findings illustrates the close relation in topography and time between the venous maturation process (from the striatal veins and transhemispheric balance set-up) and the cell migration from the germinal matrix. In conclusion: Seizures and DVAs are a complex combination (see Figs. 1.5 and 1.6). It is clearly incorrect and too simple to decline any association between the clinical problem and the imaging findings on the one hand, or to identify the DVA as the epileptogenic foci in all patients on the other. However, any DVA in a patient with seizures should guide us to look careful for cavernomas (associated with the DVA or at any other location within the brain) or any heterotopia.

There was another interesting topic in the study of Töpper et al. (1999): Among those patients referred to a private practice group, the incidence of DVA was 0.14%, among those referred to a University department of neuroradiology the incidence was 0.7%. The authors figured out that this difference can be explained by the different number of patients who undergo a contrast-enhanced MRI in a private practice to in a University department. Contrast-enhanced MRI studies increase the sensitivity of MRI for DVA significantly.

To come back to the discussion of hemorrhage in patients with DVA: A rare reason for hemorrhage around the collecting vein in DVA may be a thrombosis of the draining vein (Bouchacourt et al. 1986; Konan et al. 1999; Masson et al. 2000). There are only a few case reports in the literature about this specific problem and there is no evidence that the risk of venous occlusion is increased in DVA. But, of course, the transcerebral draining vein might have a risk of thrombosis like all other intracranial veins. It seems to be true that thrombosis of the main draining vein does cause more severe clinical problems if located in the posterior fossa. Bouchacourt et al. (1986) reported a well-documented case of thrombosis of a DVA that led to an extensive hemispheric venous infarction. Usually, the outcome is pretty good, with and without anticoagulation.

Rarely, DVAs have been reported to cause hydrocephalus or trigeminal neuralgia (Blackmore and Mamourian 1996; Numaguchi et al. 1982) due to local compression of the aqueduct or the fifth cranial nerve. There is a single case report describing the juxtaposition of capillary telangiectasia, cavernous malformation, and DVA in the brainstem (Clatterbuck et al. 2001). The authors' hypothesis is that a developmental event may disrupt local capillary-venous pattern formation.

Jung et al. (1997) described a patient with a DVA and an acute demyelination around the draining vein. However, there is no evidence that DVA may lead to any other central nervous system (CNS) disease and cases like this merely represent an occasional coincidence.

Under rare circumstances, DVA can also be associated with tumoral masses (Beers et al. 1984; Handa et al. 1984). Handa et al. (1984) reported a patient with a deep DVA combined with an intracranial varix.

Most of the DVAs are solitary, although multiple lesions might occur in the blue rubber bleb nevus syndrome, characterized by bluish discolored skin and mucocutaneous lesions. However, there are multiple DVAs in patients that do not have any syndromes or any genetic defect (see Figs. 1.8 and 1.9), but the likelihood of a coincident cavernoma seems to be increased in these patients.

1.3 Imaging

Computed tomography (CT), MRI, and angiography delineate the typical curvilinear vascular channels receiving drainage from a "Medusa head" – the typical radial pattern of small venules. The larger, central draining "collector" vein empties into a large cortical, a dural, or a subependymal vein.

The typical contrast-enhanced CT or MRI reveals the draining vein as an enhancing "dot" within the white matter of the supratentorial hemispheres or the cerebellar hemispheres.

Going up or down slice by slice, this enhancing dot is visible within a couple of slices. It depends mainly on slice thickness and on contrast resolution whether the Medusa head is visible or not. Due to the improved contrast resolution, the draining vein is usually better delineated on MRI than on CT. DVAs may be overlooked on unenhanced MRI scans, but usually the large central vein can be seen due to its linear flow void. Sometimes, the draining vein has a high signal on T1-weighted images due to slow flow rephasing phenomena. This is important to know, because otherwise some radiologists and/or clinicians misinterpret this high signal as a sign of thrombosis! There is nearly always some CSF signal around the vein. As mentioned above, this should not be interpreted as a gliotic reaction of the brain, but simply as dilated perivascular spaces.

Intravenous contrast application usually visualizes not only the draining vein, but also the Medusa head to an extent where the diagnosis can be confirmed by MRI or CT. Angiography is usually not necessary.

However, finding a DVA on MRI should always initiate a modification of the scanning protocol. This is particularly important in those patients referred because of seizures. As mentioned above, DVA can be associated with other cortical abnormalities. The theory of increased cortical disorders came up with the hypothesis that DVA might have a pathogenetic origin in a specific intrauterine phase with occlusion of one of the major venous sinus. To obtain venous drainage, one of the transmedullary draining veins is kept open; and during this vulnerable phase, other developmental problems might occur that finally cause seizures. In conclusion: if you don't find a cavernoma in seizure patients, look for heterotopia, best visualized with inversion recovery sequences.

In the majority of patients with DVA and seizures, we have to look for associated cavernomas. This association is evident; however, nobody really knows the pathogenetic background behind it. But it is also evident that we do not see all cavernomas on regular T2-weighted images, e.g., not the small ones. Therefore, in all patients with DVA (and specifically in those with seizures), a T2* gradient echo sequence has to be added to the usual protocol to be sure that there is no associated cavernoma. I am pretty sure that in the majority of patients published in the literature as having an epileptic focus in the proximity of the visible DVA (and consequently the DVA was thought to be responsible for the seizures), the diagnostic work-up was not specifically designed to rule out a cavernoma with sufficient sensitivity. Additionally, T2* sequences sometimes visualize the DVA itself pretty well with a marked hypointensity reflecting the paramagnetic deoxyhemoglobin within the venous blood.

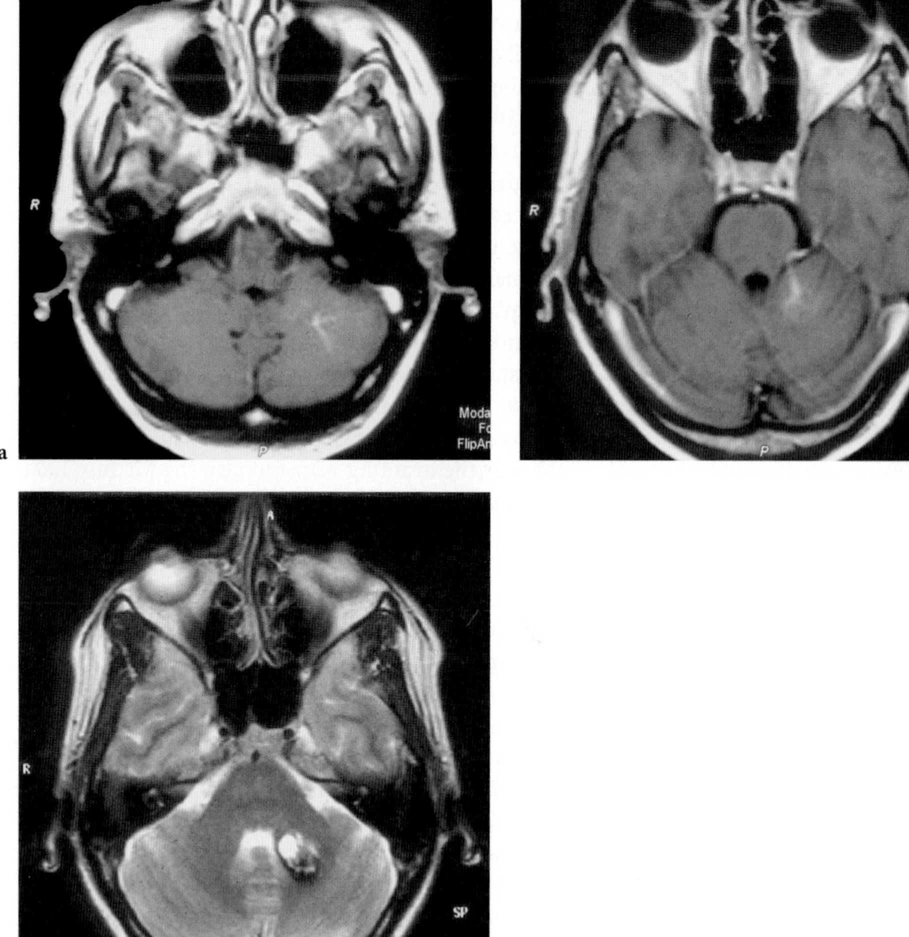

Fig. 1.9a–c. Patient with two developmental venous anomalies, one below (**a**) and one above (**b**) a cerebellar cavernoma (**c**)

There is still a debate about the usefulness of MRA in DVA. The transcerebral vein is usually visible, but MRA is clearly not necessary to confirm the diagnosis. To sum up the imaging findings: DVA is most often an incidental finding on cross-sectional imaging. If the patient is referred for symptoms like seizures or headache, the imaging protocol should include a T2*-weighted sequence to exclude an associated cavernoma.

In a nonenhanced CT scan, the transcerebral draining vein can rarely be seen as a slight hyperdense dot or band within the white matter. In enhanced scans or in source images of CT angiography, the vein is clearly visible – like in contrast-enhanced MRI (Peebles and Vieco 1997). However, if the diagnosis is based on typical MRI findings, it is not necessary to perform an additional CT scan or a CT angiography.

Angiographic characteristics include normal arterial and capillary phases, with opacification of the DVA exclusively during the venous phase and remaining opacified through the late venous phase. The only abnormal finding is the Medusa head and the abnormal transcerebral course of the collecting vein.

In general, we don't need angiography in patients with DVA. At our institution, we do perform angiography in those cases with an "atypical appearance" of the DVA, previous hemorrhage due to an associated cavernoma, or in the setting of hereditary hemorrhagic telangiectasia (with a high prevalence of true AV malformations, as well as venous anomalies).

Discussing the need for angiography in DVA, there is always somebody around with the question of ruling out an AVM. This question clearly should not be an indication for angiography in the vast majority of patients. Reports in the literature on the coincidence of DVA and true AV malformations are rare. KOMIYAMA and colleagues (1999) figured out that there are 31 patients in the literature that had a DVA with an arteriovenous shunt. They themselves saw three patients, but they did not publish any MR images.

And if you read the reports carefully and look at the illustrations, you hardly ever find a typical DVA illustration on a cross sectional image. They are always atypical: large venous convolutes, not just a single transcerebral vein and often already dilated arteries. So, the general recommendation to perform a DSA in those DVAs that have an atypical presentation on MRI can be justified; this will lead to some AVMs that on a quick view look like a DVA on cross-sectional imaging. The chance, however, of missing an AVM in a patient with a typical DVA on MRI is really low and probably much lower than the risk of performing a DSA. AKSOY and colleagues (2000) raised the question of whether MRA should be part of the diagnostic work-up of these patients. Again, it is not necessary in a typical DVA and it is probably not very helpful in an atypical one.

BOUKOBZA et al. (1996) found a specific pattern of DVAs in patients with extensive venous malformations of the head and neck. The draining veins were more tortuous and dilated and more often draining into the deep venous system. Additionally, the incidence of DVA seems to be increased in patients with slow-flow vascular malformations of the head and neck. In their series of 40 patients with head and neck venous malformations, eight had intracranial DVAs and five multiple DVAs. In the literature, multiple DVAs have been reported to occur in around 25% of cases, sometimes related to other congenital disorders and syndromes (RIGAMONTI et al. 1987; RIGAMONTI and SPETZLER 1988).

In conclusion, patients with head and neck venous malformations obviously have an increased probability of having a DVA and an increased chance of having multiple DVAs. There are no data on whether the risk of having cavernomas is also increased in this patient subgroup.

However, my personal experience is that multiple DVAs are associated with at least one, sometimes even more than one, cavernoma (Figs. 1.8 and 9).

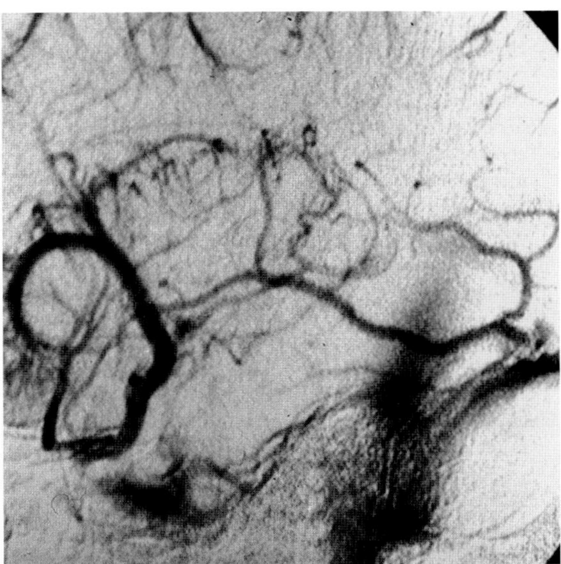

Fig. 1.10. Digital subtraction angiography (lateral view) of a developmental venous anomaly located in the right temporal lobe. Note the typical upside-down umbrella shaped transcerebral draining vein

1.4 Therapy

According to earlier literature (CABANES et al. 1979; HANDA et al. 1984; LOBATO et al. 1988; LUPRET et al. 1993; MALIK et al. 1988; MCCORMICK et al. 1968; MORITAKE et al. 1980; SADEH et al. 1982; SARWAR and MCCORMICK 1978), you will find authors recommending surgical resection of DVAs, assuming the lesion is accessible and symptomatic, e.g., presenting with hemorrhage. According to more recent literature (and what you read on the previous pages), the DVA is a functional venous channel draining normal parenchyma and the risk for venous infarction after surgery or radiosurgery is high (Fig. 1. 11). In fact, resection of the vein is associated with unacceptable morbidity and mortality (BILLER et al. 1985; MEYER et al. 1995; PAK et al. 1980; SADEH et al. 1982; SENEGOR et al. 1983). MARTIN et al. (1984) reported an episode of severe cerebellar swelling even with only temporary occlusion of the visualized draining veins requiring abortion of the operation. Similarly, radiosurgery of DVAs has a 30% complication rate, can lead to venous infarction, and nearly never leads to total venous obliteration. With the knowledge of the indolent and benign natural history of DVAs in general, MCLAUGHLIN et al. recommended observation as the primary mode of strategy. In the case of hemorrhage – assuming that the bleeding is caused by an associated cavernoma – they recommend simple clot removal with preservation of the vein

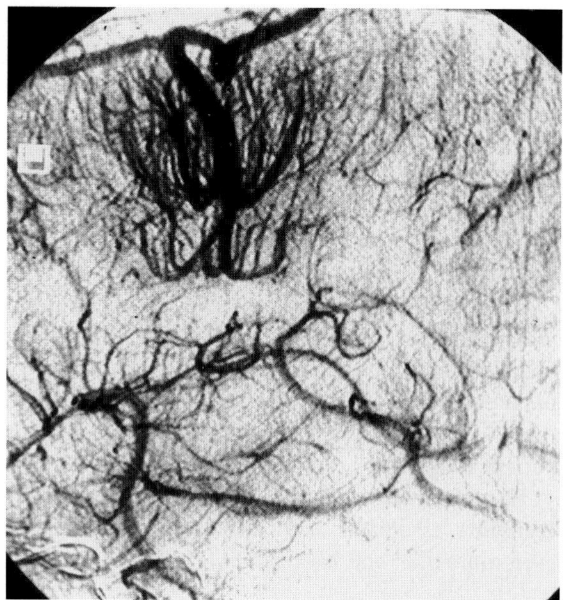
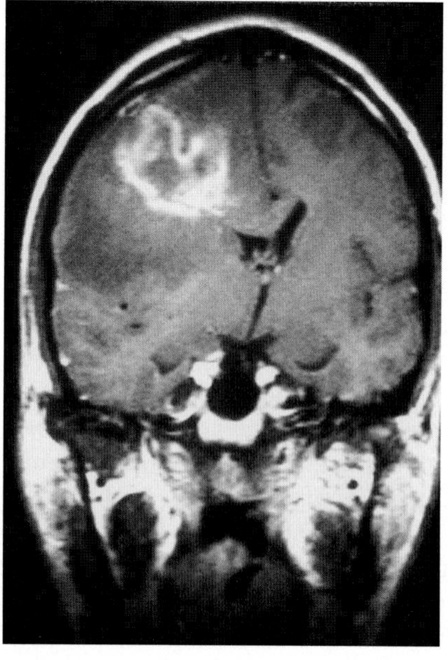

Fig. 1.11. a Digital subtraction angiography of an unusually large developmental venous anomaly of the right hemisphere. Note the doubled upside-down umbrella with two Medusa heads and a single transcerebral draining vein. For unknown reasons, the patient received stereotactic radiation therapy and came back to the hospital 9 months later. **b** The magnetic resonance image at that time revealed a massive hemispheric swelling due to a large venous infarction after radiation-induced thrombosis of the collector vein

(Fig. 1. 7). The surgeon should be alert to finding a cavernoma associated with the DVA, but the DVA itself is a "leave-me-alone" lesion.

I am not really convinced by the recommendations of McLaughlin et al. regarding pure DVA and the need for observation. If there is an adequate MRI examination, excluding a cavernoma with the highest possible probability, I would not (and in fact we don't) recommend any follow-up or observation of a patient with just a DVA. It's hard to explain that it is just a variant – and not a disease – but needs an observation over time. Our recommendation and explanation to the patient and/or the referring doctor is that it usually needs no observation, the bleeding risk is not increased, and the problem for referral is not related to the DVA.

However, if the DVA is associated with a cavernoma, the therapeutic implications are related to the cavernoma. The difference is the surgical approach: in a pure cavernoma, the goal is to remove the whole cavernoma including the hemosiderin rim. If associated with a DVA, the draining vein has to be preserved and, therefore, sometimes the cavernoma cannot be removed totally.

A final remark to those patients with an incidental finding of a DVA: Patients are not restricted in any way from normal daily activities or from pregnancy!

References

Abdulrauf SI, Kaynar MY, Awad IA (1999) A comparison of the clinical profile of cavernous malformations with and without associated venous malformations. Neurosurgery 44:41–46, discussion 46–47

Abe M, Asfora WT, DeSalles AA, Kjellberg RN (1990) Cerebellar venous angioma associated with angiographically occult brain stem vascular malformation. Report of two cases. Surg Neurol 33:400–403

Aksoy FG, Gomori JM, Tuchner Z (2000) Association of intracerebral venous angioma and true arteriovenous malformation: a rare, distinct entity. Neuroradiology 42:455–457

Barkovich AJ (1988) Abnormal vascular drainage in anomalies of neuronal migration. AJNR Am J Neuroradiol 9:939–942

Beers GJ, Carter AP, Ordia JI, Shapiro M (1984) Sinus pericranii with dural venous lakes. AJNR Am J Neuroradiol 5:629–631

Biller J, Toffol GJ, Shea JF, Fine M, Azar-Kia B (1985) Cerebellar venous angiomas. Arch Neurol 42:367–370

Blackmore CC, Mamourian AC (1996) Aqueduct compression from venous angioma: MR findings. AJNR 17:458–460

Bouchacourt E, Carpena JP, Bories J, Koussa A, Chiras J (1986) Ischemic accident caused by thrombosis of a venous angioma. Apropos of a case. J Radiol 67:631–635

Boukobza M, Enjolras O, Guichard JP, Gelbert F, Herbreteau D, Reizine D, Merland JJ (1996) Cerebral developmental venous anomalies associated with head and neck venous malformations. AJNR Am J Neuroradiol 17:987–994

Cabanes J, Blasco R, Garcia M, Tamarit L (1979) Cerebral venous angioma. Surg Neurol 11:385–389

Ciricillo SF, Dillon WP, Fink ME, Edwards MS (1994) Progression of multiple cryptic vascular malformations associated with anomalous venous drainage. Case report. J Neurosurg 81:477–481

Clatterbuck RE, Elmaci I, Rigamonti D (2001) The juxtaposition of a capillary teleangiectasia, cavernous malformation, and developmental venous anomaly in the brainstem of a single patient: case report. Neurosurgery 49:1246–50

Comey CH, Kondziolka D, Yonas H (1997) Regional parenchymal enhancement with mixed cavernous/venous malformations of the brain: case report. J Neurosurg 86:155–158

Garner TB, Del Curling O Jr, Kelly DL Jr, Laster DW (1991) The natural history of intracranial venous angiomas. J Neurosurg 75:715–722

Goulao A, Alvarez H, Garcia Monaco R, Pruvost P, Lasjaunias P (1990) Venous anomalies and abnormalities of the posterior fossa. Neuroradiology 31:476–482

Handa J, Suda K, Sato M (1984) Cerebral venous angioma associated with varix. Surg Neurol 21:436–440

Jung G, Schroder R, Lanfermann H, Jacobs A, Szelies B, Schroder R (1997) Evidence of acute demuelination around a develpomental venous anomaly: magnetic resonance imaging findings. Invest Radiol 32:575–577

Kilic T, Pamir MN, Kullu S, Eren F, Ozek MM, Black PM (2000) Expression of structural proteins and angiogenic factors in cerebrovascular anomalies. Neurosurgery 46:1179–1191, discussion 1191–1192

Konan AV, Raymond J, Bourgouin P, Laseage J, Milot G, Roy D (1999) Cerebellar infarct caused by spontaneous thrombosis of a developmental venous anomaly of the posterior fossa. AJNR Am J Neuroradiol 20:256–258

Komiyama M, Yamanaka K, Iwai Y, Yasui T (1999) Venous angiomas with arteriovenous shunts: report of three cases and review of the literature. Neurosurgery 44:1328–1334, discussion 1334–1335

Korinth MC, Moller-Hartmann W, Gilsbach JM (2002) Microvascular decompression of a developmental venous anomaly in the cerebellopontine angle causing trigeminal neuralgia. Br J Neurosurg 16:52–55

Lasjaunias P (1997) Vascular diseases in neonates, infants and children. Springer, Berlin Heidelberg New York

Little JR, Awad IA, Jones SC, Ebrahim ZY (1990) Vascular pressures and cortical blood flow in cavernous angioma of the brain. J Neurosurg 73:555–559

Lobato RD, Perez C, Rivas JJ, Cordobes F (1988) Clinical, radiological, and pathological spectrum of angiographically occult intracranial vascular malformations: analysis of 21 cases and review of the literature. J Neurosurg 68:518–531

Lupret V, Negovetic L, Smiljanic D, Klanfar Z, Lambasa S (1993) Cerebral venous angiomas: surgery as a mode of treatment for selected cases. Acta Neurochir (Wien) 120:33–39

Malik GM, Morgan JK, Boulos RS, Ausmann J (1988) Venous angiomas: an underestimated cause of intracranial hemorrhage. Surg Neurol 30:350–358

Martin NA, Wilson CB, Stein BM (1984) Venous and cavernous malformations. In: Wilson CV, Stein BM (eds) Intracranial arteriovenous malformations. Williams and Wilkins, Baltimore, pp 234–235

Masson C, Godefroy O, Leclerc X, Colombani JM, Leys D (2000) Cerebral venous infarction following thrombosis of the draining vein of a venous angioma (developmental abnormality). Cerebrovasc Dis 10:235–238

McCormick WF, Hardman JM, Boulter TR (1968) Vascular malformations ("angiomas") of the brain, with special reference to those occuring in the posterior fossa. J Neurosurg 24:241–251

McLaughlin MR, Kondziolka D, Flickinger JC, Lunsford S, Lunsford LD (1998) The prospective natural history of cerebral venous malformations. Neurosurgery 43:195–200, discusssion 200–201

Meyer B, Stangl AP, Schramm J (1995) Association of venous and true arteriovenous malformation: a rare entity among mixed vascular malformations of the brain. J Neurosurg 83:141–144

Moritake K, Handa H, Mori K, Ishikawa M, Morimoto M, Takebe Y (1980) Venous angiomas of the brain. Surg Neurol 14:95–105

Mullan S, Mojtahedi S, Johnson DL, Macdonald RL (1996) Cerebral venous malformation-arteriovenous malformation transition forms. J Neurosurg 85:9–13

Numaguchi Y, Kitamura K, Fukui M, Ikeda J, Hasuo K, Kishikawa T, Okudera T, Uemura K, Matsuura K (1982) Intracranial venous angiomas. Surg Neurol 18:193–202

Ostertun B, Solymosi L (1993) Magnetic resonance angiography of cerebral developmental venous anomalies: its role in differential diagnosis. Neuroradiology 35:97–104

Pak H, Patel SC, Malik GM, Ausmann JI (1980) Successful evacuation of a pontine hematoma secondary to rupture of a venous angioma. Surg Neurol 15:164–167

Peebles TR, Vieco PT (1997) Intracranial developmental venous anomalies: diagnosis using CT angiography. J Comput Assist Tomogr 21:582–586

Rigamonti D, Spetzler RF (1988) The association of venous and cavernous malformations: report of four cases and discussion of the pathophysiological, diagnostic, and therapeutic implications. Acta Neurochir (Wien) 92:100–105

Rigamonti D, Drayer BP, Johnson PC, Hadley MN, Zabramski J, Spetzler RF (1987) The MRI appearance of cavernous malformations (angiomas). J Neurosurg 67:518–524

Robinson JR, Brown AP, Spetzler RF (1995) Occult malformation with anomalous venous drainage. J Neurosurg 82: 311–312

Sadeh M, Shacked I, Rappaport ZH, Tadmor R (1982) Surgical extirpation of a venous angioma of the medulla oblongata simulating multiple sclerosis. Surg Neurol 17:334–337

Saito Y, Kobayashi N (1981) Cerebral venous angiomas: clinical evaluation and possible etiology. Radiology 139: 87–94

Sarwar M, McCormick WF (1978) Intracerebral venous angioma. Case report and review. Arch Neurol 35:323–325

Senegor M, Dohrmann GJ, Wollmann RL (1983) Venous angiomas of the posterior fossa should be considered as anomalous venous drainage. Surg Neurol 19:26–32

Töpper R, Jürgens E, Reul J, Thron A (1999) Clinical significance of intracranial developmental venous anomalies. J Neurol Neurosurg Psychiatry 67:234–238

Truwit CL (1992) Venous angioma of the brain: history, significance and imaging findings. AJR Am J Roentgenol 159: 1299–1307

Watanabe M, Tanaka R, Takeda N, Ikuta F, Oyanagi K (1990) Focal pachygyria with unusual vascular anomaly. Neuoradiology 32:237–240

Wilms G, Bleus E, Demaerel P, Marchal G, Plets C, Goffin J, Baert AL (1994) Simultaneous occurrence of developmental venous anomalies and cavernous angiomas. AJNR Am J Neuroradiol 15:1247–1954, discussion 1255–1257

2 Cavernomas and Capillary Telangiectasias

W. Küker and M. Forsting

CONTENTS

2.1 Cavernomas

In 1956, Crawford and Russell first coined the term "cryptic" vascular malformation in reference to small, clinically "latent vascular lesions", that resulted in either apoplectic cerebral hemorrhage or signs of growing mass lesion. Most of these vascular malformations were angiographically occult.

In 1976, Voigt and Yasargil gave a first overview of the entity of intracerebral cavernomas. At that time, these malformations were thought to be rare. Since then, diagnostic modalities have changed dramatically: not only has computed tomography (CT) become available, but magnetic resonance imaging (MRI) has proved to be the most sensitive diagnostic tool for cavernomas. And thanks to MRI, our knowledge relating to cavernomas has increased since 1976; there remain, however, several questions marks surrounding these malformations.

W. Küker, MD
Department of Neuroradiology, University Hospital Tübingen, Hoppe-Seyler Strasse 3, 72076 Tübingen, Germany
M. Forsting, MD, PhD
Institute of Diagnostic and Interventional Radiology, Department of Neuroradiology, Hufelandstrasse 55, 45122 Essen, Germany

2.1.1 Pathology

Vascular malformations of the brain are usually divided into arteriovenous malformations, capillary telangiectasias, venous malformations, and cavernous malformations. However, for a long time, the term "angiographically occult vascular malformation" or "cryptic" (Cohen et al. 1982; Dillon 1997; Wilson 1992) has been used to describe those vascular malformations that could not be visualized angiographically, but obviously were able to cause intracerebral hemorrhage.

Cavernomas, also called cerebral cavernous malformations or cavernous angiomas (CA) are characterized by endothelium lined, sinusoidal blood cavities without other features of normal blood vessels like muscular or adventitial layers (Fig. 2.1) (McCormick et al. 1968).

The diameter of the blood vessels ranges between 30–50 μm. No brain tissue is present between the blood cavities, which are embedded into connective tissue. This is from a pathological point of view the major difference between cavernomas and capillary telangiectasias. In the latter, there is intervening brain parenchyma between the vascular channels. However,

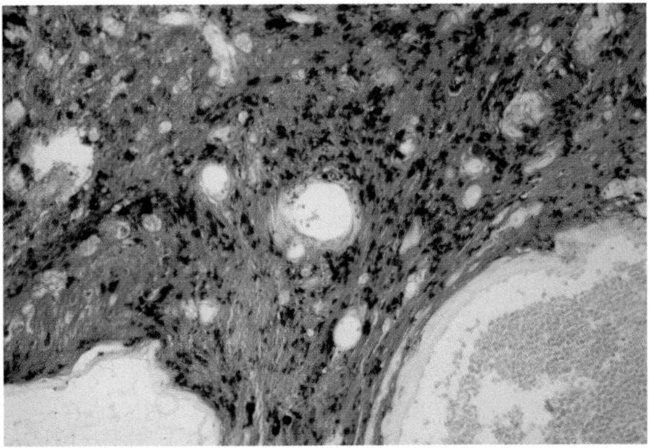

Fig. 2.1. Histology of a typical cavernoma with endothelium-lined, sinusoidal cavities without other features of normal blood vessels, such as muscular or adventitial layer

since Rigamonti et al. (1987, 1988) found a more than 30% incidence of intervening brain parenchyma in more or less typical cavernomas, there is an ongoing debate whether cavernomas and capillary telangiectasias simply represent two pathological extremes within the same vascular malformation category. The suggestion is to group them in an entity called "cerebral capillary malformation." This new way of looking at cavernomas and capillary telangiectasias is clearly of interest from a academic point of view. From a clinical point of view, it still seems reasonable to us to maintain the established classification.

Cavernomas are not encapsulated, but well separable from brain parenchyma. However, the surrounding brain usually exhibits evidence of prior microhemorrhage, hemosiderin, discoloration, and hemosiderin-filled macrophages (Maraire and Awad 1995; Russel and Rubinstein 1989). This indicates recurrent microbleedings or leakage of red blood cells. Thrombi of varying age are characteristic and are present within many of the vessels. Calcification and surrounding gliosis typify the margins of the lesion.

During follow-up, growth of cavernomas can occur, but this is exclusively related to osmotic changes or differences (as in chronic subdural hematoma) and never related to infiltration or any active growth. The sinusoidal walls may be locally thickened or hyalinized with spots of calcification. The structure of the sinusoidal walls is a unique feature of cavernomas.

The cavity of the dilated vessels may contain clotted blood in different stages of degradation. Ultrastructural examinations have disclosed a lack of tight junctions in the wall of cavernomas (Wong et al. 2000). The known propensity for growth and bleeding of cavernomas has been attributed to this rarity of tight junctions, as well as to the lack of significant subendothelial support. However, the precise reason for a macroscopic hemorrhage in these low-flow malformations without any elevated intralesional blood pressure is unclear.

The macroscopic appearance of cavernomas can be described as mulberry-, grape-, or popcorn-like with a diameter of several centimeters.

Cavernomas may occur sporadically (Kupersmith et al. 2001), after radiation therapy (Amirjamshidi and Abbassioun 2000; Olivero et al. 2000), and hereditarily (Labauge et al. 1998) following an autosomal dominant trait. Recently, genes causing cavernomas were mapped on chromosomes 7q, 7p, and 3q in a group of families. The CCM1 locus on chromosome 7q21–22 harbors the Krit1 gene, which probably encodes a tumor suppresser protein (Zhang et al. 2000; Davenport et al. 2001). The occurrence of sporadic cavernomas may be due to the functional loss of the CCM1 gene in heterozygous individuals. Further disease loci (CCM2 on chromosome 7p13–15 and CCM3 on chromosome 3q25.2–27) have been found in other families; however, the genes have not been identified as yet. Although genetic causes have been detected in familial forms of the disease, for the majority of sporadic cases the genetic contribution remains to be determined. However, because all first-degree relatives of patients with cavernomas may not be screened radiographically, the ratio of true sporadic to familial cases may be underestimated. Beside the autosomal transmission, the hallmark of the familial form is multiplicity of cavernomas within the brain (Brunereau et al. 2000).

The incidence of the familial form seems to be particularly high in individuals of Hispanic descent (Rigamonti et al. 1988; Zabramski et al. 1994).

The question as to why cavernomas predominantly occur in the central nervous system (CNS), including the spinal cord, skin, and eyes (Sarraf et al. 2000), is still unresolved. Other, rare locations include the cerebral ventricles (Reyns et al. 1999), cranial nerves (Ferrante et al. 1998), the cavernous sinus (Bristot et al. 1997), or subarachnoid space (M. Kim et al. 1997). There are also reports on an extradural location (Porter et al. 1999).

Cavernomas are frequently accompanied by developmental venous malformations (see Chap. 1) or capillary telangiectasias. According to some reports, brain-stem cavernomas are always associated with a venous abnormality (Porter et al. 1999). This has led to speculation that an impaired venous drainage may have caused the dilatation of capillary channels. However, the identification of the above-mentioned genetic defects focused the research more on the molecular level.

Finally, the pathologic descriptions of all cryptic vascular malformations have been and still are confusing. Mixtures of two and more vascular malformations within the same histologic specimen have been identified by a couple of authors (Awad et al. 1993; Chang et al. 1997; Herata et al. 1986). Wilson (1992) reported on 73 cryptic vascular malformations and classified them into cavernous angiomas, cryptic vascular malformations with arterial components, or cryptic or thrombosed arteriovenous malformations (AVMs). In addition, 40% of all cryptic vascular malformations were characterized as thrombosed AVMs. From a radiological point of view, true AVMs have an extremely low tendency towards spontaneous thrombosis, so this entity should be a rare finding.

In summary, there are many conflicting reports and interpretations in the literature regarding pathological classification of these "cryptic malformations." It is my opinion that classification of vascular malformations in the majority of patients should be done on the basis of radiological findings. Pathologists usually receive incomplete fragments of tissue, do not know anything about the flow within the lesion, and mostly do not have any correlation to radiologic findings. This is the major reason for the inconsistency that characterizes pathologic reports of cryptic malformations.

2.1.2 Clinical Presentation

There is no reliable study giving us an exact idea of the incidence and prevalence of CA; nevertheless, to get a substantial feeling about the available data: The prevalence has been estimated on the basis of autopsy or MR imaging to be 0.5%–0.7% (Del Curling et al. 1991; Robinson et al. 1991). The incidence of cavernomas has been estimated to be in the range between 0.4% and 0.9%; cavernomas account for 8%–15% of all intracranial vascular malformations (Porter et al. 1999; McCormick and Naffziger 1966; Del Curling et al. 1991; Kim et al. 1997). Over the last two decades, incidence data have been confirmed by MRI-based retrospective studies (Robinson et al. 1991; DelCurling et al. 1991). There is no male or female preponderance and up to 25% of all CA are found in the pediatric population.

Multiple cavernomas occur in up to 90% of familial cases and in around 25% of sporadic cases (Clatterbuck et al. 2000; Labauge et al. 2000). Therefore, whenever you see a single cavernoma on the MR scan of a patient, make sure that this is the only one!

On average, 20% of cavernomas occur in the posterior fossa and 80% are seen supratentorially. However, the range given for brain-stem cavernomas is 9% to 35% (Porter et al. 1999; Kupersmith et al. 2001). Spinal cord and extra-axial cavernomas are relatively rare and account for around 5% of all lesions (Clatterbuck et al. 2000).

The average size of cavernomas is between 15 and 19 mm (Kim et al. 1997; Robinson et al. 1991). However, only 10% of lesions remain stable over time: 35% increase and 55% decrease during a mean follow-up of 2 years (Clatterbuck et al. 2000). This dynamic behavior is on the one hand related to recurrent bleedings and resorption of blood products, while on the other hand related to dynamic osmotic changes (Zabramski et al. 1994).

Patients with cavernomas present with a variety of symptoms. Seizures are reported as the most common symptom, accounting for 38%–55% of patient complaints (Del Curling et al. 1991; Robinson et al. 1991; Simard et al. 1986; Brunereau et al. 2000). Other symptoms include focal neurologic deficits in 12%–45% of patients, recurrent hemorrhage in 4%–32%, and chronic headaches in 5%–52%. Brain-stem cavernomas nearly never cause seizures! Most of these patients do have typical brain-stem symptoms like diplopia, face or body sensory disturbances, or ataxia. Without imaging, this subgroup of patients with intratentorially located cavernomas can closely mimic the clinical picture of multiple sclerosis.

The majority of patients become symptomatic between the third and fifth decades, and there is no definite association between symptoms and gender. The frequency of asymptomatic cavernomas is not precisely known, but due to the reports of Zabramski et al. (1994) and Brunereau et al. (2000) it seems to be around 40%!

Hemorrhage

The central clinical problem in patients with cavernomas is the question of hemorrhage! On first view, this should be a simple question with a simple answer. However, both assumptions are wrong. The problem starts with the definition of a hemorrhage and ends with pretty individual answers for each patient.

On the one hand, hemorrhage can be defined clinically: First or sudden onset of new neurologic symptoms in a patient with a cavernoma are usually related to a new or first hemorrhagic event. But looking into the literature, you will find an amazing number of different descriptions and terms to describe cavernoma-related hemorrhages: overt hemorrhage, symptomatic hemorrhage, gross hemorrhage, microhemorrhage, intralesional or perilesional ooze or diapedesis, clinically significant hemorrhage, subclinical hemorrhage, and others (Aiba et al. 1995; Kondziolka et al. 1995b; Robinson et al. 1991; Karlsson et al. 1998). The reason for this variety of descriptions is that, sometimes, clinical events alone were used to define hemorrhage and in other studies different imaging modalities (mainly MR) had a major impact on the definition of hemorrhage. In Sect. 2.1.3, we recommend using the established Zabramski classification scheme in order to allow comparison of different patient groups and studies. However, the problem in defining a hemorrhage is a major reason for the still ongoing debate about the risk of hemorrhage and bleeding rates in patients with cavernomas.

Most estimations assume that cavernomas are present from birth and risk of hemorrhage and bleeding rates are mainly based on that assumption. In 1991, Del Curling et al. and Robinson et al. were the first to calculate the annual hemorrhage rate and figured out that it is between 0.25% and 0.7% per patient and per year. Aiba et al. (1995) analyzed their group on the basis of the initial finding: If bleeding was the initial symptom, the annualized hemorrhage rate was 22.9%; if seizures were the first symptom, the bleeding rate was calculated with 0.39% per patient and year. Kondziolka et al. (1995b) also stratified their patient group into those who had previously experienced a hemorrhage and those who had not. Patients with one previous hemorrhage had an annual 4.5% risk of hemorrhage, whereas those without a previous hemorrhage had a 0.6% annual risk. An analysis of the symptomatic bleeding risk in untreated patients who had experienced two or more hemorrhages found the rate to be approximately 30% per year (Kondziolka et al. 1995a). Other authors, usually not differentiating between initial symptoms, published hemorrhage rates of between 1.1% and 3.1% (Zambramski et al. 1994; Moriarity et al. 1999). Porter et al. reported in 1999 that brain-stem cavernomas might have a significant increased risk of hemorrhage and calculated it with 5% per person and year. In contrast, Kupersmith and coworkers found a bleeding rate of 2.46% in brain-stem cavernomas. However, the rebleeding rate – and this is quite well supported by other data – seems to be beyond 5% in brain-stem cavernomas. All studies suggest that the occurrence of a rebleeding is an indication of a higher bleeding probability of a given cavernoma. The risk of a symptomatic rebleed at least doubles in comparison to asymptomatic cavernomas (Kupersmith et al. 2001). These findings clearly should have an impact on therapeutic decisions. The bleeding incidence is higher in patients with the inherited form of cavernomatosis – not for a single given cavernoma, however, but in terms of patient years (Labauge et al. 2000).

Patients younger than 35 years of age experienced more bleeding episodes and the same was true for those with cavernomas of at least 10 mm. A number of studies addressed the increased bleeding risk among women (Robinson et al. 1991; Aiba et al. 1995; Moriarity et al. 1999); the majority of studies, however, did not find any gender difference in bleeding risks.

The main problem in all these studies is a substantial selection bias and the definition of hemorrhage. Another, but probably more important aspect for patients when discussing bleeding risks is the clinical significance of hemorrhage and the probability of a good recovery. The probability of a fatal hemorrhage is pretty low and many patients do show a complete or nearly complete recovery after the initial bleeding. In general, bleeding rates given by surgical groups tend to be higher than those observed by others.

Finally, with regard to the risk of a cavernoma for the patient, the majority of data in the literature calculate an annual risk of 0.5%–1% (which is much lower than in true AVMs) and a low risk of fatal hemorrhage (Moran et al. 1999). In the majority of patients, particularly those over 35 years of age, suffering from a single cavernoma below 10 mm of size and with seizures as the initial symptom, a wait-and-see strategy seems to be reasonable. In patients presenting with an initial hemorrhage, the repeat hemorrhage risk seems to be much higher, particularly if more than one bleeding event has already occurred.

Seizures

As mentioned above, the majority of patients with cavernomas present with seizures as the initial symptom (Moran et al. 1999). It is important to know that in the vast majority of patients these seizures are not related to acute bleeding events, but to hemosiderin deposition adjacent to neurons. Hemosiderin or ferritin is a well-known epileptogenic agent (at least in animal experiments). Being aware of the relation between seizures and hemosiderin deposition is of particular importance if surgical removal of the cavernoma is considered due to conservative not treatable seizures. It is of utmost importance not only to remove those parts of the cavernoma with blood flow, but also to remove the hemosiderin ring around the cavernoma within the adjacent brain tissue. This part of the malformation is responsible for the seizure.

Headache

Headache is a frequent reason for submitting a patient to any imaging modality. Therefore, there are always discussions whether an incidental finding like an arachnoid cyst, a small meningioma or – more relevant for this chapter – a cavernoma might be the cause of the patient's headache. However, the first and most important question is: What type of headache does the patient have? If this is a clinically typical migraine, a typical tension headache, or any other easy-to-define type, the headache is usually not related to the cavernoma. In our personal experience, there are some patients, suffering from recurrent attacks of a severe, subarachnoid hemorrhage (SAH)-like headache with cavernomas at the surface of the brain. And these cavernomas clearly have contact to the subarachnoid space and microbleeds might indeed cause headache attacks like in a SAH (warning-leak headache).

Focal Neurologic Deficits

Focal neurologic deficits like transient speech arrests, sensomotoric deficits, ataxia, visual disturbances, or eye movement disorders are nearly always related to the location of the cavernoma and hemorrhages. There are no steal mechanisms in cavernomas (this is different in real AVMs), nor are there any venous overload problems.

2.1.3 Diagnostic Imaging

Due to the slow blood flow, cavernomas are angiographically occult vascular malformations. If the lesion has hemorrhaged, an avascular area with moderate mass effect can sometimes be identified. Occasionally – in less than 10% of cases – a faint blush on the late capillary or early venous phase of high resolution angiograms can be seen (Savoiardo et al. 1983). Angiography is rarely necessary in typical cavernomas. If associated with a DVA, presurgical digital subtraction angiography (DSA) may be indicated to analyze the venous drainage pattern. The same is true for those cavernomas that do not have the typical MR appearance. In some of these, DSA can increase the diagnostic confidence.

On CT, and even more so on MRI imaging, features are more or less pathognomonic. Whereas large cavernous hemangiomas can be visible on CT, small lesions are only visible on MRI.

The CT appearance of a cavernoma depends on the amount of internal thrombosis, hemorrhage, and calcification. Examples are shown in Figs. 2.1, 2.4a, 2.7a, 2.8a, 2.10a, 2.12a, 2.13a,b. The lesions appear hyperdense compared to the adjacent brain parenchyma, but can have variable attenuation values. Because the density of blood on CT depends on clot formation, the attenuation of a thrombosed cavernoma changes with time. Calcifications do not change that much, however, cavernomas tend to calcify only partially (Figs. 2.12a,b, 2.13a,b). In patients with a recent hemorrhage, the cavernoma may be suspected on CT mainly by taking into account the site of hemorrhage and the patient's history, thus excluding other typical causes for intracerebral bleeding. Differential diagnosis must cover calcified brain tumor, mainly oligodendroglioma, which have a high tendency of intratumoral bleeding. Contrast enhancement can be observed on CT, but usually requires a substantial

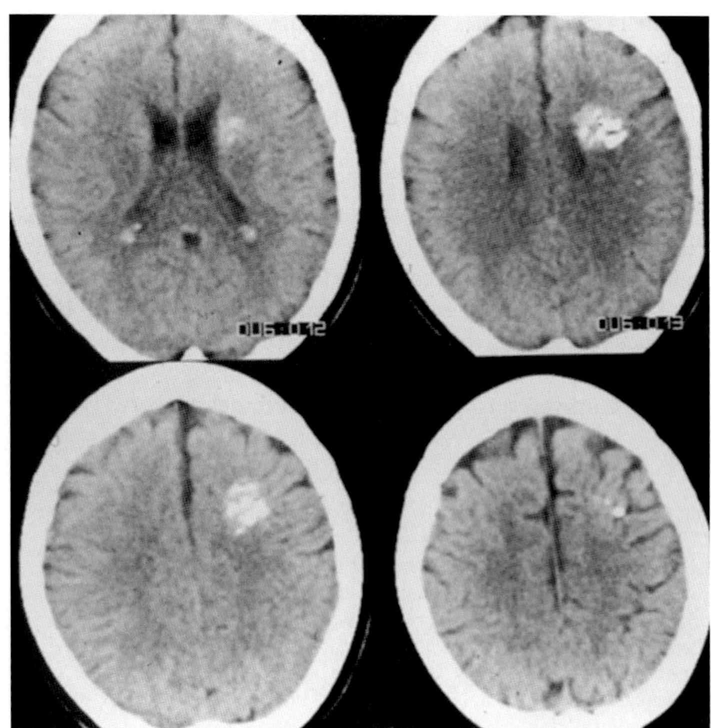

Fig. 2.2. CT of a typical, partially calcified cavernoma adjacent to the left ventricle. The missing mass effect (no compression of the ventricle, normal width of the external cerebrospinal-fluid space) is a striking argument against a true tumor (like oligodendroglioma)

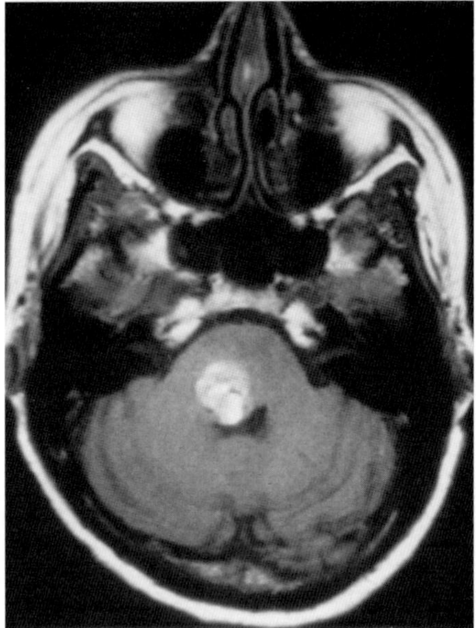

Fig. 2.3. T1-weighted magnetic resonance scan of a typical brain-stem cavernoma, bulging into the 4th ventricle

delay between contrast agent injection and scanning. But even with a standardized 10- to 15-min delay between contrast agent injection and scanning, the enhancement of a cavernoma varies from nonexistent or minimal to striking!

The imaging modality of choice is MRI. Typically, cavernomas have a popcorn-like appearance with a well-delineated complex reticulated core of mixed signal intensities representing hemorrhage in different stages of evolution and/or different velocities of blood flow. Typical is a low signal hemosiderin rim, which completely surrounds the lesion (Figs. 2.3, 2.4b, 2.5, 2.6, 2.11). The dark signal "blooms" on T2-weighted images, and is best visible on gradient-echo T2*-weighted studies (Brunereau et al. 2000). Brunereau and colleagues studied the sensitivity of T2-weighted MR versus gradient-echo (GRE) sequences in patients with the familial form of cavernomas. The mean number of lesions detected on spin-echo (SE) images versus the mean number detected

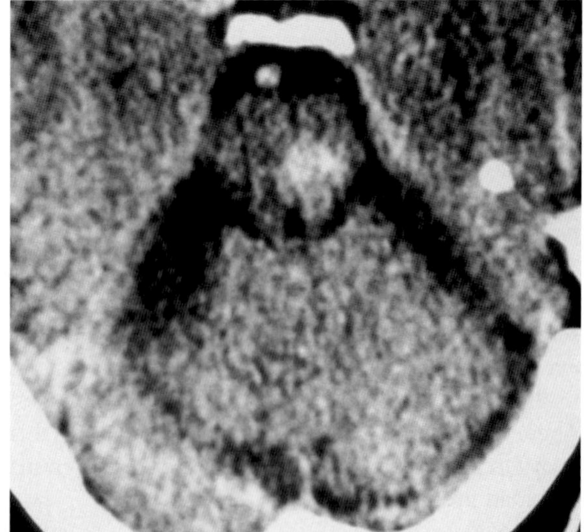

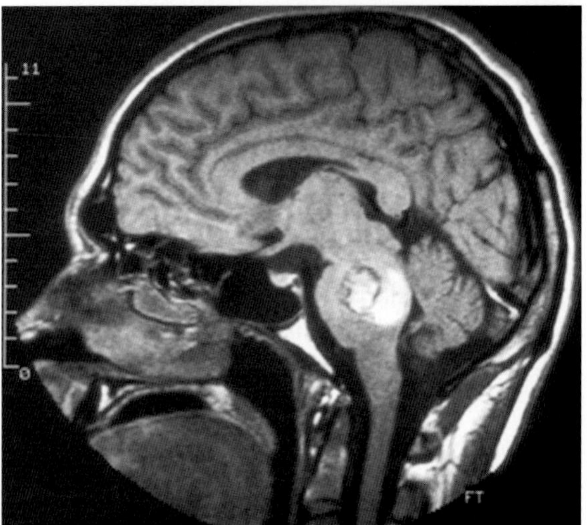

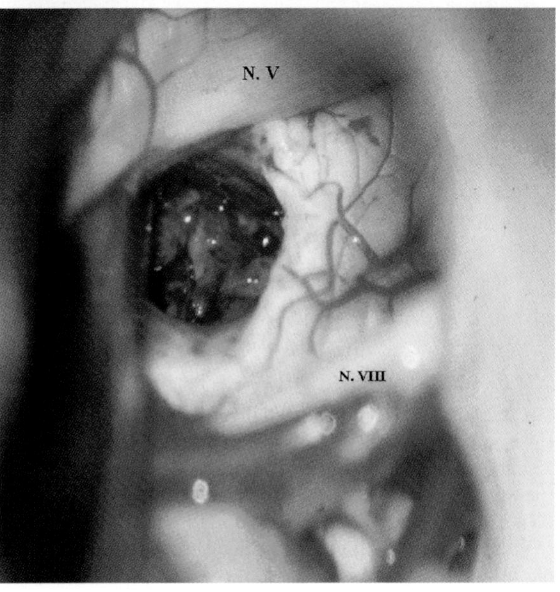

Fig. 2.4. CT (**a**) and sagittal T1-weighted magnetic resonance (MR) scan (**b**) of another brain-stem cavernoma. Due to its calcification, it is easy to see even on the CT scan. The MR nicely reveals the typical cavernoma pattern with the dark rim of hemosiderin. Note that the acute hemorrhage occurred at the dorsal aspect of the cavernoma and now facilitates easy surgical removal. **c** A view through the microscope while removing the cavernoma. Note the typical mulberry aspect of the malformation

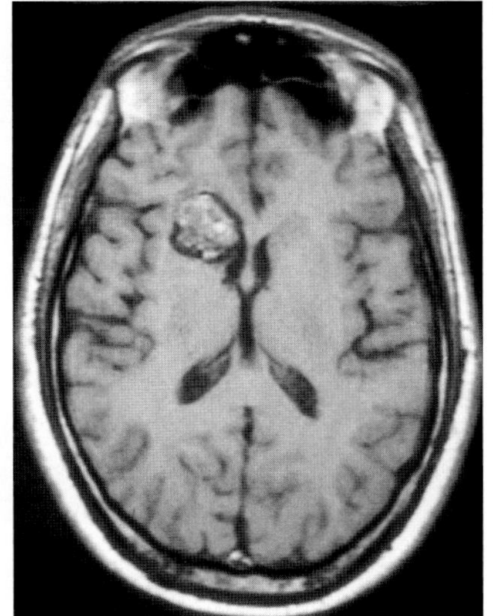

Fig. 2.5a, b. T2-weighted (**a**) and T1-weighted (**b**) magnetic resonance scan of a typical cavernoma. Note that the dark rim of hemosiderin is much more visible on the T2-weighted images. The typical mixed popcorn pattern is pathognomonic and there is no doubt about the diagnosis, even without pathological confirmation

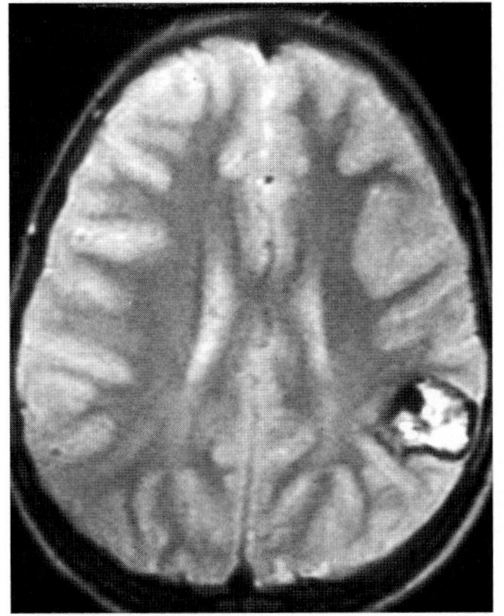

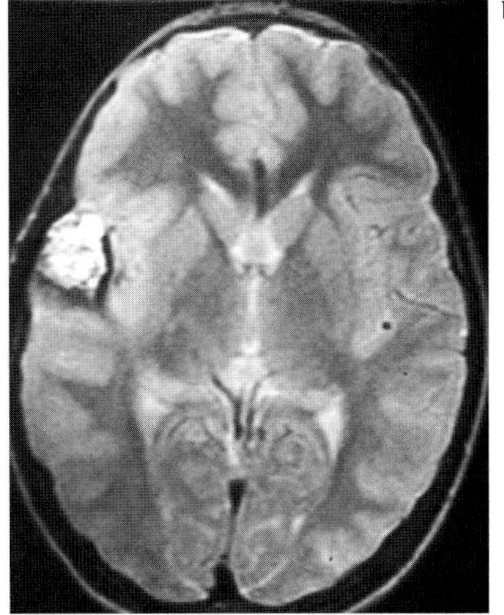

Fig. 2.6a, b. T2-weighted images of a patient who presented with recurrent attacks of severe headache. The referring clinician thought the patient had suffered from a subarachnoid hemorrhage. Magnetic resonance imaging revealed two mirror-like cavernomas, both located at the surface of the brain. The headache attacks were probably caused by repetitive microbleeds into the subarachnoid space and stopped after removal of the malformations

on GRE images was significantly different (7.2 versus 20.2 in symptomatic subjects). Owing to the blood stagnation phenomenon, or to true chronic microhemorrhages, cavernous angiomas contain deoxyhemoglobin or hemosiderin, which generate susceptibility effects and cause a decrease in signal intensity. This loss of signal intensity is much better demonstrated with T2*-weighted GRE sequences (Fig. 2.9). This sequence should be part of the imaging protocol in all patients with a positive family history of cavernoma, all patients with a suspicion of focal or generalized seizures, and in all patients with venous angiomas (there is a significant coincidence between occurrence of venous angiomas and cavernoma).

However, turbo spin-echo sequences using a long echo train, i.e. all FLAIR sequences, are very insensitive to this susceptibility effect. Furthermore, as shown in Figs. 2.11 and 2.12, even large lesions may not have a visible hemosiderin ring, if there were no relevant associated bleeding episodes (Figs. 2.11 and 2.12).

Even though T2* sequences are most sensitive for the hemosiderin ring, one should know the imaging characteristics in the remaining standard sequences. On T1-weighted images, the core of the cavernoma can be hyperintense or slightly hypointense compared to normal brain tissue, depending on the velocity of blood flow and different stages of thrombus degradation. The high signal within a cavernoma on T1-weighted sequences can cause considerable confusion if the lesion is adjacent to an artery. Time-of-flight MRA sequences are usually heavily T1-weighted. Therefore, a cavernoma can mimic an

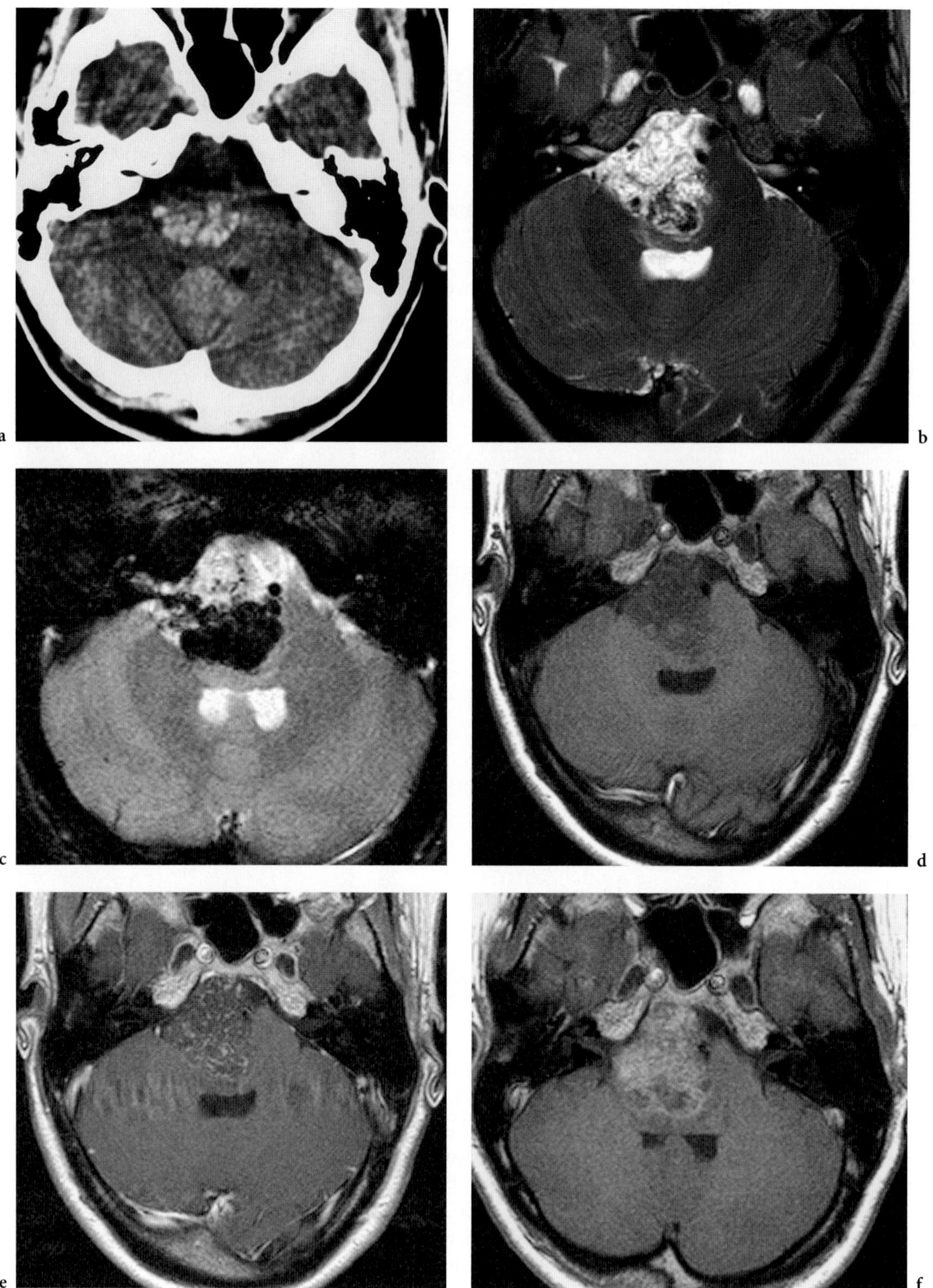

Fig. 2.7a–f. Giant, partially exophytic brain-stem cavernoma. **a** Computed tomography at the time of admission with a hyperdense lesion at the pontomedullary junction. *MRI was performed at 1.5 T*. **b** Transverse T2-weighted turbo spin-echo image at the level of the internal auditory canal. Most of the exophytic lesion is hyperintense, the dorsal part also has hypointense areas. The edema of the adjacent brain parenchyma is probably pressure-related. No blood can be seen within the brainstem itself. **c** T2*-weighted image at the same level. The marked hypointensity within the lesion represents blood degradation products. **d** T1-weighted image before contrast agent administration. The lesion is hypointense compared to brain tissue. **e** At 5 min after injection of gadolinium (0.1 mmol/kg), there is enhancement in some small areas of the mass lesion. **f** At 60 min after contrast injection, the lesion shows an extensive enhancement (pooling)

aneurysm on these images (Fig. 2.8). Most of the clinically used DWI sequences are T2*-weighted and, thus, should detect cavernomas with an increased sensitivity (Fig. 2.11).

In 1994, Zabramski and co-workers suggested establishing an MR classification of cavernomas, which in part could overcome the confusing individualized descriptions of cavernomas in the literature and the problem of defining hemorrhages (Table 2.1). The problem of this classification is the type-4 lesion. The pathologic definition of this type is totally unclear and for us it is questionable whether these lesions really represent capillary telangiectasias. Brunereau et al. (2000) found a close relationship between type-4 lesions and the familial form of cavernous angiomas. Nevertheless, despite these disadvantages, it does make sense to use an MR-based classification to describe a cavernoma and, thus, give somebody in the future the opportunity to compare the results of different authors.

Contrast enhancement has not been described as a characteristic feature of cavernomas of the CNS in the CT era. Because of the improved contrast resolution of MRI (compared to CT), contrast enhancement is much more visible. However, MRI does not overcome the problem created by the slow blood exchange between the normal blood and the dilated cavernous vessels. Specifically with fast T1-weighted sequences it is necessary to delay the interval between contrast agent injection and the start of the scanning procedure. However, contrast injection is usually not necessary (T2 and T2* are diagnostic in the majority of patients).

Whereas a typical cavernoma can usually be identified using MRI, it may be problematic to identify it within an acute hematoma. Our recommendation is: If there is suspicion of an underlying cavernoma in an acute intracerebral hemorrhage (ICH), MR should be performed as early as possible. If the early MR reveals any hemosiderin, former bleeding episodes are evident and the probability of an underlying cavernoma is high (Fig. 2.10).

If MR is performed as a presurgical planning procedure, it is of the utmost importance to scan with thin slices in order to demonstrate the relationship of the cavernoma to the surface of the brain. Particularly in brain stem cavernomas, this relationship is crucial for balancing the risk of the disease against the risk of therapy.

2.1.4 Therapy

Treatment options in cavernomas depend mainly on the natural course of the lesion, as well as its location and surgical accessibility. The latter depends on the skill of the surgeon and the position of the lesion

Table 2.1. Magnetic resonance (MR) imaging classification of cavernous angioma (Zabramski et al. 1994)

Classification and MR sequence	MR imaging features	Histopathologic features
Type 1		
T1-weighted SE	Hyperintense core	Subacute hemorrhage
T2-weighted SE	Hyper- or hypointense core	Subacute hemorrhage
Type 2		
T1-weighted SE	Reticulated mixed core signal	Lesions with hemorrhages and thromboses of different age
T2-weighted SE	Mixed core, dark rim	
Type 3		
T1-weighted SE	Iso- or hypointense	Chronic hemorrhage with hemosiderin staining in and around lesion
T2-weighted SE	Hypointense lesion with dark rim	
Type 4		
T1-weighted SE	Not visible	Tiny lesion or telangiectasia
T2-weighted SE	Not visible	Tiny lesion or telangiectasia
GRE images	Punctate hypointense lesion	Tiny lesion or telangiectasia

SE, spin echo; *GRE*, gradient echo

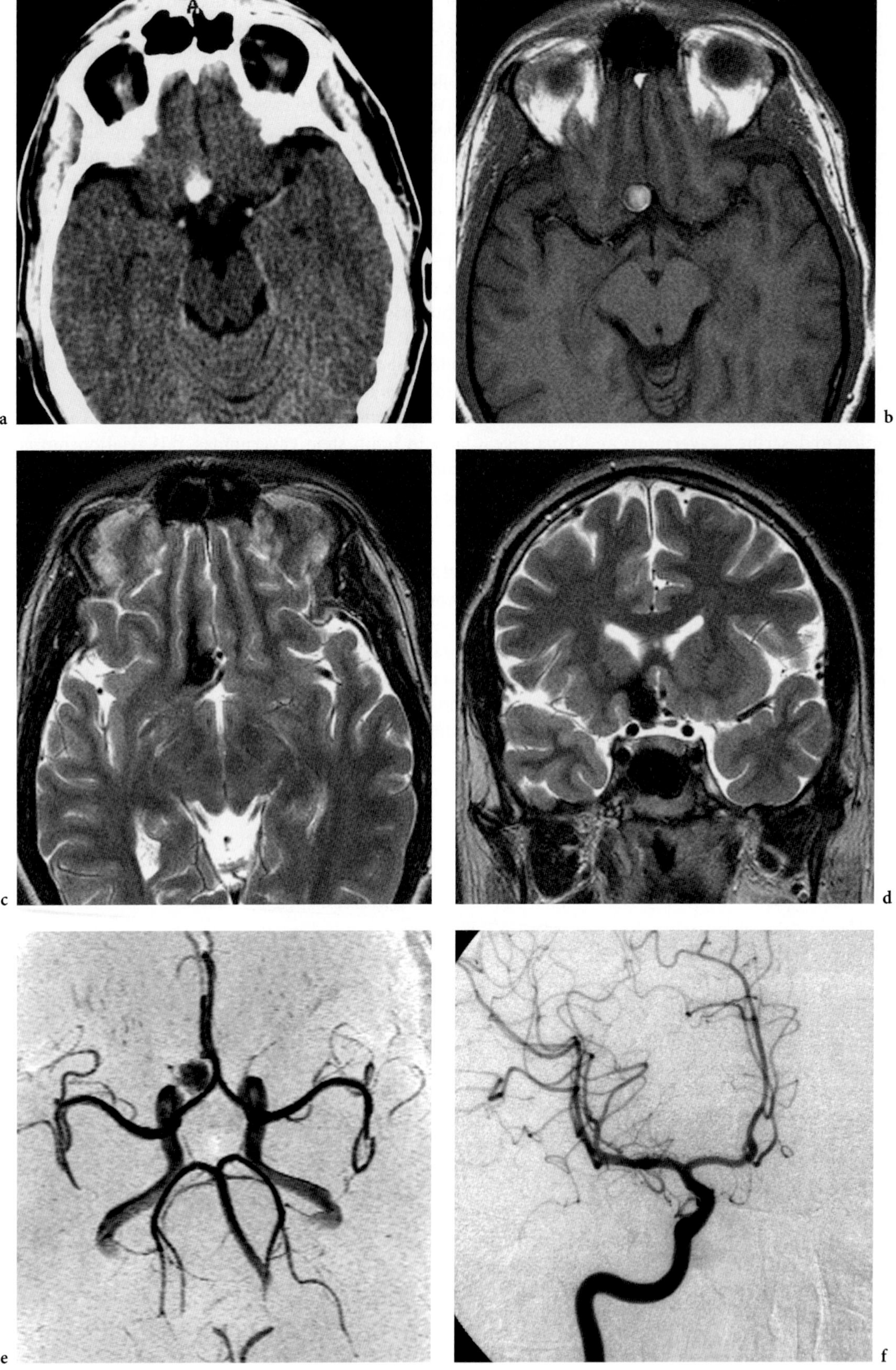
A
a
b
c
d
e
f

Fig. 2.8a–f. Cavernoma mimicking an arterial aneurysm on magnetic resonance angiography (MRA). **a** The non-enhanced computed tomography (CT) scan reveals a hyperdense lesion in the straight gyrus adjacent to the optic nerve and right anterior cerebral artery. **b** T1-weighted MR image without contrast enhancement reveals a hyperintense and well circumscribed lesion. There was no contrast enhancement after injection of gadolinium (not shown). **c** Axial T2-weighted image reveals a dark lesion with an extensive hypointense area. This dark area represents hemosiderin deposition resulting from old hemorrhage. Note that the hemosiderin is within the white matter, but not on the surface of the brain. There is no communication between the anterior cerebral arteries in the interhemispheric fissure and the lesion in the straight gyrus. **d** Coronal T2-weighted image also demonstrates the hemosiderin deposition within the white matter and not on the surface of the brain. **e** This maximum-intensity projection of a time-of-flight MRA shows a structure adjacent to the anterior cerebral arteries. This is due to the high T1 signal of the cavernoma, indistinguishable from the flow signal in a T1-weighted FISP-MRA sequence. This phenomenon can be misinterpreted as an aneurysm. **f** Intraarterial digital subtraction angiography to rule out an aneurysm. The wall of the anterior cerebral artery is smooth and without any hint of an aneurysm, patent or thrombosed

relative to eloquent areas of the brain. In general, therapeutic strategies include:

- Observation of patients with asymptomatic or inaccessible lesions
- Surgical excision of symptomatic and accessible lesions
- Radiosurgery for progressively symptomatic but surgically inaccessible lesions.

Patients presenting without gross hemorrhage, seizures, or other specific symptoms are clearly candidates for clinical observation. For us, it is questionable whether this patient group does need repeat imaging, if the clinical condition remains unchanged.

Surgical resection is recommended for cavernomas presenting with symptomatic (or repeat symptomatic) hemorrhage and located in an accessible and noneloquent area of the brain.

If the lesion is surgically inaccessible or does not present with bleeding episodes, the treatment options are less clear. In a recently published review (Moran et al. 1999), the results after surgical removal of cavernomas causing seizures were analyzed. After removal of the cavernoma, 84% of the patients were seizure-free and 8% were improved. A total of 6% of the patients did not have any change of their status, and in only 2% of patients was there deterioration. In cases of medically intractable seizures in which surgery is technically feasible and the seizures can be localized to the region of the cavernoma, surgery is a reasonable option. However, in nonintractable cases, it is unclear whether early surgery is advantageous. It is plausible that a longer duration of epilepsy may prejudice the outcome of any surgery ultimately performed. Kindling effects may play a role in increasing intractability and this may be a theoretical basis

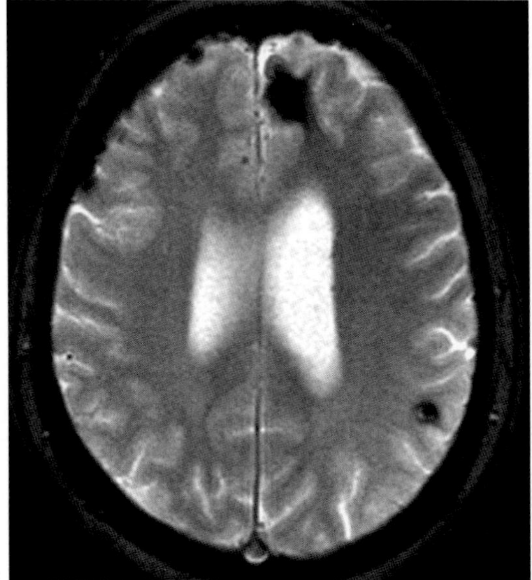

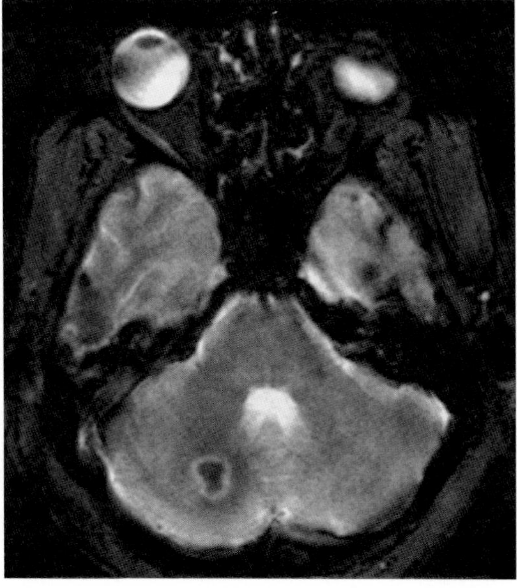

Fig. 2.9a, b. Multiple cavernomas. T2*-weighted gradient echo sequence. There are multiple cavernomas in both cerebral hemispheres and the cerebellum. The T2* sequence is particularly sensitive to hemosiderin depositions indicative of cavernomas

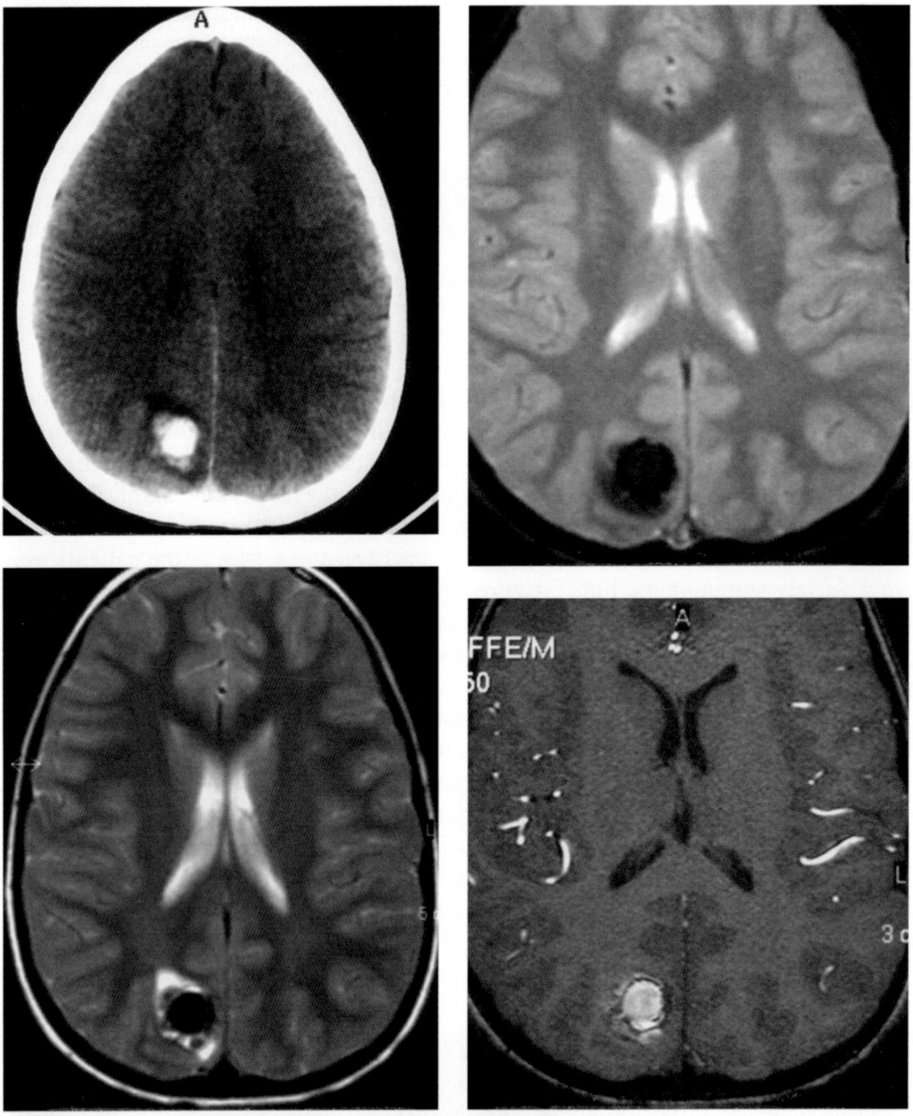

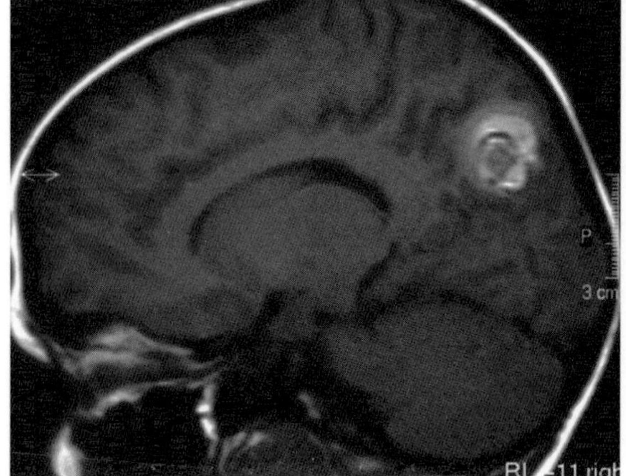

Fig. 2.10a–e. Cavernoma with signs of recent hemorrhage in a 9-year-old child. **a** Computed tomography scan reveals a hyperdense lesion in the right occipital lobe with perifocal edema. The lesion has a heterogeneous density with a very dense core and reduced attenuation values at the peripheral zone. **b** T2*-weighted gradient-echo image displays the lesion as a dark spot. **c** The T2-weighted turbo spin-echo image shows a dark center with a bright rim of edema. **d** This flow-sensitive gradient-echo sequence demonstrates a bright core with a pseudocapsule. A maximum-intensity projection of this sequence will display arterial vessels and the bright hemorrhage, giving rise to a misinterpretation of the cavernoma as an aneurysm. **e** T1-weighted spin-echo image shows the cavernoma core with surrounding subacute hemorrhage located in the cuneus adjacent to the calcarine fissure

for early surgery. However, there are no data on this problem in the literature.

The main indication for surgical removal of a cavernoma is prevention of hemorrhage. Therefore, many surgical groups recommend surgical removal of a cavernoma if it is located in a noneloquent brain area and easily accessible. However, as mentioned above, it is quite difficult to predict the natural course of an individual cavernoma and, therefore, it is impossible to balance the individual bleeding risk of the individual patient against the morbidity and mortality of a surgical procedure. It seems to be more appropriate to limit surgical excision to those patients with at least one hemorrhagic episode – based on clinical and imaging findings and never alone on MR – or those with intractable seizures. Brain-stem cavernomas are clearly a specific subgroup. Over the years, neurosurgical techniques and knowledge about different approaches to the brain stem increased, enabling the excision of many lesions without significant morbidity and mortality. The necessity for removal of brain-stem cavernomas is mainly based on some reports suggesting that the bleeding rates in brain-stem cavernomas is significantly higher than in those located supratentorially (Porter et al. 1999). In contrast, Kupersmith recommended a more conservative approach, because he found that brain-stem cavernomas do not have a relevant elevated risk of hemorrhage. Finally, there is no definite answer to the question of how to handle brain-stem cavernomas! In experienced hands, it seems to be reasonable to remove them, but it is also not a mistake to wait and just observe the patient.

Recently, Hasegawa and colleagues (2002) reported their results after stereotactic radiosurgery of cavernomas. The authors found that before radiosurgery, the annual rehemorrhage rate was 33.9%, whereas after radiosurgery, the rehemorrhage rates were 12.3% for the first 2 years and 0.76% for years 2–12 after radiosurgery. More than 50% of the cavernomas decreased in size after radiosurgery. The theory behind this therapeutic option is that radiosurgery even in cavernomas leads to progressive hyalinization with thickening of the endothelium-lined vessels and eventual closure of the lumen. These results seem striking and lead the authors to conclude that radiosurgery offers a dramatic reduction in the risk of rehemorrhage in high-risk patients. Treatment morbidity was 13%. The major drawback of this study, however, is that there is no control group and therefore it was not possible to perform a true risk-to-benefit analysis. Nevertheless: if the lesion is really not surgically removable and the patient is at high risk of rehemorrhage (more than two previous bleeding episodes), radiosurgery can be a treatment option. Radiosurgery is clearly not an established therapeutic option and should not be used instead of surgery in surgically accessible lesions.

To optimize therapeutic approaches to CNS cavernomas, a randomized multicenter trial dedicated to different therapeutic options would be necessary.

2.2 Capillary Telangiectasia

2.2.1 Pathology

Capillary telangiectasias are a distinct category of cerebral vascular malformations, consisting of localized collections of multiple thin-walled vascular channels interposed between normal brain parenchyma. They were first described in 1959 (Russell and Rubinstein 1989) and are characterized by small capillaries with a maximum diameter of 30 µm. In contrast to cavernomas, brain parenchyma is located between the dilated vessels. There is still some disagreement in literature as to whether the vessels of a capillary telangiectasia have a normal wall (Ferszt 1989) or not (Okazaki 1989). Growth and bleeding have not been observed so far, however, hemosiderin may be seen rarely in the surrounding tissue (Küker et al. 2000).

The true incidence of capillary malformations or telangiectasias of the brain is difficult to discern because the vast majority are obviously clinically asymptomatic. Estimates from autopsy series suggest they are not uncommon, representing approximately 16%–20% of all CNS vascular malformations (Chaloupka and Huddle 1998). Capillary telangiectasias, although known to occur throughout the brain and spine, are most frequently found within the striate pons and are the most frequent incidental vascular malformation of the pons at autopsy (Russell and Rubinstein 1959; McCormick et al. 1968). Other locations are the basal ganglia, where they usually cause confusion because of their enhancement and the lack of mass effect (Castillo et al. 2001).

Several authors found an association with cavernomas in their patients (Küker et al. 2000), or suggested that both vascular abnormalities have a common origin (Rigamonti et al. 1991). However, in contrast to cavernomas, the occurrence of capillary telangiectasia seems to be mainly sporadic. No hereditary

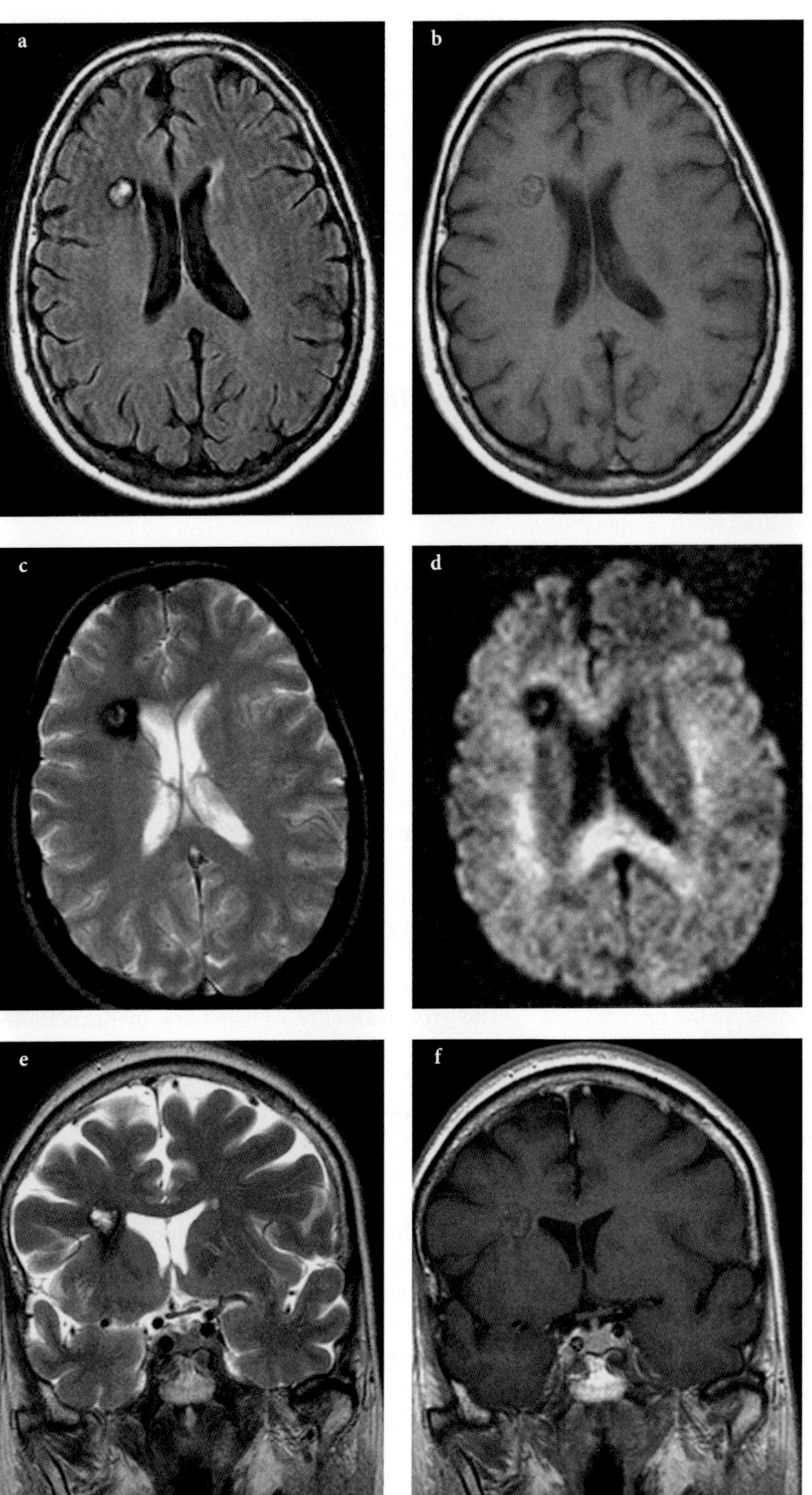

Fig. 2.11a–f. Synoptical presentation of a cavernoma in standard magnetic resonance sequences at 1.5 T. **a** T2-weighted FLAIR sequence. There has been no scientific evaluation of FLAIR for cavernomas to date. In our experience, a hyperintense center is well depicted; however, due to the long echo train lengths, the hemosiderin wall is usually not well depicted. **b** In T1-weighted spin-echo sequences the cavernoma may have the same signal intensity as the adjacent brain parenchyma. In particular, small cavernomas can easily be missed. **c** T2*-weighted gradient echo sequences are the gold standard for cavernoma depiction, due to the susceptibility effect of the hemosiderin rim. Because the hemosiderin rim may be much larger than the cavernoma core, gradient-echo images should always be applied in doubtful cases and to look for additional cavernomas. **d** Diffusion-weighted echo planar imaging (EPI) sequence. Diffusion imaging is not routinely used for the evaluation of cavernomas. However, these sequences are mostly T2*-weighted and the contrast should be like in the T2*-weighted non-EPI gradient echo images. Due to the matrix size, the spatial resolution of DWI is usually lower. **e** T2-weighted turbo spin-echo image. The bright core is well depicted as is the dark rim, less apparent in the FLAIR sequence [compare to (**a**)]. A problem may arise, if the cavernoma is close to the cerebrospinal-fluid space. **f** T1-weighted image after contrast administration (0.1 mmol Gd-DTPA/kg). Even on this scan performed 10 min after contrast injection, there is very little contrast enhancement visible. Higher doses or delayed scanning for the demonstration of "pooling" may be necessary

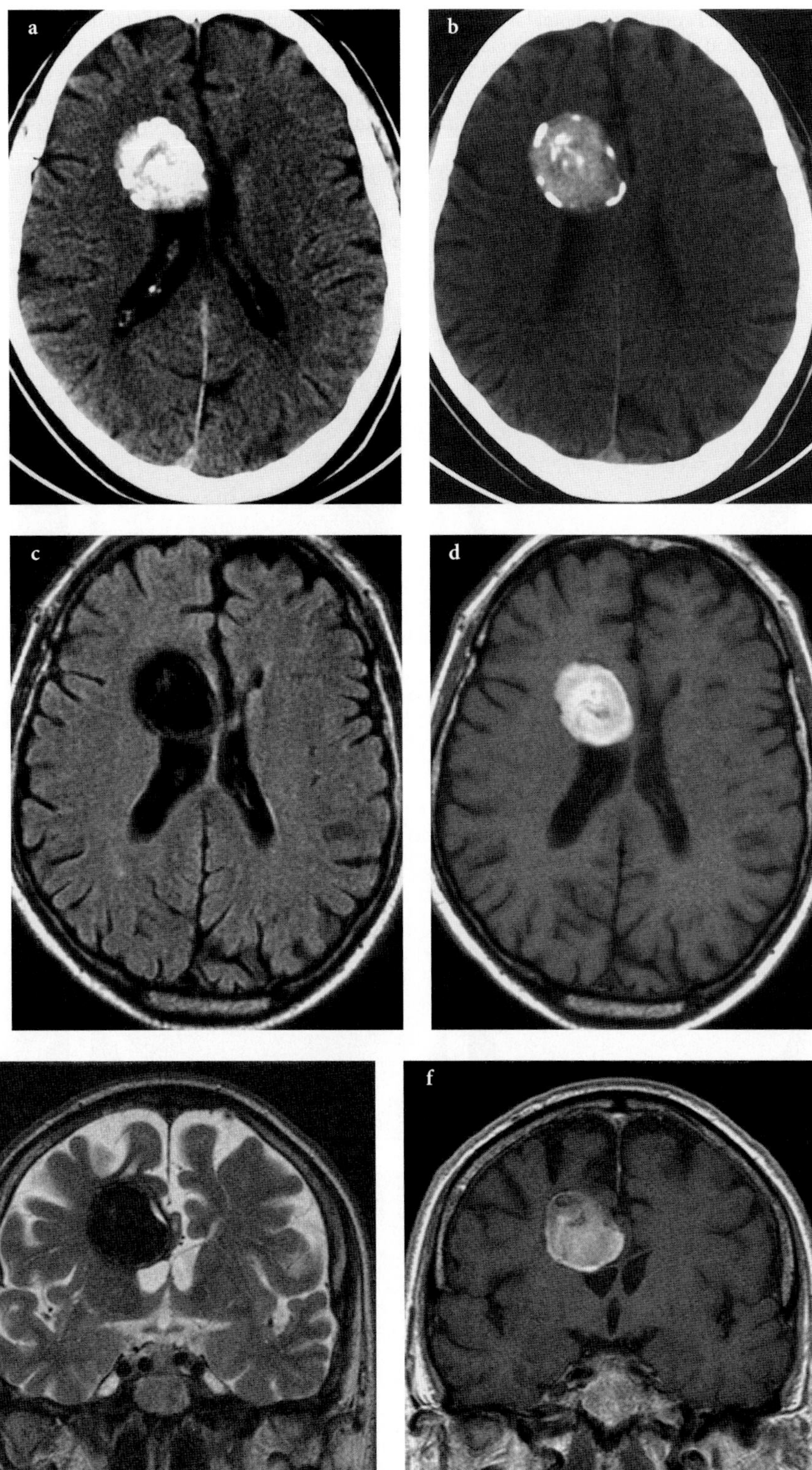

Fig. 2.12a–f. Supratentorial giant cavernoma as an incidental finding. **a** Computer tomography scan without intravenous contrast. The large, hyperdense lesion in the white matter adjacent to the lateral ventricle is not surrounded by edema, nor is there any blood in the ventricle itself. **b** In this window setting, calcified areas of the wall and parts of the inner structures are clearly visible. **c** The T2-weighted FLAIR sequence shows a dark mass lesion protruding into the ventricle. There is no perifocal edema. **d** T1-weighted spin-echo sequence without contrast reveals the lesion as hyperintense. **e** T2-weighted image in the coronal plain reveals a mostly hypointense, sharply demarcated lesion in the right cingulate gyrus, protruding into the interhemispheric fissure. There is no dark rim, edema, or any other signs of recent or older extralesional hemorrhage. **f** The cavernoma is mostly hyperintense on this T1-weighted image after contrast administration (Gd-DTPA 0.1 mmol/kg). Contrast enhancement could not be demonstrated

Fig. 2.13a–n. Familial cavernomatosis: **a, b** Computed tomography (CT) scans at different levels. Multiple lesions of high density are visible in the cerebral parenchyma. The lesions are of inhomogeneous density. There is no perifocal edema. **c, d** The T2*-weighted gradient-echo sequence (FLASH) clearly shows the large cavernomas, mostly hypointense with bright foci. However, there are many more dark areas in both hemispheres which were not visible on the CT scan. These lesions are also cavernomas. The T2*-gradient-echo sequence is most sensitive to susceptibility effects of hemosiderin deposits and therefore a screening ▷▷

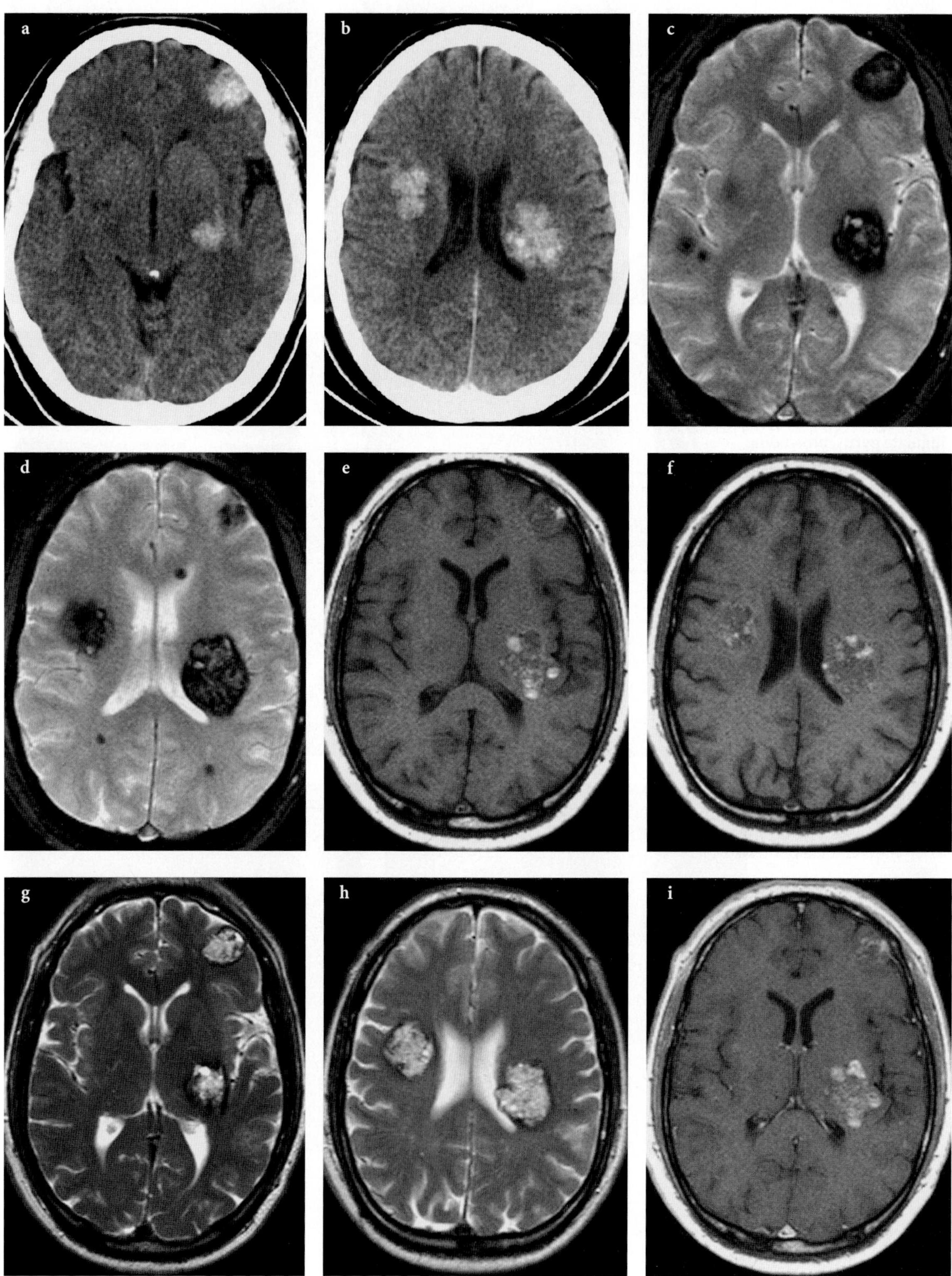

sequence for small cavernomas. It should always be added to the imaging protocol. **e, f** T1-weighted spin-echo images. Cavernomas are of inhomogeneous signal intensity. There are some areas of high signal intensity in this sequence, but large parts of the cavernomas are isointense to the adjacent brain. The small cavernomas are not visible with this sequence. **g, h** T2-weighted turbo spin-echo sequence. The large cavernomas are mainly hyperintense with a small dark rim due to hemosiderin deposits. The small lesions, which were clearly visible in the T2*-weighted images, are not apparent on these slices. There is no perifocal edema. This sequence demonstrates the relation to the brain surface. The cortex over the cavernoma is slightly displaced and contains hemosiderin. Therefore, the location of the cavernoma will be visible intraoperatively. **i, j** T1-weighted spin-echo image 3 min after administration of gadolinium (0.1 mmol/kg). The increase in signal intensity is very subtle compared to the images prior to contrast injection. The enhancement is inhomogeneous. **k** T2-weighted turbo spin-echo image in a coronal view. Large cavernomas are visible in the basal ganglia on both sides with an inhomogeneous signal pattern. There is a peripheral zone of hypointensity due to hemosiderin. The absence of a perifocal edema is a hint at recent enlargement or bleeding. The displacement of adjacent structures is small for the size of the lesions. **l** T1-weighted image 15 min after administration of contrast. The signal appears higher than in (**i**) and (**j**). **m** This T2-weighted coronal view shows a large cavernoma in the basal ganglia with moderate mass effect and slight compression of the internal capsule. The patient had no neurological symptoms. **n** T1-weighted image 15 min after administration of contrast. The lesion also displays a delayed enhancement of a typical pattern. The cavernoma extends from the brain surface in the Sylvian fissure to the lateral ventricle

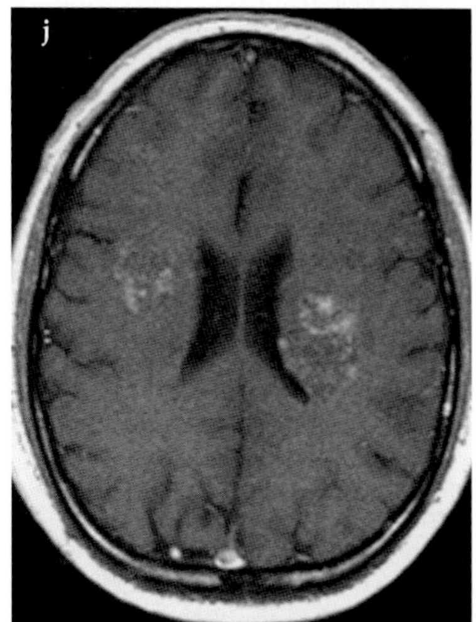

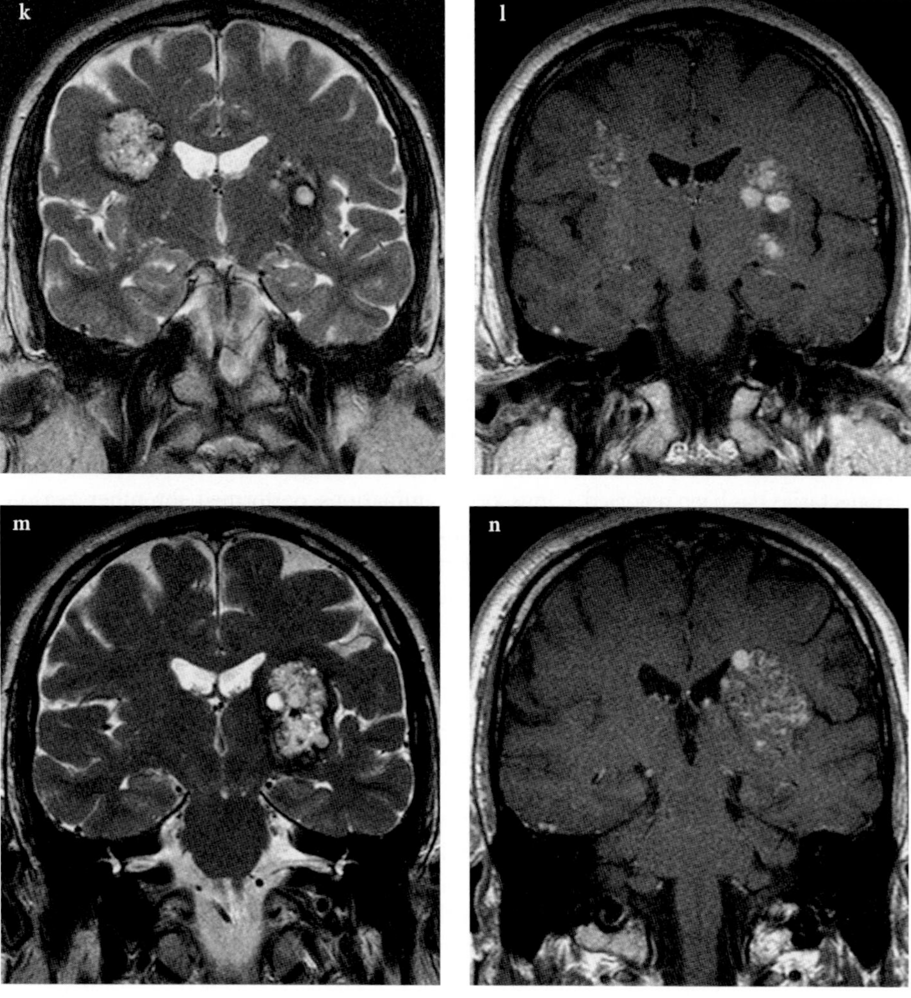

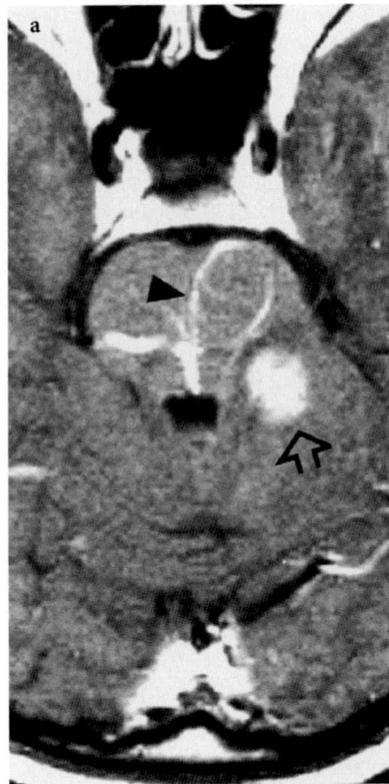

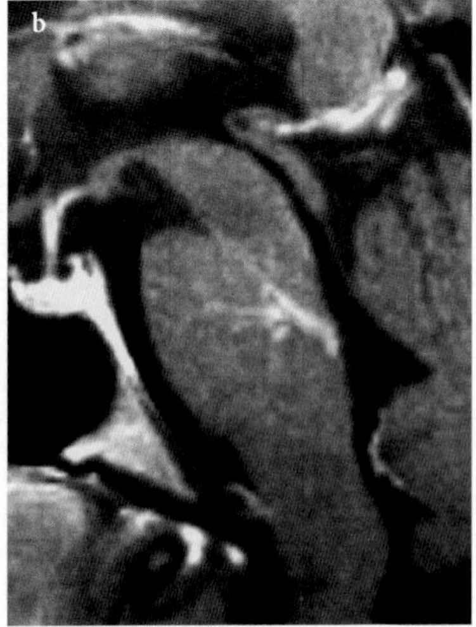

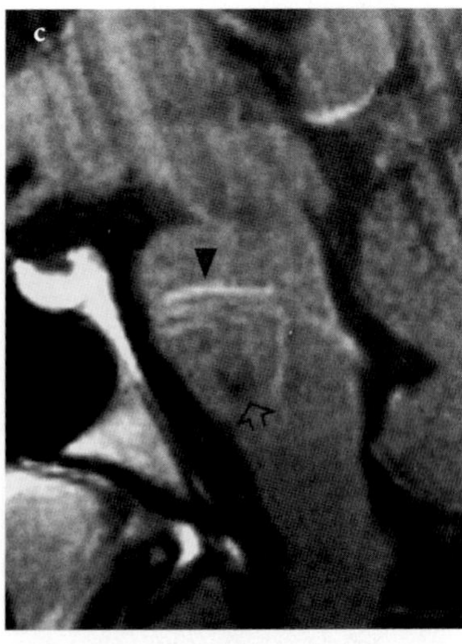

Fig. 2.14a–c. Combination of brainstem cavernoma and capillary telangiectasia. **a** This T1-weighted transverse image after contrast administration at the level of the upper pons shows a cavernoma (*open arrow*) and transparenchymal venous vessels (*arrowhead*), belonging to a capillary telangiectasia. **b** This midline sagittal T1 image after contrast injection shows the venous tributary of the capillary telangiectasia, a typical sign of capillary malformations. **c** This T1 image slightly off the midline demonstrates the draining veins of the capillary telangiectasia (*arrowhead*), as well as a second cavernoma (*open arrow*)

forms have been reported and no underlying genetic abnormality were identified in this specific form of vascular abnormality. However, genetic defects may be responsible for the occurrence of cerebral venous malformations in general (Korpelainen et al. 1999; Vikkula et al. 1996).

It has been suggested that they have a common origin with cavernous hemangiomas (Rigamonti et al. 1991; Awad et al. 1993). Therefore, hemorrhagic complications may be due to associated cavernomas and not to bleeding of the capillary telangiectasia. However, in some large groups of cavernomas, no association with capillary telangiectasias has been reported (Mull et al. 1995). It remains undetermined to date whether capillary telangiectasias change with time or are developmental abnormalities, i.e., small DVA.

The rarity of in vivo histologic verification indicates that the benign clinical behavior and the critical anatomic localization of brain-stem capillary telangiectasias do not allow stereotactic biopsy on a regular basis. The earlier case reports depended on histologic examinations of cadaver specimens.

Hereditary hemorrhagic telangiectasia (Rendu-Osler disease) is not associated with cerebral capillary telangiectasia, but with other forms of cerebral vascular malformations (Maher et al. 2001), mainly true pial arteriovenous malformations, dural arteriovenous malformations, and, rarely, cavernomas.

2.2.2 Clinical Presentation

Capillary telangiectasias are vascular malformations of unknown origin and unknown clinical significance (Rigamonti et al. 1991; Awad et al. 1993). In vivo diagnosis is only possible with MRI because these lesions are so small that they are undetectable by either angiography or CT (Barr et al. 1996). Furthermore, slow blood flow may also contribute to the lack of angiographic opacification.

Most capillary telangiectasia are incidental findings on examinations performed for other reasons than brain-stem symptoms. In general, the clinical manifestations related to capillary malformations are variable, although typically they are regarded as quiescent lesions occasionally presenting with headaches, confusion, weakness, dizziness, visual changes, vertigo, tinnitus, or seizures (Barr et al. 1996; Lee et al. 1997).

However, there is evidence of a possible symptomatic subgroup of capillary telangiectasia (Huddle et al. 1999; Scaglione et al. 2001). One of our patients (Fig. 2.9) also presented with symptoms attributable to a vascular malformation of the brain-stem, which best fits into the category of capillary telangiectasia. Whereas the patients reported by Scaglione et al. (2001) had only minor complaints with disputable cause due to the capillary telangiectasia, the patient

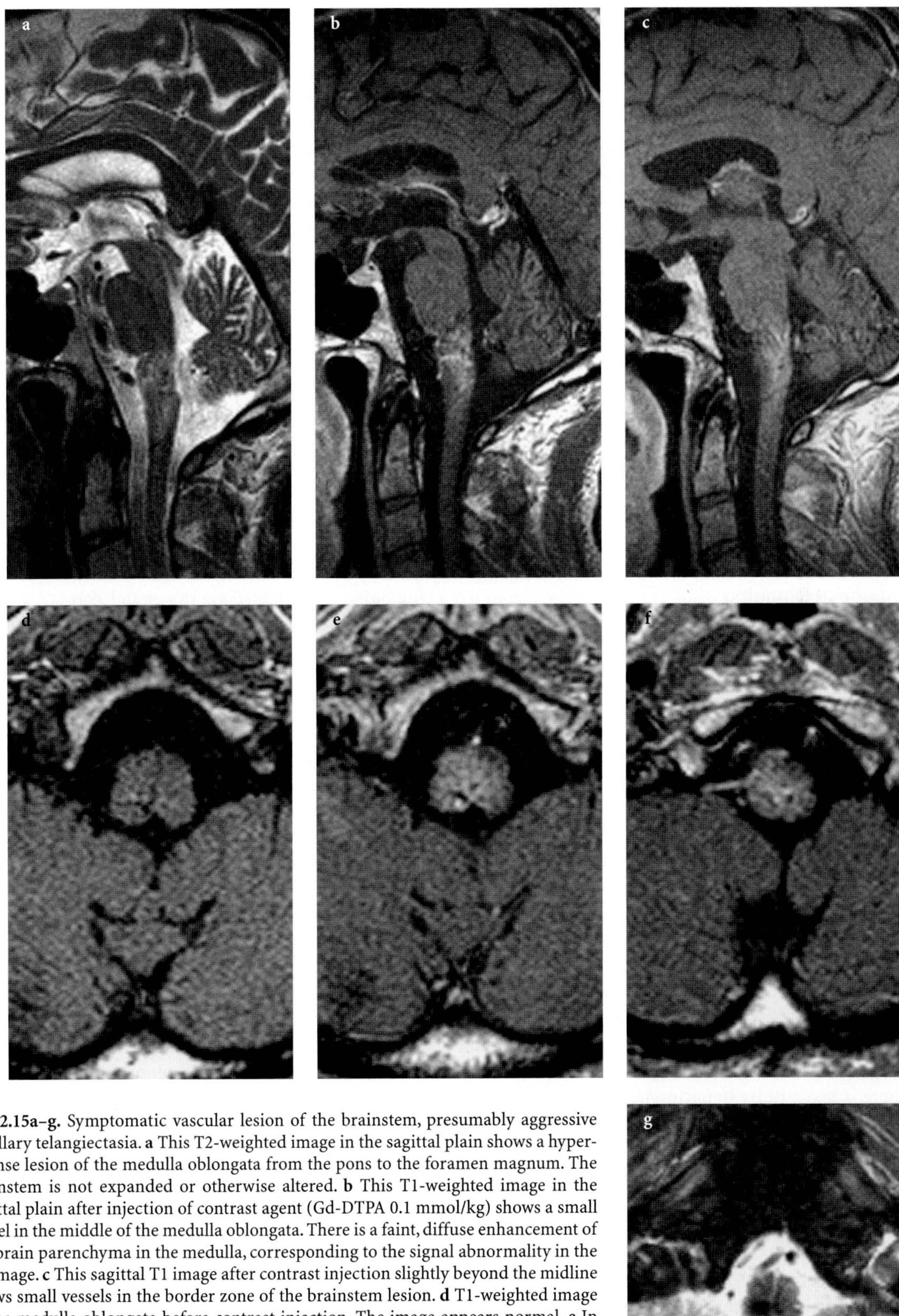

Fig. 2.15a–g. Symptomatic vascular lesion of the brainstem, presumably aggressive capillary telangiectasia. **a** This T2-weighted image in the sagittal plain shows a hyperintense lesion of the medulla oblongata from the pons to the foramen magnum. The brainstem is not expanded or otherwise altered. **b** This T1-weighted image in the sagittal plain after injection of contrast agent (Gd-DTPA 0.1 mmol/kg) shows a small vessel in the middle of the medulla oblongata. There is a faint, diffuse enhancement of the brain parenchyma in the medulla, corresponding to the signal abnormality in the T2 image. **c** This sagittal T1 image after contrast injection slightly beyond the midline shows small vessels in the border zone of the brainstem lesion. **d** T1-weighted image of the medulla oblongata before contrast injection. The image appears normal. **e** In the same position, there is diffuse enhancement of the medulla and a small vessel can be seen near to the dorsal surface of the brainstem. **f** This T1-weighted transverse slice in a more caudal position shows a blood vessel in the cerebrospinal-fluid space on the right of the medulla. The absence of a flow void suggests a draining vein. However, the vertebral arteries are also hyperintense. **g** This T2*-weighted image shows a hypointense lesion in the medulla, predominately on the right. An arteriovenous malformation was ruled out by intraarterial angiography and the lesion was stable on follow-up magnetic resonance imaging

reported by Huddle et al. (1999) had severe neurologic symptoms and died presumably due to the ensuing brain-stem dysfunction. Both severely symptomatic patients showed an extensive T2 signal abnormality of the affected parts of the brain stem. Furthermore, for us there is an association of tinnitus and pontine capillary telangiectasia. Many of our tinnitus patients had a long history of doctor-hopping and were at least once in their life considered to be mentally ill.

This is in contrast to most other cases, who are asymptomatic or have very little symptoms. Further observations will be necessary to establish whether there is in fact a severely symptomatic, aggressive subform of capillary telangiectasia.

Up to now, there has been no pertinent hypothesis for a possible pathomechanism for the ensuing symptoms.

2.2.3 Diagnostic Imaging

The number of observations of presumed brain-stem capillary telangiectasias is limited. There are only two reports of MRI features in a larger group of patients (Barr et al. 1996; Lee et al. 1997). These 30 cases seem to have very similar imaging findings. With two exceptions, all were located in the brain stem with a predominance of the mid pons.

MRI is the imaging modality of choice for the evaluation of brain-stem lesions in general (Küker et al. 2000), but is the only tool capillary telangiectasias can be visualized with during life.

Capillary telangiectasia are usually first discovered on T1-weighted images after contrast injection (Fig. 2.14). Depending on slice thickness and individual appearance, the characteristic picture is dominated by small radiating venous vessels, converging on a small collecting vein. In other patients, there is just a fluffy hyperintensity without apparent individual vessels. In these cases, the radiating vessels are so small that even thin section MRI is not able to discriminate between them. In such conditions, the vascular malformation appears as a homogenous, somewhat irregularly contoured lesion (Küker et al. 2000; Barr et al. 1996; Lee et al. 1997).

In contrast to cavernous hemangiomas or other brain-stem lesions, the contrast enhancement of capillary telangiectasia is only of short duration. In typical cases, it will not last longer than 20 min. Dynamic MRI, therefore, will reveal a fast signal increase and a substantial signal decrease after 20 min. In some patients, brain-stem metastasis might be a reasonable differential diagnosis. And, usually, metastatic disease accumulates contrast agent over time and will reach a peak enhancement somewhere between 15 and 30 min following administration. Dynamic MRI is a nice tool to differentiate between both entities.

A highly suggestive feature of a capillary telangiectasia is the presence of a larger, easily detectable draining vein (Küker et al. 2000; Barr et al. 1996).

Because capillary telangiectasias are usually dark on T2*-weighted images, the use of GRE sequences for differential diagnosis has been strongly advocated (Fig. 2.15). Lee et al. (1997) reported that most lesions in their series were not detectable on either the T1- and T2- weighted images, but were consistently identified as regions of pronounced loss of signal on the GRE images, which they considered essential for making the diagnosis. Macroscopic hemorrhage and calcifications are rare in capillary telangiectasia, suggesting that the finding on T2*-weighted images are probably related to the presence of deoxyhemoglobin in the slow-flowing blood (Auffray-Calvier et al. 1999)

A dark lesion on GRE images, which is not visible on conventional T2, is usually not a cavernoma, but a capillary malformation. Edema, gliosis, or signs of previous hemorrhage are usually absent. Follow-up images have never revealed any change in capillary malformations.

Curiously, about two thirds of capillary telangiectasias show an enlarged vessel believed to represent a draining vein. This observation has led some authors to consider the concept of "transitional malformations" (Rigamonti et al. 1991).

Angiography is not required for diagnostic work-up in typical cases.

The exact nature of pontine lesions classified as capillary malformations will remain speculative in the vast majority of patients. Aside from vascular malformations, the differential diagnosis of an enhancing pontine lesion might include neoplasm, demyelinating disease, infection, infarction, or, rarely, central pontine myelinolysis. The absence of mass effect or significant T2 prolongation, however, argues strongly against each of these entities. In particular, the distinction from neoplasm must be reinforced to avoid unnecessary biopsy in these patients. A relatively common misinterpretation is that of a pontine glioma; and again: capillary malformations do not exhibit a mass effect and do not change over time! In addition: Decreased signal on GRE images is not a typical feature of pontine gliomas.

Although thought to be typical of the brain stem (Figs. 2.16 and 2.17), close scrutiny of high quality MR images discloses similar abnormalities in other locations as well. Capillary telangiectasias may be located

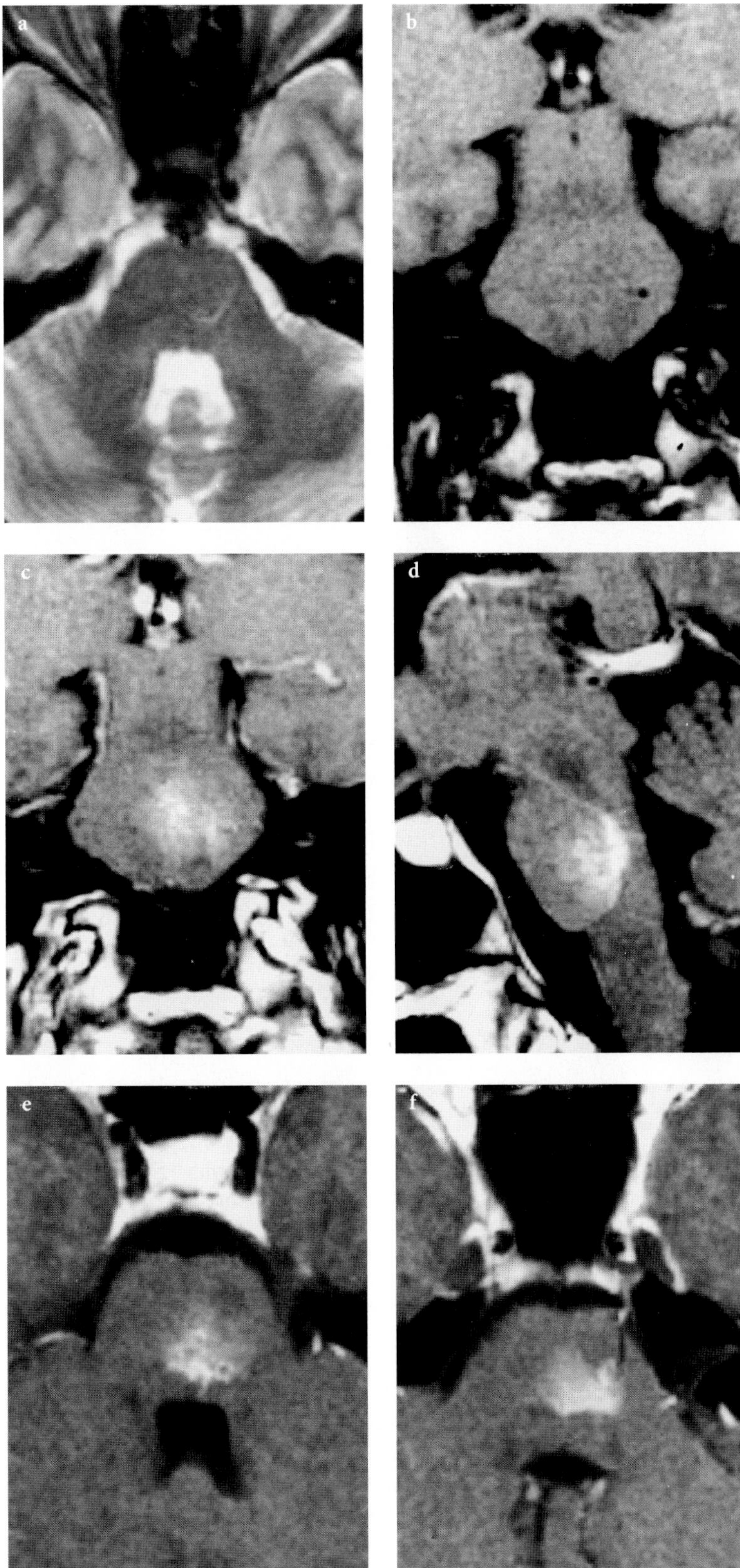

Fig. 2.16a–f. Asymptomatic capillary telangiectasia of the pons with normal T2 appearance. **a** This transverse, thin-section T2 image of the pons is normal. **b** The T1 image of the brain stem in the coronal view before administration of contrast agent shows an abnormal vessel in the pons on the left, but is otherwise normal. **c** T1-weighted image in the coronal plain. After contrast administration (Gd-DTPA 0.1 mmol/kg), there is a diffuse enhancement in the pons, more pronounced on the left and in the center. **d** The T1 image in the sagittal plain after contrast injection shows the typical aspect of a large capillary telangiectasia. **e** Transverse T1-weighted image after contrast injection. Even in this 3-mm slice, the tiny vessels can not be separated. **f** Apart from a more homogenous enhancing area, there is a small vessel displaying flow void on the left border of the pons

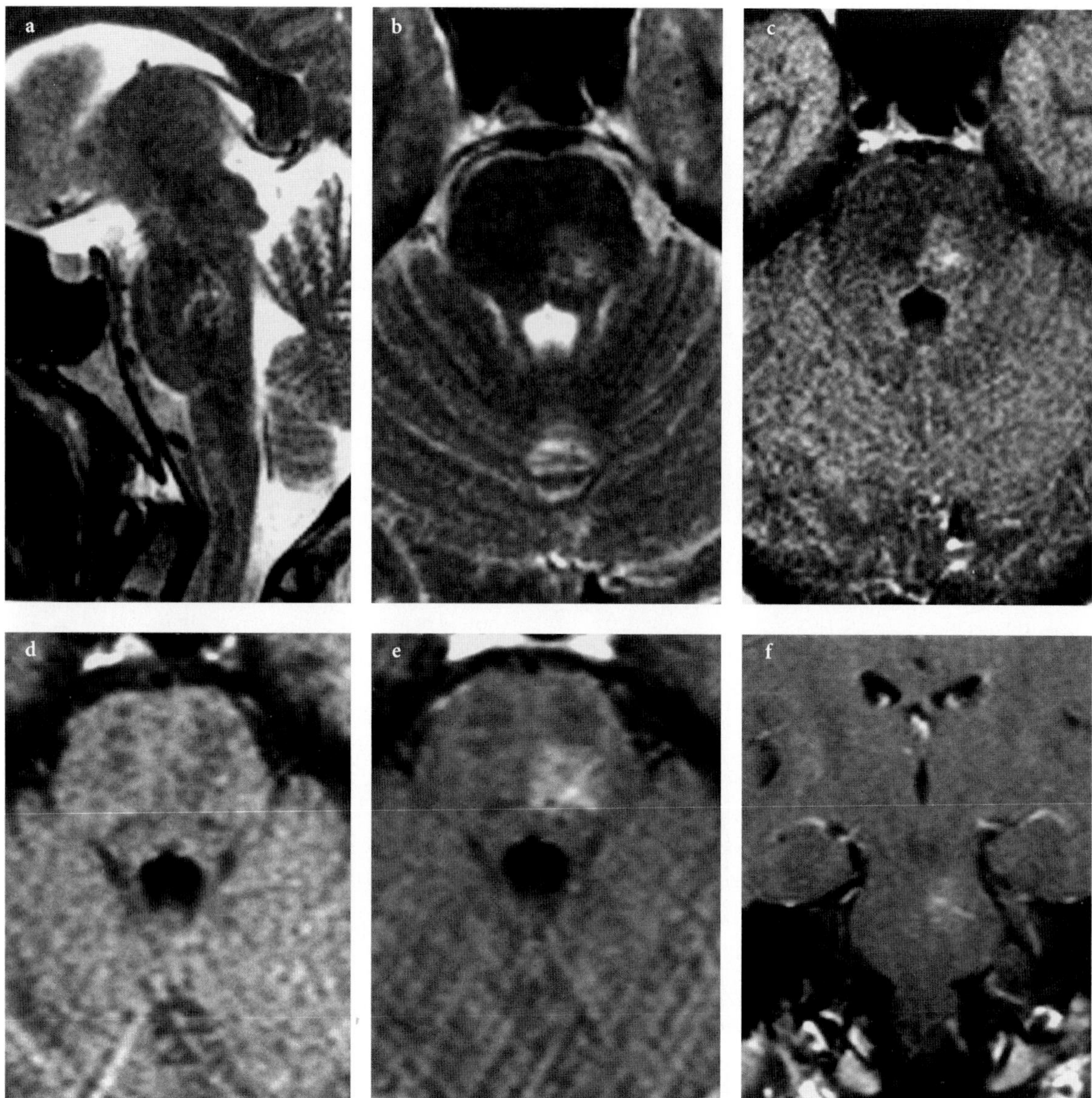

Fig. 2.17a–f. Asymptomatic pontine capillary telangiectasia with T2-signal abnormality. **a** Sagittal T2-weighted image. There is a abnormal structure in the pons with a tree-like appearance. **b** The thin-section, T2-weighted turbo spin-echo image shows a signal abnormality on the left side of the pons. **c** The lesion is also apparent on this T2-weighted FLAIR image. **d** The T1-weighted image before contrast injection is normal. **e** After administration of contrast agent (Gd-DTPA, 0.1 mmol/kg), there is an enhancing lesion in the brain stem, corresponding to the area of abnormal T2 signal. **f** The T1 image in the coronal plain also shows the typical capillary telangiectasia

in the cerebral hemispheres and in the basal ganglia. This should always be kept in mind prior to embarking on surgery or biopsy (Castillo et al. 2001).

Because of its benign clinical course and the lack of therapeutic options, invasive diagnostic procedures like biopsy or angiography must be avoided. However, it is still unclear whether these patients are at increased risk for hemorrhage or the development of cavernous angiomas (Barr et al. 1996).

2.2.4 Therapy

No therapy is available, nor is it usually required. It is not even established practice to perform any follow-up imaging (unless you want to confirm the diagnosis). If the diagnosis seems to be established, there is no need for further follow-up.

References

Aiba T, Tanaka R, Koike T, Kamayama S, Takeda N, Komata T (1995) Natural history of intracranial cavernous malformations. J Neurosurg 83:56–59

Amirjamshidi A, Abbassioun K (2000) Radiation-induced tumors of the central nernous system occurring in childhood and adolescence. Four unusual lesions in three patients and a review of the literature. Childs Nerv Syst 16:390–397

Auffray-Calvier E, Desal HA, Freund P, Laplaud D, Mathon G, de Kersaint-Gilly A (1999) Capillary teleangiectasias: angiographically occult vascular malformations – MRI symptomatology apropos of 7 cases. J Neuroradiol 26: 257–261

Awad IA, Robinson JR, Mohanty S, Estes ML (1993) Mixed vascular malformations of the brain: clinical and pathogenetic considerations. Neurosurgery 33:179–188

Barr RM, Dillon WP, Wilson CB (1996) Slow-flow vascular malformations of the pons: capillary telangiectasias? AJNR Am J Neuroradiol 17:71–78

Bristot R, Santoro A, Fantozzi L, Delfini R (1997) Cavernoma of the cavernous sinus: case report. Surg Neurol 48:160–163

Brunereau L, Labauge P, Tournier Lasserve E, Laberge S, Levy C, Houtteville JP (2000) Familial form of intracranial cavernous angioma: MR imaging findings in 51 families. French Society of Neurosurgery. Radiology 214:209–216

Castillo M, Morrison T, Shaw JA, Bouldin TW (2001) MR imaging and histologic features of capillary telangiectasia of the basal ganglia. AJNR Am J Neuroradiol 22:1553–1555

Chaloupka JC, Huddle DC (1998) Classification of vascular malformations of the central nervous system. Neuroimaging Clin North Am 8:295–321

Chang SD, Steinberg GK, Rosario M, Crowley RS, Hevner RF (1997) Mixed arteriovenous and capillary teleangiectasia: a rare subset of mixed vascular malformations. J Neurosurg 86:699–703

Clatterbuck RE, Moriaritiy JL, Elmaci I, Lee RR, Breiter SN, Rigamonti D (2000) Dynamic nature of cavernous malformations: a prospective magnetic resonance imaging study with volumetric analyses. J Neurosurg 93:981–986

Cohen HC, Tucker WS, Humphreys RP, Perrin RJ (1982) Angiographically cryptic histologically verified cerebrovascular malformations. Neurosurgery 10:704–714

Crawford J, Russell D (1956) Cryptic arteriovenous and venous hamartomas of the brain. J Neurol Neurosurg Psychiatry 19:1–11

Davenport WJ, Siegel AM, Dichgans J, Drigo P, Mammi I, Pereda P, Wood NW, Rouleau GA (2001) CCM1 gene mutations in families segregating cerebral cavernous malformations. Neurology 56:540–543

Del Curling O, Kelly DL, Elster AD, Craven TE (1991) An analysis of the natural history of cavernous angiomas. J Neurosurg 75:702–708

Dillon WP (1997) Cryptic vascular malformations: controversies in terminology, diagnosis, pathophysiology, and treatment. AJNR Am J Neuroradiol 18:1839–1846

Ferrante L, Acqui M, Trillo G, Antonio M, Nardacci B, Celli P (1998) Cavernous angioma of the VIIIth cranial nerve. A case report. Neurosurg Rev 21:270–276

Ferszt R (1989) Kreislaufstörungen des Nervensystems. In: Cervos-Navarro J, Ferszt R (eds) Klinische Neuropathologie. Thieme, Stuttgart, p 112

Hasegawa T, McInerney J, Kondziolka D, Lee JYK, Flickinger JC, Lunsford LD (2002) Long-term results after stereotactic radiosurgery for patients with cavernous malformations. Neurosurgery 50:1190–1198

Herata Y, Matsukado Y, Nagahiro S, Kuratsu J (1986) Intracerebral venous angioma with arterial blood supply: a mixed angioma. Surg Neurol 25:227–232

Huddle DC, Chaloupka JC, Sehgal V (1999) Clinically aggressive diffuse capillary telangiectasia of the brain stem: a clinical radiologic-pathologic case study. AJNR Am J Neuroradiol 20:1674–1677

Karlsson B, Kihlstroem L, Lindquist C, Ericson K, Steiner L (1998) Radiosurgery for cavernous malformations. J Neurosurg 88:293–297

Kim DS, Park YG, Choi JU, Chung SS, Lee KC (1997) An analysis of the natural history of cavernous malformations. Surg Neurol 48:9–18

Kim M, Rowed DW, Cheung G, Ang LC (1997) Cavernous malformation presenting as an extra-axial cerebellopontine angle mass: case report. Neurosurgery 40:187–190

Kondziolka D, Lunsford LD, Flickinger JC, Kestle JRW (1995a) Reduction of hemorrhagic risk after stereotactic radiosurgery for cavernous malformations. J Neurosurg 83:825–831

Kondziolka D, Lunsford LD, Flickinger JC (1995b) The natural history of cerebral cavernous malformations J Neurosurg 83:820–824

Korpelainen EI, Karkkainen M, Gunji Y, Vikkula M, Alitalo K (1999) Endothelials receptor tyrosine kinases activate the STAT signaling pathway: mutant Tie-2 causing venous malformations signals a distinct STAT activation response. Oncogene 18:1–8

Küker W, Nacimiento W, Block F, Thron A (2000) Presumed capillary telangiectasia of the pons: MRI and follow-up. Eur Radiol 10:945–950

Kupersmith MJ, Kalish H, Epstein F, Yu G, Berenstein A, Woo H, Jafar J, Mandel G, De Lara F (2001) Natural history of brainstem cavernous malformations. Neurosurgery 48:47–53

Labauge P, Laberge S, Brunerau L, Levy C, Tournier Lasserve E (1998) Hereditary cerebral cavernous angiomas: clinical and genetic features in 57 French families. Societe Francaise de Neurochirurgie. Lancet 352:1892–1897

Labauge P, Brunereau L, Levy C, Laberge S, Houtteville JP (2000) The natural history of familial cerebral cavernomas: a retrospectice MRI study of 40 patients. Neuroradiology 42:327–332

Lee RR, Becher MW, Benson ML, Rigamonti D (1997) Brain capillary telangiectasia: MR imaging appearance and clinicohistopathologic findings. Radiology 205:797–805

Maher CO, Piepgras DG, Brown RD, Friedman JA, Pollock BE (2001) Cerebrovascular manifestations in 321 cases of hereditary hemorrhagic telangiectasia. Stroke 32:877–882

Maraire JN, Awad IA (1995) Intracranial cavernous malformations: lesion behavior and management strategies. Neurosurgery 37:591–605

Mc Cormick WF, Nofzinger JD (1966) "Cryptic" vascular malformations of the central nervous system. J Neurosurg 24: 865–875

Mc Cormick WF, Hardman JM, Boulter TR (1968) Vascular malformations ("angiomas") of the brain, with special reference to those occuring in the posterior fossa. J Neurosurg 28:241–251

Moran NF, Fish DR, Kitchen N, Shorvon S, Kendall BE, Stevens JM (1999) Supratentorial cavernous haemangiomas and epilepsy: a review of the literature and case series. J Neurol Neurosurg Psychiatry 66:561–568

Moriarity JL, Wetzel M, Clatterbuck RE, Javedan SJ, Sheppard JM, Hoenig-Rigamonti K, Crone NE, Breiter SN, Lee RR, Rigamonti D (1999) The natural history of cavernous malformations: a prospective study of 68 patients. Neurosurgery 44:1166–1173

Mull M, Reinhardt J, Bertalanffy H, Thron A (1995) Pre- and postoperative findings in cavernomas of the CNS-diagnostic limiations and pitfalls. Neuroradiology 37 [Suppl 1]:49

Okazaki H (1989) Cerebrovascular disease. In: Okazaki H (ed) Fundamentals of neuropathology. Igaku-Shoin, New York, pp 27–94

Olivero WC, Deshmukh P, Gujrati M (2000) Radiation-induced cavernous angioma mimicking metastatic disease. Br J Neurosurg 14:575–578

Porter PJ, Willinsky RA, Harper W, Wallace MC (1997) Cerebral cavernous malformations: natural history and prognosis after clinical deterioration with or without hemorrhage. J Neurosurg 87:190–197

Porter RW, Detwiler PW, Spetzler RF, Lawton MT, Baskin JJ, Derksen PT et al (1999) Cavernous malformations of the brainstem: experience with 100 patients. J Neurosurg 90: 50–58

Reyns N, Assaker R, Louis E, Lejeune JP (1999) Intraventricular cavernomas: three cases and review of the literature. Neurosurgery 44:648–654

Rigamonti D, Drayer B, Johnson P, Hadley M, Zabramski J, Spetzler R (1987) The MRI appearance of cavernous malformations (angiomas). J Neurosurg 67:518–524

Rigamonti D, Spetzler RF (1988) The association of venous and cavernous malformations. Report of four cases and discussion of the pathophysiological, diagnostic and therapeutic implications. Acta Neurochirur (Wien) 92:100–105

Rigamonti D, Hadley MN, Drayer BP, Johnson PC, Hoenig-Rigamonti K, Knight JT, Spetzler RF (1988) Cerebral cavernous malformations. Incidence and familial occurence. N Engl J Med 319:343–347

Rigamonti D, Johnson PC, Spetzler RF, Hadley MN, Drayer BP (1991) Cavernous malformations and capillary telangiectasie: a spectrum within a single pathological entity. Neurosurgery 28:60–64

Robinson JR, Awad IA, Little JR (1991) Natural history of the cavernous angioma. J Neurosurg 75:709–714

Russel DS, Rubinstein LJ (1989) Tumours and hamartomas of the blood vessels. In: Russel DS, Rubinstein LJ (eds) The pathology of tumours of the nervous system, 5th edn. Arnold, London, pp 727–790

Sarraf D, Payne AM, Kitchen ND, Sehmi KS, Downes SM, Bird AC (2000) Familial cavernous hemangioma: An expanding ocular spectrum. Arch Ophthalmol 118:969–973

Savoiardo M, Strada L, Passerini A (1983) Intracranial cavernous hemangioma: neuroradiologic review of 36 operated cases. Am J Neuroradiol AJNR 4:945–950

Scaglione C, Salvi F, Riguzzi P, Vergelli M, Tassinari CA, Mascalchi M (2001) Symptomatic unruptured capillary telangiectasia of the brain stem: report of t hree cases and review of the literature. J Neurol Neurosurg Psychiatry 71:390–393

Simard JM, Garcia-Bengochea F, Ballinger WE, Mickle JP, Quisling RG (1986) Cavernous angioma: a review of 126 collected and 12 new clinical cases. Neurosurgery 18:162–172

Vikkula M, Boon LM, Carraway KL, Calvert JT, Diamonti AJ, Goumnerov B, Pasyk KA, Marchuk DA, Warman ML, Cantley LC, Mulliken JB, Olsen BR (1996) Vascular dysmorphogenesis caused by an activating mutation in the receptor tyrosine kinase TIE2. Cell 87:1181–1190

Voigt K, Yasargil MG (1976) Cerebral cavernous haemangiomas or cavernomas. Neurochirurgia 19:59–68

Wilson CB (1992) Cryptic vascular malformations. Clin Neurosurg 38:49–84

Wong JH, Awad IA, Kim JH (2000) Ultrastructural pathological features of cerebrovascular malformations: a preliminary report. Neurosurgery 46:1454–1459

Zabramski JM, Wascher TM, Spetzler RF, Johnson B, Golfinos J, Drayer BP, Brown B, Rigamonti D, Brown G (1994) The natural history of familial cavernous malformation: results of an ongoing study. J Neurosurg 80:422–432

Zhang J, Clatterbuck RE, Rigamonti D, Dietz HC (2000) Mutations in KRIT1 in familial cerebral cavernous malformations. Neurosurgery 46:1272–1277

3 Pial Arteriovenous Malformations

C. Cognard, L. Spelle, and L. Pierot

CONTENTS

C. Cognard, MD
Service de Neuroradiologie, Hôpital Purpan, Place du Dr Baylac, 31059 Toulouse Cedex, France
L. Spelle, MD
Département de Neuroradiologie interventionnelle et fonctionnelle, Fondation A. de Rothschild, 25-29 Rue Manin, 75940 Paris Cedex 19, France
L. Pierot, MD
Service de Radiologie, Hôpital Maison-Blanche, 45 rue Cognacq-Jay, 51092 Reims Cedex, France

3.1 Introduction

Arteriovenous malformations of the brain (brain AVMs) correspond to congenital cerebrovascular anomalies, also known as intracerebral or pial AVMs. First of all, it is important to stress the fact that this is not a neoplastic lesion and therefore not an "angioma", which is obviously an inappropriate though commonly used term (Rosenblum et al. 1996).

Clinically, brain AVMs are an increasingly recognized cause of death and long-term morbidity, mostly due to intracranial hemorrhage and epilepsy; however, they may remain silent over a long period of time, even over an entire life. Anatomically speaking, they are constituted by a complex, tangled web of afferent arteries and draining veins linked by an abnormal intervening capillary bed – the so-called nidus – which may or not harbor direct arteriovenous shunts (Challa et al. 1995; Rosenblum et al. 1996; The Arteriovenous Malformation Study Group 1999), of which two categories must be recognized: AV malformations (AVMs) and AV fistulas (AVFs) (Lasjaunias and Berenstein 1993a).

- AVMs are composed of a network of channels interposed between feeding arteries and draining veins, without any direct shunt. Two different anatomic types of nidus may be more or less differentiated: *compact* nidus, constituting a tumor-like well-circumscribed network, and *diffuse* nidus, with sparse, abnormal AV channels spread within normal brain parenchyma (Chin et al. 1992).
- AVFs are formed by direct communication between an enlarged artery and vein without

interposed nidus. Lack of a capillary bed in the AVM nidus results in direct arteriovenous communication, which may be unique or multiple (Stapf and Mohr 2000). AVFs are much more rare than AVMs (2%, Lasjaunias and Berenstein 1993a) and are always located on the brain surface. They may be present within an AVM nidus as a direct AV shunt surrounded by the network of arteriovenous channels.

AVMs may be situated in any region of the brain, lying mostly within the distribution of the middle cerebral arteries and involving the hemispheric convexities in continuity with the adjacent leptomeninges; however, they can be restricted to the dura or choroid plexus. They vary in size from cryptic lesions, which remain invisible even on angiographic studies and are discovered on anatomic studies of surgically removed hematomas, to giant AVMs, which can involve a whole hemisphere.

Feeding arteries may be one or numerous. They may be very enlarged or present an almost normal diameter. High flow may produce either (a) saccular aneurysm formation, located at the level of the circle of Willis or the feeding arteries or within the nidus (Cunha e Sa et al. 1992; Ogilvy et al. 2001; Lasjaunias et al. 1988; Meisel et al. 2000; Redekop et al. 1998; Thompson et al. 1998; Turjman et al. 1994), or (b) high-flow angiopathy with progressive stenosis and eventual occlusion of feeding arteries (Mawad et al. 1984).

Draining veins as well may be one or numerous, deep or cortical. Direct shunting of blood at arterial pressure causes dilatation and tortuosity in the involved veins. High flow may also produce localized stenosis, frequently at the level where the veins cross the dura to reach the sinus (Mansmann et al. 2000; Miyasaka et al. 1992) and secondary venous aneurysmal dilatation (Nataf et al. 1997).

3.2 Pathology

3.2.1 Epidemiology

There is very little information in the literature about the ***prevalence*** of AVMs, i.e., the proportion of a population living with the diagnosis of AVM at a single point in time. Because of the rarity of the disease and the existence of asymptomatic patients, establishing a true prevalence rate is difficult and probably not feasible (Stapf et al. 2000). Considering unselected populations, Al-Shahi and Warlow (2001) found a prevalence of AVMs in a retrospective study in a region of Scotland of 15 per 100,000 living adults over 16 years of age. In this series, prevalence is obviously underestimated, since it does not consider asymptomatic AVMs. Only large post-mortem studies in the general population could give a more accurate estimation of the prevalence of both symptomatic and clinically silent AVM. However, such a series does not exist. Only few hospital-based post-mortem studies are available, in which the prevalence of AVMs was found to be between 400 and 600 per 100,000 (Al-Shahi and Warlow 2001; Berman et al. 2000; Jellinger 1986). This huge discrepancy is obviously due to the fact that the prevalence in living subjects is underestimated, first because of the lack of diagnosed cases being filed in a registry in retrospective studies, and second because the entire group of nonsymptomatic AVMs are not included in the counting because they are not detected. Berman et al. (2000) have provided a very interesting paper in which they reviewed all of the relevant original literature. They conclude that "the estimates for AVM prevalence that are published in the medical literature are unfounded". For these authors, the most reliable estimate for the occurrence of the disease is the detection rate for symptomatic lesions: 0.94 per 100,000 persons per year.

Incidence corresponds to the proportion of a population newly diagnosed with an AVM. Population-based incidence data are also very difficult to evaluate; only two population-based studies of AVM incidence are available (Brown et al. 1996a; Jessurun et al. 1993), and both are retrospective. Over a 10-year-period (between 1980 and 1990) in the Netherlands Antilles, the annual incidence of symptomatic AVMs was 1.1 per 100,000 per year (Jessurun et al. 1993).

In a second study, using the comprehensive Mayo Clinic medical records linkage system over a 27-year period from 1965 to 1972 in Olmsted County (USA), the incidence of symptomatic AVMs was 1.84 per 100,000 per year (Brown et al. 1996). Interestingly, the incidence rate increased over time, probably due to the use of more advanced brain imaging modalities. Obviously, a prospective study would give a more accurate estimate of AVM incidence and a better description of the population affected by the disease, but such a study is currently lacking.

Where *other demographic characteristics* of patients with brain AVMs are concerned, mean age at diagnosis is between 30 and 40 years (HOFMEISTER et al. 2000; JESSURUN et al. 1993, THE ARTERIOVENOUS MALFORMATION STUDY GROUP 1999) and it affects both sexes in nearly equal proportions (HOFMEISTER et al. 2000; THE ARTERIOVENOUS MALFORMATION STUDY GROUP 1999).

Even though brain AVMs are considered to be a congenital disorder, nonsystematized familial AVMs are extremely rare and very few familial cases have been reported in the literature (ABERFELD and RAO 1981; HERZIG et al. 2000; KAMIRYO et al. 2000; YOKOYAMA et al. 1991). No genetic predisposition was found and the occurrence of brain AVMs in two members of the same family could be purely accidental.

Autopsy data showed that only 12% of AVMs become symptomatic during life (THE ARTERIOVENOUS MALFORMATION STUDY GROUP 1999), and intracranial hemorrhage is the most common clinical presentation (AL-SHAHI and WARLOW 2001; HOFMEISTER et al. 2000; THE ARTERIOVENOUS MALFORMATION STUDY GROUP 1999).

AVMs typically present as solitary lesions. Multiple brain AVMs occur in approximately 0.3%–3.2% of all cases. Surprisingly enough, WILLINSKY et al. (1990) reported 11 cases of multiple AVMs among 203 patients (6%). Although multiple AVMs may occur spontaneously, they are frequently associated with cutaneous or extracranial vascular anomalies (SALCMAN et al. 1992), such as Rendu-Osler-Weber disease and Wyburn-Mason syndrome. However, the clinical mode of presentation, age and sex of the patient, and anatomic distribution of the lesions are the same as those in patients with single arteriovenous malformations:

Rendu-Osler-Weber disease – also known as hereditary hemorrhagic telangiectasia (HHT) – is a rare autosomal dominant angiodysplastic disorder with a prevalence estimated at between 2 and 40 per 100,000 people (GUTTMACHER et al. 1995). Rendu-Osler-Weber disease is characterized by multisystemic vascular dysplasia and recurrent hemorrhage of the nose, skin, lung, brain, and gastrointestinal tract. It includes: (a) multiple capillary telangiectasias of the skin and mucosa, and (b) arteriovenous malformations and fistulas located in the liver (30% of the cases) (RALLS et al. 1992), the lungs (15 to 20%), the brain (28%) or the spine (8%). Epistaxis is the most frequent symptom, present in 85% of the patients (GUTTMACHER et al. 1995; PORTEOUS et al. 1992).

The prevalence of brain AVMs in patients presenting with Rendu-Osler-Weber disease is estimated to be between 4% and 13% (PORTEOUS et al. 1992; ROMAN et al. 1978; WILLINSKY et al. 1990). They have no specific characteristics, especially regarding location and angioarchitecture. However, multiple AVMs in this syndrome are more frequent than in the general population, with a frequency estimated at around 30% (AESCH et al. 1991; HASEGAWA et al. 1999; JELLINGER 1986; JESSURUN et al. 1993; MATSUBARA et al. 2000; PUTMAN et al. 1996; ROMAN et al. 1978; Sobel and NORMAN 1984; WILLEMSE et al. 2000; WILLINSKY et al. 1990). A recent study of 196 patients with Rendu-Osler-Weber disease (WILLEMSE et al. 2000) showed that 12% had a brain AVM, and 96% of these were low grade (Spetzler-Martin grade I or II). The risk of bleeding has been estimated to be lower than in non-Rendu-Osler-Weber disease brain AVMs, ranging from 0.4 to 0.72 per year (KJELDSEN et al. 1999). For some families, linkage has been established to a mutated gene located on chromosome 9q, which induces abnormality in endoglin, a transforming growth factor beta-binding protein expressed on endothelial cells (CHEIFETZ et al. 1992; MCALLISTER et al. 1994, SHOVLIN et al. 1997); other linkage studies have established another locus at chromosome 12q, resulting in a mutation in the activin receptor-like kinase gene ("ALK-1" gene), also predominantly expressed on endothelial cells and also related to the same TGF-b receptor system (BERG et al. 1997; JOHNSON et al. 1996).

The very rare *Bonnet-Blanc-Dechaume syndrome* – also called Wyburn-Mason syndrome, neuroretinal angiomatosis, or mesencephalo-oculo-facial angiomatosis – corresponds to the association of unilateral retinal angiomatosis and a cutaneous hemangioma in an ipsilateral trigeminal distribution with an AVM located in the midbrain (PATEL and GUPTA 1990; ROSENBLUM et al. 1996; WILLINSKY et al. 1990). In the 25 cases reported by THERON et al. (1974), the lesions involved the optic nerve, then followed the optic track as a unique continuous nidus or as multiple focal AVMs.

3.2.2
Pathology, Genetics, and Hemodynamics

3.2.2.1
Pathology

In macroscopic pathology, brain AVMs are composed of (a) clustered and abnormally muscularized feeding arteries, which may also show changes such as duplication or destruction of the elastica, fibrosis of the media, and focal thinning of the wall; (b) arterialized veins of varying size and wall thickness; (c) structurally ambiguous vessels formed, solely of fibrous tissue or displaying both arterial and venous characteristics; and (d) intervening gliotic neural parenchyma (Jellinger 1986; Mandybur and Nazek 1990; McCormick 1966; Rosenblum et al. 1996) (Fig. 3.1). They anastomose with normal cerebral vessels. Critical to the distinction of the true brain AVM from normal leptomeningeal vessels that may assume the appearance of a malformation in neurosurgical material as a result of artifactual compaction are the former's conspicuous mural anomalies. Chief among these are striking fluctuations in medial thickness, architectural disarray, or focal disappearance of the media altogether, or its separation into inner and outer coats by a seemingly aberrant elastic lamina. Numerous abnormalities of the muscular layer were identified, including partially developed media, two layers of the media separated by a well-formed internal elastic membrane, total or partial disarray of the muscle coat, and partial absence of the media (Mandybur and Nazek 1990). Previously described large capillaries proved to be postcapillary venules by virtue of having a distinct muscular layer. Mandybur et al. performed serial sectioning, indicating that the previously described "polypoid projections" of the media are mostly artifacts, and the concept of "arterialization of veins in arteriovenous malformations" could not be substantiated (Mandybur and Nazek 1990; Rosenblum et al. 1996).

Ultrastructural pathological features of brain AVMs were also studied but consist only in the disorganization of collagen bundles within nidal vessels' walls (Wong et al. 2000).

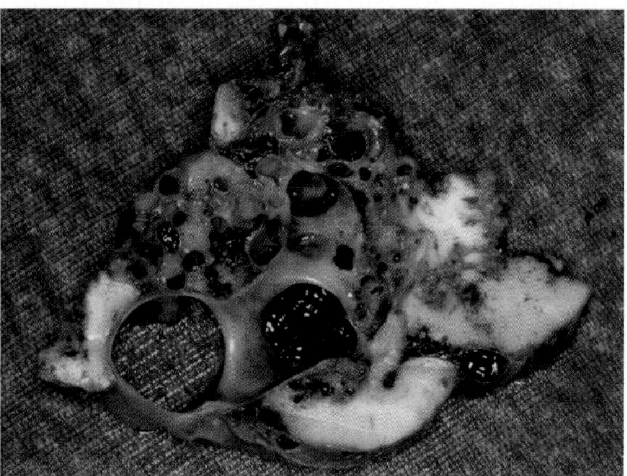

Fig. 3.1. Macroscopic view of a surgically resected brain AVM depicts enlarged feeding arteries and draining veins with arteriovenous shunts. Normal brain surrounds the AVM with partially necrosed areas. (Courtesy of Pr. Mikol, Neuropathology Department, Lariboisière, Paris, France)

Embolization results in endothelial cell disruption with preservation of the underlying subendothelial vessel wall (Wong et al. 2000). Lesions subjected to embolization with bucrylate or polyvinyl alcohol (Germano et al. 1992; Vinters et al. 1986) exhibit a foreign-body response and may undergo focal necrosis. Entrapped neuropil usually manifests dense astrogliosis, neuronal depopulation, and ferruginous encrustation of included neuroglial elements. Within interstices of AVM, oligodendroglioma-like regions may be encountered that may be intrinsic to the underlying misdevelopment process or the result of abnormal oligodendroglial aggregation caused by the ischemic contraction of entrapped white matter (Lombardi et al. 1991; Nazek et al. 1988; Rosenblum et al. 1996).

3.2.2.2 Genetics

The majority of AVMs are believed to be congenital, although it is possible that some lesions are acquired. Thus, even though they are developmental anomalies, it is likely that a combination of congenital predisposition and extrinsic factors lead to their generation (Challa et al. 1995; Chaloupka et al. 1998). The vast majority of cases are sporadic, in which no familial association is observed, and no specific gene mutations have been reported for these AVMs.

Although familial brain AVMs are rare, elective screening of individuals with a family history of AVM is recommended (Aberfeld and Rao 1981; Amin-Hanjani et al. 1998). An exception is the rare setting of Rendu-Osler-Weber disease, mapped to the endoglin gene on chromosome 9q, or the activin receptor-like kinase gene on chromosome 12q, both expressed on endothelial cells and related to the TGF-beta receptor system. It is presumed that the genetic defects in this disease result in a signaling-pathway abnormality, potentially affecting vascular assembly and remodeling. It is not yet known why abnormal vascular morphology is limited to focal AVM lesions and whether more common sporadic AVMs also reflect similar mechanisms of dysmorphogenesis (Hademenos et al. 2001).

3.2.2.3 Hemodynamics

The velocity of blood flow is considerably higher through AVMs than through normal brain parenchyma. As a result of the abnormal hemodynamic condition, feeding arteries and draining veins become progressively dilated and tortuous. The hemodynamic effects of shunt flow through an AVM on the surrounding brain have been implicated in the pathogenesis of pretreatment neurological deficits. In fact, AVMs could be compared to vascular "sponges", which consume large volumes of blood, depriving the brain of normal circulation (Barnett 1987; Duckwiler et al. 1990; Jungreis et al. 1989; Spetzler et al. 1992; Young et al. 1994b). A decrease in the perfusion pressure may place these neighboring vascular territories below the lower limit of autoregulation by a combination of arterial hypotension and venous hypertension. Focal neurological deficits have been attributed to this phenomenon of "cerebral steal" (Fink 1992; Manchola et al. 1993; Marks et al. 1991; Nornes and Grip 1980); its reported clinical frequency varies widely but is probably much lower than was previously thought (Mast et al. 1995). Moreover, in the same prospective series, Mast et al. demonstrated that there was no relation between feeding artery pressure or flow velocity and the occurrence of focal neurological deficit.

3.2.3 Physiopathology and Biology

The pathogenesis of brain AVMs is currently unknown, but recent work suggests that their genesis and development may be linked to aberrant vasculogenesis or angiogenesis (Shalaby et al. 1995). Indeed, in embryos, vascular morphogenesis is a two-stage process: The first stage – *vasculogenesis* – corresponds to the differentiation of angioblasts into endothelial cells to form the primary vascular plexus. During the second stage – *angiogenesis* – this primary vascular plexus undergoes remodeling and organization including recruitment of periendothelial cell support (Hashimoto et al. 2001). In both processes, blood vessels are established and remodeled by protein ligands that bind and modulate the activity of transmembrane receptor tyrosine kinases. Recent studies have clarified two main systems of angiogenesis growth factor and the endothelial cell-specific protein tyrosine kinase (Hanahan 1997). The high-affinity binding receptors of the vascular endothelial growth factor (VEGF-R1 and VEGF-R2) appear to mediate various facets of endothelial cell proliferation, migration, adhesion, and tube formation (Uranishi et al. 2001). A recently discovered group of cytokines, the angiopoietins 1 and 2, and their receptors Tie-1 and Tie-2, play an important role at later stages of vascular development (Sato et al. 1995).

More precisely, when VEGF binds to VEGF-R2 during embryogenesis, endothelial cells are created and caused to proliferate. When VEGF binds to VEGF-R1, endothelial cells interact and capillary tubes are formed (Fong et al. 1995; Shalaby et al. 1995). When angiopoietin-1 binds to Tie-2, periendothelial support cells are recruited and caused to associate with endothelial cells (Patan 1998). When angiopoietin-2 binds to Tie-2, kinase activation in endothelial cells is blocked and vessel structures become loosened.

Experimental embryos that are deficient in Tie-2 produce the formation of abnormal enlarged vessels without intervening normal capillaries (Sato et al. 1995), and these abnormal vessels resemble human brain AVMs. Embryos that are deficient in Tie-1 fail to establish the structural integrity of vascular endothelial cells, resulting in vascular leakage, edema, and breakthrough hemorrhage. Targeted disruption of angiopoietin-1 in the embryo is lethal, and associated vascular defects resemble those in the tie-2-deficient model. Angiopoietin-2 has been shown to be a naturally occurring antagonist for angiopoietin-1 and Tie-1. Transgenic overexpression of angiopoietin-2 disrupts blood vessel formation in the mouse embryo (Maisonpierre et al. 1997).

Interestingly, it has been proven that endothelial cell expression of VEGF-R and angiopoietin receptors in endothelial cells is significantly higher in patients with surgically resected brain AVMs than in controls (Hashimoto 2001; Uranishi et al. 2001). The significant up-regulation of VEGF and Tie in AVMs may indicate some ongoing angiogenesis, possibly contributing to the slow growth and maintenance of the AVM, and could be of potential use in the therapeutic targeting of these lesions.

However, it is currently difficult to attribute abnormal VEGF-R expression to specific pathophysiological features of AVMs. It is likely that biological alterations reflect not only the specific mechanisms that triggered lesion genesis but also subsequent nonspecific changes attributable to flow hemorrhage, and other injury responses.

3.3 Clinical Presentation

The most frequent clinical presentations of brain AVMs are hemorrhage, seizure, chronic headache, and focal deficits not related to hemorrhage (Mast et al. 1995).

3.3.1 Natural History

Brain AVMs are lesions that are not affected by important anatomic modifications over time. However, as was outlined by BERENSTEIN et al. (1992), AVMs are dynamic, i.e., they undergo continuous subtle anatomic and hemodynamic changes. A cerebral AVM becomes clinically evident when the host's capacity to effectively compensate has reached its threshold. Cerebral AVMs are often symptomatic in young adults, typically before the age of 40 (HOFMEISTER et al. 2000).

From an anatomic point of view, the natural history of brain AVMs may rarely include enlargement, decrease, or regression (MINAKAWA et al. 1989; CHEN et al. 1991; KRAPF et al. 2001). Surprisingly, in a small series of 20 patients followed up by angiography for periods of 5–28 years, MINAKAWA observed an increase in size of the AVM in four patients, a decrease in four, and total regression in four. Enlargement of brain AVMs is observed in young patients (under 30 years of age), and especially in childhood (KRAYENBUHL 1977; MENDELOW et al. 1987; MINAKAWA et al. 1989).

Spontaneous obliteration of cerebral AVMs is rare; only 50 cases have been reported in the literature. Factors predisposing an AVM to regression by thrombosis are those that affect the venous hemodynamic state of the AVM: anatomy of the AVM, surgical manipulation of the lesion, compression of the AVM by surrounding mass lesions (CHEN et al. 1991). Most often, the thrombosis of the AVM nidus will occur secondary to an intracerebral or subarachnoid hemorrhage. In this case, the mass effect of the blood clot may alter the dynamic of the AVM and decrease blood flow, probably by compression of draining veins to the extent that thrombosis may occur. Surgical intervention, including evacuation of a blood clot or placement of a shunt, has been associated with regression of AVMs explained by compression of the veins from bleeding or swelling. Spontaneous regression may also occur (KRAPF et al. 2001). Several factors appear to be associated with spontaneous occlusion of cerebral AVM: single draining vein (84% of cases of spontaneous occlusion), solitary arterial feeder (30%), small size of the nidus (<3 cm in 50%) (KRAPF et al. 2001).

3.3.2 Intracranial Hemorrhage

Intracranial hemorrhage is the most common clinical presentation of brain AVM, with a frequency of between 30% and 82% (MAST et al. 1995). Identification of factors increasing the risk of bleeding of a brain AVM is very important with regard to the treatment strategy. However, two difficulties are encountered in an analysis of the literature:

- There is a lack of consistency in the terminology used to describe clinical and radiographic features of brain AVMs. Recently, the Joint Writing Group of the Technology Assessment Committee, American Society of Interventional and Therapeutic Neuroradiology, Joint Section on Cerebrovascular Neurosurgery, Section of Stroke and Section of Interventional Neurology of the American Academy of Neurology (OGILVY et al. 2001) proposed a uniform terminology for clinical and radiographic description of brain AVMs.
- The identification of factors affecting the bleeding risk of brain AVMs is difficult, because anatomic and hemodynamic factors are often not independent, and a precise analysis has to be performed (MANSMANN et al. 2000).

3.3.2.1 Factors Increasing the Risk of Bleeding

Several factors may increase the risk of a first hemorrhage in case of brain AVM:

Anatomic Factors

Many factors have been studied to evaluate their influence on the bleeding rate of brain AVMs (MARKS et al. 1990; HOUDART et al. 1993; SPETZLER et al. 1992; KADER et al. 1994; TURJMAN et al. 1995a; POLLOCK et al. 1996a; NATAF et al. 1997; MANSMANN et al. 2000).

Feeding Vessels

Arterial Aneurysms

The prevalence of arterial aneurysms is estimated at between 2.7% and 22.7%, with a mean of about 10%.

Several classifications of arterial aneurysms associated with brain AVMs have been proposed. According to HOUDART et al.(1993), three groups of aneurysms associated with brain AVMs have to be defined according to their site: type I, proximally on a large artery; type II, distally on a large feeding artery; type III, intra- or juxtanidal. CUNHA E SA et al. (1992) have proposed another classification: type I, proximal on ipsilateral major artery feeding the AVM; type Ia, proximal on major artery related but contralateral to the AVM; type II, distal on superficial artery feeding the AVM; type III, proximal or distal on deep artery feeding the AVM; type IV, on artery unrelated to the AVM. In fact, the most useful classification of aneurysms associated with brain AVMs is probably that proposed by the Joint Writing Group (OGILVY et al. 2001). Aneurysms are categorized as flow related, non-flow related, nidal, proximal, and distal. Flow-related aneurysms are located on a pathway supplying the brain AVM shunt. Aneurysms are defined as saccular luminal dilatations of the parent feeding vessel. Nidal is defined as contiguous with the nidus. Proximal aneurysms would be located on the vessel or branch points of the circle of Willis or proximal to it. Distal refers to locations beyond the circle of Willis. A similar classification was recently used in a series dealing with brain AVMs associated with arterial aneurysms (REDEKOP et al. 1998). PIOTIN et al. (2001) also define proximal, distal, and intranidal aneurysms but do not distinguish between flow-related and non-flow-related aneurysms.

As outlined by HOUDART et al.(1993), the depiction of intranidal aneurysms is difficult; it is often performed at the time of superselective angiography. Moreover, true arterial intranidal aneurysms have to be distinguished from pseudoaneurysms, which are at the point of rupture of the nidus or of the venous drainage.

The significance of aneurysms associated with brain AVMs in the occurrence of bleeding is unclear. POLLOCK et al. (1996) find no association between proximal or nidal associated aneurysms and intracranial bleeding. The univariate and multivariate analysis performed by MANSMANN et al. (2000) in a large series of patients revealed no association between aneurysms in the feeders or intranidal aneurysms and intracranial hemorrhage. In other series, arterial aneurysms and intranidal aneurysms are associated with a high prevalence of hemorrhage (MARKS et al. 1990; TURJMAN et al. 1995; THOMPSON et al. 1998; REDEKOP et al. 1998; PIOTIN et al. 2001).

In the series of CUNHA E SA et al. (1992) the site of rupture was the aneurysm in 46% of cases, the AVM in 33% of cases, and undetermined in 21% of cases. In other series (BATJER et al. 1986; PIOTIN et al. 2001), the source of hemorrhage in patients harboring brain AVMs and associated aneurysms was identified as an aneurysm in approximately 80% of cases.

Thus, we can postulate with BERENSTEIN et al. (1992) that intranidal aneurysms represent a weakness of the angioarchitecture and should influence treatment strategy. This is probably also true for other associated aneurysms.

A higher percentage of multiple aneurysms has been reported in the population of patients with brain AVMs (BATJER et al. 1986; BROWN et al. 1990; CUNHA E SA et al. 1992; THOMPSON et al. 1998), but this feature seems not to be associated with a higher risk of hemorrhage (PIOTIN et al. 2001).

Feeders from the External Carotid Artery

Some brain AVMs are fed by branches of external carotid arteries, and the significance of this anatomic situation is uncertain. Is there an intradural compartment of the AVM? Or is there a vascularization of the nidus through arterial anastomosis coming from external branches? Whatever, it seems that the incidence of bleeding is not increased when the brain AVM is fed by branches of the external arteries.

Others

TURJMAN et al. (1995a) have shown an increased risk of bleeding in case of feeding by perforators and by the vertebrobasilar system. As outlined by TURJMAN, perforators are involved in the supply of deep AVMs, such as corpus callosum and basal ganglia AVMs, and it is difficult to evaluate which feature is the most important for determination of the bleeding risk.

Regarding feeders coming from the vertebrobasilar system, the discussion is the same as for the location of AVMs (see below).

Nidus

Size

A relationship between the size of an AVM and its tendency to rupture has been suggested. In the series of GRAF et al. (1983), the risk of hemorrhage at 5 years was 10% for large AVMs (>3.0 cm in diameter) and 52% for small AVMs (<3 cm in diameter). In the series of SPETZLER et al. (1992), 82% of patients with small AVMs (less than 3 cm), 29% of patients with medium-sized AVMs (3–6 cm), and 12% of patients with large AVM (greater than 6 cm) presented with hemorrhage. The same relation between nidus size and bleeding was found by other authors (ITOYAMA et al. 1989; KADER et al. 1994; DUONG et al. 1998). The multivariate analysis performed in the large series of patients studied by MANSMANN et al. (2000) also identified AVM size of more than 3 cm as a factor negatively associated with intracranial hemorrhage.

However, the absolute risk of spontaneous intracranial hemorrhage from small and large brain AVMs is still a matter of controversy. In the series of CRAWFORD et al. (1986), 21% small and 18% large AVM rebled within 5 years. Small and large AVMs may have the same risk of bleeding. Large AVMs can more often present in other ways than hemorrhage (seizures, progressive deficits, headache), and this may lead to an overestimation of the rate of bleeding of small AVMs. In this case, age at the time of presentation would be higher in the group of patients with hemorrhage than in the group without. However, age at the time of presentation is the same in both groups (Kader et al. 1994), supporting the idea that small AVMs have a higher risk of hemorrhage. Moreover, by measuring the feeding artery pressure intraoperatively, Spetzler et al. (1992) demonstrated that the pressure is higher in small brain AVMs, which could explain the higher rate of bleeding of small AVMs (see below).

Hematoma size seems to be inversely related to the size of the AVM (Spetzler et al. 1992).

Location

The risk of bleeding of brain AVMs depending on their location has not been evaluated systematically. Some authors suggest that AVMs in deep locations, such as in the basal ganglia or in the periventricular or intraventricular space, have an increased risk of bleeding (Marks et al. 1990; Turjmann et al. 1995). Willinski et al. (1988) concluded that hemorrhage is more likely to occur in deep lesions and posterior fossa AVMs. However, Crawford et al. (1986) showed that the depth of the AVM had no influence on the risk of hemorrhage. Moreover, the high prevalence of hemorrhage in deep-seated AVMs identified in some series may be partially explained by the fact that the patients are less likely to present with focal neurologic deficits or seizure disorders.

The results published by Stapf et al. (2000) suggest that an arterial border zone location of brain AVMs is an independent determinant of lower risk of incident AVM hemorrhage.

Angiogenesis

This factor was defined as transdural anastomosis or secondarily acquired perilesional angiogenesis (Mansmann et al. 2000). When it is combined with arterial stenosis or dural venous stenosis, this factor may increase the risk of intracranial hemorrhage.

Venous Drainage

Deep Venous Drainage

Deep venous drainage is associated with a higher risk of bleeding (Marks et al. 1990; Miyasaka et al. 1992; Kader et al. 1994; Nataf et al. 1997; Duong et al. 1998). Superficial and deep venous drainage are different from an anatomic point of view. The veins of the central drainage have one final common pathway which is the vein of Galen and the straight sinus. On the other hand, superficial veins have more connections and may drain posteriorly via the superior sagittal sinus and anteriorly via the sylvian vein. The superficial venous system is probably more flexible in adaptation to the hemodynamic situation created by the presence of the AVM.

Venous Stenosis

The presence of a stenosis on the venous drainage of a brain AVM is associated with an increased risk of bleeding (Miyasaka et al. 1992; Nataf et al. 1997), probably due to proximal venous hypertension. This factor was also identified in the large series of patients analyzed by Mansmann et al. (2000), but venous stenosis was not statistically associated with intracranial hemorrhage for cortical AVMs. Venous dilatation was correlated to an increased risk of hemorrhagic presentation in dural arteriovenous fistulas (Cognard et al. 1995).

The suggested mechanisms for venous stenosis in AVMs are varied: endovascular proliferation in reaction to increased venous flow or pressure (Fry 1968), congenital extrinsic anatomic narrowing of the lumen as it traverses the dura mater or curves around bone (Crawford et al. 1986; Willinsky et al. 1988), kinking in ectatic veins (Nataf et al. 1997).

Others

The presence of a single draining vein may be associated with an increased risk of bleeding (Miyasaka et al. 1992; Pollock et al. 1996).

Venous reflux into a sinus or a deep vein seems to be positively correlated with the risk of hemorrhage (Nataf et al. 1997), but this feature has seldom been studied. In contrast, venous recruitment seems to be protective against bleeding.

Venous ectasia may be intra- or paranidal and the sign of a previous hemorrhage. Venous ectasia may also be remote from the nidus. The link between venous ectasia and bleeding is unclear (Nataf et al. 1997).

Hemodynamic Factors

Feeding Artery Pressures

In a relatively small series of patients, Spetzler et al. (1992) evaluated the perfusion pressure of AVM arterial feeders. The difference between mean arterial blood pressure and the feeding artery pressure was higher in ruptured than in non-ruptured AVMs. Moreover, smaller AVMs had significantly higher feeding artery pressure than larger AVMs and were associated with larger hematomas. These results were partially confirmed by Kader et al. (1994), who found that patients presenting with hemorrhage had higher feeding artery pressure than patients in the nonhemorrhage group. The feeding artery pressure was only weakly related to the size of the lesion, but measurements were performed only in medium and large-sized AVMs.

In a large series of patients, Duong et al. (1998) also found that feeding arterial pressure was positively correlated with the occurrence of bleeding.

In the study performed by Norbash et al. (1994), feeding arterial pressure was not statistically different in the hemorrhage and nonhemorrhage groups and was not related to the size. A non-statistically significant trend to decreasing feeding arterial pressures from AVMs having a central venous drainage to those having peripheral venous drainage was observed. Moreover, the feeding arterial pressure was lower when the feeding artery was longer, and the length of the feeding artery was also correlated to the type of venous drainage (deep or superficial).

Draining Vein Pressures

The draining vein pressure did not differ between patients with hemorrhage and those without (Kader et al. 1994).

3.3.2.2 Factors Decreasing the Risk of Bleeding

Very few studies have evaluated anatomic factors decreasing the risk of bleeding of a brain AVM. Two factors were identified on the arterial side as having a protective effect against bleeding (Mansmann et al. 2000):

- Arterial stenosis, which is defined as a reduction in arterial caliber and could be intrinsic (concentric narrowing by intraluminal protrusions related to high-flow angiopathy) or extrinsic (bony, dural or venous compression)
- Arterial angioectasia, which is defined as segmental arterial capillary dilatation in the collateral system in the vicinity of the AVMs (with recruitment and enlargement of leptomeningeal and subependymal anastomoses) and hemodynamic enlargement of preexisting feeding arteries

These two factors probably contribute to the decrease of the pressure inside the nidus.

Arteriovenous fistulas, defined as large arteriovenous communications between the arterial and venous components of AVMs with high flow velocity and a visible shunting transition, seem to be also associated with a lower risk of bleeding (Mansmann et al. 2000).

In summary, several factors have been identified which potentially modify the risk of bleeding of brain AVMs. However, there is clearly a general bias in many studies regarding the evaluation of bleeding rates. Indeed, some anatomic characteristics identified as increasing the risk of bleeding are also related to a less frequent nonhemorrhagic presentation such as epilepsy or focal deficit, e.g., small size of the AVM, deep location, and deep venous drainage. If a group of brain AVMs can be only asymptomatic or hemorrhagic, then the percentage of bleeding in this group will be 100%, except if asymptomatic AVMs are detected for any reason by CT or MRI.

3.3.2.3 Annual Rate of Bleeding

The natural history of brain AVMs has been studied in different series of untreated patients (Graf et al. 1983; Fults and Kelly 1984; Crawford et al. 1986; Brown et al. 1988; Itoyama et al. 1989; Ondra et al. 1990). There are a number of biases in these different studies:

- Generally, studies were conducted at centers specialized in the treatment of cerebrovascular disorders, thus creating a recruitment bias.
- The number of patients included in these series is usually small (50 to 343 patients).
- In the majority of series, natural history was studied in the group of patients managed nonsurgically, and this is a very important recruitment bias.
- Most studies are retrospective.

For all these reasons, we have to be careful with the data provided by these series.

Graf et al. (1983) reported a series of 191 patients presenting with unruptured or ruptured AVMs. The average yearly risk of bleeding was estimated to be between 2% and 3%. Crawford et al. (1986) reported a series of 217 patients harboring AVMs who were managed without surgery with a mean follow-up period of 10.4 years. There was 42% risk of hemorrhage, 29% risk of death, 18% risk of epilepsy, and 27% risk of having a neurological handicap at 20 years after diagnosis.

Brown et al. (1988) reported a series of 168 patients with unruptured AVMs followed for a mean period of 8.2 years. The mean risk of hemorrhage was estimated to 2.2% per year. The risk of death from rupture was 29%.

The series of Ondra et al. (1990) included 166 patients with a mean follow-up of 24 years (Ondra et al. 1990). The annual rate of bleeding was 4% per year and the mortality was 1% per year. The combined rate of major morbidity and mortality was 2.7% per year. Overall, the percentages are relatively close between the different series, with annual rates of bleeding between 2% and 4% (Jomin et al. 1993).

The occurrence of a first hemorrhage seems to be associated with an increased risk of subsequent hemorrhage (Graf et al. 1983; Itoyama et al. 1989; Mast et al. 1997). In the series of Graf et al., patients with ruptured AVMs had a 6% risk of rebleeding in the first year after hemorrhage and 2% thereafter (Graf et al. 1983). Itoyama et al. found relatively similar results (Itoyama et al. 1989). The incidence of rebleeding after a first hemorrhage is 6.9% in the first year, 1.9% per year after 5 years and 0.9% after 15 years.

Pregnancy does not appear to significantly increase the likelihood of hemorrhage from an AVM (Finnerty et al. 1999). In a large retrospective study of 451 women (Horton et al. 1990), the hemorrhage rate for pregnant and nonpregnant women of childbearing age with an unruptured AVM was respectively 0.035 per person-year and 0.032 per person-year. Women with an AVM have a 3.5% risk of hemorrhage during pregnancy. In this series, none of the hemorrhages occurred during labor, vaginal delivery, or cesarean section. Thus, the route of delivery should be based on obstetric considerations (Horton et al. 1990; Dias and Shekhar 1990).

3.3.2.4 Severity of the Hemorrhage

On the basis of retrospective analysis, the rupture of brain AVMs is estimated to be less severe than that of intracranial aneurysms, with mortality between 10% and 15% and an overall morbidity of less than 50% (The Arteriovenous Malformation Study Group 1999). Hemorrhages of brain AVMs are subarachnoidal (30%), parenchymal (23%), intraventricular (16%), and in combined locations in 31% of cases (Hartmann et al. 1998). Parenchymal hemorrhages were most likely to result in a neurological deficit (52%). Overall, in the series of Hartmann et al. (1998), 47% of patients had a good outcome after the bleeding and an additional 37% of patients were independent in their daily life.

In fact, as was shown by Hillman (2001), the rupture of an AVM is as devastating as that of an aneurysm. While aneurysm rupture is more lethal than AVM rupture (21% versus 9%), a good outcome is obtained less frequently in AVM than in aneurysm ruptures (49% versus 56%), due to the high incidence of parenchymal hematoma.

3.3.3 Epilepsy

Seizures are the initial symptom in 16%–53% of patients, with a mean of 34% (Mast et al. 1995). In the majority of cases, seizures are partial or partial complex (Osipov et al. 1997). Grand mal seizures are encountered in 27%–35% of cases (Osipov et al. 1997).

Cortical AVMs are more often associated with seizures (Turjman et al. 1995). In a large number of cases antiepileptic drugs provide good control of seizures (Osipov et al. 1997).

3.3.4 Headache

Chronic headache is the initial symptom in 7%–48% (mean: 31%) of cases (Mast et al. 1995). The relation between headache, migraine, and arteriovenous malformations is unclear. In a large review of the literature, Frishberg concluded that "while most patients with AVM who have headache have it on the side of the AVM, migraine patients with strictly unilateral location of headache are very unlikely to have an AVM" (Frishberg 1997).

There is no feature such as frequency, duration, or severity suggesting the diagnosis of AVM (The AVM Study Group 1999).

3.3.5 Focal Neurologic Deficits

Focal neurologic deficits without hemorrhage are the initial symptom in 1%–40% of patients (Mast et al. 1995). In fact, this clinical presentation is probably infrequent (The AVM Study Group 1999). As outlined by Mast et al. (1995), focal neurologic deficits encountered in patients harboring brain AVMs may be progressive, stable, or reversible. Reversible focal neurologic deficits are questionable regarding their mechanism, since a post-ictal etiology cannot be ruled out. The progression of neurologic deficit may have different explanations: steal phenomenon (Carter and Gumerlock 1995), venous hypertension, or mass effect (Miyasaka et al. 1997). The relevance of the steal phenomenon is in fact very difficult to demonstrate in patients presenting with progressive neurologic deficits (Mast et al. 1995). Indeed, positron emission tomography studies (Fink 1992; Kaminaga et al. 1999) showed a decrease of cerebral blood flow in brain tissues surrounding AVMs, but without increase in parenchymal blood volume or modifications of glucose and oxygen extraction fractions.

Mass effect is detected in a relatively high percentage of nonhemorrhagic cases (44%, Miyasaka et al. 1997). Cortical sulci obliteration and lateral ventricle displacement are frequently observed. Mass effect could be related to the size of the AVM itself or to the presence of large dilated venous sacs or ectatic veins. White-matter edema is rarely the cause of mass effect.

3.4 Diagnostic Imaging

3.4.1 Goals of Imaging

Imaging has several roles and goals:

1 To establish the diagnosis of brain AVM in various clinical situations
2 To make a pretherapeutic evaluation of the AVM to help in decision-making
3 To treat the AVM as a sole therapy or in association with surgery or radiosurgery
4 To perform post-therapeutic evaluation

3.4.2 Imaging Modalities

3.4.2.1 CT Scan

In patients with a sudden-onset of a neurological deficit, a CT scan is usually the first imaging modality used, mainly to rule out hemorrhage (Ducreux et al. 2001). CT is able to show very early parenchymal, subarachnoid, and intraventricular bleeding. The diagnosis of brain AVM should be discussed when the patient is young, if the parenchymal hematoma has a lobar topography, and if calcifications or spontaneously hyperdense serpiginous structures are visible (Fig. 3.2).

In case of unruptured AVM, non-contrast-enhanced CT scans can be normal. However, in some patients slightly hyperdense serpiginous structures can be seen (Fig. 3.3). Parenchymatous calcifications are observed in 20% of cases, related to intravascular thrombosis or evolution of an old hematoma. Contrast agent injection is absolutely mandatory to depict the brain AVM (Figs. 3.4, 3.5) on CT. Abnormalities of the parenchymal density are visible in approximately 25% of cases, related to the presence of gliosis or an old hematoma. Abnormalities of the ventricular system can be observed: focal dilatation in case of associated parenchymal atrophy; compression of the ventricular system in case of mass effect caused by the AVM. Hydrocephalus can be observed in case of previous hemorrhage or if the ventricular system is compressed by enlarged draining veins of the AVM.

The role of CT angiography in the diagnostic workup of brain AVMs is not precisely defined. Aoki et al. (1998) showed that 3D CT angiography provided precise anatomic information on nidus and draining veins but did not demonstrate small feeders.

In patients with a large hematoma for which emergency evacuation is necessary, CTA may be useful to detect a brain AVM preoperatively and thus give the surgeon some idea about the surgical strategy to be followed. However, small AVMs can be misdiagnosed by this technique.

3.4.2.2 MR

Patients presenting with ruptured AVMs are usually examined in the acute phase by a CT scan. MRI is currently used in case of unruptured AVM or to find the underlying lesion in case of lobar hematoma, generally days or weeks after the bleeding.

Given the different sequences available in MR imaging, MRI is able to give three levels of analysis of the AVM:

- Anatomic analysis using conventional sequences
- Vascular analysis using MR angiography
- Functional analysis using fMRI

Anatomic Analysis

Conventional sequences (T_1, T_2, T_1 with gadolinium) enable a very precise analysis of the brain AVM (Smith et al. 1988b). On T_1- and T_2-weighted images, circulating vessels have no signal because of the flow void phenomenon (Fig. 3.5). On T_1-weighted images with gadolinium, vessels are enhanced.

The size and the anatomic location of the nidus are precisely delineated by MRI (Figs. 3.4, 3.6). Smith et al. (1988) showed that the size of the nidus was

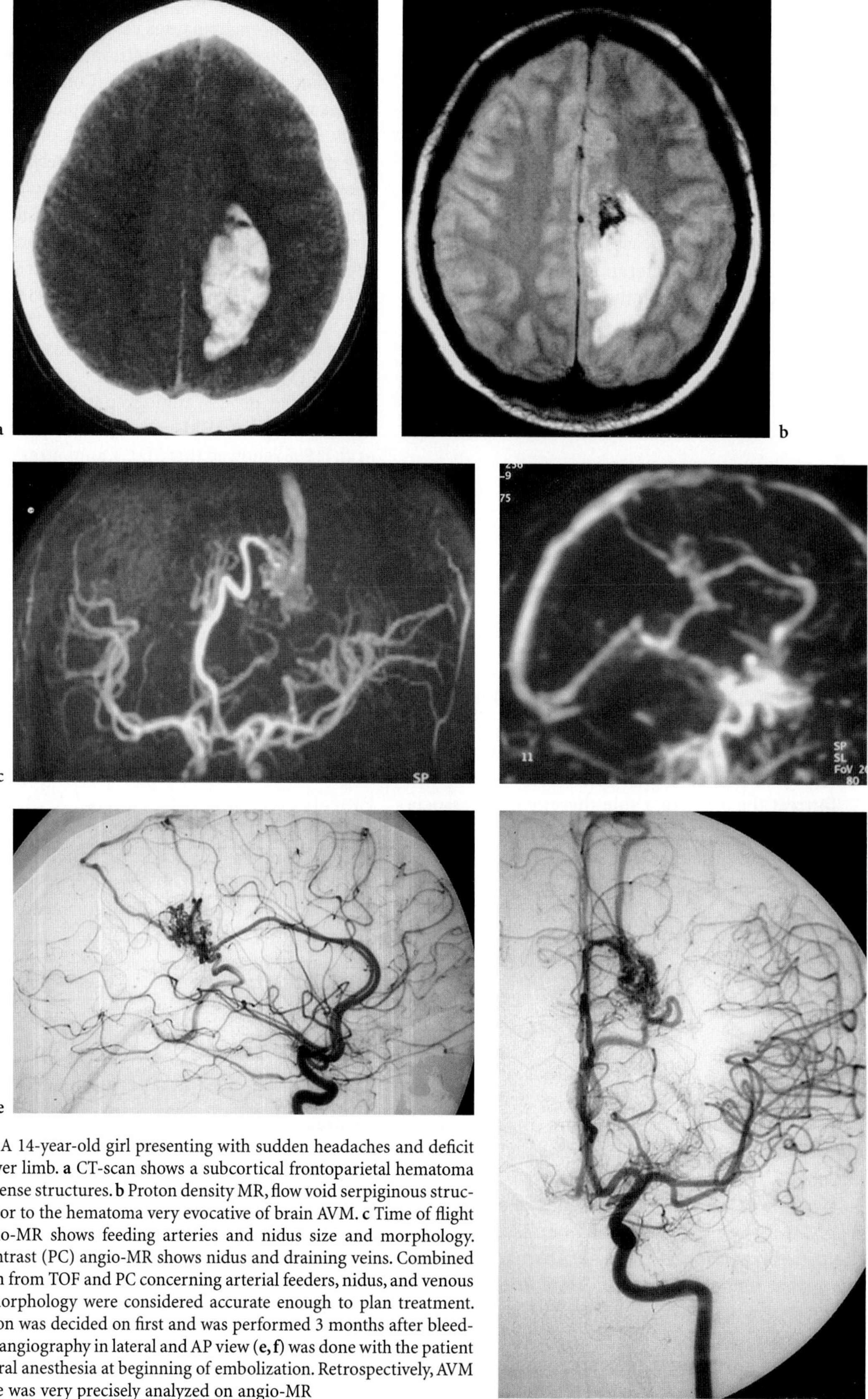

Fig. 3.2a–f. A 14-year-old girl presenting with sudden headaches and deficit of right lower limb. **a** CT-scan shows a subcortical frontoparietal hematoma with hypodense structures. **b** Proton density MR, flow void serpiginous structures anterior to the hematoma very evocative of brain AVM. **c** Time of flight (TOF) angio-MR shows feeding arteries and nidus size and morphology. **d** Phase contrast (PC) angio-MR shows nidus and draining veins. Combined information from TOF and PC concerning arterial feeders, nidus, and venous drainage morphology were considered accurate enough to plan treatment. Embolization was decided on first and was performed 3 months after bleeding. Digital angiography in lateral and AP view (**e, f**) was done with the patient under general anesthesia at beginning of embolization. Retrospectively, AVM architecture was very precisely analyzed on angio-MR

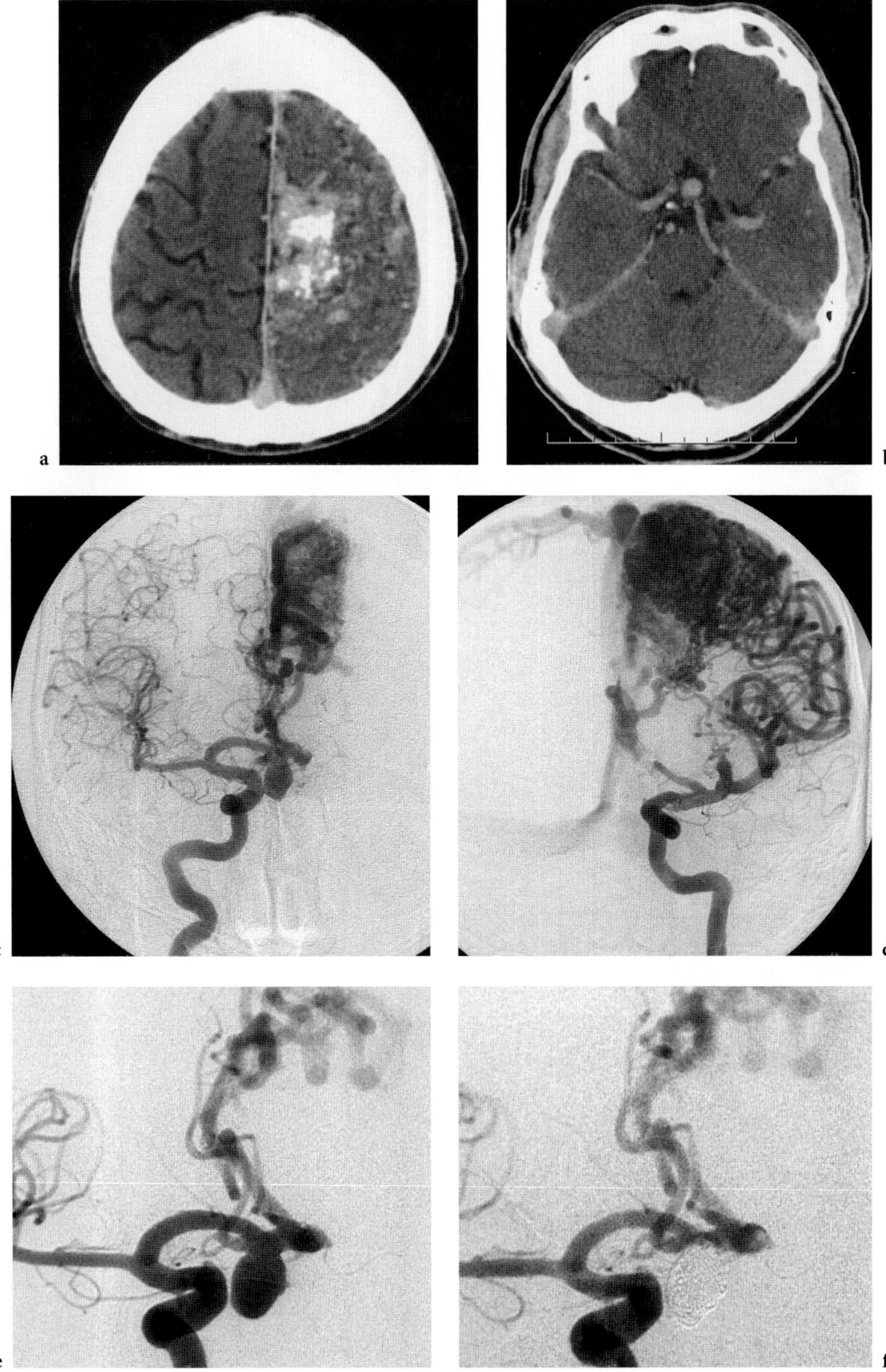

Fig. 3.3a–f. A 46-year-old man who presented with a parenchymal frontal hematoma in 1976, resulting in a slight residual right hemiparesis predominating at the level of the lower limb. The patient came to our department in 2000 complaining of progressive worsening of the deficit, confirmed by repeated clinical examination during the preceding 6 months. Contrast CT scan shows an AVM of the left medial frontal lobe with calcifications (**a**) and an aneurysm of the anterior communicating (Acom) artery (**b**). Digital angiography shows Acom aneurysm and huge frontoparietal AVM fed by both anterior and middle cerebral artery branches and deeply involving the white matter (**c, d**). Acom aneurysm was considered the weakest point and treated first (**e, f**). Treatment was difficult due to aneurysm neck size and high flow. Oversized coils were necessary to keep them in the aneurysm cavity. The AVM is still under an embolization protocol with the aim of reducing AVM volume and flow to improve progressively worsening symptoms

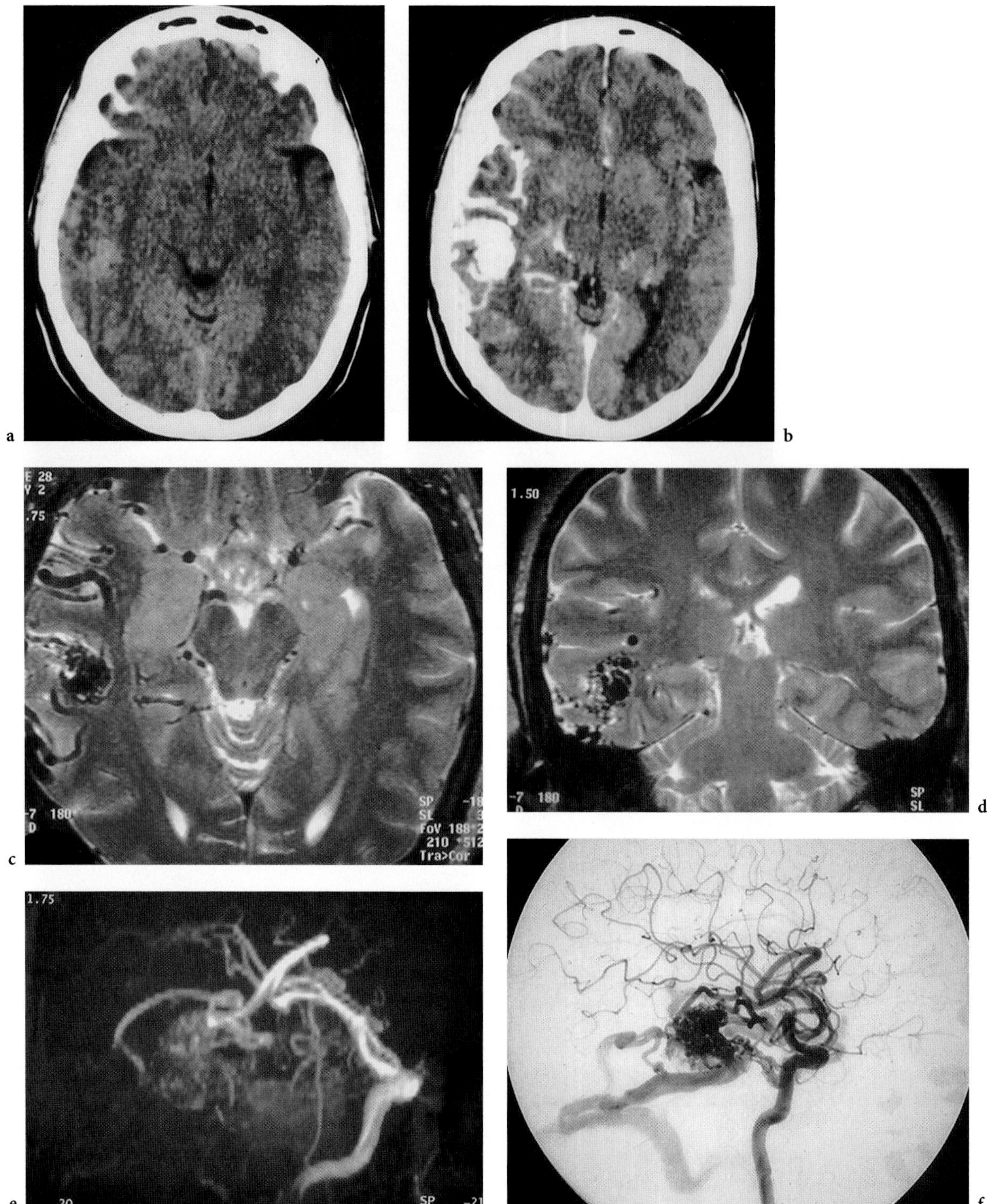
a
b
1.50
SP
SL
d
Tra>Cor
c
1.75
20
SP -21
e
f

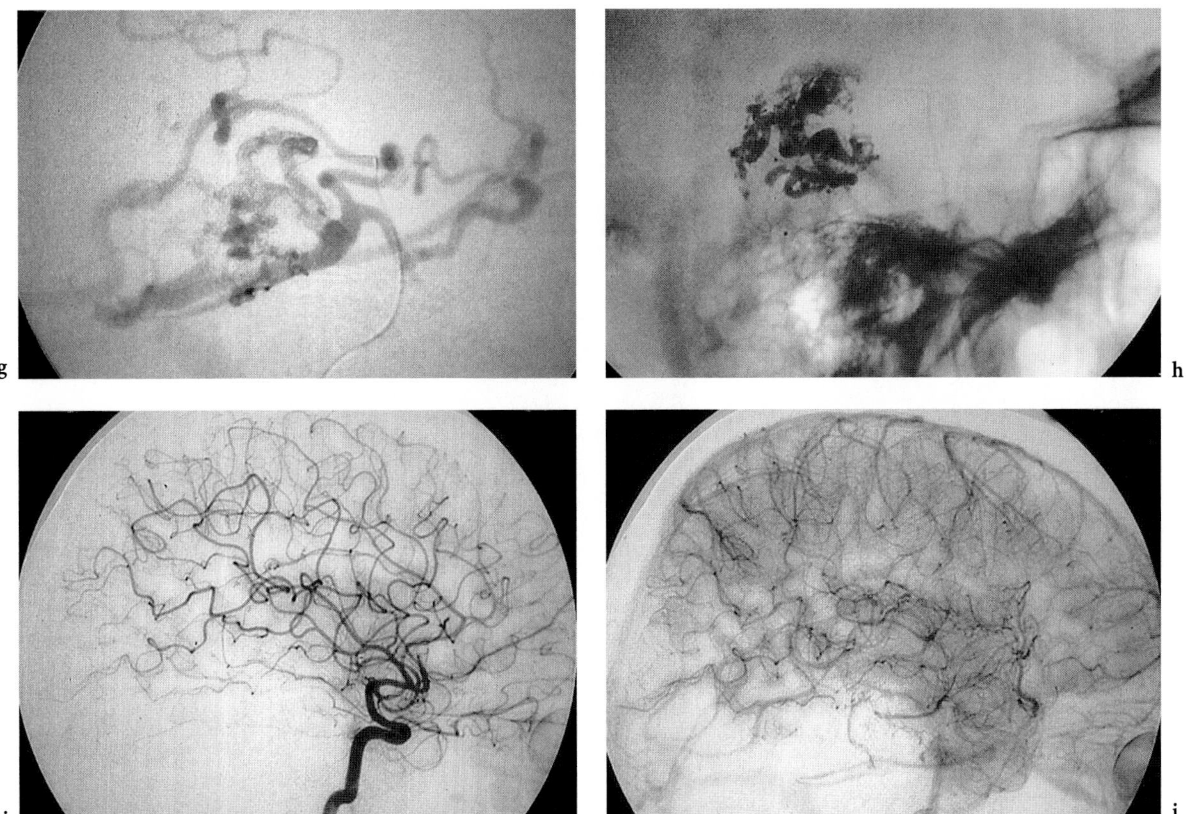

△

◁ **Fig. 3.4a–j.** A 42-year-old woman presenting with two episodes of seizures. Pre- and post-contrast CT scans (**a, b**) show a right temporal AVM. A slightly hyperdense structure is visible before and, strongly enhanced, after injection. Frontal and axial T_2 images perfectly localize the AVM within the white matter of the right temporal lobe, but determination of the nidus border is difficult (**c, d**). 3D TOF image does not show the nidus limits precisely and affords poor understanding of the AVM architecture (**e**). Digital angiography performed during embolization shows the arterial feeders, nidus size and venous drainage much better (**f**). Superselective injection during embolization allows a much better understanding of nidus arteriovenous architecture. Distal catheterization shows immediate opacification of draining veins (**g**). Such arteriovenous anatomy allows very efficient embolization with easy gluing of origin of draining veins (**h**). Three and 18 months after second embolization, follow-up angiography showed complete occlusion (**i, j**)

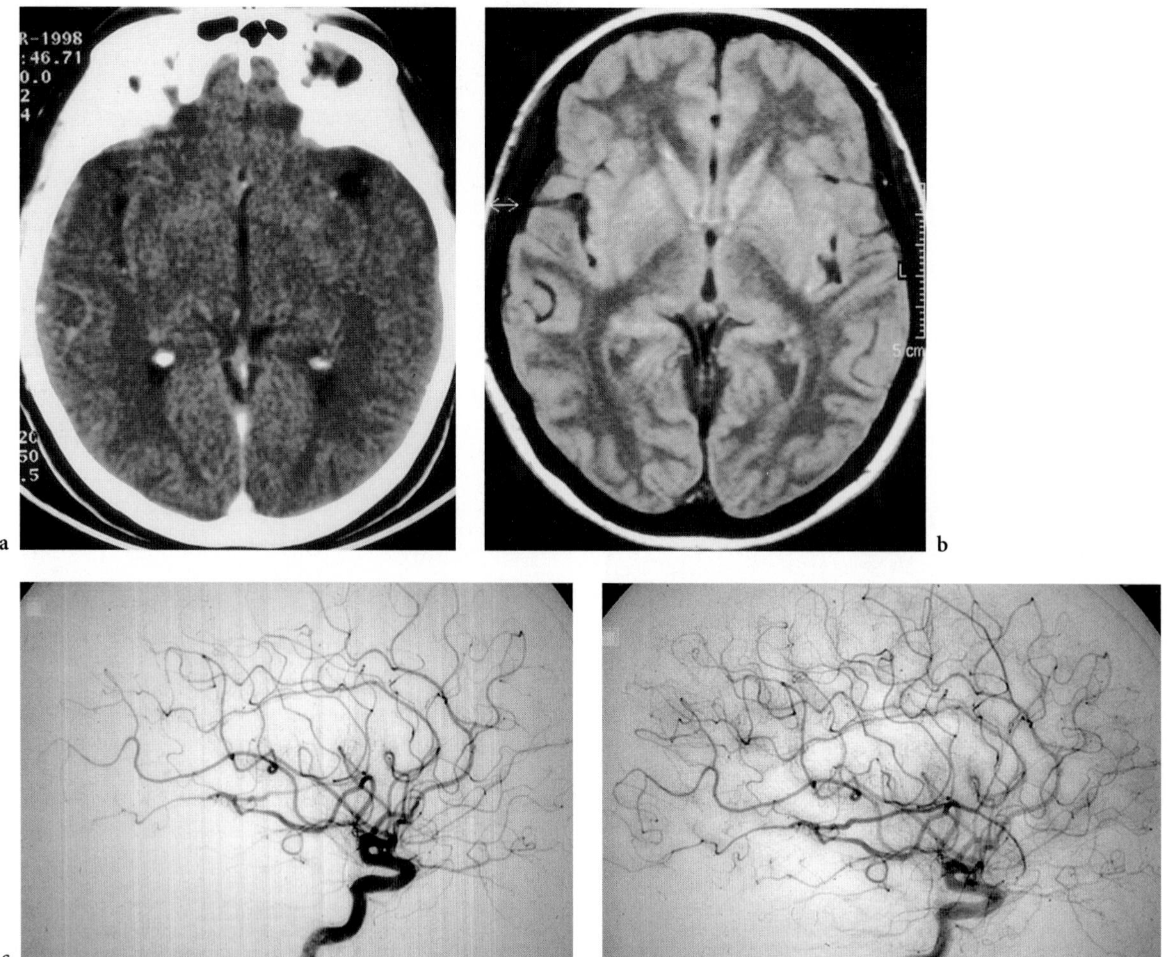

Fig. 3.5a–d. A 63-year-old woman presenting with common headaches. Post-contrast CT scan shows an abnormal vessel within the right temporal lobe (**a**). Axial proton density image shows enlarged flow void vessel (**b**). Digital angiography depicts a very small superficial temporal AVM draining into a single, slightly dilated, superficial vein (**c, d**). AVM is supplied by very short "en passage" feeders. Due to patient's age, absence of symptoms, and AVM morphology no therapy was planned

Fig. 3.6a–f. A 27-year-old man presenting with a small deep hematoma with ventricular hemorrhage. Axial proton density MR image shows a left temporopolar small brain AVM (**a**) and the hematoma in a remote, more posterior location at the medial aspect of the left temporal lobe (**b**). Internal carotid injection shows the temporal AVM with a deep venous drainage (**c**). An intranidal aneurysm or false aneurysm is visible; this must be considered the most likely cause of the bleeding and should be the first target of embolization. Superselective catheterization of the lenticulostriate artery harboring the aneurysm allowed gluing of both aneurysm and AVM (**d**). Final follow-up angiography after four embolizations showed incomplete obliteration of the AVM with disappearance of any nidus but persistent early venous drainage (**e, f**)

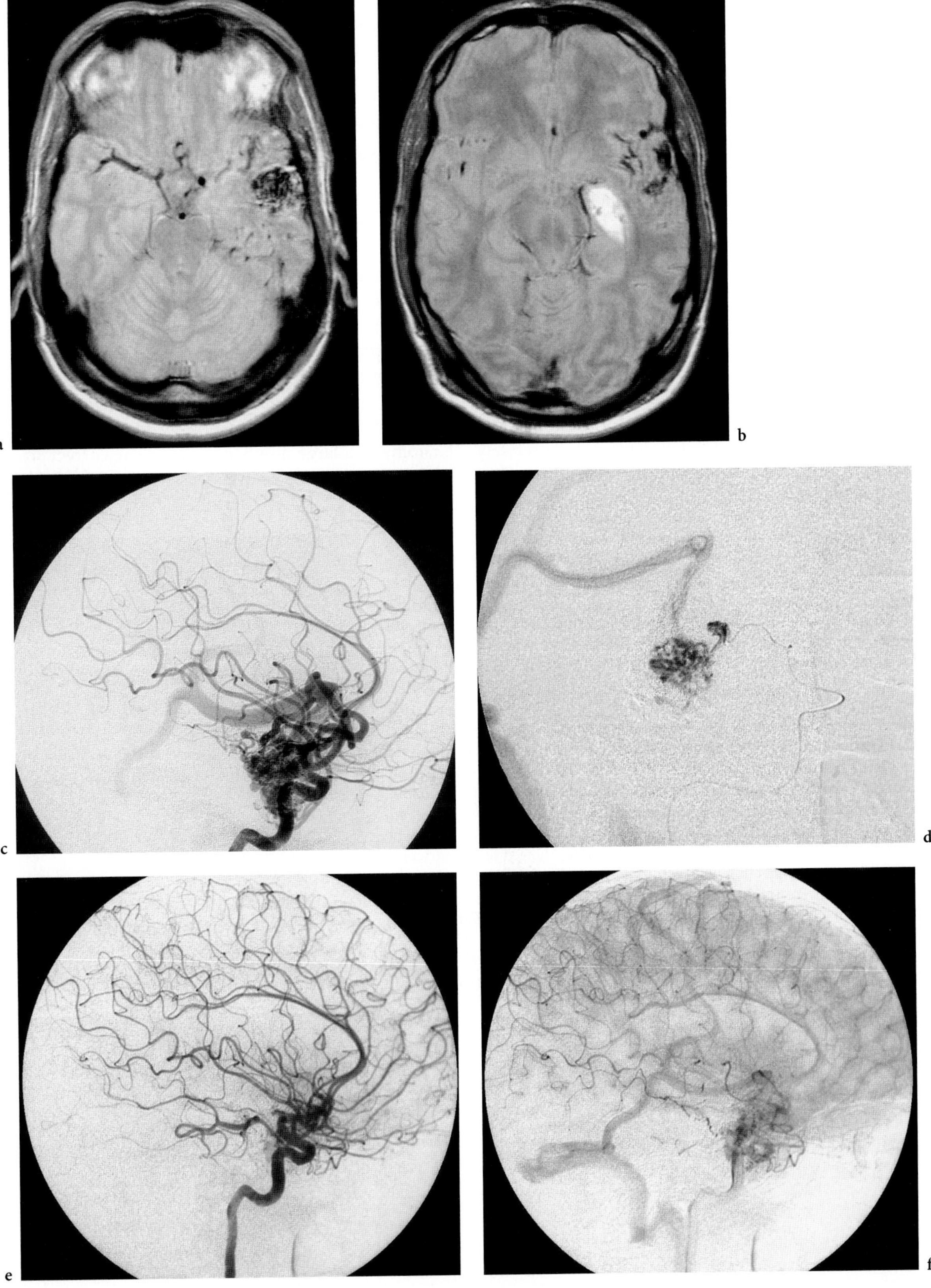
a
b
c
d
e
f

more precisely shown by MRI than by conventional angiography. Anatomic location was always better defined by MRI than by angiography. Depiction of arterial feeders and draining veins is often incomplete with conventional sequences.

MRI is also a good tool to clearly demonstrate parenchymal lesions caused by the AVM. Because of the high sensibility to hemosiderin, MR is able to depict a recent, but also an old hematoma (Fig. 3.7). However, the presence of a recent hematoma may mask a small AVM leading to a false-negative MR (Fig. 3.8). In the absence of hemorrhage, perinidal abnormalities of signal, particularly hypersignal on T_2-weighted images, can be evidence of perinidal ischemic changes or gliosis. Fluid-attenuated inversion-recovery sequence (FLAIR) seems to be superior to the conventional T_2-weighted fast spin-echo sequences in the assessment of intralesional and perilesional gliosis (Essig et al. 2000). More precisely than CT, MR is able to depict either morphological changes induced by the AVM itself or its parenchymal or ventricular consequences: parenchymal atrophy with focal dilatation of the ventricular system; compression of the ventricular system in case of mass effect caused by the AVM; hydrocephalus in case of previous hemorrhage or if the ventricular system is compressed by enlarged draining veins of the AVM.

Vascular Analysis

Until recently, only phase-contrast and time-of-flight techniques were available to study the vascular system (Fig. 3.2). These have been demonstrated to be of value in providing three-dimensional representations of AVM vascular architecture (Marchal et al. 1990). However, these techniques have limited anatomic coverage and are not able to adequately depict the precise anatomy in a large number of cases: The correct size of the nidus cannot be assessed (Fig. 3.4); intranidal

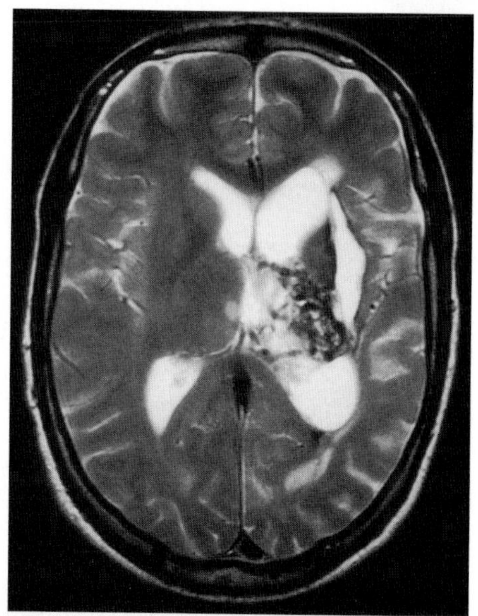

a

Fig. 3.7a–i. A 34-year-old man who presented with a first episode of bleeding in 1985 from a deep brain AVM. The patient was treated with radiosurgery. He presented a new hemorrhage in 1987, with major clinical consequences (right severe hemiparesis and aphasia). **a** Axial T_2 image performed in 1998 shows deep paraventricular AVM with old hematoma of right striatum and posterior limb of internal capsule. 3D TOF angio-MR in sagittal and frontal views (**b**, **c**) allows good delineation of nidus limits and angioarchitecture evaluation. Digital angiography by internal carotid injection in AP view (**d**) and vertebral injection in sagittal view (**e**) provide same information about feeders, nidus shape and architecture, and drainage. Very early phase of vertebral injection depicts a small intranidal aneurysm or false aneurysm of distal thalamo-perforating artery; this was considered a weak point of the malformation and treated first (**f**). Superselective catheterization of posterolateral choroidal arteries performed immediately after thalamo-perforating artery and aneurysm gluing showed intranidal wedge positioning of catheter tip (**g**). Late venous phase of this injection showed intraventricular hemorrhage. Glue injection was performed immediately after bleeding was recognized (**h**). Post-embolization CT scan confirmed intraventricular hemorrhage but no parenchymal hematoma (**i**). External ventricular shunting was performed just after embolization. Patient was awakened 3 days later and showed moderate worsening of initial symptoms. At 3-month follow-up examination he had completely recovered his initial clinical status

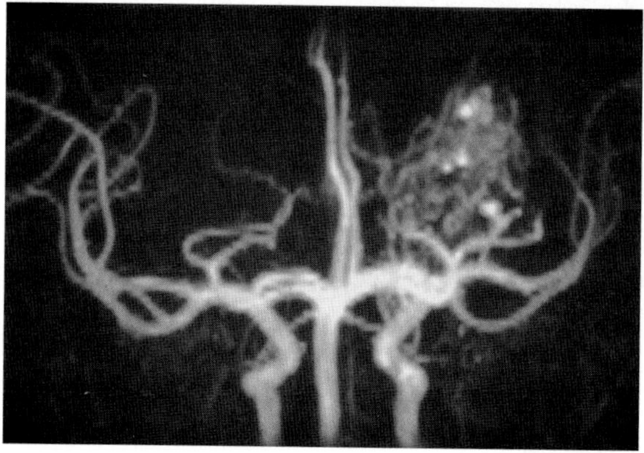

b

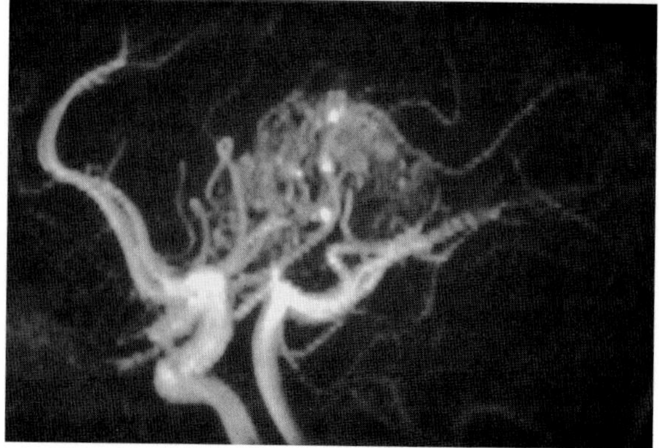

c

▷

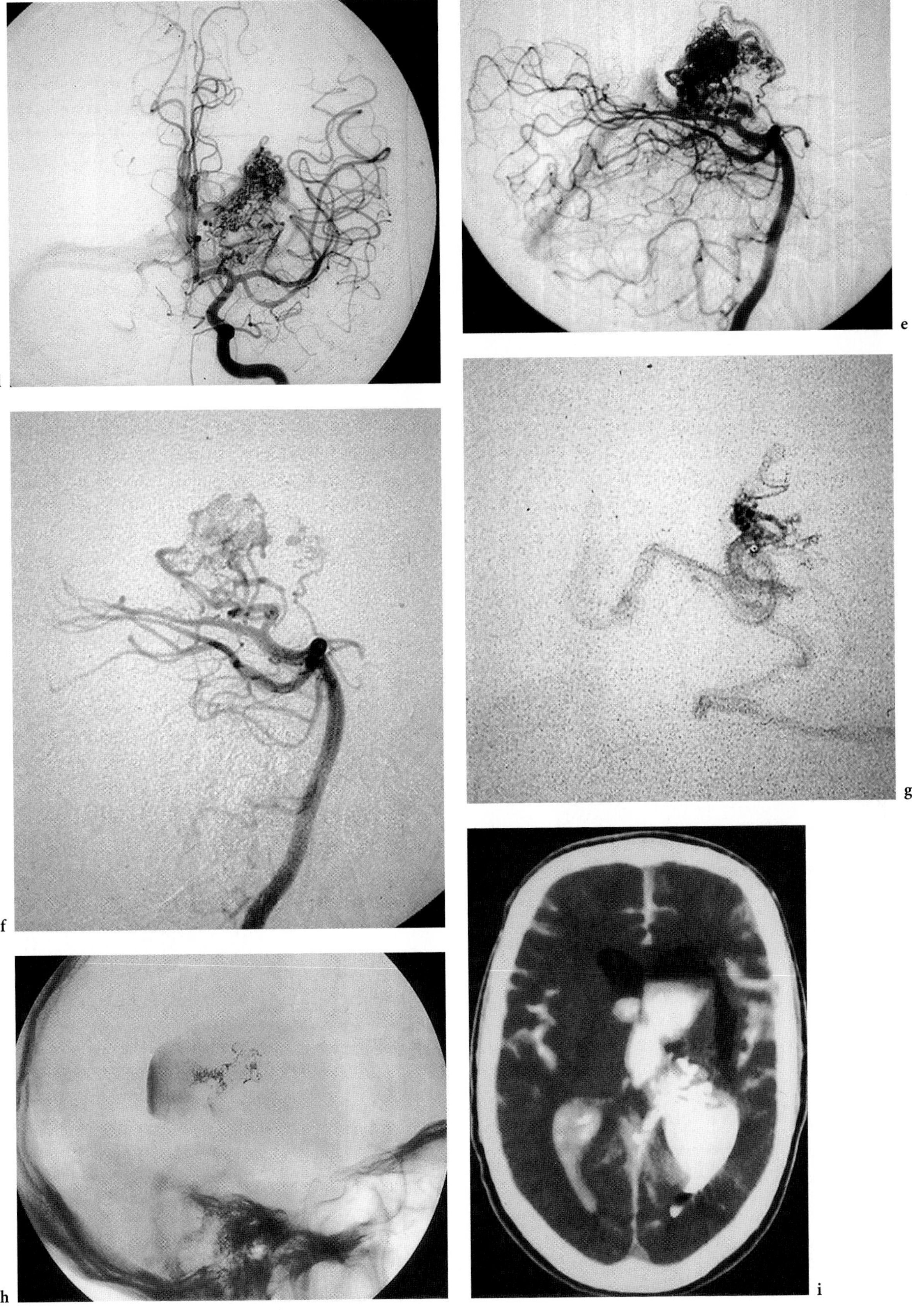
d
e
f
g
h
i

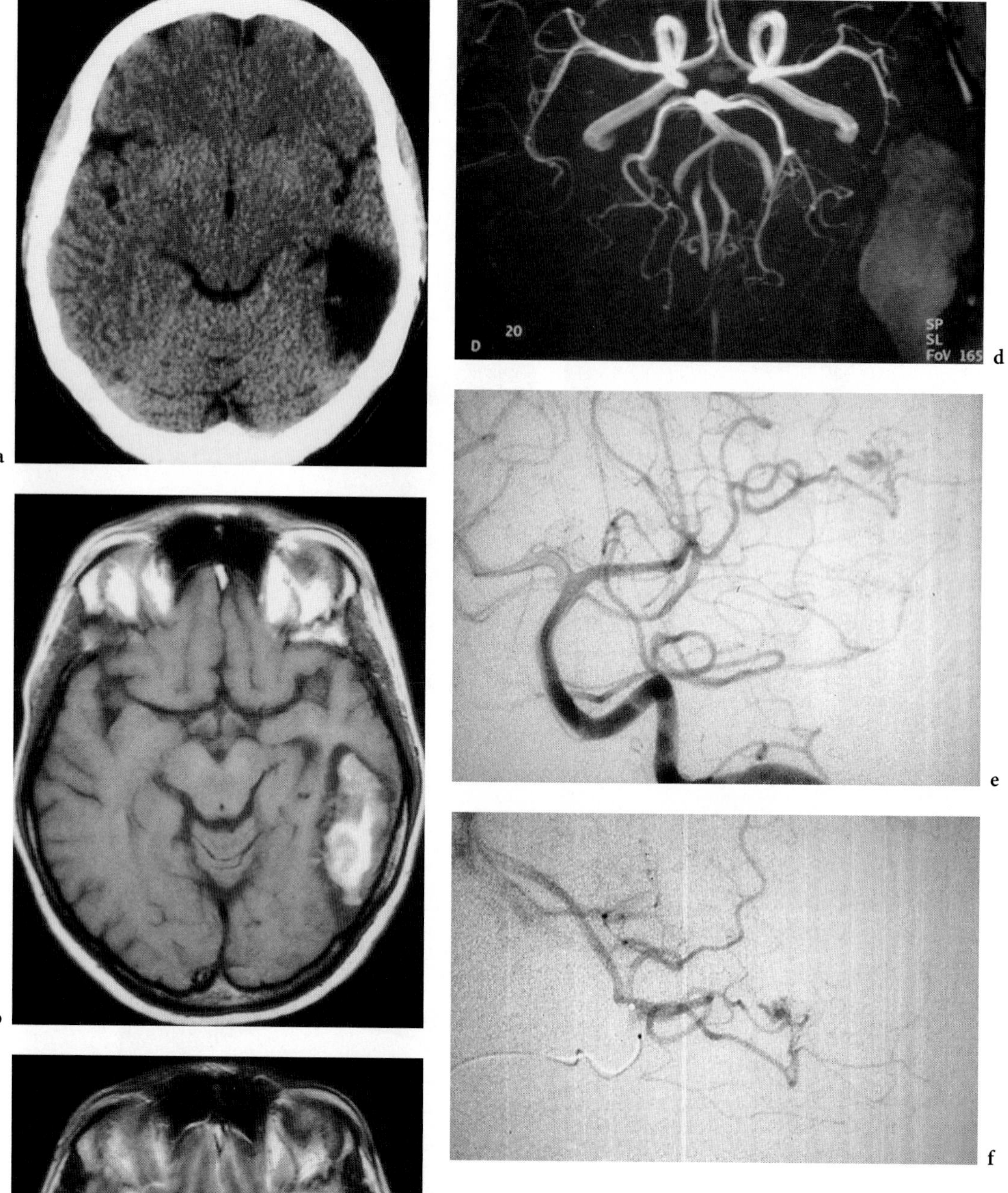

Fig. 3.8a–f. A 42-year-old woman who presented with sudden headaches and aphasia at 7 months of pregnancy. CT scan showed a left temporal hematoma. Digital angiography was performed and considered normal (not available). Pregnancy was carried out to term and cesarean delivery was performed. She progressively recovered and came to our institution3 months later. CT-scan and MR were performed at that time. CT scan shows chronic hypodense hematoma (**a**). MR T_1 and T_2 axial images show hyperintense signal within the hematoma due to extracellular methemoglobin (**b, c**). 3D TOF MIP reconstruction is normal (**d**). Both axial conventional images and angio-MR were considered not accurate enough to rule out a small AVM. Digital angiography depicts a small left temporal micro-AVM (**e**). Superselective catheterization allowed more precise understanding of nidus morphology (**f**). More distal catheterization did not obtain wedge positioning of catheter tip and good control of the flow. Consequently, embolization was not performed and the patient was treated with radiosurgery

aneurysms are frequently not visible (Fig. 3.7); depiction of the draining veins is inconsistent (Fig. 3.9); small-caliber vessels and regions of slow blood flow cannot be consistently revealed (Fig. 3.9) (Edelman et al. 1989; Marchal et al. 1990; Nüssel et al. 1991). Moreover, dynamic information is not provided by these sequences.

Multiple overlapping thin-slab acquisition time-of-flight MR allows greater anatomic coverage and produces better signal-to-noise ratio and higher resolution than conventional MR angiography, but slab boundary artifacts represent a major limitation (Liu and Rutt 1998; Warren et al. 2001).

New gadolinium-enhanced MRA techniques are currently in development which are superior to TOF MR angiograms but still inferior to DSA images for depiction of AVM components because of limitations in both temporal and spatial resolution (Takano et al. 1999; Griffiths et al. 2000; Warren et al. 2001; Farb et al. 2001).

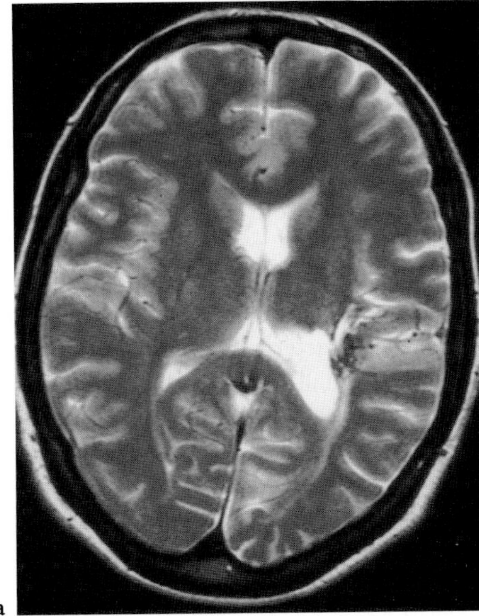
a

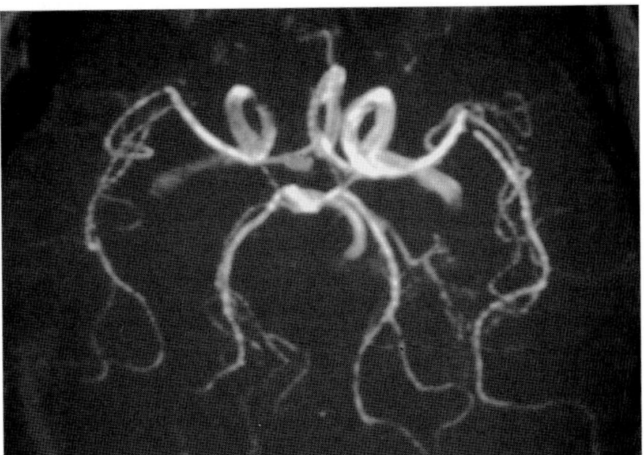
b

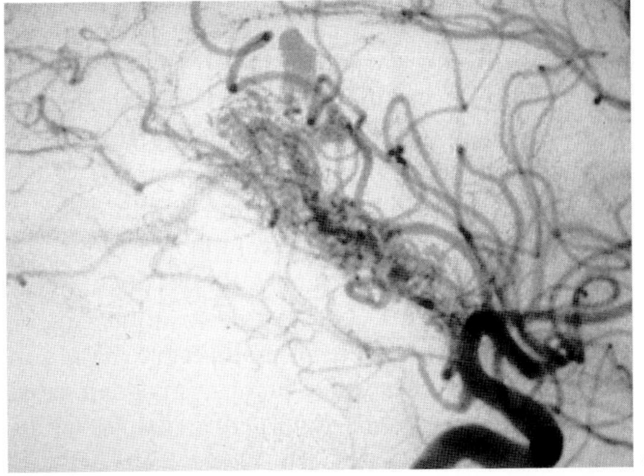
c

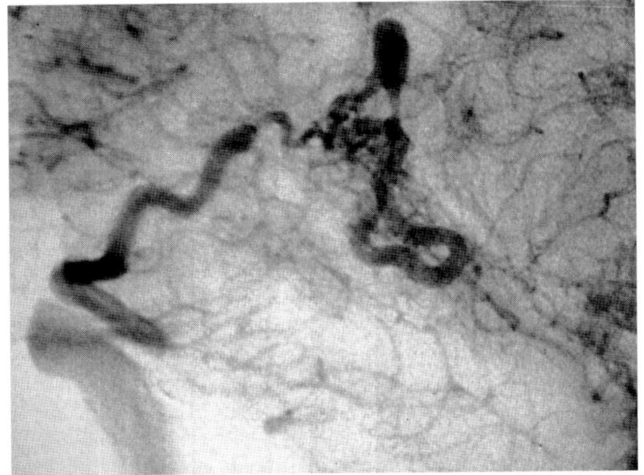
d

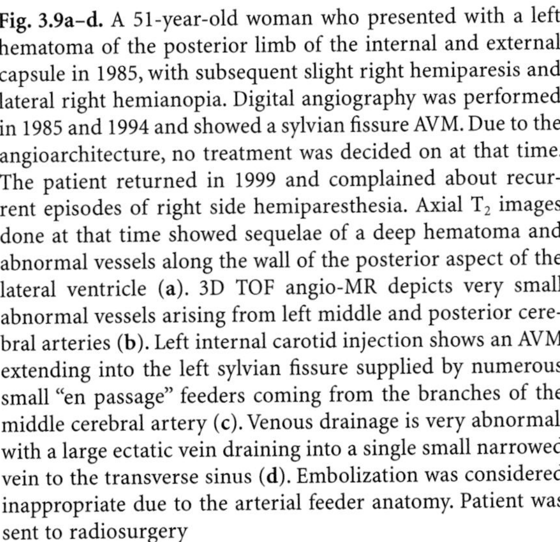
Fig. 3.9a–d. A 51-year-old woman who presented with a left hematoma of the posterior limb of the internal and external capsule in 1985, with subsequent slight right hemiparesis and lateral right hemianopia. Digital angiography was performed in 1985 and 1994 and showed a sylvian fissure AVM. Due to the angioarchitecture, no treatment was decided on at that time. The patient returned in 1999 and complained about recurrent episodes of right side hemiparesthesia. Axial T_2 images done at that time showed sequelae of a deep hematoma and abnormal vessels along the wall of the posterior aspect of the lateral ventricle (**a**). 3D TOF angio-MR depicts very small abnormal vessels arising from left middle and posterior cerebral arteries (**b**). Left internal carotid injection shows an AVM extending into the left sylvian fissure supplied by numerous small "en passage" feeders coming from the branches of the middle cerebral artery (**c**). Venous drainage is very abnormal, with a large ectatic vein draining into a single small narrowed vein to the transverse sinus (**d**). Embolization was considered inappropriate due to the arterial feeder anatomy. Patient was sent to radiosurgery

Functional Analysis

Functional MRI (fMRI) includes perfusion and diffusion imaging and study of brain function.

The role of DWI has to be determined (Ducreux et al. 2001). The nidus has usually a low signal with a large and homogeneous increase of the apparent diffusion coefficient (ADC). However, to date DWI does not play a major role in AVMs.

Perfusion MRI is an additional new tool, but its role in brain AVMs is also unclear. It may be possible to evaluate hemodynamic characteristics of different AVMs, but no scientific data are currently available.

Functional MRI activation has been studied largely in patients with brain AVMs (Latchaw et al. 1995; Maldjian et al. 1996; Schlosser et al. 1997; Vikingstad et al. 2000; Lazar et al. 2000; Alkadhi et al. 2000; Carpentier et al. 2001). fMRI activation is a potentially very interesting tool to depict functional areas of the brain, when a brain AVM is located in an eloquent area, particularly sensorimotor, visual, and language cortex. Bold sequences used for the performance of fMRI activation are based primarily on the detection of hemodynamic changes in the cortex during the performance of a task. Given the huge hemodynamic modifications induced by the AVM in the perinidal parenchyma, there is some doubt regarding fMRI activation patterns.

In the great majority of cases, no activation is detected inside the nidus during the performance of a task. This could be related to the absence of functional tissue within the nidus, but the detection of subtle and minor activation within an AVM could also be obscured by the complex relationships between the BOLD effect and AVM circulatory patterns (Vikingstad et al. 2000). Activation can be observed in the cortical regions adjacent to AVMs. In the majority of cases where brain AVMs are located in eloquent areas, a shift of the activated areas with a frequent interhemispheric transfer is observed.

A recent study showed a discrepancy between the superselective Wada test and fMRI activation in a patient with a left frontal brain AVM (Lazar et al. 2000). An area which was activated during fMRI was not detected as a language area by the Wada test.

Thus, fMRI activation has a potential for the study of brain function in brain AVMs, but larger series are necessary to evaluate the liability of this technique.

3.4.2.3 *Selective and Superselective Angiography*

As shown in Sect. 3.3.2.1, many anatomic factors have to be analyzed to evaluate the risk of rupture of an AVM and to decide which treatment is appropriate. Despite recent developments, CTA and MRA are currently not sufficient to obtain a precise description of the AVM from an anatomic and hemodynamic point of view. Selective angiography is still always necessary to make a decision regarding the treatment. In summary: the diagnosis of an AVM nowadays is usually based on CT or MR; the exact and therapeutically relevant anatomic and functional information still has to be obtained by angiography.

Technically, selective angiography has to be performed according to a rigorous protocol. To assess as precisely as possible the anatomic components of the AVM, it is important to selectively inject the internal and external carotid arteries and vertebral arteries. Analysis of the arterial feeders, nidus, and venous drainage is obtained by performing multiple projections (anteroposterior, lateral, and oblique). Three-dimensional angiography may be helpful.

However, even excellent angiograms are often inadequate for reaching correct therapeutic decisions (Nakstad and Nornes 1994). The exact anatomy of large feeding arteries may be obscure with selective injections. Small feeding arteries are sometimes not visible on selective angiograms. Although the size of the nidus is generally well evaluated by selective angiography, intranidal aneurysms (Fig. 3.7) and direct intranidal AV fistulas are often misdiagnosed. The venous drainage of the AVM is generally well studied by selective angiography, but the compartments of the AVM and their venous drainage are often not depicted because the AVM is injected as a whole (Fig. 3.4).

For all these reasons, superselective angiography often gives a more detailed analysis of the AVM and may become more important in making the diagnosis. Superselective angiography is performed by manual injection of each separate arterial feeder. It is usually the first step of embolization.

3.4.3 Imaging Strategy

Imaging strategy is closely related to the clinical presentation (rupture of the AVM or not) and the clinical status of the patient.

3.4.3.1 *Ruptured AVM*

In this situation, the patient has the clinical presentation of a parenchymal hematoma or a subarachnoid hemorrhage or both. The first examination is the CT scan, which has a high sensibility to detect intracranial hemorrhage in the acute phase with a high specificity.

Contrast-enhanced CT scan and CT angiography are currently not useful. Indeed, small AVMs may be mistaken by CTA and the anatomic data provided by this technique are often not sufficient to make a therapeutic decision. Only in patients with a large space-occupying hematoma CTA can be performed to try to indicate to the neurosurgeon whether a brain AVM is the underlying cause of bleeding, before emergency surgery is performed.

With the exception of this specific situation, the next step after the diagnosis of the hemorrhage is selective angiography. In case of isolated subarachnoid hemorrhage or when a brain hematoma may be related to a ruptured aneurysm, it has to be performed emergently. In other cases, the time to perform angiography is a matter of debate. When an intraparenchymal hematoma is present it can compress the AVM, leading in some cases to a false-negative diagnosis. For the same reasons, anatomic analysis in the acute phase may be erroneous. Therefore, selective angiography should probably be delayed. However, angiography is often performed at the acute phase of bleeding to obtain a definite diagnosis and to have all the information at hand concerning the AVM in case the patient's clinical status should worsen, requiring prompt surgery. Moreover, when the cause of bleeding is unclear (AVM or associated aneurysm), angiography is also important to determine if an associated aneurysm is present, and in such instances angiographic criteria combined with CT or MR findings may be helpful to determine the site of bleeding (Fig. 3.6).

After the acute phase of bleeding, the therapeutic approach to the AVM will be defined on the basis of anatomic data provided by MRI and selective angiography (Figs. 3.2, 3.7).

3.4.3.2
Unruptured AVM

For an unruptured AVM CT is not indicated; the first step is MRI and MRA to obtain all the information needed to make a therapeutic decision. In a great number of cases, clinical data, MRI, and MRA are sufficient to make a decision regarding therapeutic options: – in some cases, it is clear that treatment should be conservative, and in this situation selective angiography is not needed; in other cases, the AVM has to be treated and the next step depends on the therapeutic strategy. If embolization is the first step of treatment, there is no reason to perform first a selective angiogram and then superselective angiography and embolization. In this situation, complete information has to be given to the patient and selective, superselective angiography and the first embolization have to be performed at the same time. If surgery is the modality of choice, selective angiography has to be performed first. If radiosurgery is indicated as the sole treatment, selective angiography has to be performed immediately before treatment for stereotactic localization of the AVM.

In some cases, the therapeutic decision is not clear after MRI and MRA, and selective angiography is performed to make a decision.

3.4.4
Classification of Brain AVMs

Several systems have been designed to classify patients with brain AVMs regarding surgical risk (Spetzler et al. 1992) and individual hemorrhagic risk (Nataf et al. 1998).

3.4.4.1
Classification of Spetzler and Martin

The Spetzler and Martin (1986)classification was established to grade AVMs according to their degree of surgical difficulty and the risk of surgical morbidity and mortality. To assign an AVM grade, the size, the venous drainage, and the eloquence of the adjacent brain are determined from angiography, computed tomography, and MRI. A numerical value is assigned for each of the categories:

- Size of the AVM: small (<3 cm): 1; medium (3–6 cm): 2; large (>6 cm): 3
- Eloquence of adjacent brain: noneloquent: 0; eloquent: 1
- Pattern of venous drainage: superficial only: 0; deep: 1

The grade of the lesion is obtained by summing up the points assigned for each category. As previously outlined, the Spetzler-Martin grading system is clearly a surgical one and is of little value for interventional neuroradiologists and radiotherapists (Mansmann et al. 2000).

3.4.4.2
Classification of Nataf et al.

Based on a retrospective study of 250 consecutive patients treated by radiotherapy, the classification of Nataf et al. (1998) was established to individually evaluate the risk of hemorrhage. Five angiographic parameters were considered to be determinants of the bleeding risk, leading to a four-grade classification.

Grade I: no risk factor
  Ia: with venous recruitment
  Ib: without venous recruitment
Grade II: venous stenosis or venous reflux
Grade III: deep venous drainage only
Grade IV: intra- or juxtanidal aneurysm

In the series mentioned, there were 13% of hemorrhages in grade Ia, 38% in grade Ib, 48% in grade II, and 90% in grades III and IV.

3.5 Therapy

3.5.1 Neurosurgery

Neurosurgery may be indicated in emergency to remove a large life-threatening hematoma. Only superficial AVMs, more easy to control, may be removed with the hematoma. When surgery of a brain AVM is difficult, the hematoma may be removed and the treatment strategy may then be decided without hurry regarding AVM location, size, and architecture. Treatment of AVM is then performed later, after the patient has recovered. Very few papers report patient outcome after early surgical treatment of intracerebral hemorrhage caused by AVMs (Lamy et al. 1990; Jafar and Rezai 1994; Puzzilli et al. 1998). The numbers of patients are too small to allow any firm conclusions. In the largest series of 24 operated patients there were 53% good results, 25% comatose patients, and 21% deaths (Lamy et al. 1990).

Elective Surgery. In a non-emergent situation surgery is elective, by the standard microsurgical technique with an operating microscope (Ogilvy et al. 2001). Usually, the arterial feeders are attacked first, followed by the nidus, and only at the very end of treatment the draining veins (Yasargil 1988). The goal of surgery is complete cure, which should be proven by intraoperative and postoperative angiography. In case of residual AVM a new surgical approach should be considered immediately to avoid subsequent bleeding that may be favored by subtotal occlusion of the nidus. Radiosurgery or embolization of postoperative residual AVM may be considered even if the first carries a risk of bleeding until complete occlusion.

Outcome of Direct Surgery. A recently published meta-analysis reviewed all series of more than 50 patients published since 1990 (25 series, 2452 patients) (Castel and Kantor 2000). The clinical presentation was hemorrhage in 57% of cases. Global mortality varied from 0% to 15%, mean 3.3% (68 of the 2452 patients). It was below 5% in 81% of the reported cases. Postoperative global morbidity was 1.5%–18.7%, mean 8.6%. Hamilton and Spetzler made a prospective study of 120 consecutive patients who underwent complete microsurgical excision of their AVM, with or without previous embolization, to evaluate correlation between the Spetzler-Martin grade and postoperative clinical complications (Hamilton and Spetzler 1994). Permanent major morbidities were 0% for grades I–III, 21.9% for grade IV, and 16.7% for grade V. Deficit related to surgery and evaluated 6 weeks after operation was 0% in grade I, 4.2% in grade II, 2.8% in grade III, 31% in grade IV, and 50% in grade V. Mortality directly related to surgery was 0%. Risk of surgery is quite well estimated by the Spetzler-Martin grading system, with a favorable outcome in 92%–100% grade I, 95% grade II, 88% grade III, 73% grade IV, and 57% grade V (Spetzler and Martin 1986; Heros et al. 1990). Series in which patients were examined before surgery, postoperatively, and over the long term by independent neurologists showed less good results: 124 prospective patients were studied by Hartmann et al. (2000). Postoperatively, 41% of the patients had new neurological deficits, 15% disabling and 26% non-disabling. At long-term follow up 38% of patients had surgery-related deficits, 6% disabling and 32% non-disabling. Morgan et al. (1993) reported a series of 112 Patients with 44 small (<2 cm), 43 medium, and 25 large (>4 cm) AVMs. There was 3.6% mortality and 18% morbidity. Comparing their results with others, the authors stressed the considerable variation of results published in the literature, i.e., 0%–12.5% mortality and 3%–30% morbidity. This variation may be explained by selection criteria for surgery as well as by methods of analysis. One example highlighted by Morgan was the 1.5% mortality in the series of Davis and Symon (1985), which would have been 10% if seven patients who died postoperatively and who had a poor neurological grade on admission had been included. In the series of Morgan the major cause of mortality and severe morbidity were neurological deficits unrelated to hemorrhage or edema, normal pressure perfusion breakthrough, and intraoperative hemorrhage. Batjer et al. defined hyperemic complications as "unexpected brain swelling or hemorrhage unrelated to technical error or concealed ventricular hemorrhage, CT evidence of edema associated with neurological deficits not related to inadvertent proximal vascular occlusion or intraoperative brain retraction, or hemorrhage after angiographically proven complete AVM resection" (Batjer et al. 1989a). They reported 13 cases (21%) in 62 patients operated on (seven dead or severely disabled). Spetzler et al. (1987), as well as Andrews and Wilson (1987), considered this complication to be sufficiently frequent in large AVMs that they proposed performing staged surgical resection. Another series confirmed the correlation between size, deep venous drainage, and the Spetzler-Martin scale (Schaller et al. 1998). In this series, 150 operated patients presented with 15.3% surgical morbidity and early new deficits in 39.3%, permanent new deficits in 10.6%, being significant in 7.3%. There was statistical evidence of a trend to risk of poor surgical outcome across three categories: noneloquent, less eloquent (ex: visual cortex), and highly eloquent (ex: brainstem, basal ganglia, precentral cortex). The authors emphasized that "eloquence of Spetzler-Martin classification should be divided in two categories of less eloquent and highly eloquent, which is important for risk analysis of the treatment of asymptomatic and deep-seated AVMs and for future trials comparing various treatment modalities".

Small superficial AVMs may be operated on with a very low morbidity (1.5%–9.7%) (Pik and Margan 2000; Schaller et al. 1998; Sisit et al. 1993). In contrast, morbidity of deep-seated lesions is much higher, at 9% in 22 patients (Lawton et al. 1995), 17% in 18 patients (De Oliveira et al. 1997), 20% in 22 patients (Sasaki et al. 1998), and 25% in 16 patients (U et al. 1992). Lawton et al. (1995) emphasized the role of preoperative embolization. Sasaki did not report any cases of surgical treatment of deep-seated lesion since 1990 and advised a multimodality approach. Surgery of posterior fossa AVMs is supposed to be more dangerous. In the series of Drake, eight (19.5%) of 41 patients operated on died (Drake et al. 1986). In the series of 30 patients of Batjer and Sansom mortality was 7% and permanent morbidity was 13% (Batjer et al. 1986).

Surgery may be helped by two imaging facilities: In 8%–19% intraoperative angiography showed residual AVMs not suspected during surgery (Munshi et al. 1999; Pietila et al. 1998). Nevertheless, the risk of cerebral angiography performed under difficult conditions during brain surgery should be taken into account. Computer-assisted resection for nidus definition and depiction was described (Muacevic and Steiger 1999). It may allow a better understanding of AVMs and their relationship with adjacent brain structures as well as a better surgical approach.

Many papers have described the risk of recurrence of cerebral AVMs after complete AVM occlusion confirmed by postoperative angiography (Sano et al. 1978; Kader et al. 1996; Lanzino et al. 1997; Fox 1997; Patil 1997; Freudenstein et al. 2001). Kondziolka et al. (1992) reported two recurrences in 70 patients who had undergone complete AVM resection, and two patients presented 3 years later with recurrent hemorrhage. True regrowth of brain AVM can be considered only in children. Postoperative vasospasm, thrombosis of arteries and veins, and, above all, delayed recruitment of collateral arteries are the more likely explanations for the so-called recurrences. This emphasizes the role of delayed postoperative angiography, which should be performed 6 months to 1 year after surgery to assess a definitively complete cure.

3.5.2 Radiosurgery

The concept of radiosurgery is to obtain a progressive obliteration of nidal vessels by focusing a high radiation dose. It has proven to be equally safe and effective whatever the device used, gamma knife, cyclotron, or linear accelerator (Colombo et al. 1989; Kjellberg 1989; Steiner 1988; Lundsford et al. 1991). Nataf et al. (2001a) recently reported a series of 705 patients treated by radiosurgery alone or in combination with embolization or surgery. The overall complete obliteration rate (OR) was 55%. The OR was correlated to size: 77% for nidus <15 mm, 62% for nidus between 15 mm and 25 mm, 44% for nidus >25 mm; dose at reference isodose; minimal dose; and morphological parameters: presence of meningeal feeders, AV fistulas, plexiform angioarchitecture, arterial steal, arterial recruitment, deep exclusive drainage, venous ectasia, confluence or reflux. Presence of a dural component with meningeal feeders decreased the OR from 58% to 33%. Embolization was reported to be a "confusion factor not associated with OR". At multivariate analysis only minimal dose and complete coverage of the AVM were correlated to OR. Mortality in that series was 1.6%, due mainly to recurrent bleeding, which occurred in 6.5% of the cases. Rate of recurrent bleeding was 2.98%/year/patient. Neurological deficits related to radiosurgery and not related to hemorrhage were observed in 5.37% of the cases and were permanent in 1.46% of the cases. This series summarizes well the current results of radiosurgery and major issues concerning rate of obliteration, factors related to success or failure, and complication rate.

A meta-analysis of the literature is difficult to perform because of (a) the different techniques used, e.g., most teams nowadays use a high single dose at least for small AVMs, but the minimum target dose, treated volume, and target definition may vary from one team to another; (b) very different patient selection with various AVM sizes, locations (lobar, deep, brain stem, choroidal or ventricular), and symptoms (bleeding or not); (c) different patient follow-up strategy for evaluation of obliteration rate: up to 2 years, 3 years or more, on angiography or MR, systematic or not. NATAF et al. (2001a) highlighted the fact that the rate of patients followed is very variable from one series to another: 55.6% for KJELLBERG (1986), 42%–64% for STEINER et al. (1992, 1993), 51.5% for COLOMBO et al. (1994), and 20.3% for LUNDSFORD et al. (1991).

Factors Influencing the Obliteration Rate. An evaluation of overall obliteration rate (OR) in the recent literature shows very different results, OR being 22% (KJELLBERG 1986), 80% (LUNDSFORD et al. 1991), 79% to 86.5% (STEINER et al. 1992, 1993), 88.9% (AOKI et al. 1996), or 64% (SCHLIENGER et al. 2000). These differences are explained mainly by selection criteria.

- ***AVM volume***: The AVM volume is certainly the main factor determining AVM cure (BETTI and MUNARI 1992; LUNDSFORD 1993; COLOMBO et al. 1994). FRIEDMAN et al. (1995) reported an OR of 70% in 37 of 57 patients with small AVMs. OR was 90% at 2 years for AVMs <2.5 cm (COLOMBO et al. 1994), 82% for AVMs <2.2 cm (KONDZIOLKA et al. 1993), and 94% for AVMs <2 cm (BETTI and MUNARI 1992). POLLOCK et al. (1996b) documented angiographic obliteration of only 27 (42%) of 65 Spetzler-Martin grade I and II AVMs. In the series of STEINBERG et al. (1993), the OR was 94% at 2 years and 100% at 3 years for AVMs with a volume <4 cc (20 mm diameter), 75% at 2 years and 95% at 3 years for volumes between 4 cc and 25 cc, and 42% at 2 years and 73% at 3 years for volumes >25 cc. Results concerning treatment of large AVMs were specifically studied (PAN et al. 2000; FRIEDMAN et al. 1996; YAMAMOTO et al. 1995; NATAF et al. 2001b). PAN et al. (2000= reviewed 240 treated AVMs, classified as small (<3 cc), medium (3–10 cc), and large (>10 cc). Evaluated using the Kaplan-Meier method, the actual complete OR was 75% at 40 months. Complete ORs for small, medium, and large AVMs were 92%, 80%, and 50%, respectively. In the group of large AVMs the OR was 77% for nidus of 10–15 cc and 25% for nidus >15 cc. The latency for complete obliteration was significantly longer for large AVMs. There was no significant correlation between AVM size and the occurrence of neurological complications. FRIEDMAN et al. (1996) reported an OR of 69% for AVMs larger than 10 cc. In the series of NATAF, in 112 patients with an AVM >10 cc the OR was 39%. MIYAWAKI et al. (1999) reported an OR of 23% for AVMs >14 cc. None of the AVMs which received a minimal dose below 14 Gy were cured, but induced radionecrosis necessitated surgical excision in 22% of patients who received more than 16 Gy.
- ***Target determination***: The main factor associated with successful radiosurgery and rapid decrease of bleeding risk is irradiation of the entire nidus (GALLINA et al. 1998). In the series of COLOMBO, among 180 patients who underwent radiosurgery, 153 (85%) were treated as usual with the entire nidus receiving the prescribed radiation dose, while for 27 (15%) only part of the nidus was covered with a dose adequate for obliteration (COLOMBO et al. 1994). In totally irradiated cases, bleeding risk decreased from 4.8% in the first 6 months to 0% after 12 months. In partially irradiated cases bleeding risk decreased to 10%–12% from 6 to 18 months and 5.5% from 18 to 24 months after treatment. Overall incidence of bleeding was 5% in the 153 patients with total irradiation and 26% in the 27 patients with partial irradiation. Inadequate nidus definition is known to be the major cause of treatment failure (Y. KWON et al. 2000; GALINA et al. 1998; POLLOCK et al. 1998). Stereotactic angiography is known to be not completely accurate in evaluation of nidus shape and size. The combined use of CT scan or MR and stereotactic angiography for target determination were evaluated. BLAT et al. (1993) showed that determination of nidus diameter and isocenter may be different depending on whether enhanced stereotactic CT scan or stereotactic angiography is used. MR images and CT scan were said to be "superior" to angiography in determining different structures of the AVM (SMITH 1988a). Stereotactic MR angiography was compared with stereotactic angiography in 28 cases (KONDZIOLKA et al. 1994): in 24 cases the two techniques were similar, in three cases MR was shown to be "superior", and in one case

angiography determined nidus shape better. In 45 patients who underwent repeated radiosurgery for residual nidus, incomplete original angiographic definition of AVM nidus was the most frequent definite cause of initial radiosurgery failure (26/45 cases, 58%) (Yamamoto et al. 1995). The authors claimed that the risk of poor nidus shape evaluation is reduced when stereotactic MR images are included in the dose-planning database. However, stereotactic angiography is still the best examination for delineating small AVMs. The combination of different imaging modalities such as 3D angiography, MR cross-sections, and angio-MR performed with three-dimensional acquisition will probably allow much better delineation of nidus shape, feeders, nidus and veins.

- ***Angioarchitecture and hemodynamics:*** A small number of draining veins was correlated with better OR (Pollock et al. 1998). In the same study, presence of direct AV fistula was a negative predictor of successful radiosurgery. The same conclusion that high-flow AV shunt decreases the chance for complete cure was shown in other series (Nataf et al. 2001a; O.K. Kwon et al. 2000). Preradiosurgical embolization was a negative predictor of success in several series (Pollock et al. 1998; O.K. Kwon et al. 2000). Recanalization of compartments of the nidus previously presumed to be occluded by embolization was responsible for nidus recurrence. Failure of radiosurgery was then attributed to failure of embolization. Such recanalization is not surprising, in view of the technique used for presurgical embolization at that time. Great strides have been made in the embolization technique for brain AVMs with the development of intranidal embolization using permanent liquid embolic agents (see chapter 3.5.3 on embolization) have completely modified the goal and results of embolization. Consequently, series reporting a bad influence of preradiosurgical embolization should not be considered today in treatment decision-making because results of particle injection in pedicle feeders and intranidal definitive gluing cannot be compared.
- ***AVM location:*** Hemispheric location of the AVM was correlated to better OR (Pollock et al. 1998). There is more risk of clinical complications with radiosurgery of brain-stem AVMs than of superficial AVMs (Karlsson et al. 1996). A recent series reported the results in 45 patients with brain-stem AVMs (Regis et al. 2001). The overall OR was 82%. Complications were neurological deficit in three patients (two permanent) and recurrent hemorrhage in two. Choroidal and cisternal AVMs seem to be less radiosensitive, with an OR of 47.6% (Nataf et al. 2001d).

Rate of Complications: The American Stroke Association estimated that there is a 5%–7% risk of treatment-related complications with radiosurgery and, in addition, a 3%–4% risk per year of hemorrhage prior to obliteration. Over a 3-year period the patient has a 14%–19% risk of complications or hemorrhage (The AVM Study Group 1999).

- The rate of rebleeding (RR) is probably increased during the first 3 years after radiosurgery. In the large series of Nataf et al. (2001a), bleeding recurred in 6.5% of the cases and was responsible for a mortality of 1.6%. The RR was 2.98%/year/patient. Steiner et al. (1992) reported an actuarial RR of 1.9%–6.5% up to 60 months after radiosurgery. The overall RR was even higher in another series at 12.5% (Betti et al. 1989). It was 7.7% during the first 8 months after radiosurgery in grade I and II AVMs (Pollock et al. 1994), 6.6% in AVMs <10 cc (Yamamoto et al. 1995), and 9.2% in AVMs >10 cc (Pan et al. 2000). Hemorrhage occurring in the latency period before complete obliteration of the AVM is responsible for a high rate of severe clinical complications. The rate of death after hemorrhage was 50% (Yamamoto et al. 1995) and 40% in patients with grade I and II (Pollock et al. 1994).
- Neurologic deficits related to radiosurgery and not related to hemorrhage were observed in 5.37% of the cases and were permanent in 1.46% (Nataf et al. 2001a). In a recent series of 240 patients, the rate of permanent deficit was 3.9% in AVMs >10 cc, 3.8% in AVMs between 10 and 3 cc, and 2.4% in AVMs <3 cc (Pan et al. 2000). Brain parenchyma reactions due to radiosurgery, so-called radionecrosis (RN), have been known since 1930 (Fisher and Er 1930). RN was classified as acute, subacute, or late (Jellinger 1977). According to this series, there was a correlation between dose of radiosurgery and delay of RS appearance. MR parenchymal lesions associated with RN may be classified into four grades (Nataf et al. 1997): grade I, no anomalies; grade II, hypersignal (HyperS) T_2; grade III, grade II-associated homogeneous contrast (gadolinium) enhancement on T_1; grade IV, central hyposignal T_1 and heterogeneous peripheral contrast enhancement, rim of hypoS T_1 and T_2 (hemosiderin). In the series of (Nataf et al. 2001c), the size of the AVM was the only factor correlated to the appearance of these parenchy-

mal lesions. Presence of a grade-IV MR lesion was the only factor correlated to neurologic deficit. On the other hand, the appearance of T_2 hyperintensity was correlated to radiosurgery efficacy and achieved 72% sensitivity in predicting successful treatment response (Mobin et al. 1999). The formation of cystic lesions has been described in the long-term MR follow-up of irradiated AVMs (Yamamoto et al. 1998).

Re-irradiation after Radiosurgery Failure: In the series of Pollock et al. (1996), 21% of the 210 AVMs irradiated underwent re-irradiation. Karlsson et al. (1998) reported the most important series about re-irradiation including 115 patients previously irradiated from 1976 to 1994. The mean delay between the two radiosurgical treatments was 3.6 years. The OR was 65%, the rate of clinical complications 14%. The authors concluded that the OR following gamma-knife surgery for previously irradiated AVM is similar to that after primary surgery, but that complication rate increases with the amount of radiation previously given. Very similar results were shown in a series of 39 patients who were re-irradiated (Schlienger et al. 2001). The OR was 60.7% and the rate of complications was 14.7%.

Risk of Recurrence: AVMs may reappear after having been completely occluded after radiosurgery (Yamamoto et al. 1992). In the series of Lindquist et al. (2000), covering 48 patients who underwent angiograms more than 4 years after their AVM had been proven to be occluded, ten (21%) patients developed clinical symptoms attributable to the AVM. There was evidence of residual AVM nidus in four cases. Three of the recurrent AVMs were revealed by hemorrhage. It is well known that the risk of recurrence after radiosurgery and surgery is higher in young patients. Kader et al. (1996) reported a 3.5% rate of hemorrhage in 141 patients less than 18 years of age who were thought to have been cured by surgery. The imaging strategy for follow-up varies greatly from one center to another. Most authors consider that irradiated AVMs must be followed up with MR and MRA, but that only angiograms can assess a complete cure. A recent series showed that important AVM changes seen on early angiograms are highly predictive of radiosurgical success (Oppenheim et al. 1999). Nevertheless, we are of the opinion that repeated angiograms increase the overall morbidity and cost of the radiosurgery, and that the information provided by these early repeated angiograms does not justify their practice. We advise the performance of MR each year after radiosurgery to follow AVM changes on MRA and parenchymal anomalies on cross-sections. Final angiography should be performed 3 years after radiosurgery to evaluate the final efficacy of the treatment. In case of complete AVM obliteration, another follow-up angiogram should be performed several years later in children or young adults to monitor the long-term efficacy of radiosurgery.

3.5.3 Embolization

3.5.3.1 *General Considerations*

Endovascular treatment of brain AVMs is still controversial for several reasons:

- The goal of the treatment itself, which can be regarded as an invasive technique to prevent a likely risk of bleeding in patients presenting few or no symptoms
- The availability of alternative therapeutic options
- The variety of techniques, embolic agents, and even basic treatment concepts from one team to another and then from one publication to another, making evaluation of the results extremely difficult
- The lack of uniformity of interventional training and very different levels of specialization
- The absence of large series and accurate evaluation of clinical and angiographic results, and clinical complications

Fundamental rules must be followed:

- Therapeutic decision should ever be taken by a multidisciplinary team of neurologists, neurosurgeons, radiotherapists, and neuroradiologists. Embolization must be performed as one step in the global therapeutic approach and as an associated technique.
- Specialists must determine the goal of the treatment concerning:
  - The angiographic result: complete occlusion or targeted and partial occlusion
  - Clinical results: prevention of bleeding or improvement of clinical symptoms (intractable seizures, neurologic deficit, headaches)
- The strategy, goal of treatment, and practical organization of the different steps and procedures should be explained in detail to the patient and, if possible, to his or her relatives.

- The neurointervention itself should be performed by a qualified neuroradiologist, a neuroanesthesiologist, and a technical team, starting with the pre-procedural planning, continuing through the procedural organization, and including post-procedural care. Medical treatment necessitated by the embolization before, during, and after the procedure should be decided on by the neuroradiologist.
- The patient should be monitored within an intensive care unit for 24 h after the procedure. A neurosurgeon must be available to provide shunting if necessary, or emergent surgery for hematoma evacuation.
- The anesthetic procedure: Most embolizations today are performed with the patient under general anesthesia with endotracheal intubation. There are at least two reasons for this tendency:
  - The duration of the procedure (2–4 h) with no possibility of movement makes embolization very uncomfortable and painful for the patient when local anesthesia is used.
  - Total immobility of the head is mandatory to allow safe catheterization and embolic agent injection under road-mapping.

Some teams are still performing brain AVM embolization using local anesthesia, mainly because this allows clinical testing during selective catheterization with the superselective Amytal test to predict neurologic dysfunction before embolization. Intra-arterial injection of Amytal (amobarbitol) was described by WADA and RASMUSSEN (1960) to evaluate brain function within the vascular distribution of the injected artery. This technique is still performed for presurgical evaluation in patients with intractable seizures to determine which cerebral hemisphere is dominant. However, fMRI is progressively replacing the Wada test in this indication (BINDER et al. 1996). Superselective Amytal injection prior to embolization was described and used in large series of patients (PURDY et al. 1991b; RAUCH et al. 1992a,b). In their original paper concerning the method, RAUCH et al, (1992a) concluded that the injection of 30 mg Amytal into a vessel can produce transient neurologic deficits if normal brain tissue is supplied by the vessel; that the test is safe, with no long-term adverse effect; and that EEG testing is mandatory, because in 50% of the cases no clinical symptoms were associated with EEG disturbances. In the second paper concerning the clinical use in brain AVMs on 30 patients who underwent 147 embolizations, the authors reported the following: None of the patients with a negative Amytal test had clinical or EEG changes; the test was positive in 20% of cases; in the few cases where patients were embolized despite a positive test the rate of neurologic complications was very high (40%); using fractionated embolization with multiple procedures, the rate of clinical complications was significantly higher (8%) in cases where a series of embolizations were performed after a single Amytal test as compared with a single embolization performed after an Amytal test. This means that the Amytal test performed during the initial procedure cannot be considered an accurate method for predicting the risk of further procedures.

For many years the Amytal test was considered to be mandatory before brain AVM embolization. In 1997, DEBRUN et al. still claimed that "Amytal testing continues to have extremely important medico-legal implications, and most experts who would be asked to review a case of severe complications occurring during an embolization of brain AVM with acrylate glue would criticize the interventionalist for not having performed the Amytal test" (DEBRUN et al. 1997). However the recently published recommendations for the management of brain AVMs (OGILVY et al. 2001) concluded that there was no evidence that either general anesthesia or intravenous sedation is associated with a lower rate of complications (level IV evidence).

In our own experience, all the patients underwent embolization under general anesthesia, and in almost all French centers the Amytal test has not been performed for many years. The main reason is that principle of brain AVM embolization has been completely modified in the past 10 years owing to the great strides made in catheter and guidewire capabilities. Our current technique is intranidal wedged injection. The tip of the catheter is placed in the most distal arterioles and the glue is injected within the nidus itself, so that no normal brain is threatened. Obviously, there is still some risk of normal artery occlusion and consequent neurologic deficit. This may be due either to reflux of glue along the tip of the catheter or to opening of the arterio-arterial anastomosis within the nidus and reflux in normal arteries. However, an Amytal test would not be able to predict these inadvertent embolizations.

Bladder catheters help with fluid management as well as patient comfort at the end of the procedure. Careful management of coagulation is required to prevent thromboembolic complications during the procedure. In our teams, intravenous heparin is given with the aim of obtaining activated clotting time at twice the normal value throughout the procedure.

In comparison, during endovascular treatment of intracranial aneurysms the anticoagulation therapy aims at keeping the ACT at four to six times above the normal value. The risk of embolic complications is indeed much less important in treatment of brain AVMs due to the high-flow arteriovenous shunt that protects against clot formation and distal artery occlusion. Heparin is stopped at the end of the procedure, and the femoral sheath is removed immediately thereafter.

Hypertension may be induced during the procedure to help distal catheter progression and nidus approach (Picard et al. 2001). However, recent tremendous advances in catheter technology now provide considerable capabilities for catheterization of very distal and tortuous arteries, and hypertension is much less is use. In contrast, profound deliberate systemic hypotension during glue injection has been proposed (Ogilvy et al. 2001) to slow the flow within the pedicle and provide more controlled glue deposition in arterial, nidal, and venous compartments of the AVM. Hypotension can be provoked by either vasoactive agents, general anesthetic, or – in some rare instances – adenosine-induced cardiac pause (Pile-Speelman et al. 1999). This technique is used today only in case of high-flow direct fistulas, where glue injection is very tricky and risky. Otherwise, it is seldom useful due to improvements in the technique of glue injection and choice of concentration.

3.5.3.2 Technique

The first embolization was performed by Luessenhop and Spence in 1959 using Silastic spheres (Luessenhop and Spence 1960). The later advances include transfemoral embolization of brain AVMs (Krichef et al. 1972), use of detachable balloons (Serbinenko 1974; Debrun et al. 1978), and the calibrated-leak balloon (Kerber 1976; Pevsner 1977). At the beginning of the 1990s, many authors reported results of preoperative embolization with polyvinyl alcohol (PVA) particles (Purdy et al. 1990; Fox et al. 1990; Schumacher and Horton 1991; Nakstad et al. 1992). Nevertheless, there are many drawbacks related to PVA embolization: PVA particles do not afford long-term occlusion of embolized arteries and nidus and recanalization is more frequent; migration of particles in normal adjacent branches is much more likely because catheterization is less distal; because very different arteriovenous shunt size may be observed within the nidus with direct fistula, most of the particles may reach the venous side in some instances and produce either no embolization efficacy or, on the contrary, inadvertent venous occlusion. We feel that this kind of embolization should no longer be performed because it carries more risk and is much less efficient than glue embolization. Microcoils were also used to treat brain AVMs in order to increase the effectiveness of occlusion by PVA (Nakstad et al. 1992). Such embolization consists in a proximal occlusion of the feeding arteries which, in the long term, favors the recruitment of arterio-arterial anastomosis. Therefore, the treatment is not efficient to reduce the nidus because occlusion is too proximal and the nidus size remains the same even if the AVM is fed by collateral channels. Furthermore, coil occlusion shuts the door to further embolization, which cannot be performed through an arterio-arterial anastomosis. For these reasons, coil occlusion should be performed only in case of direct AV fistulas in which the AV junction itself may be occluded by the coils. Other agents have been used for brain AVM treatment, such as silk sutures (Deveikis et al. 1994), pure ethanol (Yakes et al. 1997), or Ethibloc. Their efficacy and safety have never been assessed in large series and their use has been more or less abandoned. Cyanoacrylates were first used at the end of the 1970s for preoperative embolization (Debrun et al. 1982; Picard et al. 1984; Vinuela et al. 1984, 1986, 1991; Wallace et al. 1995; Jafar et al. 1993); the results were compared with those obtained with PVA for that indication. Due to the great strides made in catheter and guidewire technology, the technique and goal of embolization progressively switched from proximal feeding artery occlusion as the preoperative goal to intranidal occlusion for definitive treatment.

Intranidal Embolization with Cyanoacrylates

Principles

The concept of embolization with cyanoacrylates is to occlude the nidus and the draining veins. The arteries should be occluded only at the level of very distal arterioles. The principle of intranidal embolization consists in placing the catheter in a wedge position in those very small arterioles close to the origin of the draining veins. The catheterization has to be as distal as possible (Figs. 3.4, 3.10). In this position the injection of contrast medium during a run or under subtracted fluoroscopy showed a stagnation of the contrast medium in the pedicle, from the tip of the catheter to the nidus or vein. Arterial flow is almost completely stopped by the catheter.

Following a pre-embolization test injection a reflux of contrast along the tip of the catheter within the distal artery should be looked for carefully. This often predicts a very rapid reflux of glue along the catheter and risk of gluing normal adjacent arteries or gluing the catheter. When a wedge position is obtained, the glue may progress slowly without arterial flow contamination and finally reach the origin of the veins, or enter another part of the nidus, and even reflux into other feeding arteries through the nidus. The progression of the glue has to be followed under subtracted fluoroscopy. Biplane equipment is mandatory to follow this progression in two different projections. Two major issues should be addressed prior to gluing: What is the course of the feeding artery (which is revealed by the catheter), and were is the origin of the draining vein? Indeed, before injecting the glue the operator should understand the anatomy perfectly and be able to determine as soon as possible when the glue begins to reflux along the tip of the catheter, and when the glue penetrates the origin of the draining vein, in order to predict to what point the glue has to be pushed. These two arterial and venous limits of gluing should be decided prior to the injection. It is mandatory to find the best projections to separate: (a) the course of the feeding arteries from the nidus and the veins and avoid overlapping of the structures which need to be occluded (nidus and veins) and the one which should not (feeding artery), and (b) the nidus from the vein (Figs. 3.4, 3.6, 3.10). Biplane equipment makes it possible to follow the injection and progression of glue by looking alternately at the two screens. As soon as the injection begins the operator should carefully look at the distal tip of the catheter to see the slow progression of the glue. The injection must be very slow when glue comes out of the catheter to avoid the formation of multiple little drops of glue exiting too rapidly and spreading quickly in the veins. On the contrary, the first kernel of glue should be pushed very gently from the tip of the catheter to the distal artery and nidus. The penetration of the glue in the origin of the draining vein is recognized by an enlargement of this kernel (Fig. 3.4). The injection must be stopped for a few seconds and then resumed. If the glue again progresses in the vein or enters another vein, the injection is stopped again for 4–5 s and then resumed. Here again, the operator should decide before performing the injection whether the goal of the injection is to occlude the vein completely or just to reach its origin, keeping it patent. In case of large AVMs with multiple feeders, the aim of each injection from the first to the last procedure should be the occlusion of the draining veins (Figs. 3.10, 3.11). In case of a small AVM, with only one draining vein, the operator should decide before injecting whether the goal is to occlude all the nidus and the draining vein in one shot or to occlude just one part of the nidus, to enter the origin of the vein with glue but keep the vein patent. In the first strategy the operator has to foresee, during the injection, whether it will be possible or not to occlude all the nidus before deciding to completely occlude the vein. In the last strategy, the injection has to be stopped as soon as the glue penetrates the vein. Within a few minutes the kernel of glue will progressively laminate the walls of the vein, producing a reduction of the flow (Fig. 3.10). At the end of the injection the operator must aspirate back the glue with the syringe, then rapidly pull the microcatheter into the guiding catheter to avoid inadvertent migration of some drops of glue in the normal circulation. Before the development of the glide microcatheter, both the microcatheter and the guiding catheter were abruptly pulled out of the femoral sheath to avoid rupture of the microcatheter body or gluing tip. Very smooth microcatheters can be pulled out alone and the guiding catheter can be left in place.

The technique of intranidal embolization with Histoacryl requires tremendous experience on the part of the operator, because the injection is fast (from a few seconds to 1–2 min) and clinical consequences or improper gluing are disastrous.

Material

A 5- or 6-F guiding catheter is placed through the femoral sheet into the internal carotid or vertebral artery. The tip of the catheter should be placed high enough to facilitate microcatheterization by allowing the possibility of pushing more on the microcatheter and guidewires. However, too distal catheterization may induce a spasm of the artery which may decrease the flow and may, on the contrary, render the microcatheterization more difficult. Nimodipine may be injected in the guiding catheter to treat vasospasm induced by the guiding catheter. Two milligrams of nimodipine (10 cc) may be slowly injected two or three times. Nimodipine has very little effect on the systemic blood pressure. Its efficacy lasts throughout the procedure.

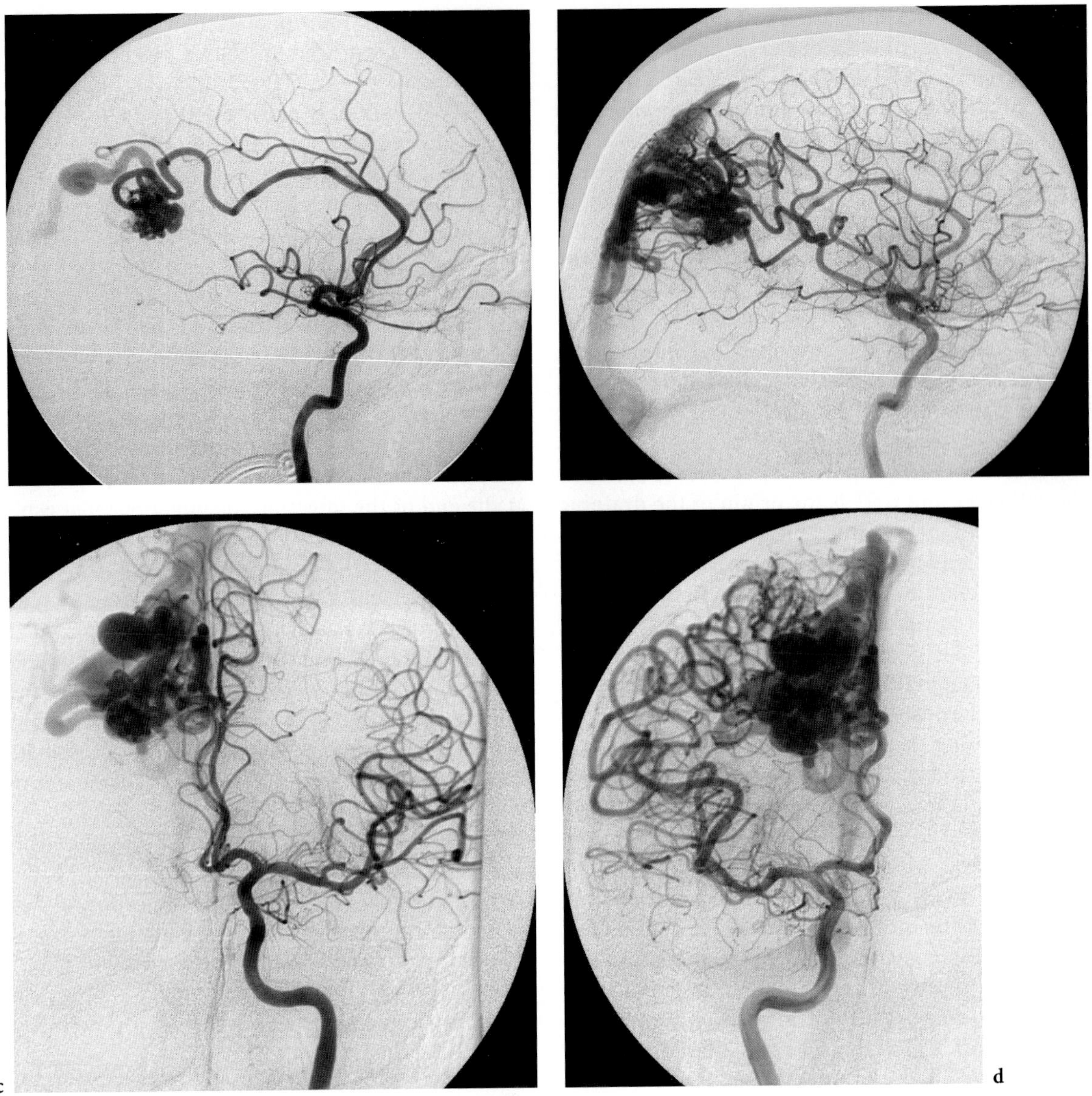

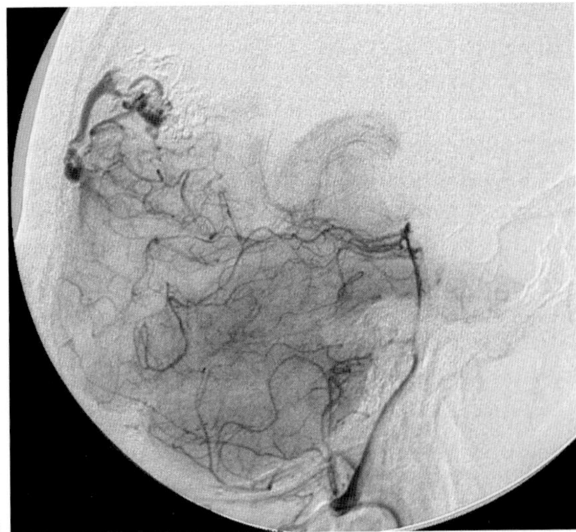

Fig. 3.10a–k. A 32-year-old man presenting with seizures. Left internal carotid (**a, b**), right internal carotid (**c, d**), and vertebral (**e**) injections show a right compact parietal AVM fed by parietal distal branches of anterior, middle, and posterior cerebral arteries. Determination of size of the nidus itself and nidus limits is difficult due to the presence of multiple, very dilated draining veins. First and second superselective catheterization during first embolization showed favorable angioarchitecture with very good access to the origin of the draining veins (**f, g**). A 20% mixture of Histoacryl and Lipiodol was injected in both cases. Gluing of the origin of the draining vein obtained after the first injection is visible (**g**). Cast of glue at the end of the two sessions of embolization delineates the exact size of the nidus itself and origin of veins (**h**). Right internal carotid injection in AP (**i**) and frontal (**j**) views and right vertebral injection (**k**) performed 3 months later confirm complete cure

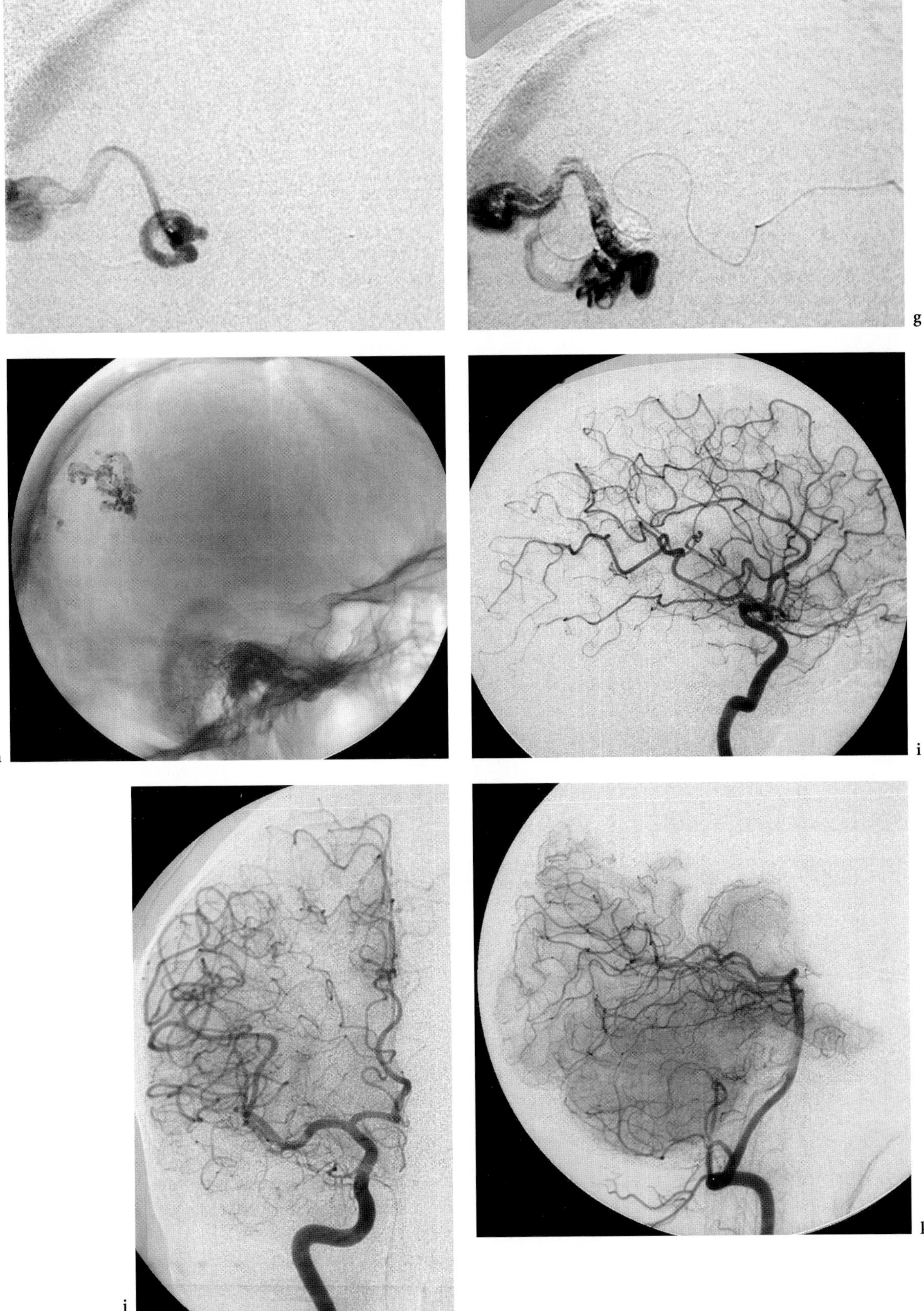
f
g
h
i
j
k

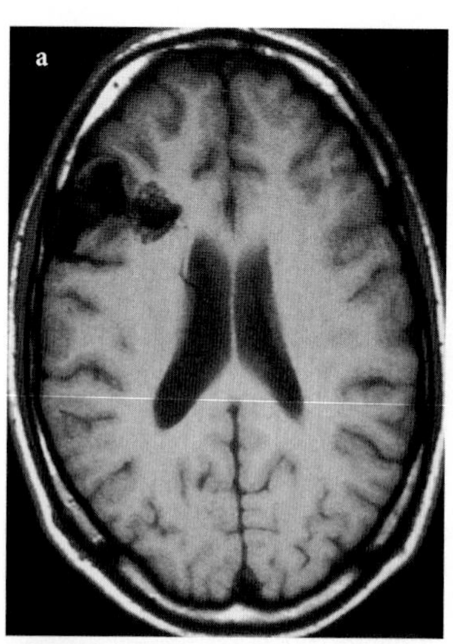

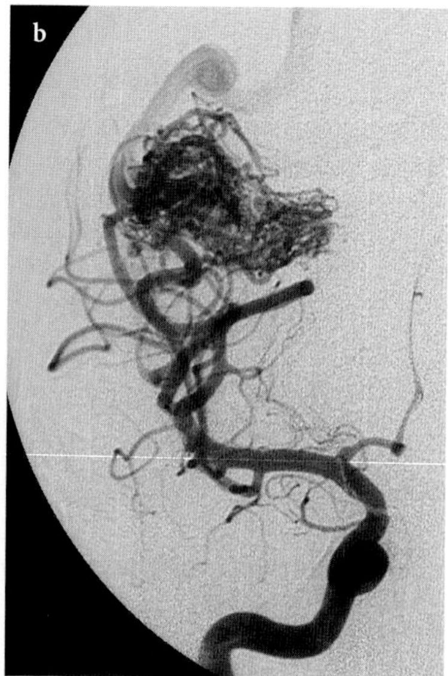

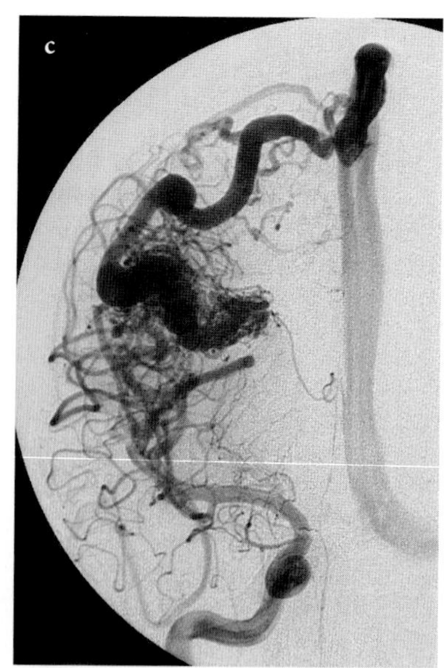

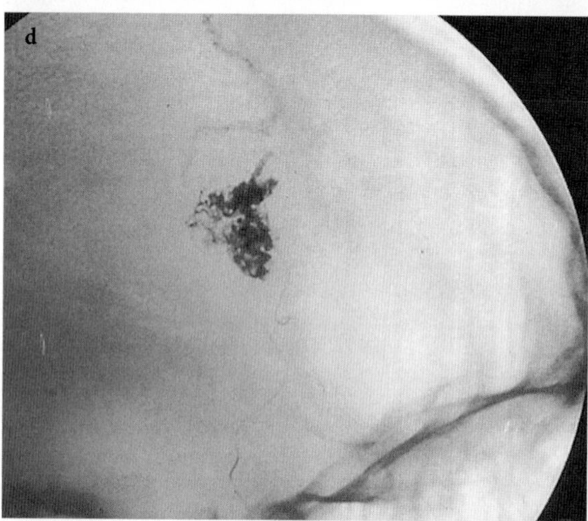

Fig. 3.11a–f. A 27-year-old man presenting with a frontal AVM revealed by seizures. Axial T_1 image precisely localizes the frontal AVM at the surface of the cortex and extending partially within the white matter (**a**). Poor understanding of AVM architecture, nidus shape and limits, and determination of **venous** compartment are obtained with this axial image. Right internal carotid injection in the early arterial (**b**) and venous phase (**c**) shows type of arteriovenous shunt better, with a compact nidus and a single dilated vein. During the second embolization the microcatheter broke during retrieval at the end of glue injection (**d**), outside of the patient, approximately 20 cm from the hub. It was cut at the level of the skin of the groin. Patient was treated for 2 weeks with low-molecular-weight heparin and for 3 months with aspirin. This technical complication had no clinical consequences. Four embolizations resulted in incomplete occlusion with residual nidus draining into a small collateral vein which was visible on pre-treatment angiography (**e, f**). Radiosurgery was performed

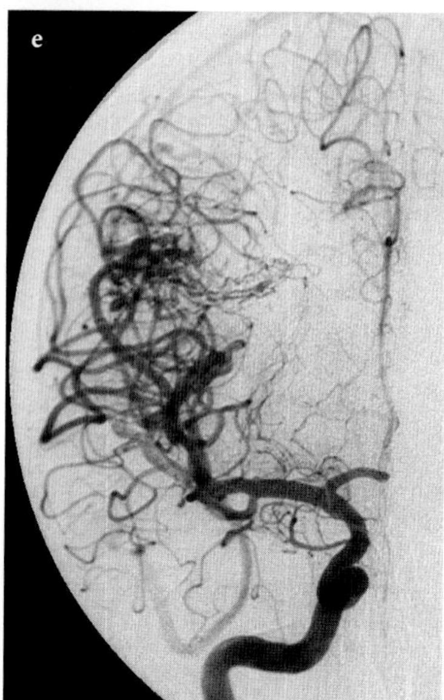

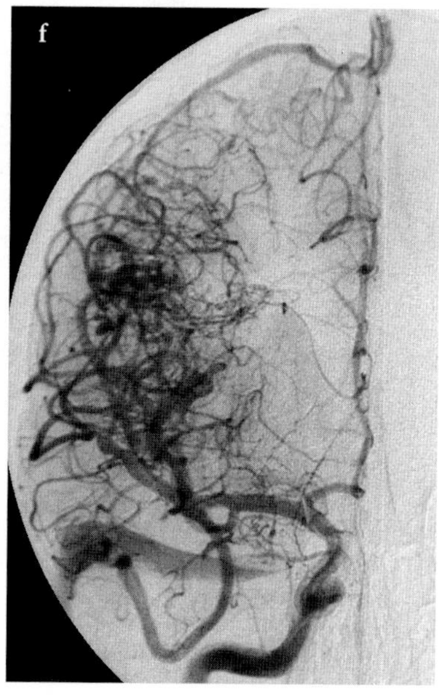

Types of Catheters

Microcatheterization is performed today with two different types of catheters:

- The true flow-guided catheter (Magic 1.8, 1.5- or 1.2-F, Balt Extrusion, Montmorency, France; Elite 1.8, 1.5-F, Target therapeutic, Fremont, Calif., USA). Diluted contrast medium is injected through the catheter under subtracted fluoroscopy to select the desired pedicle. Although these catheters are supposed to navigate with the flow, they frequently enter normal, not dilated, branches instead of being aspirated by the flow into dilated arteries feeding the AVM. Catheterization of the desired branch is then performed by flushing pure saline or a mixture of saline and contrast medium within the microcatheter with a different pressure. That way, the tip of the catheter tends to go back (depending on the pressure produced on the syringe) and to vibrate. This makes it possible to guide the tip (which was previously shaped as a small curve) from one artery to another. If the catheter fails to progress one can use a micro guidewire in the flow-guided catheter to provide more stiffness and increase "pushability". The wire is pushed almost up to the tip of the catheter, but extreme caution should be used to keep the guidewire from extending beyond the tip of the catheter. The catheter and guidewire are then pushed together and the guidewire is very quickly removed. The catheter usually progresses in the last step when the wire is pulled back. This procedure is repeated until no more progression of the tip is achieved.
- The intermediate-flow-guided/over-the-wire catheter (Flowrider and Ultraflow 1.8- or 1.5-F, Micro-therapeutics, Irvine, Calif., USA). These catheters do not navigate without a guidewire. The very floppy guidewire is placed within the catheter almost at its tip. Both catheter and guidewire are pushed simultaneously, making distal catheterization very easy and fast. The guidewire may be pushed outside the tip of the catheter into the desired branch of a bifurcation or in order to navigate into distal acute curves. The catheter progresses very easily with the guidewire. In contrast, a true flow-guided catheter does not navigate over the wire when the wire is pushed outside its tip. Thus, these new catheters behave as intermediate-flow-guided/over-the-wire catheters. The disadvantage is that they are more rigid because of the guidewire than true flow-guided catheters. They may modify the course of the catheterized artery, and they may induce spasm or arterial damage during abrupt removal. The risk of very distal catheterization may be higher.

Concentration of the Glue Mixture

Superselective angiography precedes each embolization. Since 1988, NBCA (N-butyl cyanoacrylate) has replaced IBCA (I-butyl cyanoacrylate). Histoacryl (B. Braun, Melsungen, Germany) was the only glue available in Europe for many years. This glue is still not approved by the European Community for the indication of intracranial arterial embolization. Nevertheless, it was used for more than 10 years in thousands of patients and is considered by all the experts to be safe. A new glue has recently been approved by the Food and Drug Administration in the USA (Trufill n-BCA Liquid embolic system, Cordis, Miami) and another one in Europe (Glubran, GEM, Viareggio, Italy).

Histoacryl is mixed with Lipiodol (Guerbet, Aulnay sous Bois, France) in concentrations varying from 17% to 100%. Tantalum powder (Nycomed Ingenor, Paris, France) was previously used as a contrast agent to enhance the visibility of the mixture. Due to tremendous new improvements made in angiography rooms, however, the mixture is now very well visible under subtracted fluoroscopy. The best concentration of glue/Lipiodol is very difficult to determine and the choice depends on the operator's experience and knowledge of glue embolization in brain AVMs. The choice is purely subjective and is made on the basis of the pre-embolization superselective angiograph. In case of a wedge position within the nidus without very early venous drainage, a dilution of 17% (1 cc Histoacryl in 4.5 cc Lipiodol) allows very slow and long injection and progression within the nidus without a major risk of gluing the catheter. This concentration may be increased from 17% to 20%, 25%, or 33% (respectively, 1 cc Histoacryl in 4 cc, 3 cc, or 2 cc Lipiodol). Various situations call for the use of these more concentrated mixtures – when the origin of a vein which should not be occluded is very close to the catheter tip (Fig. 3.4), for instance, or when the "security distance" from the tip of the catheter to normal arteries is short and reflux along the tip of the catheter must be perfectly controlled. This is particularly true during embolization of perforating arteries (lenticulostriate, anterior choroidal, posterolateral and posteromedian choroidal, thalamo-perforating arteries). They are also necessary when a direct arteriovenous fistula without interposed arterioles induces a risk of not being able to control the glue, some drops of which may flow through the shunt into the venous system. Highly concentrated mixtures are rarely used: 50% (1 cc Histoacryl in 1 cc Lipiodol), - 66% (1 cc Histoacryl in 0.5 cc Lipiodol), and pure Histoacryl is extremely rare. These concentrations are used only in large-caliber direct fistulas in which the catheter tends to be aspirated into the vein. In this situation the tip of the catheter has to be pulled back into the arterial side of the shunt. The glue should be injected as slowly as possible to obtain the formation of a kernel stuck at the tip of the catheter, which can be progressively inflated to obtain slow occlusion of the shunt from the artery to the vein. The operator should not give slack to the catheter, which might be aspirated by the kernel in the flow and reach the vein. Although the glue is very concentrated, there is a risk the column of glue will detach prior to polymerization and rapidly migrate into the distal veins, sinus, or extracranial veins. This is why it is necessary to wait several seconds for glue polymerization before pulling the catheter.

3.5.3.3 Complications

Technical Complications

Gluing the Tip of the Catheter. In some instances the catheter may be stuck within the nidus during its rapid removal at the end of gluing (Fig. 3.11). A Magic catheter may rupture at the level of one of the distal junctions, or the body of the catheter may not rupture but elongate. No endovascular mechanical maneuver to retrieve the catheter should be done. Neurosurgery aimed at removing the catheter tip should be proscribed as not useful and dangerous. Clinical complications due to the presence of a broken catheter within intracranial arteries, the internal carotid or vertebral artery, or the aorta are very rare. In such instances we recommend anticoagulation treatment for the patient for 1 week with low-molecular-weight heparin and for 3 months with aspirin. In case of distal rupture the risk is related to progressive migration of the broken distal portion into intracranial distal arteries. When the catheter is not ruptured, it may be cut at the level of the skin and left in the iliac artery. With more resistant catheters the risk of tearing the nidus when pulling back the catheter is probably higher. The catheter does not rupture, and even very elastic catheters may stretch the feeding artery and damage the nidus with eventual bleeding. Different steps must be followed to minimize the risk of gluing the catheter (Debrun et al. 1997): wedge position on preembolization angiography with no reflux of contrast on catheter tip; good projection of work to separate the tip of the catheter from nidus and vein on subtracted fluoroscopy; removal of any loop in the microcatheter before injection of glue; use of diluted mixture (17%–33%); aspiration with the syringe before pulling the catheter.

Catheter Rupture: During difficult distal and tortuous navigation the catheter may be perforated by the guidewire due to repeated "push and pull" maneuvers in acute curves. The major problem is to depict this rupture during superselective preembolization angiography or during contrast medium injection before injecting the glue. In such cases, the contrast medium opacifies the parent artery at the same time as the distal artery downstream of the catheter tip. The operator can sometimes feel less resistance during injection. The risk of injecting glue through the perforation of the catheter within the parent artery is extreme, and clinical consequences related to occlusion of major vessels may be disastrous. In any case where the operator suspects a likely perforation, he should remove the catheter and not inject glue.

Polymerization Within the Catheter. Prior to injection of glue, the dead space of the catheter and hub must be filled with 5% dextrose solution to avoid polymerization of the glue within the catheter. In some cases, however, this unexplained rapid polymerization may happen. The main reason is probably poor quality control of Histoacryl or Lipiodol. The operator should always push the glue slowly through the microcatheter and follow its progression at the level of its distal tip. If the glue does not exit the tip of the catheter, and even if there is no increased resistance to pressure on the syringe, the operator should never increase the injection pressure. The major risk is catheter rupture and major artery occlusion or embolization of distal normal arteries.

Clinical Complications

The major risk of brain AVM embolization is acute postembolization hemorrhage (APEH). APEH is both the most frequent and the most neurologically devastating complication of embolization. Ischemic complications due to inadvertent embolization of normal arteries feeding adjacent brain parenchyma is much more rare and is associated with better a neurologic outcome.

APEH may be due to multiple causes and can be more or less predictable. Many groups have studied retrospectively the angioarchitectural characteristics correlated with hemorrhagic presentation of brain AVMs (Kader et al. 1994; Marks et al. 1990; Nataf et al. 1997; Turjman et al. 1995; Thompson et al. 1998; Meisel et al. 2000; Piotin et al. 2001). Various architectural and hemodynamic factors may increase the risk of APEH. Other studies addressed the cerebral hemodynamic of brain AVM before, during, and after embolization to provide a theoretical basis for a possible physiopathology of APEH (NORNES and GRIP 1980; BARNET et al. 1987; HANDA et al. 1993; AL-RODHAN et al. 1993; YOUNG et al. 1994; SORIMACHI et al. 1995; YOUNG et al. 1996; GAO et al. 1997; KAMINAGA et al. 1999; MASSOUD et al. 2000). The different causes of APEH are: occlusion of the draining vein with glue, delayed venous thrombosis, normal perfusion pressure breakthrough, intranidal aneurysm rupture, and vessel wall tearing during microcatheter retrieval. The only causes of APEH that may be accurately recognized are occlusion of the draining vein with glue or delayed venous occlusion. In others instances the cause is only putative (Fig. 3.7).

Occlusion of the Draining Vein with Glue and Delayed Venous Thrombosis. These complications involve the so-called occlusive hyperemia syndrome. This term was introduced by AL-RODHAN and co-workers to describe another mechanism of APEH related to impaired venous drainage due to AVM resection or embolization (AL-RODHAN et al. 1993). Secondary to embolization, impaired venous drainage can result from gluing of the draining vein; delayed venous thrombosis may be due to occlusion of substantial arteries and nidus. Progressive and extensive thrombosis of the residual nidus and draining vein has been described (VINUELA et al. 1983b; PURDY et al. 1991a; DUCKWILER et al. 1992; PICARD et al. 2001). PURDY et al. (1991a) reported three hemorrhages in the week after embolization with PVA foam particles and platinum microcoils. They believed that hemorrhages were related to venous thrombosis due to stasis caused by substantial obliteration of AVM, which slowed the flow in the enlarged venous channel, rather than by direct occlusion of the vein by embolic material. Nevertheless, inadvertent embolization with sudden complete occlusion of the veins is probably the most frequent cause of APEH. DERUTY et al. (1996) reported five cases of APEH in 40 patients (12.5%) in the week after embolization. In four of these five cases occlusion of the main venous drainage was demonstrated. Continued inflow into the malformation with impaired outflow is a very high risk situation for rupture and hemorrhage. Partial occlusion of the draining vein with glue, associated with decreased arterial flow, may favor further complete venous thrombosis and hemorrhage. The time course of the complications may indicate the etiology of the problem: Inadvertent venous occlusion causes immediate or early postprocedural complications, while delayed venous thrombosis causes delayed complications.

Normal Perfusion Pressure Breakthrough. This concept of normal perfusion pressure breakthrough (NPPB) was first described by SPETZLER et al. (1978), who assessed that the normal brain parenchyma surrounding brain AVMs is subjected to the chronic vascular steal phenomenon by the AVM and disturbed vascular autoregulation. The acute reduction of flow after resection of an AVM reestablishes a normal flow in the surrounding brain; the lack of autoregulation results in disruption of local capillary beds and produces subsequent brain edema or hemorrhage. There is experimental evidence for the theory that vasomotor regulation can be seriously impaired due to the long period of arteriole inactivity (NORNES and GRIP 1980). With intraoperative measurements of cerebral vascular reactivity to CO_2 in the cortex surrounding the AVM, BARNETT et al. (1987) showed that impaired reactivity was associated with APEH. FOLKOW et al. (1971) showed an adaptive structural change of the resistance vessels in chronically hypotensive beds with reduction of the media and greatly increased lumina. The maximal contractile strength and steepness of the resistance curve were decreased. The hemodynamics of AVMs and surrounding brain have been debated for years. Pre- and postoperative cerebral blood flow was studied using various techniques: thermodilution (BARNETT et al. 1987; SPETZLER et al. 1987), -xenon CT scan (SPETZLER et al. 1987), single photon emission computerized tomography (BATJER 1988; TAKEUCHI et al. 1987; HACEIN-BEY et al. 2001), and positron emission tomography (KAMINAGA et al. 1999). Intraoperative vascular pressure measurements were performed with either direct puncture (BARNETT et al. 1987; HASSLER and STEINMETZ 1987; SPETZLER et al. 1987; YOUNG et al. 1994) or Doppler ultrasonography. They showed that the pressure is reduced in the pedicle feeding the AVM and that obliteration markedly elevates the pressure after AVM occlusion. Similar changes were measured during catheterization and embolization (HANDA et al. 1993; JUNGREIS et al. 1989; SORIMACHI et al. 1995). YOUNG et al. (1994) showed that the transnidal pressure gradients were lower in larger AVMs. In the experience of SORIMACHI et al., the pressure was higher in pedicles feeding both the AVM and normal adjacent brain (SORIMACHI et al. 1995). This is due to the fact that brain-supplying arteries have a higher resistance than AVM-feeding vessels. The authors concluded that the lower the feeder pressure, the more likely complications are to occur, due to tremendous postembolization hemodynamic alterations. In contrast, DUCKWILER et al. (1990), who performed pressure measurements in more than 250 pedicles in 100 patients, did not find any direct correlation between pressure changes and risk of hemorrhage. The observation of pressure gradients >40 mmHg between feeding arteries and cervical arteries was highly suggestive of the presence of direct fistula associated with the AVM nidus. The hemodynamic changes expected from obliteration of different-sized AVM shunt flows were estimated using a computational model (Gao et al. 1997). Three important issues became evident: First, the nonlinearity of the arterial pressure increase that occurs with gradual occlusion of the shunt at the feeding artery level can be expressed as the percentage of occlusion at half maximal pressure (% of flow reduction to increased feeding artery pressure from baseline pretreatment level to a level mid-way to the final vascular pressure expected with complete occlusion of the shunt flow). The percentage of occlusion at half maximal pressure increase was 92% for a large and 71% for a medium AVM model. This suggests that there might be a higher risk of increased pressure gradients (a) during final stages of embolization, (b) in the presence of a small AVM remnant post embolization or surgery, (c) during the final stage of radiosurgery. Second, pressure changes are relatively minor near the circle of Willis and much more profound approaching the nidus as the flow shunt is decreased. Third, at a fixed flow there is a buffering effect of direct fistula, such that higher-flow fistulas are exposed to smaller variations in intravascular pressure during manipulation of systemic arterial pressure. This means that the pressure changes to be expected in distal vascular structures close to the nidus will be proportionally less than changes in systemic pressure; the degree of proportionality depending on the magnitude of AVM shunt flow.

Intranidal Aneurysm Rupture. An APEH may happen due to the rupture of an intranidal aneurysm or false aneurysm after partial occlusion of the AVM. The likely increase in blood pressure in the feeding artery and part of the nidus not embolized is probably responsible for the APEH in some cases. This is why it is mandatory to precisely analyze the angioarchitecture of the nidus before deciding on the embolization strategy. First embolizations should focus on the weakest compartment of the AVM. Small false aneurysms must be systematically researched on selective and superselective angiography and compared with CT scan and MRI (Figs. 3.6, 3.7).

Tearing of Vessel Wall During Microcatheter Retrieval. Arteries may be damaged during microcatheter retrieval. Several conditions may favor the tearing and bleeding of vessel walls: very distal and tortuous catheterization, vasospasm of the catheterized pedicle, reflux of glue along the tip of the catheter, very small arterial feeders, choroidal feeders, looping of the catheter within artery. Such arterial damage is very rarely encountered with floppy flow-guided catheters. The safety of the use of intermediate catheters (good gliding properties but more rigid) has to be evaluated.

Frequency of Acute Postembolization Hemorrhage. In the very early period of brain AVM embolization, procedures involved injection of Silastic spheres or silicone rubber. Kvam et al. (1980) were the first to report on postembolization hemorrhage. At the same time they made the excellent suggestion of staging the embolization in several steps to avoid abrupt dramatic changes in blood pressure. This recommendation should be kept in mind by all interventional neuroradiologists as the main way to decrease the rate of bleeding. Picard et al. (2001) did a recent review of the literature and presented the largest series ever published on APEH. In 18 series of brain AVM embolizations in which cases of spontaneous APEH were reported there were 58 (4.8%) APEHs among 1206 patients. These series involved very different embolization techniques and embolic materials (pellets, IBCA, silk suture, PVA, NBCA). Considering only series with glue embolization, there were 31 (8.2%) APEH in 379 patients (Bank et al. 1981; Debrun et al. 1982, 1997; Deruty et al. 1996; Fournier et al. 1991; Jafar et al. 1993; Lawton et al. 1995; Merland et al. 1986; Wallace et al. 1995). However, these publication are very inhomogeneous and almost obsolete in view of the tremendous changes in embolization techniques and devices seen in recent years. Debrun et al. (1997) reported a risk of 3.9% APEH per embolization (6/152) and 11% per patient. In a series of 283 patients, the risk of post-embolization subarachnoid hemorrhage and intraparenchymal hematoma was, respectively, 3.1% and 2.1% (Vinuela 1992). The most recent publication from Picard et al. gives probably the most up-to-date rate of hemorrhagic complications using the intranidal injection technique as described above (Picard et al. 2001). They report a series of 564 patients with brain AVMs; 492 (87%) were treated with intranidal injection in a total of 1569 procedures, with a mean embolization of three pedicles per procedure. The rate of APEH was 1% per embolization (15/1569) and 3% per patient (15/492). Of these 15 patients, only three had previously bled prior to treatment. Four patients were asymptomatic after hemorrhage (incidental discovery on systematic third-day CT scan), seven had excellent or good outcomes, two had fair outcomes, and two died. Severe morbidity and mortality combined was 0.8% (4/492 patients).

Basic Rules for Avoiding APEH. Several recommendations for minimizing the risk of APEH may be highlighted: Treatment should always be staged, except for grade I AVMs, in which all the feeders as well as the origins of draining veins can be occluded in one session. When the vein has to be preserved, the venous passage should be controlled by pausing for a few seconds when the glue reaches the vein before continuing to fill the nidus. Reflux along the tip of the catheter should be avoided. First embolizations should focus on weak points (intranidal aneurysms). Floppy flow-guided catheters should be used in tortuous thin arteries.

Management of APEH. Like spontaneous hemorrhage, APEH may present with either no symptoms (incidental discovery on systematic post-embolization CT scan), headaches, or more aggressive symptoms with neurologic deficit or coma. APEH may occur during the procedure or within the following days. Prompt surgical evacuation of the hematoma is mandatory in case of mass effect and risk of herniation (Jafar and Rezai 1994). Some angiographic features may predict an increased risk of APEH: (a) occlusion or very slow flow of one of the major draining veins, (b) stagnation of contrast within the nidus, (c) almost complete occlusion of a small AVM with persistent tiny residual nidus, (d) occlusion of a large direct fistula within a nidus. In these instances it is necessary to treat the patient with antihypertensive drugs for several days after the procedure in the intensive care unit. The ability of induced systemic hypotension to prevent nidus rupture was analyzed by Massoud et al. (2000), using a theoretical model. The authors distinguished five hypothetical mechanisms for nidus hemorrhage: intranidal rerouting of blood pressure due to occlusion of direct fistula, extranidal rerouting of blood pressure (NPPB), occlusion of a draining vein, delayed thrombosis of draining veins, and excessively high injection pressure during superselective catheterization. These different mechanisms had the same capacity to generate surges in intranidal hemodynamic parameters, resulting in nidus rupture. Using their theoretical model, the authors showed that inducing systemic hypotension reduced the risk of hemorrhage whatever the mechanism involved.

3.5.3.4
Particular Instances

AVM and Aneurysms. The association of brain AVMs and aneurysms has been discussed for many years in numerous papers. However, management of these cases is still controversial. The incidence of aneurysms associated with brain AVM reported in the literature ranges from 2.7% to 58% (Batjer et al. 1986; Brown et al. 1990; Cunha e Sa et al. 1992; Deruty et al. 1990; Nakahara et al. 1999; Redekop et al. 1998; Thompson et al. 1998; Turjman et al. 1994). This great discrepancies is due to the lack of uniformity in aneurysm classifications. In the series of Turjman et al. (1995b), 58 of 100 consecutive patients presenting with brain AVM had associated aneurysms. They were classified as intranidal aneurysms (INA) in 25 cases and feeding artery aneurysms (FAA) in 38 cases. Many systems have been proposed to classify aneurysms associated with brain AVM, but a widely accepted system of classification based on their anatomic and pathophysiological relationship to the AVM has yet to be developed and validated. According to Redekop et al., aneurysms may be classified as intranidal or flow related when located along the course of arteries that eventually supply the nidus. These aneurysms were classified as proximal, if located at the usual topography of typical aneurysms, or as distal, if above the MCA bifurcation, anterior communicating, or first segment of posterior cerebral arteries. They are unrelated to AVM if occurring on arteries not supplying the AVM. Due to the absence of any reliable factors to assess whether the aneurysm is flow related or not, Piotin et al. (2001) simply classified aneurysms (except for intranidal aneurysms) depending on their location as proximal or distal. Basically, it is necessary to differentiate between feeding artery aneurysms (FAA) and intranidal aneurysms (INA).

Feeding Artery Aneurysms. Three major papers reported the rate of FAA. The numbers of patients exhibiting FAA were 45 of 600 (7.5%) (Thompson et al. 1998), 71 of 632 (12%) (Redekop et al. 1998), and 30 of 270 (11%) (Piotin et al. 2001). Among the 45 patients of Thompson et al., 23 (51%) presented with bleeding. Bleeding occurred from the AVM in 15, from the aneurysm in five, and the source of bleeding could not be determined in three. Among the 71 patients of Redekop et al. (1998), 15 (21%) presented with bleeding from the AVM and 12 (17%) from the aneurysm. Among the 30 patients of Piotin et al. (2001), 15 (50%) presented with bleeding, which occurred from the AVM in three and from aneurysm in 12. In this last series, only 66 of the 240 patients (27.5%) without aneurysm bled. The coexistence of AVM and aneurysms correlated significantly with intracranial hemorrhage at presentation. Similarly, Cunha e Sa et al. (1992) identified the source of hemorrhage as the aneurysm in 18 (46%) of 39 patients and as the AVM in 13 (33%). According to Batjer et al. (1986), there were nine (41%) of 22 patients with hemorrhage and the aneurysm was thought to be responsible for it in seven (78%) of these cases. Thus it is now obvious that in patients with both AVM and aneurysm either one may be the source of hemorrhage. However, Meisel et al. (2000) reported opposite results in a large series of 662 patients with brain AVMs, in which 305 (46%) of them had either FAA or INA. Pretreatment hemorrhage occurred in 54.8% of the patients with aneurysms (56.8% in case of only FAA and 44% in case of FAA and INA). The bleeding rate among patients without aneurysm was 55%, suggesting that FAA are not the primary source of bleeding. The therapeutic strategy of the authors was based on a hypothesis stated in 1998 (Lasjaunias et al. 1988) and consisted in targeting the embolization on AVM compartments harboring INA or compartments fed by arteries harboring FAA. Partial targeted embolization was performed in 450 (68%) of the 662 patients; 138 (30.7%) of them had at least one FAA. Follow-up of 83 patients with 149 FAAs showed 100% FAA shrinkage in 12 cases (8.1%), and more than 50% in 33 of the 149 FAAs (22%). No shrinkage was observed in 40 of the 102 (39%) FAAs with AVM occlusion of less than 50% and in 26 of 47 (55.3%) FAA with AVM occlusion of more than 50%. The authors concluded that because the FAAs shrink and do not rupture during targeted AVM treatment they should be considered as indicators of high-flow angiopathic changes and that there is no evidence that they should be treated prior to AVM treatment.

Because there is no consensus concerning treatment of AVM and associated aneurysms, we propose the following practical strategy:

- In case of subarachnoid hemorrhage or parenchymal hematoma obviously related to FAA rupture, the aneurysm should be treated in emergency.
  - If the aneurysm is proximal on the arterial feeder it should be treated with coils as a regular aneurysm (Fig. 3.3). Treatment of these aneurysms may be very tricky because of a large neck, high arterial flow, and very dysplastic, enlarged feeders. The remodeling technique described by Moret et al. (1997) may be very useful in these instances to ease coiling, control possible peroperative rupture, and perform dense packing of the neck. All pre-, per-, and postoperative care should be exactly the same as for regular aneurysms not associated with brain AVM, except for anticoagulation, which may be less deep due to less risk of thromboembolic complications.
  - If the aneurysm is distal on the arterial feeder treatment may be performed either with coils or with glue. Intra-aneurysmal glue injection was described for treatment of distal aneurysms without associated brain AVM (Cognard et al. 1999). This technique may aim at occluding both the aneurysm and feeding artery or only the aneurysm, preserving the patency of the parent artery. There are several advantages to aneurysm glue occlusion compared with coiling: very distal catheterization is much easier and safer with a flow-guided catheter than with a catheter for coil delivery, and the risk of aneurysm rupture during embolization is very low, primarily because the glue is injected very slowly into the aneurysm and secondarily because no manipulation is required as it is for coiling. The major drawback of this technique is parent artery occlusion, which hinders further AVM embolization. We advocate the use of this technique only in cases of very distally located aneurysm in which occlusion of the parent vessel is not critical. To allow simultaneous treatment of both the aneurysm and the AVM, the treatment can be achieved by intranidal glue injection until there is a reflux along the tip of the catheter into the arterial feeder and aneurysmal sac.
- In cases where the hemorrhage is clearly due to AVM rupture the treatment is aimed primarily at the AVM. The first embolization procedure may be performed after the acute phase, as for ruptured brain AVM not associated with aneurysms.
- In case the subarachnoid hemorrhage or parenchymal hematoma cannot be obviously ascribed to FAA or AVM rupture, the aneurysm should be treated in emergency (Pucheu). The treatment should indeed focus on the lesion presenting the more important risk of rebleeding and likely more severe clinical consequences.
- In cases without hemorrhage, indications for treating first the aneurysm or the AVM are highly controversial. FAA may be regarded as a risk factor of bleeding that should be treated first, owing to the severe clinical consequences, or as high-flow angiopathic changes that may disappear after AVM occlusion. Two options may be proposed:
  - AVM nidus-staged, stepwise embolization. If this option is considered, the first embolization procedure should be targeted at compartments of the nidus fed by arteries harboring the aneurysm. Cases in which the aneurysm has not shrunk at follow-up, despite complete occlusion of the AVM, could be treated with coils. At this point, the treatment decision is as difficult to make as for unruptured regular aneurysm and depends basically on the aneurysm size.

- Selective aneurysm treatment to be performed first (Fig. 3.3), the rationale for this option being that the morbidity and mortality associated with aneurysm hemorrhage are greater than those associated with AVM, and that the presence of the AVM downstream of the aneurysm protects against thromboembolic complications which could occur during aneurysm treatment, rendering the coiling very safe.

In fact, it is not possible to elaborate a strategy of treatment based on a theoretical approach and treatment planning should be determined in each individual depending on many factors such as aneurysm location, size, neck, and morphology and nidus size and architecture.

- Intranidal aneurysms (INA) are located within or in the immediate vicinity of the AVM nidus. They should be differentiated from "false or pseudoaneurysms" observed after an AVM rupture (Figs. 3.12–3.14).

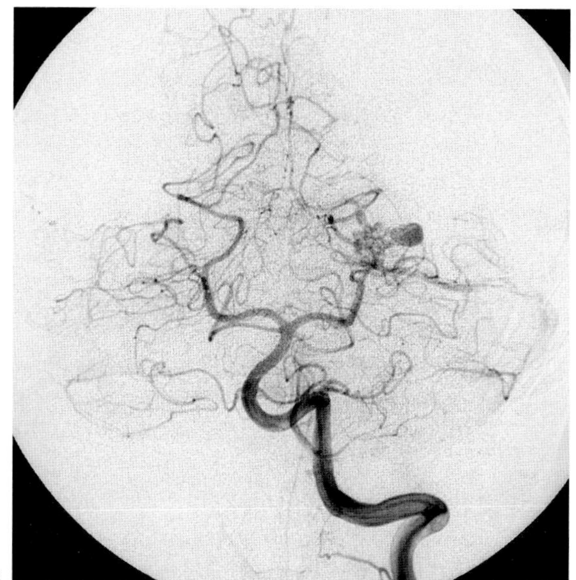
a

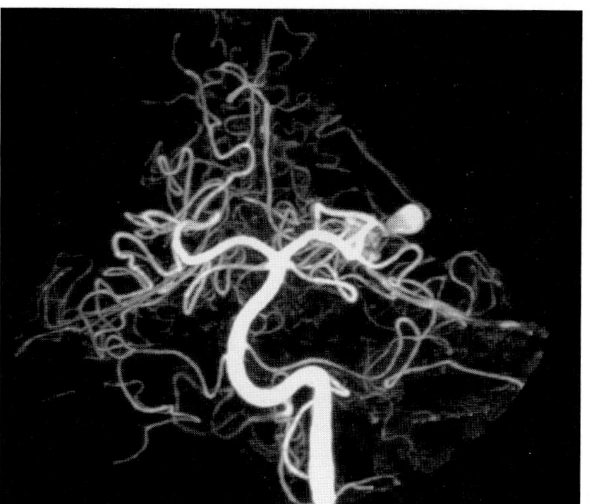
b

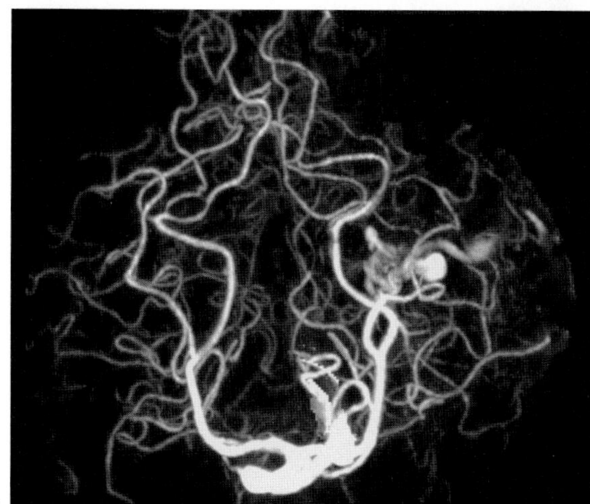
c

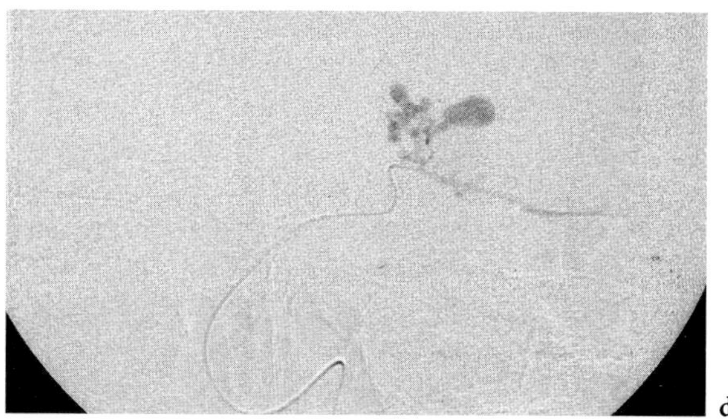
d

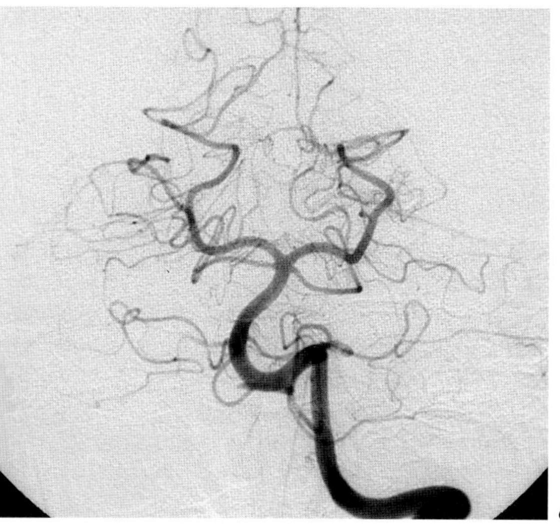
e

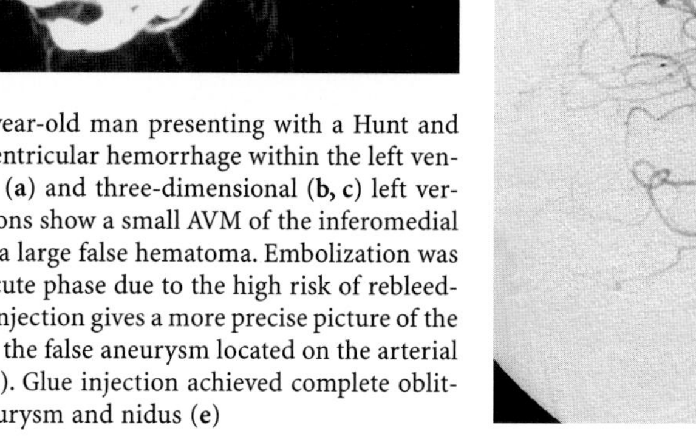

Fig. 3.12a–e. A 30-year-old man presenting with a Hunt and Hess grade I intraventricular hemorrhage within the left ventricular horn. Two- (**a**) and three-dimensional (**b, c**) left vertebral artery injections show a small AVM of the inferomedial temporal lobe with a large false hematoma. Embolization was performed in the acute phase due to the high risk of rebleeding. Superselective injection gives a more precise picture of the angioanatomy, with the false aneurysm located on the arterial side of the nidus (**d**). Glue injection achieved complete obliteration of both aneurysm and nidus (**e**)

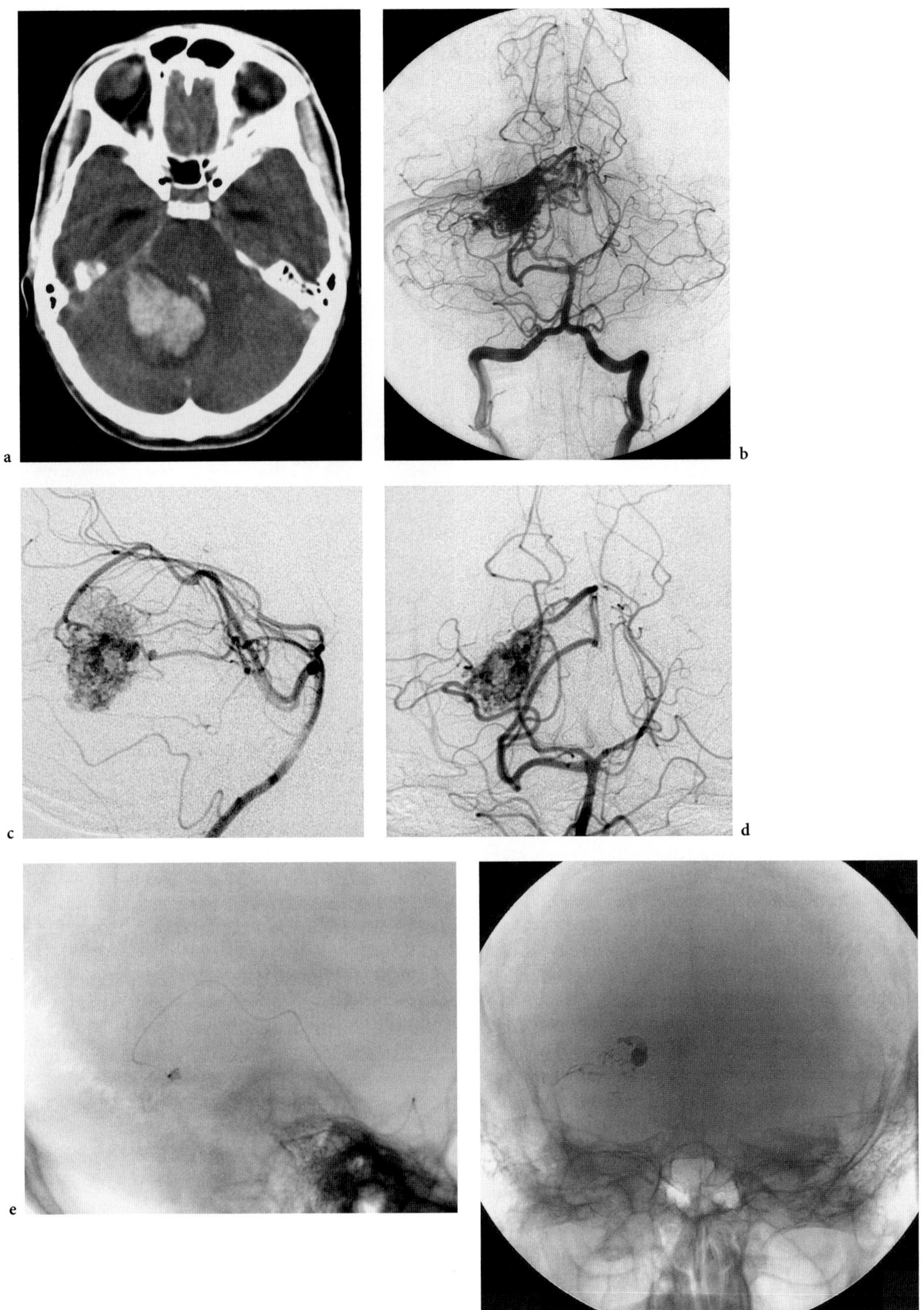
a
b
c
d
e
f ▷

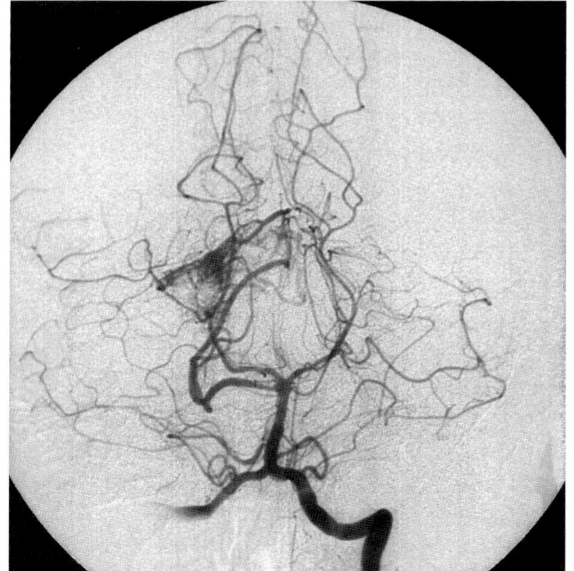
g

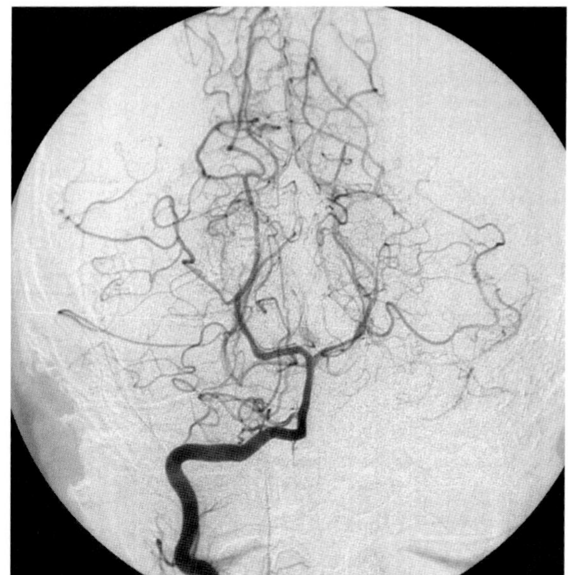
h

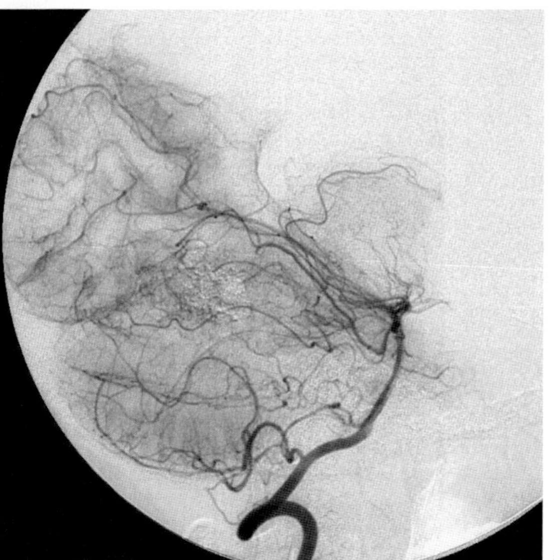
i

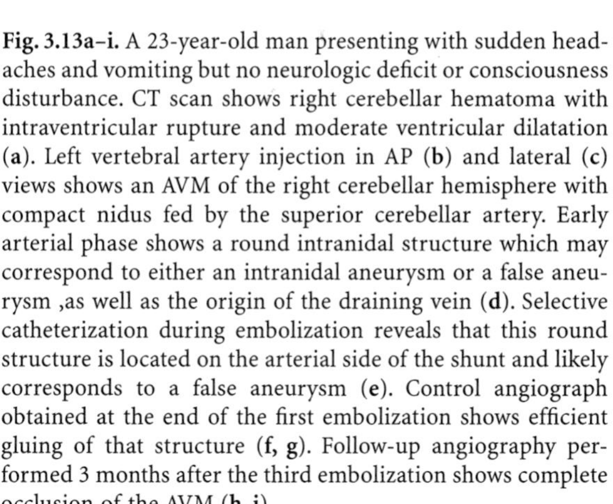
Fig. 3.13a–i. A 23-year-old man presenting with sudden headaches and vomiting but no neurologic deficit or consciousness disturbance. CT scan shows right cerebellar hematoma with intraventricular rupture and moderate ventricular dilatation (**a**). Left vertebral artery injection in AP (**b**) and lateral (**c**) views shows an AVM of the right cerebellar hemisphere with compact nidus fed by the superior cerebellar artery. Early arterial phase shows a round intranidal structure which may correspond to either an intranidal aneurysm or a false aneurysm ,as well as the origin of the draining vein (**d**). Selective catheterization during embolization reveals that this round structure is located on the arterial side of the shunt and likely corresponds to a false aneurysm (**e**). Control angiograph obtained at the end of the first embolization shows efficient gluing of that structure (**f, g**). Follow-up angiography performed 3 months after the third embolization shows complete occlusion of the AVM (**h, i**)

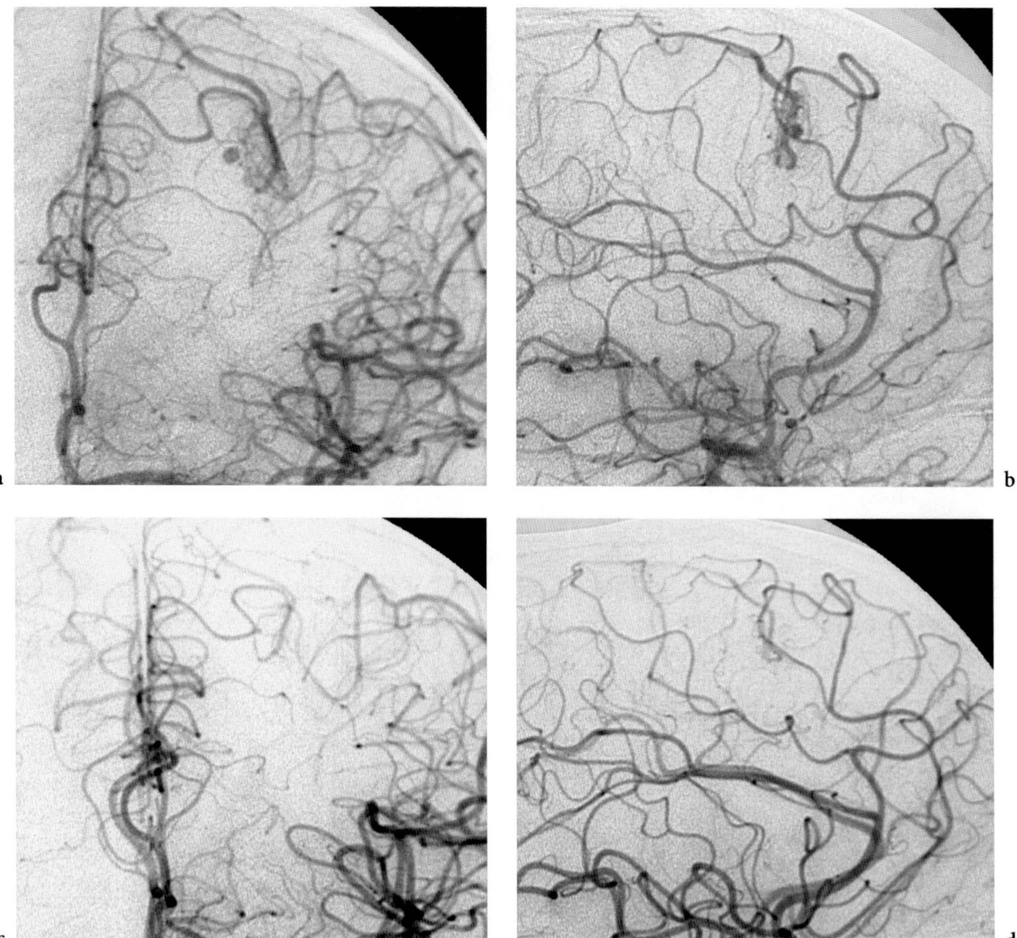

Fig. 3.14a–d. A 43-year-old man presenting with an internal frontal hematoma with no neurologic deficit, only headaches and apraxia. Digital angiography in AP (**a**) and sagittal (**b**) projections performed 2 days after the hematoma occurred showed a small frontal superficial AVM fed by very small branches arising from the "en passage" posteromedial frontal artery. A small aneurysm is visible in the medial aspect of the nidus. Due to the unfavorable angioarchitecture no embolization was performed. Due to the large size of the hematoma and very small size of the AVM, surgery was not considered in the acute phase considering the likely difficulty of finding the AVM. At follow-up 2 months later, angiography in AP (**c**) and sagittal (**d**) projections showed disappearance of the aneurysm. Such spontaneous aneurysm regression is consistent with the diagnosis of false aneurysm

These pseudoaneurysms are supposed to correspond to an unclotted portion of the hematoma still communicating with the vessel lumen. Pseudoaneurysms should be suspected in the presence of a vascular cavity, usually of irregular shape, within or at the periphery of the hematoma (Fig. 3.6). Nevertheless, it is impossible to accurately determine in the case of AVM rupture whether the lesion is a true or a false aneurysm. Garcia-Monaco et al. (1993) reported 15 cases of pseudoaneurysm in a population of 189 patients with brain AVMs. Eight of the nine cases not treated by embolization or surgery had resolved at follow-up angiography. None of the pseudoaneurysms was confirmed histologically. Marks et al. (1992) reported 15 patients with INA detected after AVM rupture. In two of the three patients operated on the aneurysms were located in the pathological specimens. Histological evaluation demonstrated these aneurysms to be thin-walled vascular structures rather than pseudoaneurysms due to AVM rupture. In fact, the acquired nature of a pseudoaneurysm secondary to AVM rupture can be asserted only when comparison with available pre-hemorrhage angiography confirms the aneurysm as a new angioarchitectural feature. However, even though it is almost impossible to differentiate between INA and pseudoaneurysms, both lesions should be considered risk factors for acute rebleeding. That risk was 11% in a small series of supposed pseudoaneurysms (Garcia-monaco et al. 1993) and 11% in a large series of INA (Meisel et al. 2000). The therapeutic planning concerning INA may be the following:

- Where a pseudoaneurysm or a false aneurysm is responsible for the hemorrhage, the first step of embolization must be performed in the acute phase and should focus on aneurysm occlusion (Figs. 3.12, 3.13). Superselective angiography performed with the flow-guided catheter must be done to understand which feeding artery is supplying the compartment of the nidus harboring the INA (Fig. 3.6). Catheter progression within the desired vessel should be performed as usual but with minimal injection of contrast material (Garcia-Monaco et al. 1993). Overinjection of fluid may exert a significant strain on the false aneurysm and increase the risk of rupture. A wedge position of the tip of the catheter may produce rebleeding as well, because the injection force is directly transmitted to the pseudoaneurysm (Lasjaunias et al. 1988). Glue embolization is performed as usual, with the aim of occluding the nidus and aneurysm at the same shot.
- In case of unruptured AVM associated with INA or ruptured AVM with INA not responsible for the bleeding, there is no need to perform the treatment in the acute phase. The first embolization procedure should be performed several weeks after bleeding and must be targeted at the compartment of the AVM harboring the INA.

Direct Arteriovenous Fistulas. Direct communication between arteries and veins without interposed nidus may be observed. Two types of direct AVF must be distinguished, pial AVF and AVF within a brain AVM nidus.

The two major types of pial AVF are vein of Galen aneurysmal malformations (VGAMs) located in the subarachnoid space, and direct AVF (brain AVFs) between cortical arteries and pial veins located in the subpial space (Lasjaunias and Berenstein 1993b). VGAMs are encountered mainly in neonates and children and correspond to a separated entity with specific embryology, physiopathology, clinical presentation, and treatment strategy. Therefore, they will not be treated in this chapter. Brain AVFs may present in children with systemic manifestation due to high-flow shunt with congestive heart failure or failure to thrive. They may also present in adults with the same symptoms as brain AVMs. Because they are very rare, there is no large series published in the literature concerning their rate of bleeding and rebleeding and specific treatment. Nevertheless, treatment consists in occluding the arteriovenous shunt itself. This may be attained by glue injection or parent artery coil occlusion. The best therapeutic option is shunt gluing, because it allows complete occlusion of the AV communication from the arterial side to the origin of the vein. Catheterization is often easy with regard to the dilatation of the feeding vessel, even though the shunt is very distal. The tip of the catheter is aspirated in the venous system and has to be pulled back in the arterial side if possible, in a curve of the feeding artery, to obtain better control of the glue injection. The operator should not give too much slack to the catheter, which could, under these conditions, progress during the injection of glue into the veins and result in total absence of control of glue deposition, with no arterial embolization but venous occlusion and consequent bleeding. The injection of a concentrated mixture of glue and Lipiodol has to be as slow as possible to avoid formation of small drops of glue flowing into the veins. After progressive inflation of the kernel of glue from the artery to the foot of the vein, the operator should stop the injection and wait several seconds for glue polymerization before withdrawing the catheter. Removal of the catheter too early may result in more or less fast progression of the kernel of glue to the veins. This technique, however, requires experience with glue injection and may be dangerous if uncontrolled. This is why in some instances the shunt may be occluded with coils. A floppy catheter with a very small diameter should be used to avoid arterial damage (Fig. 3.15). Small three-dimensional soft coils should be used to perform dense packing on a short arterial segment and avoid occlusion of normal adjacent arteries.

Intranidal Direct Fistulas. The angioarchitecture of brain AVM may sometimes associate usual nidus and direct fistulas. True AVFs are recognized when the tip of the catheter reaches the origin of the vein during superselective catheterization (Fig. 3.16). In contrast, very rapid opacification of the foot of the vein after opacification of a very short arterial segment should not be considered as an AVF but as a very distal intranidal catheterization (Figs. 3.4, 3.10). When a true AVF is encountered within a brain AVM nidus the problem is to determine which compartment should be the first target of the treatment. The abrupt occlusion of an intranidal fistula may result in rerouting of significantly high shunting blood flow through delicate plexiform portions of the nidus and subsequent immediate rupture (Fig. 3.16). The hypothesis that partial nidus embolization causes

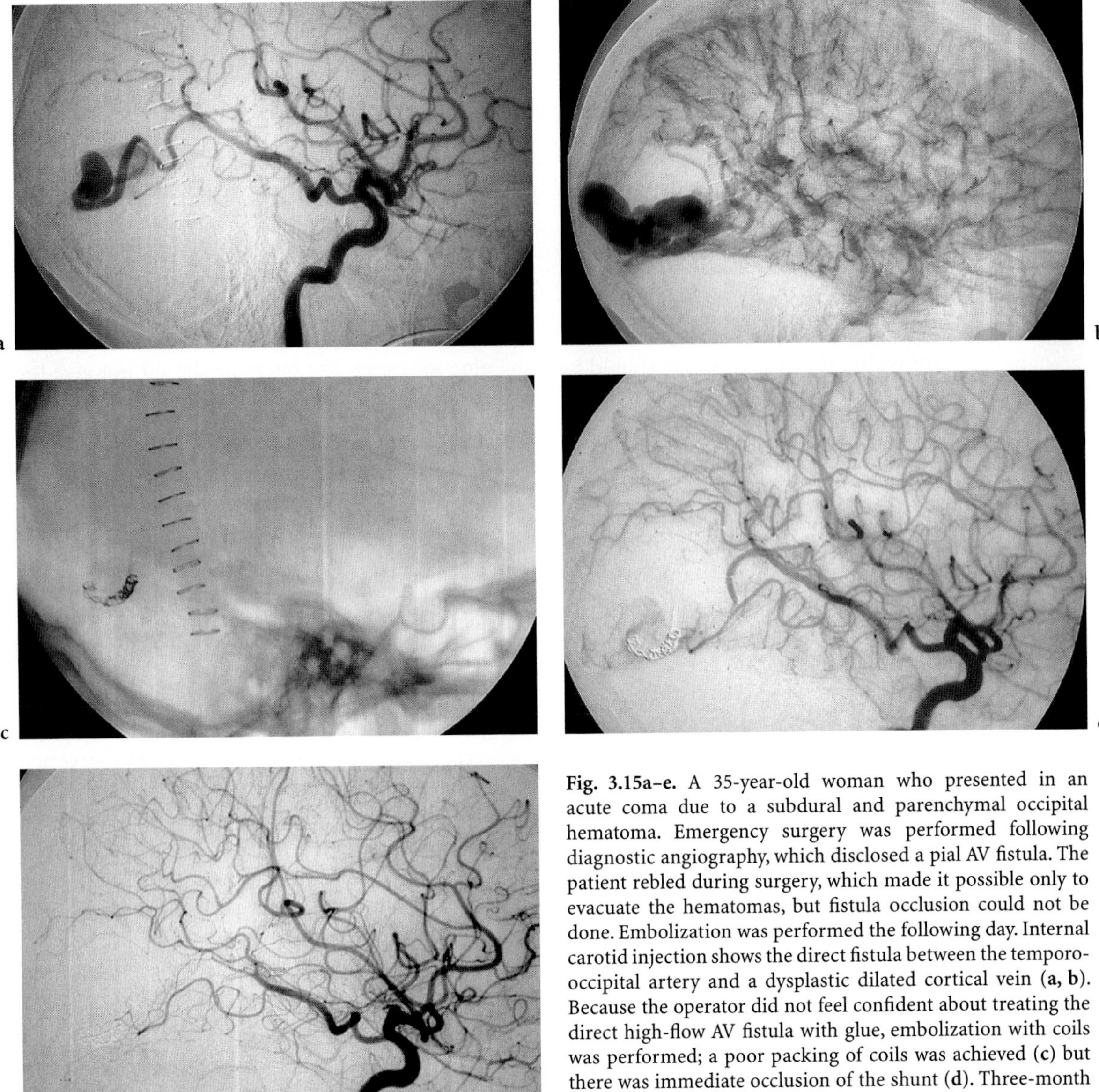

Fig. 3.15a–e. A 35-year-old woman who presented in an acute coma due to a subdural and parenchymal occipital hematoma. Emergency surgery was performed following diagnostic angiography, which disclosed a pial AV fistula. The patient rebled during surgery, which made it possible only to evacuate the hematomas, but fistula occlusion could not be done. Embolization was performed the following day. Internal carotid injection shows the direct fistula between the temporo-occipital artery and a dysplastic dilated cortical vein (**a, b**). Because the operator did not feel confident about treating the direct high-flow AV fistula with glue, embolization with coils was performed; a poor packing of coils was achieved (**c**) but there was immediate occlusion of the shunt (**d**). Three-month follow-up angiography confirmed the complete occlusion (**e**)

Fig. 3.16a–i. A 57-year-old man who presented with a frontal hematoma (grade II, Hunt and Hess). Left internal carotid angiography in lateral (**a, b**) and AP (**c, d**) views done on day 2 after bleeding showed a large brain AVM with very dilated feeding arteries and draining veins. Such dilatation of the feeding arteries indicates the presence of direct AV fistula shunts within the nidus. Superselective catheterization was performed, showing multiple direct fistulas but no true nidus (**e**). Injection of glue in these very high flow shunts was considered too hazardous. Catheterization of the origin of the feeding vessels with a nondetachable balloon catheter allowed much better control of the glue injection by balloon inflation (**f**). Two injections were performed, which occluded several direct shunts (**g, h**). The patient awoke from anesthesia in the same clinical status as before treatment. Three hours later he became hemiplegic, then comatose. CT scan showed a wide, deep, left hematoma with ventricular rupture (**i**). The patient died several hours later. Dramatic modification of the hemodynamics due to sudden occlusion of several fistulas with increased pressure in residual feeders and shunts is the most likely explanation for such bleeding. Nevertheless, although the nidus should theoretically be considered the first target in case of direct AV fistula, recognition and catheterization of the nidus itself is almost impossible because the catheter is systematically aspirated through the direct fistula

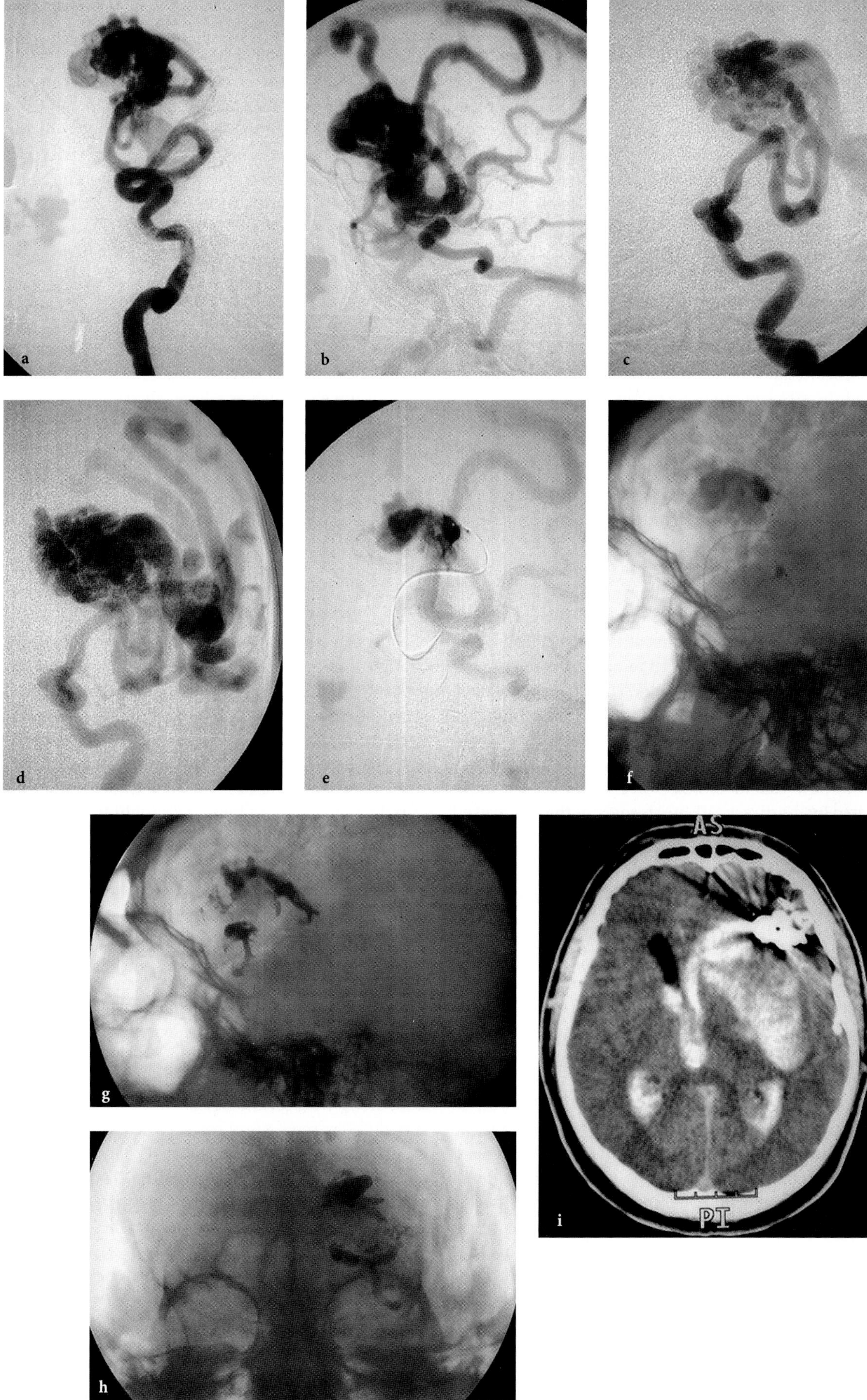

a
b
c
d
e
f
g
h
AS
PI
i

upstream pressure elevation in arterial feeders and that pressure increase is transmitted to persistently unobliterated portions of the nidus producing a risk of nidus rupture was evaluated with a theoretical model (Massoud et al. 2000). Intranidal rerouting of blood pressure due to occlusion of a direct fistula generated surges in intranidal hemodynamic parameters, resulting in nidus rupture. In the same way, a computational model analysis showed that direct fistulas have a buffering effect, so that their abrupt occlusion may produce an increased pressure gradient in the nonembolized arteries and related nidus (Gao et al. 1997). There is a theoretically higher risk of occluding a direct fistula before nidus occlusion, and the strategy might be to focus in the first embolization procedure on the nidus and keep the direct AVF open until the end of the treatment. The other reason for this strategy is that, by definition, direct AVFs give access to the vein, and if a direct AVF is embolized at the end of nidus embolization it may allow venous gluing and complete cure of the AVM. In contrast, if the AVF is treated first there is an important risk of inadvertent venous gluing and occlusion with a major risk of nidus rupture. The major drawback of this strategy is that it is sometimes almost impossible to understand the angioarchitecture of the nidus when a direct AVF is associated with it. The occlusion of a direct AVF first rapidly clarifies the angioarchitecture of the nidus. Besides, because pedicles feeding AVFs are larger and have a higher flow, flow-guided catheters are systematically aspirated by the direct AVF and feeders of the nidus itself are almost impossible to catheterize.

3.5.3.5 Goals and Results

Goals

The goal of treating brain AVMs is first to eliminate the risk of hemorrhage and then to completely eliminate the AVM. Complete cure must be defined as complete disappearance of the nidus and absence of early venous drainage (Figs. 3.4, 3.10, 3.12, 3.13, 3.15). To attain that goal a multidisciplinary strategy must be decided on by the neuroradiologist, neurosurgeons, and the radiotherapist. If embolization is considered as the first step of the therapeutic strategy, its goal is to occlude the AVM or to decrease its size as much as possible, because occlusion and complication rates after radiosurgery are closely related to the size of the residual AVM. Embolization should aim obtaining a single residual nidus and avoid spreading the AVM in multiple separated residual nidus compartments (Fig. 3.11). For this reason, each embolization should be targeted at specific compartments of the nidus to try to occlude the AVM from the periphery to the center. We consider the embolization completed when further catheterization and glue injection is no more possible (too thin or tortuous pedicles, or pedicles feeding the AVM through arterio-arterial anastomosis). At that time, depending on the final result of embolization, radiosurgery or surgery is performed to obtain complete occlusion of the AVM.

In some instances, complete cure is deemed impossible despite a combined technique. Partial treatment can yet be indicated in some cases: (a) to cure a weak point of the AVM such as a false aneurysm, intranidal aneurysms, or large feeding artery aneurysms (Fig. 3.6); (b) to improve the clinical symptoms in case of a large AVM presenting with progressive neurologic deficits (Fox 1997).

The efficacy of partial embolization to improve the condition of patients with intractable seizures has never been proved, and such embolization should not be performed owing to the risk induced by repeated embolization with no evidence of benefits. In the same way, the efficacy of partial embolization to reduce the risk of bleeding has not been proved. On the contrary, the computational model from Gao et al. suggests that there might be a higher risk of increased pressure gradients and subsequent risk of bleeding during final stages of embolization (Gao et al. 1997). Partial embolization with the aim of reducing the risk of bleeding should therefore not be performed.

Results

Several factors make it impossible to accurately evaluate the results of brain AVM embolization:(a) the tremendous variety of embolic agents used; (b) considering only glue embolization, the extreme variety of techniques used (pedicle versus intranidal embolization) and the very rapid evolution of catheter technology and changes in operator experience and skill, along with technological improvement; (c) the very different methods of patient selection (nonsurgical brain AVMs with series reporting only grade III–V AVM, versus series in which embolization is indicated as the first treatment step before surgery or radiosurgery); (d) the different goals of treatment (presurgical embolization aimed at reducing the flow, versus curative embolization aimed at definitely occluding the AVM). Neurosurgeons are right when they claim that no large series with good methodology can accurately evaluate the results of current brain AVM embolization. In a meta-analysis, FRIZZEL and co-workers reviewed the past 35 years of brain AVM embolization (32 series, 1246 patients) (FRIZZEL and FISHER 1995). This study having been published in 1995, all the reviewed papers concerned almost obsolete embolization techniques and certainly do not reflect the current embolization techniques and results. Embolization resulted in AVM cure in only 5%. Permanent morbidity was 9% and mortality 2%–1%. Ten years ago, complete occlusion of a brain AVM was supposed to be possible only in case of a small single pedicle AVM (PELZ et al. 1988; BERTHELSEN et al. 1990). In addition, these authors reported a case of complete obliterated AVM with a later recanalization, suggesting what is still in the mind of many neurosurgeons – that glue embolization does not provide long-term occlusion of brain AVMs. More recent, though still obsolete, series reported cure rates of 10%–20% including large lesions (BERENSTEIN and CHOI 1988; GRZYSKA et al. 1993; GUO et al. 1993). A cure rate of 70% has been reported for small lesions (BERENSTEIN and CHOI 1988). Three small series reported much better results with cure rates of more than 50% (SAMSON et al. 1981; NAKSTAD et al. 1992; WILMS et al. 1993). Nevertheless, these results are quite surprising with regard to the embolization material used and no details are available concerning AVM characteristics. WIKHOLM et al. (1996) reported, for 150 patients treated, a cure rate of 13% with a mortality of 1.3% and severe morbidity of 6.7%. However, in this series the referred patients were selected by the neurosurgeons, creating a recruitment bias favoring left side and eloquent-located AVMs as well as high Spetzler-Martin grades (85% of the AVMs were grade III–V). Much better but still unpublished results include an obliteration rate by embolization alone of 33% (138/419 patients) (PICARD et al. 1999).

The long-term stability of nidus occlusion with glue has been a matter of debate for many years; some authors have raised questions about the danger of revascularization. This concern was based on two different observations: (a) that revascularization of a nidus may occur after incomplete occlusion of large brain AVM (VINTERS et al. 1986; VINUELA et al. 1986), (b) the long-term resorption of cyanoacrylate cast (RAO et al. 1989). The first finding of revascularization of the nidus due to development of extensive collaterals after incomplete occlusion of large brain AVM has been correlated to the proximity of the deposition of the embolic material (VINUELA et al. 1986; FOURNIER et al. 1990). This phenomenon is well recognized today as being secondary to too proximal occlusion of the feeding vessel without intranidal gluing. The proximal occlusion favors extensive collateral recruitment to supply the nidus, which may be misinterpreted as recanalization due to poor long-term efficacy of the glue itself (Fig. 3.17). However, it is certain today that when complete occlusion is obtained by intranidal injection the result is permanent (WIKHOLM et al. 1995). However, complete disappearance of any nidus and draining vein immediately after embolization does not always predict definitive occlusion, which can be ascertained only on angiography at several months' follow-up (Fig. 3.18). The second observation, concerning resorption of the glue at follow-up angiography (RAO et al. 1989) is a constant phenomenon (Fig. 3.19). Long-term follow-up of embolized brain AVM, whatever the result (cured or not cured), always shows a progressive disappearance of the cast of glue. The reason why the glue is less and less visible over years is still not clear. A chronic inflammatory response with varying degrees of collagenization, fibrosis, and mild lymphohistiocytic infiltrates with an indistinct layer of normal vessel walls were observed on light microscopy (KISH et al. 1983; VINTERS et al. 1985). The giant cell reaction is confined to the vessel lumen, without any reaction in the media or adventitia (FREENY et al. 1979; VINTERS et al. 1986). The most likely mechanism to explain the progressive decreased density of the cast is intracellular phagocytosis of bucrylates or Lipiodol.

3.5.3.6
Intranidal Embolization with Nonadhesive Liquid Embolic Agents

A nonadhesive liquid polymer was recently developed (Onyx, Micro Therapeutics, Inc., Irvine, Calif.) (TAKI et al. 1990; MURAYAMA et al. 1998). Onyx is made of a mixture of ethylene-vinyl alcohol copolymer (EVOH) and dimethyl sulfoxide (DMSO). EVOH is a copolymer of polyethylene and polyvinyl alcohol. Polyethylene was used for artificial joint implantation and polyvinyl alcohol constituted the particles of PVA used for embolization. The EVOH is dissolved in the DMSO at three different concentrations: 6% (with 6% copolymer and 94% solvent), 6.5%, and --8%. A low concentration (6%) is less viscous and can allow more distal nidal penetration. The mixture is made opaque with tantalum powder. Onyx is supplied in prepared vials that must be kept on a specific shaker for at least 20 min prior to its injection to avoid tantalum settlement and poor opacity. Only catheters compatible with DMSO can be used (Flowrider, Ultraflow, Micro Therapeutics, Inc., Irvine, Calif.). The main advantage of a nonadhesive liquid is that it theoretically eliminates the risk of gluing the cath-

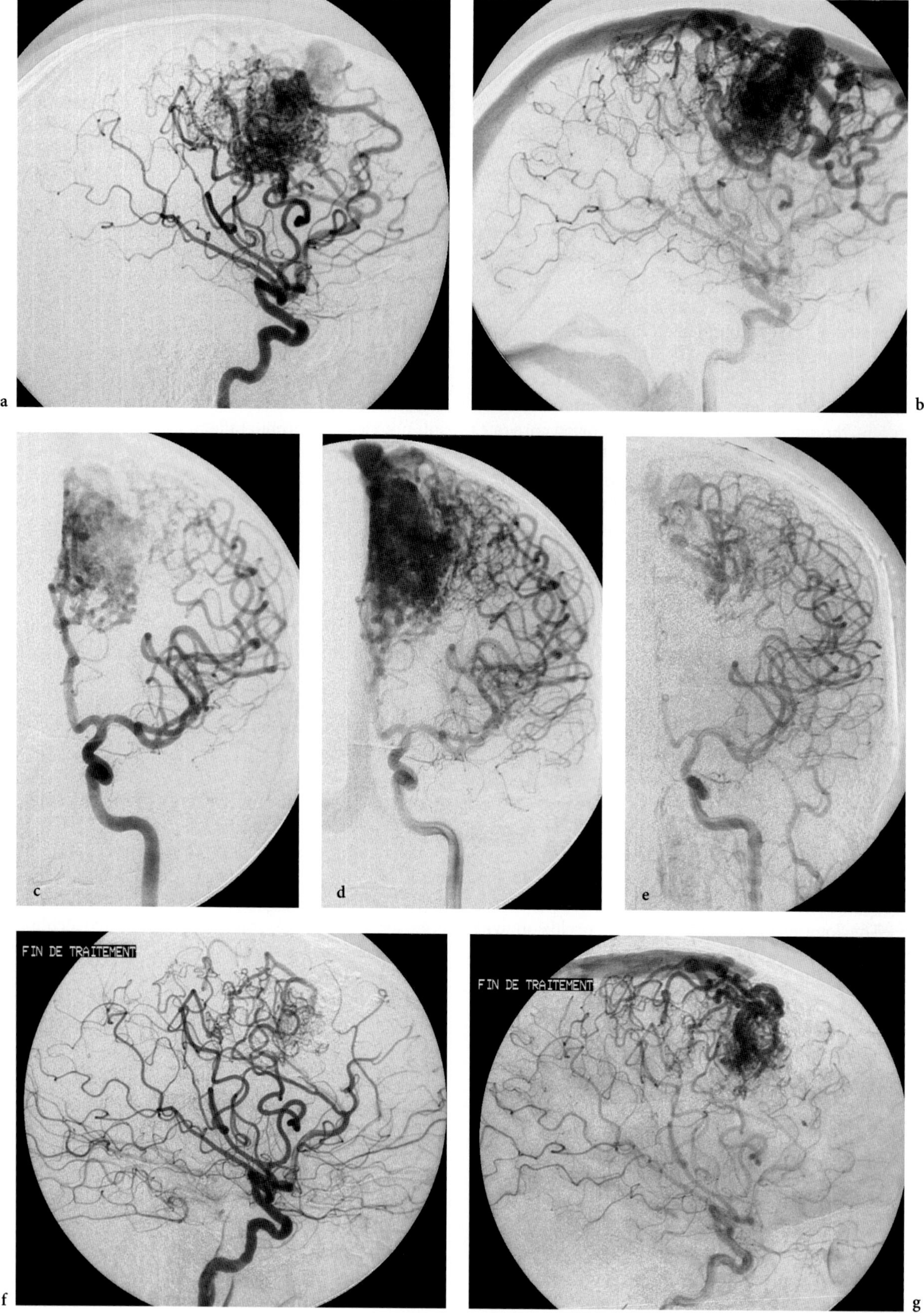
a
b
c
d
e
FIN DE TRAITEMENT
f
FIN DE TRAITEMENT
g

Fig. 3.17a–g. An 18-year-old woman presenting with a 3-year history of intractable seizures despite adapted therapy. Right internal carotid injection in lateral (**a, b**) and AP (**c, d**) views show a large frontoparietal medial AVM, fed mainly by frontal branches of the anterior cerebral artery, as well as by a leptomeningeal anastomosis arising from distal branches of middle cerebral arteries. Final angiography obtained after four procedures shows important nidus remnant due to too proximal embolization of feeding pedicles from the anterior cerebral artery branches and opacification of the distal aspect of these embolized arteries by the pial anastomosis from middle cerebral artery branches (**e–g**). Embolization through these anastomoses should never be performed in view of the certain subsequent neurologic deficit

eter and makes it possible to perform a more durable injection, with a larger amount of agent delivered in a single injection. Taki et al. first described the use of Onyx in cerebral AVM (Goto et al. 1991; Taki et al. 1990; Terada et al. 1991; Yamashita et al. 1994; Murayama et al. 1999). Onyx was used in 23 patients, achieving an average of 63% volume reduction after a total of 129 arterial feeder embolizations (Jahan et al. 2001). Morbidity was 4% permanent deficits and no death. No complete cure was obtained. Eleven patients were subsequently operated on. Histopathologic study showed inflammatory changes as well as angionecrosis of embolized vessels in two cases. Onyx has some advantages and some drawbacks to its use in AVMs:

Advantages

The major advantage to the use of Onyx compared with cyanoacrylates is the ease of injection. The catheter should be placed in the same wedge situation as for intranidal glue injection. The injection should be very slow, as well. It may be stopped for a few seconds or minutes to wait for precipitation of Onyx, and then resumed. Control angiography may be performed during Onyx injection for a better understanding of material progression and of nidus and vein occlusion. Onyx always behaves as a column, and the formation of small drops flowing into the vein that may be seen when glue is injected too fast never occurs. The injection may last for several minutes or even tens of minutes. The total amount of Onyx injected at one time in one single pedicle may therefore be more important than with glue. It may reduce the number of catheters used and the total number of procedures needed to achieve a complete cure of the AVM. The other major advantage is that because injection is more prolonged and the decision to stop or continue the injection does not have to be made immediately, as it does for glue injection, the training of young neuroradiologists to perform Onyx injection is much easier than the mastering of glue injection.

Disadvantages

The toxicity of DMSO has been discussed in a few reports (Chaloupka et al. 1994; Sampei 1996; Murayama et al. 1998; Chaloupka et al. 1999). The first paper of Chaloupka et al. emphasized the risk of severe vasospasm after injection of 0.8 ml EVOH and DMSO in the swine rete mirabile with subsequent infarction. Injection of 0.5 ml resulted in delayed (7–14 days) subarachnoid hemorrhage with angionecrosis on histology and arterial microaneurysms. Two other studies reexamined this toxicity and concluded that the two major points are contact time with the arterial wall and volume of injection (Murayama et al. 1998; Chaloupka et al. 1999). Finally, it has been proved that injection of 0.3 ml for 40 s produced neither vasospasm nor angionecrosis. The protocol of injection is as follows: Prior to injection the microcatheter is flushed with 5 ml normal saline. Then 0.25 ml DMSO is injected over more than 40 s for dead space catheter filling. Onyx is then injected slowly (Jahan et al. 2001). Nevertheless, despite the fact that this protocol was used in all the 23 patients treated, histology showed angionecrosis of many vessels in two of four patients operated on 1 day after embolization. Consequently, there is still some question of a likely toxicity of DMSO. One issue may be that because of the wedge position of the catheter, there might be a stagnation of DMSO in the pedicle and nidus, with prolonged contact of DMSO with the vessel wall and risk of necrosis.

At the beginning of injection there is frequently a reflux of Onyx along the tip of the catheter. The injection must be stopped and resumed a few seconds or minutes later until a progression within the nidus is observed. As soon as it has precipitated around the tip of the catheter, the Onyx tends to open different compartments of the nidus and the injection may be prolonged. This technique carries two risks: the occlusion of an adjacent normal branch due to reflux of Onyx in the feeding pedicle; gluing of the tip of the catheter because of a very prolonged injection. Although the Onyx is not adhesive, catheter with-

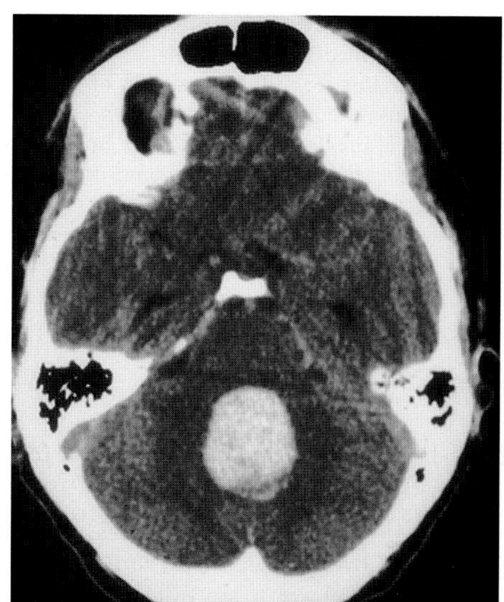

a

Fig. 3.18a–g. A 28-year-old who presented with a huge cerebellar hematoma with headaches, diplopia, and consciousness disturbances but no deficit (**a**). Right vertebral injection shows a vermian AVM fed by both superior cerebellar arteries with a compact nidus draining into a single vermian vein presenting extensive ectasia, probably corresponding to the rupture site (**b, c**). Control angiography obtained at the end of the two sessions of embolization showed the cast of Histoacryl (**d, e**) and complete occlusion of the AVM (**f**). Follow-up angiography at 3 months showed a residual nidus and early venous drainage (**g**). The patient was treated with radiosurgery

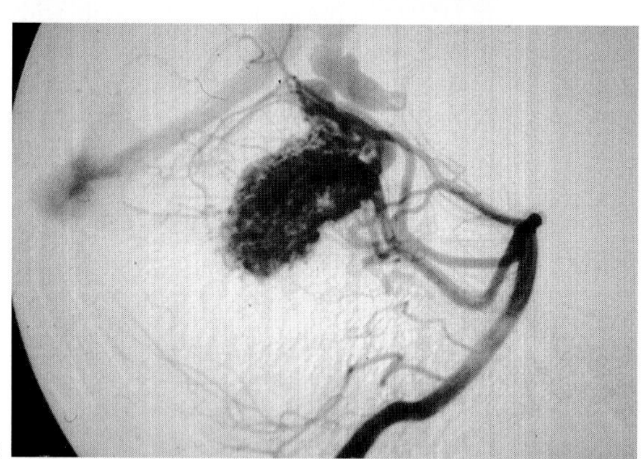

b

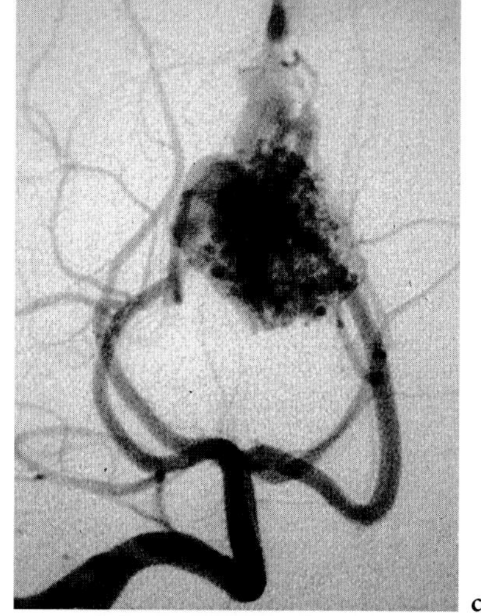

c

▷▷

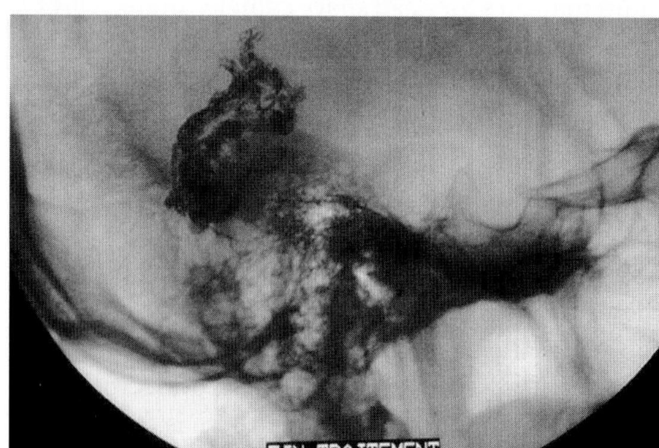

d

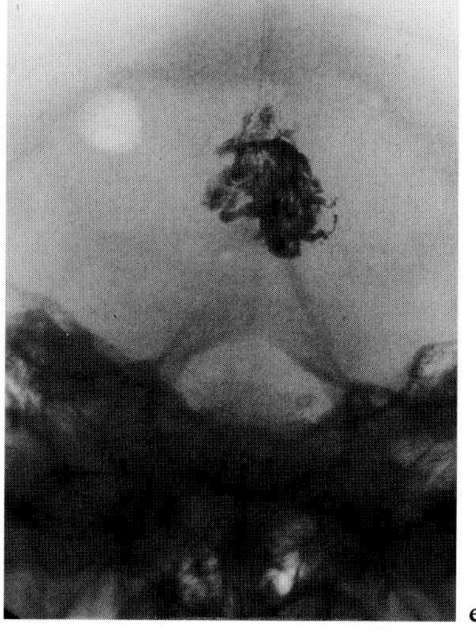

e

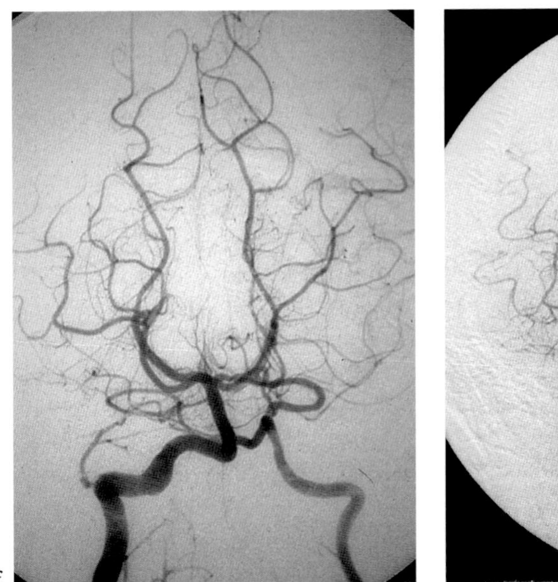

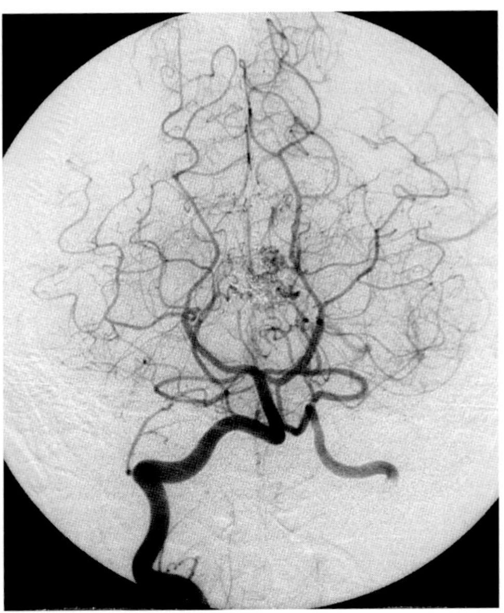

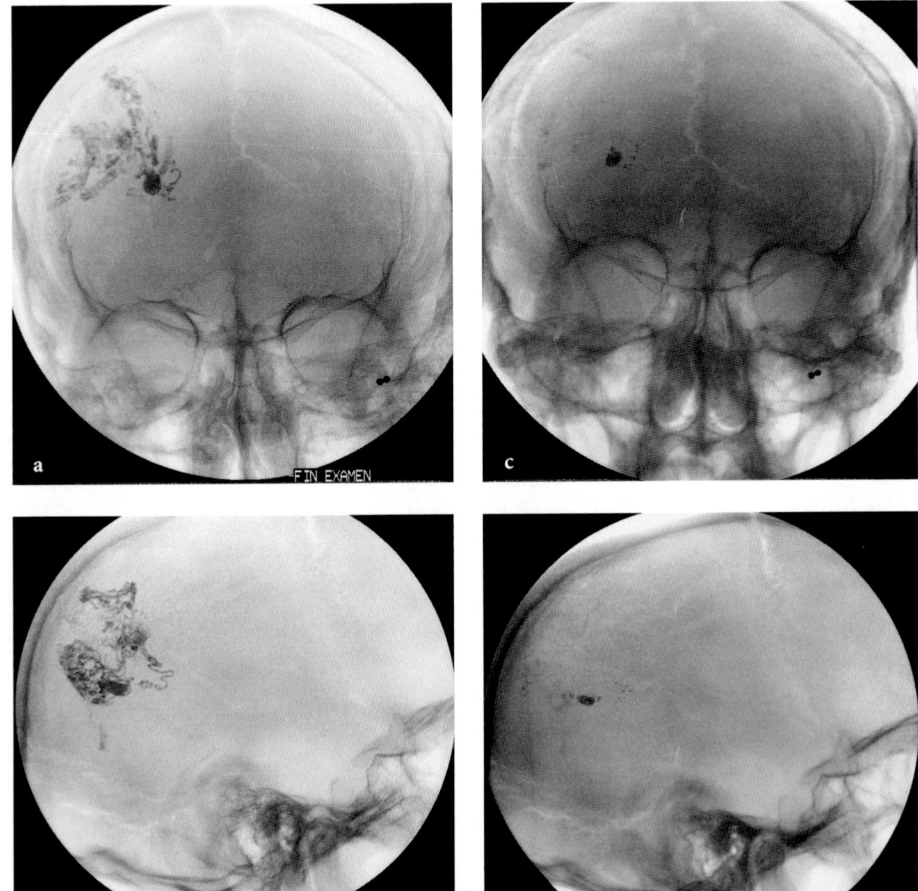

Fig. 3.19a–d. Large parietal AVM. Cast of glue obtained after two embolizations, AP and lateral view (**a, b**). The patient was lost to follow-up for 3 years. Nonsubtracted images obtained at the beginning of the third procedure of embolization show almost complete resorption of the cast of glue (**c, d**)

drawal may be difficult and result in either gluing or breaking of the catheter, or stretching and rupture of the AVM and artery. Very prolonged injection with serious reflux along the catheter tip should be unconditionally avoided.

One of the major advantages of Onyx is that a large volume may be introduced in one single catheter injection. However, there is a risk of hemorrhage. The operator may be temped to occlude a very large portion of the nidus in one procedure. Many years ago it was proven that staged embolization aimed at reducing the nidus in several sessions is mandatory to progressively modify the flow dynamic. Very sudden and large-scale occlusion of the nidus surely increases the risk of postprocedural hemorrhage, as discussed above.

There are still two situations in which Onyx should not be used today: direct fistula, in which the Onyx cannot occlude a high-flow large shunt because it is not adhesive, and a feeding pedicle "en passage", in which reflux on the tip of the catheter is not allowed due to major risk of normal vessel occlusion.

3.5.4 Therapeutic Strategy

It is extremely difficult to establish a therapeutic algorithm for brain AVM. The indication for treatment basically depends on:

- Clinical presentation (hemorrhage or not)
- Patient age
- Natural risk, roughly evaluated by the presence or not of likely risk factors of bleeding (associated aneurysm or false aneurysm, venous stenosis or ectasia)
- AVM size, location (superficial or deep, eloquent or not) and angioarchitecture (compact or diffuse)

The goal of treatment may be:

- Definitive complete obliteration to protect from hemorrhage
- Partially targeted treatment (embolization) to eliminate risk factors of bleeding/rebleeding (feeding artery aneurysms, intranidal aneurysms, false aneurysms)
- Partial treatment in case of AVM presenting with worsening neurologic deficits (although the efficacy of such treatment is yet to be proven)

Partial treatment should not be performed to:

- Decrease bleeding risk, because even subtotal therapy does not confer protection from hemorrhage
- Improve seizures, because of treatment-induced risks and unproved efficiency

The indication for treatment, goal of treatment, and therapeutic strategy should be decided on by an experienced multidisciplinary team in agreement with the patient, who has been precisely informed of natural and therapeutic risks. Multimodality treatment is frequently performed – either as a planned maneuver, typically with embolization followed by radiosurgery or surgery, or as an unplanned maneuver when one modality fails and a second modality is required for complete obliteration. Goals of the different modalities should be clear at the outset. In our experience, embolization is the first-intention approach in the vast majority of the patients, followed by either surgery or radiosurgery. Nevertheless, because of the extreme variability of resources available in any one area of the country or world, as well as very different skills and experience on the part of neurosurgeons and interventional neuroradiologists, it is impossible to draft any recommendations about strategy itself. Because there is almost never a need for brain AVM treatment in emergency (as opposed to aneurysm treatment), patients with brain AVMs should be sent to very specialized and experienced centers that can afford the most up-to-date multimodality therapy.

Acknowledgements. Acknowledgments go to Drs. Zhang Peng and Zhu Fengshiu for their major contribution to the bibliographic research.

References

Aberfeld DC, Rao KR (1981) Familial arteriovenous malformation of the brain. Neurology 31:184–186

Aesch B, Lioret E, deToffel B, et al (1991) Multiple cerebral angiomas and Rendu-Osler-Weber disease: case report. Neurosurgery 29:599–602

Alkadhi H, Kollias SS, Crelier GR, et al (2000) Plasticity of the human motor cortex in patients with arteriovenous malformations: a functional MR imaging study. AJNR Am J Neuroradiol 21:1423–1433

Al-Rodhan NRF, Sundt TM jr, Piepgras DG (1993) A theory for the hemodynamic complications following resection of intracerebral arteriovenous malformations. J Neurosurg 78:167–175

Al-Shahi R, Warlow C (2001) A systematic review of the frequency and prognosis of arteriovenous malformations of the brain in adults. Brain 124:1900–1926

Amin-Hanjani S, Robertzon R, Arginteanu MS, Scott RM (1998) Familial intracranial arteriovenous malformations. Case report and review of the literature. Pediatr Neurosurg 29:208–213

Andrews BT, Wilson CB (1987) Staged treatment of arteriovenous malformations of the brain. Neurosurgery 21: 314–323

Aoki Y, Nakasawa K, Tago M, et al (1996) Clinical evaluation of Gamma knife radiosurgery for intracranial arteriovenous malformations. Radiat Med 14:265–268

Aoki S, Sasaki Y, Machida T, et al (1998) 3D-CT angiography of cerebral arteriovenous malformations. Radiat Med 16: 263–271

Bank WO, Kerber CW, Cromwell LD (1981) Treatment of intracerebral arteriovenous malformations with isobutyl 2-cyanoacrylate: initial experience. Radiology 31:1

Barnett GH, Little JR, Ebrahim ZY, Jones SC, Friel HT (1987) Cerebral circulation during arteriovenous malformation operation. Neurosurgery 20:836–842

Batjer HH, Suss RA, Samson D (1986) Intracranial arteriovenous malformations associated with aneurysms. Neurosurg 18:29–35

Batjer HH, Devous MD Sr, Meyer YJ, Purdy PD, Samson DS (1988) Cerebrovascular hemodynamics in arteriovenous malformation complicated by normal perfusion pressure breakthrough. Neurosurgery 22:503–509

Batjer HH, Devous MD sr, Seibert GB, et al (1989a) Intracranial arteriovenous malformation: relationship between clinical factors and surgical complications. Neurosurgery 24:75–79

Batjer HH, Purdy PD, Giller CA, Samson DS (1989b) Evidence of redistribution of cerebral blood flow during treatment for an intracranial arteriovenous malformation. Neurosurgery 25:599–605

Berenstein A, Choi IS (1988) Surgical neuroangiography of intracranial lesions. Radiol Clin North Am 26: 1143–1151

Berenstein A, Lasjaunias P (1992) Classification of brain arteriovenous malformations. In: Surgical neuroangiography, vol 4. Springer, Berlin Heidelberg New York, pp 1–86

Berg JN, Gallione CJ, Stenzel T, et al (1997) The activin receptor-like-kinase 1 gene: genomic structure and mutations in hereditary hemorrhagic telangiectasia type 2. Am J Hum Genet 61:60–67

Berman MF, Sciacca RR, Pile-Spellman J, et al (2000) The epidemiology of brain arteriovenous malformations. Neurosurgery 47:389–396

Berthelsen B, Lofgren J, Svendsen P (1990) Embolization of cerebral arteriovenous malformations with bucrylate: experience in a first series of 29 patients. Acta Radiol 31: 13–21

Betti OO, Munari C (1992) Traitement radiochirurgical avec accélérateur linéaire des «petites» malformations artérioveineus intra-craniennes. Neurochirurgie 38:27–34

Betti OO, Munari C, Rosler R (1989) Stereotactic radiosurgery with linear accelerator: treatment of arterio-venous malformations. Neurosurgery 24:311–321

Binder JR, Swanson SJ, Hammeke TA, et al (1996) Determination of language dominance with fMRI: a comparison with the Wada test. Neurology 46:978–984

Blat DR, Friedman WA, Bova FJ (1993) Modifications based on computed tomographic imaging in planning the radiosurgical treatment of arterio-venous malformations. Neurosurgery 33:588–595

Brown RD, Wiebers DO, Forbes G, et al (1988) The natural history of unruptured intracranial arteriovenous malformations. J Neurosurg 68:352–357

Brown RD, Wiebers DO, Forbes GS (1990) Unruptured intracranial aneurysms and arteriovenous malformations and relationship of lesions. J Neurosurg 73:859–863

Brown RD jr, Wiebers DO, Torner JC O'Fallon WM (1996a) Incidence and prevalence of intracranial vascular malformations in Olmsted County, Minnesota, 1965 to 1992. Neurology 46:949–952

Brown RD jr, Wiebers DO, Torner JC, et al (1996b) Frequency of intracranial hemorrhage as a presenting symtom and subtype analysis: a population-based study of intracranial vascular malformations in Olmsted Country, Minnesota. J Neurosurg 85:29–32

Carpentier AC, Constable RT, Schlosser MJ, et al (2001) Patterns of functional magnetic resonance imaging activation in association with structural lesions in the rolandic region: a classification system. J Neurosurg 94:946–954

Carter LP, Gumerlock MK (1995) Steal and cerebral arteriovenous malformations. Stroke 26:2371–2372

Castel JP, Kantor G (2000) Postoperative morbidity and mortality after microsurgical exclusion of cerebral arteriovenous malformations. Current data and analysis of recent literature. Neurochirurgie 47:369–383

Challa VR, Moody DM, Brown WR (1995) Vascular malformations in the central nervous system. J Neuropathol Exp Neurol 54:609–621

Chaloupka JC, Vinuela F, Vinters HV, Robert J (1994) Technical feasibility and histopathologic studies of ethylene vinyl copolymer (EVAL) using a swine endovascular embolization model. AJNR Am J Neuroradiol 15:1107–1115

Chaloupka JC, Huddle DC, Alderman JJ, et al (1998) classification of vascular malformations of the central nervous system. J Neuropathol Exp Neurol 54:609–621

Chaloupka JC, Huddle DC, Alderman J, et al (1999) A reexamination of the angiotoxicity of superselective injection of DMSO in the swine rete embolization model. AJNR Am J Neuroradiol 20:401–410

Cheifetz S, Bellon T, Calles C,Vera S, et al (1992) Endoglin is a component of the transforming growth factor-beta receptor system in human endothelial cells. J Biol Chem 267: 19027–19030

Chen JW, Kerber C, Hoi-Sang U (1991) Spontaneous regression of large bilateral basal ganglia arteriovenous malformations. AJNR Am J Neuroradiol 12:835–837

Chin LS, Raffel C, Gonzalez-Gomez I, Giannotta SL, McComb JG (1992) Diffuse arteriovenous malformations: a clinical, radiological and pathological description. Neurosurgery 31:863–868

Cognard C, Weill A, Tovi M, Castaings L, et al (1999) Treatment of distal aneurysms of the cerebellar arteries by intraaneurysmal injection of glue. AJNR Am J Neuroradiol 20: 780–784

Colombo F (1989) Linear accelerator radiosurgery. A clinical experience. J Neurosurg Sci 33:123–5

Colombo F, Benedetti A, Pozza F, et al (1989) Linear accelerator radiosurgery of cerebral arteriovenous malformations. Neurosurgery 24:833–840

Colombo F, Pozza F, Chierego G, et al (1994) Linear accelerator radiosurgery of cerebral arteriovenous malformations: an update. Neurosugery 34:14–21

Crawford M, West CR, Chadwick, et al (1986) Arteriovenous malformations of the brain: natural history in unoperated patients. J Neurol Neurosurg Psychiatry 49:1–10

Cunha e Sa MJ, Stein BM, Solomon RA, et al (1992) The treatment of associated intracranial aneurysms and arteriovenous malformations. J Neurosurg 77:853–859

Davis C, Symon L (1985) The management of cerebral arteriovenous malformations. Acta Neurochir (Wien) 74:4–11

Debrun G, Lacour P, Caron JP, et al (1978) Detachable balloon and calibrated leak balloon techniques in the treatment of cerebral vascular lesions. J Neurosurg 49:635–649

Debrun G, Vinuela F, Fox A, et al (1982) Embolization of cerebral arteriovenous malformations with bucrylate. J Neurosurg 56:615–627

Debrun GM, Aletich V, Ausman JI, et al (1997) Embolization of nidus of brain arteriovenous malformations with n-butyl cyanoacrylate. Neurosurgery 40:112–121

De Oliveira E, Tedeschi H, Siqueira MG, et al (1997) Arteriovenous malformations of the basal ganglia region: rationale for surgical management. Acta Neurochir 139:487–506

Deruty R, Mottolese C, Soustiel JF, Pelissou-Guyotat I (1990) Association of cerebral arteriovenous malformation and cerebral aneurysm. Diagnosis and management. Acta Neurochir (Wien) 107:133–139

Deruty R, Pelissou-Guyotat I, Mottolese C, Amat D, et al (1996) Therapeutic risk in multidisciplinary approach of cerebral arteriovenous malformations. Neurochirurgie 42:35–43

Devekis JP, Manz HJ, Luessenhop AJ, et al (1994) A clinical and neuropathologic study of silk suture as an embolic agent for brain arteriovenous malformation. AJNR Am J Neuroradiol 15:263–271

Dias MS, Sekhar LN (1990) Intracranial hemorrhage from aneurysms and arteriovenous malformations during pregnancy and the puerperium. Neurosurg 27:855–866

Drake CG, Friedman AH, Peerless SJ (1986) Posterior fossa arteriovenous malformations. J Neurosurg 64:1–10

Duckwiler GR, Dion JE, Vinuela F, Jabour B, Martin N, Bentson J (1990) Intravascular microcatheter pressure monitoring: experimental results and early clinical evaluation. AJNR Am J Neuroradiol 11:169–175

Duckwiler GR, Dion JE, Vinuela F, et al (1992) Delayed venous occlusion following embolotherapy of vascular malformations in the brain. AJNR Am J Neuroradiol 13:1571–1579

Ducreux D, Trystram D, Oppenheim C, et al (2001) Imagerie diagnostique des malformations artério-veineuses cérébrales. Neurochirurgie 47:190–200

Duong DH, Young WL, Vang MC, et al (1998) Feeding artery pressure and venous drainage pattern are primary determinants of hemorrhage from cerebral arteriovenous malformations. Stroke 29:1167–1176

Edelman RR, Wentz KU, Mattle HP, et al (1989) Intracerebral arteriovenous malformations: evaluation with selective MR angiography and venography. Radiology 173:831–837

Essig M, Wenz F, Schoenberg SO, et al (2000) Arteriovenous malformations. Assessment of gliotic and ischemic changes with fluid-attenuated inversion-recovery MRI. Invest Radiol 35:689–694

Farb RI, McGregor C, Kim JK, et al (2001) Intracranial arteriovenous malformations: real-time auto-triggered elliptic centric-ordered 3D gadolinium-enhanced MR angiography – initial assessment. Radiology 220:244–251

Fink GR (1992) Effects of cerebral angiomas on perifocal and remote tissue: a multivariate positron emission tomography study. Stroke 23:1099–1105

Finnerty JJ, Chisholm CA, Chapple H, et al (1999) Cerebral arteriovenous malformation in pregnancy: presentation and neurologic, obstetric, and ethical significance. Am J Obstet Gynecol 181:296–303

Fischer AW, Er H (1930) Lokales Amyloid im Gehirn. Eine Spätfolge von Roentgenbestrahlungen. Dtsch Z Chir 227: 475–483

Folkow B, Gurevich M, Hallbach M, Lundgren Y, et al (1971) The hemodynamic consequences of regional hypotension in spontaneously hypertensive and normotensive rats. Acta Physiol Scand 83:532–541

Fong GH, Rossant J, Gertsenstein M,Breitman ML (1995) Role of the Flt-1 receptor tyrosine kinase in regulating the assembly of vascular endothelium. Nature 376:66–70

Fournier D, Terbrugge K, Rodesch G, et al (1990) Revascularization of brain arteriovenous malformations after embolization with bucrylate. Neuroradiology 32:497–501

Fournier D, Terbrugge K, Willinsky R, et al (1991) Endovascular treatment of intracerebral arteriovenous malformations: experience in 49 cases. J Neurosurg 75:228–233

Fox AJ (1997) Recurrent AVMs after negative angiography. J Neurosurg 86:170–171

Fox AJ, Pelz DM, Lee DH (1990) Arteriovenous malformations of the brain: recent results of endovascular therapy. Radiology 177:51–57

Freeny PC, Mennemeyer R, Kidd CR (1979) Long-time radiographic pathologic follow-up of patients treated with visceral transcatheter occlusion using isobutyl 2-cyanoacrylate (bucrylate). Radiology 132:51–60

Freudenstein D, Duffner F, Ernemann U, et al (2001) Recurrence of a cerebral arteriovenous malformation after surgical excision. Cerebrovasc Disc 11:59–64

Friedman WA, Bova FJ, Mendenhall WM (1995) Linear accelerator radiosurgery for arterio-venous malformations. The relationship of size to outcome. J Neurosurg 82:180–189

Friedman WA, Blatt DL, Bova FJ, et al (1996) The risk of hemorrhage after radiosurgery for arterio-venous malformations. J Neurosurg 84:912–919

Frishberg BM (1997) Neuroimaging in presumed primary headache disorders. Semin Neurol 17:373–382

Frizzel RT, Fisher WS (1995) Cure, morbidity, and mortality associated with embolization of cerebral arteriovenous malformations: a review of 1246 patients in 32 series over a 35-year period. Neurosurgery 37:1031–1040

Fry D (1968) Acute vascular endothelial changes associated with increased blood velocity gradients. Circ Res 22: 165–197

Fults D, Kelly DL (1984) Natural history of arteriovenous malformations of the brain: a clinical study. Neurosurg 15:658–662

Gallina P, Merienne L, Meder JF, et al (1998) Failure in radiosurgery treatment of cerebral arteriovenous malformations. Neurosurgery 2:996–1004

Gao E, Young WL, Pile-Spellman J, et al (1997) Cerebral arteriovenous malformations feeding artefact aneurysms: a theoretical model of intravascular pressure changes after treatment. Neurosurgery 41:1345–1356

Garcia-Monaco R, Rodesch G, Alvarez H, et al (1993) Pseudoaneurysms within ruptured intracranial arteriovenous malformations: diagnosis and early endovascular management. AJNR Am J Neuroradiol 14:315–321

Garretson HD (1985) Intracranial arteriovenous malformations. In: Wilkins RH, Rengachary SS (eds) Neurosurgery. McGraw-Hill, New York, pp 1448–1457

Germano IM, Davis RL, Wilson CB, Hieshima GB (1992) Histopathological follow-up study of 66 cerebral arteriovenous malformations after therapeutic embolization with polyvinyl alcohol. J Neurosurg 76:607–614

Goto K, Uda K, Ogata N (1991) Embolization of cerebral arteriovenous malformations (AVMs): material selection, improved technique, and tactics in the initial therapy of cerebral AVMs. Neurol Med Chir (Tokyo) 33 Suppl:193–199

Graf CJ, Perret GE, Torner JC (1983) Bleeding from cerebral arteriovenous malformations as part of their natural history. J Neurosurg 58:331–337

Griffiths PD, Hoggard N, Warren DJ, et al (2000) Brain arteriovenous malformations: assessment with dynamic MR digital subtraction angiography. AJNR Am J Neuroradiol 21:1892–1899

Grzyska U, Westphal M, Zanella F, Freckmann N, Herrmann HD, Zeumer H (1993) A joint protocol for the neurosurgical and neuroradiologic treatment of cerebral arteriovenous malformations: indications, technique, and results in 76 cases. Surg Neurol 40:476–484

Guo WY, Wikholm G, Karlsson B, Lindquist C, Svendsen P, Ericson K (1993) Combined embolization and gamma knife radiosurgery for cerebral arteriovenous malformations. Acta Radiol 34:600–606

Guttmacher AE, Marchuk DA, White RIJ (1995) Hereditary hemorrhagic telanciectasia. N Engl J Med 33:918–924

Hacein-Bey L, Nour R, Pile-Spellman J, et al (2001) Adaptive changes in autoregulation to chronic cerebral hypotension with arteriovenous malformations: an acetazolamide-enhanced single-photon emission CT study. AJNR Am J Neuroradiol 199516(9):1865–1874

Hademenos GJ, Alberts MJ, Awad I, Maiberg M, et al (2001) Advances in the genetics of cerebrovascular disease and stroke. Neurology 56:997–1008

Hamilton MG, Spetzler RF (1994) The prospective application of a grading system for arteriovenous malformations. Neurosurgery 34:2–7

Hanahan D (1997) Signaling vascular morphogenesis and maintenance. Sciences 277:48–50

Handa T, Negoro M, Miyachi S, et al (1993) Evaluation of pressure changes in feeding arteries during embolization intracerebral arteriovenous malformations. J Neurosurg 79:383–389

Hartmann A, Mast H, Mohr JP, et al (1998) Morbidity of intracranial hemorrhage in patients with cerebral arteriovenous malformation. Stroke 29:931–934

Hartmann A, Stapf C, Hofmeister C, et al (2000) Determinants of neurological outcome after surgery for brain arteriovenous malformations. Stroke 31:2361–2364

Hasegawa S, Hamada JI, Morioka M, Kai Y, Takaki S, Ushio (1999) Multiple cerebral arteriovenous malformations (AVMs) associated with spinal AVM. Acta Neurochir (Wien) 141:315–319

Hashimoto N (2001) Microsurgery for cerebral arteriovenous malformations: a dissection technique and its theoretical implications. Neurosurgery 48:1278–1281

Hashimoto N, Emala CW, Joshi S, Mesa-Tejada R, et al (2001) Abnormal pattern of Tie-2 and vascular endothelial growth factor receptor expression in human cerebral arteriovenous malformations. Neurosurgery 47:910–918

Hassler W, Steinmetz H (1987) Cerebral hemodynamics in angioma patients: an intraoperative study. J Neurosurg 67:822–831

Henkes H, Nahser HC, Berg-Dammer E, et al (1998) Endovascular therapy of brain AVMs prior to radiosurgery. Neurol Res 20:479–492

Heros RC, Korosue K,Diebold PM (1990) Surgical excision of cerebral arteriovenous malformations: late results. Neurosurgery 26:570–578

Herzig R, Burval S, Vladyka V, et al (2000) Familial occurrence of cerebral arteriovenous malformation in sisters: case report and review of the literature. Eur J Neurol 7:95–100

Hillman J (2001) Population-based analysis of arteriovenous malformation treatment. J Neurosurg 95:633–637

Hofmeister C, Stapf C, Hartmann A, et al (2000) Demographic, morphological, and clinical characteristics of 1289 patients with brain arteriovenous malformation. Stroke 31: 1307–1310

Horton JC, Chambers WA, Lyons SL, et al (1990) Pregnancy and the risk of hemorrhage from cerebral arteriovenous malformations. Neurosurgery 27:8 67–872

Houdart E, Gobin YP, Casasco A, Aymard A, Herbreteau D, Merland JJ (1993) A proposed angiographic classification of intracranial Arterio-venous fistulae and malformations Neuroradiol 35: 381–385

Itoyama Y, Uemura S, Ushio Y, et al (1989) Natural course of unoperated intracranial arteriovenous malformations: study of 50 cases. J Neurosurg 71:805–809

Jafar JJ, Rezai AR (1994) Acute surgical management of intracranial arteriovenous malformations. Neurosurgery 34:8–13

Jafar JJ, Daviss AJ, Berenstein A (1993) The effect of embolization with n-butyl cyanoacrylate prior to surgical resection of cerebral arteriovenous malformations. J Neurosurg 78:60–69

Jahan R, Murayama Y, Gobin YP, et al (2001) Embolization of arteriovenous malformations with Onyx: clinicopathological experience in 23 patients. Neurosurgery 48:984–997

Jellinger K (1977) Human central nervous system lesions following radiation therapy. Zentralbl Neurochir 38:199–200

Jellinger K (1986) Vascular malformations of the ventral nervous system: a morphological overview. Neurosurg Rev 9: 177–216

Jessurun GA, Kamphuis DJ, van der Zande FH, Nossent JC (1993) Cerebral arteriovenous malformations in the Netherlands Antilles. High prevalence of heridatary hemorrhagic telangiectasia-related single and multiple cerebral arteriovenous malformations. Clin Neurol Neurosurg 95: 193–198

Johnson Dw, Berg JN, Baldwin MA, Gallione CJ, et al (1996) Mutations in the activin receptor-like kinase 1 gene in hereditary haemorrhagic telangiectasia type 2. Nat Genet 13:189–195

Jomin M, Lejeune JP, Blond S (1993) Histoire naturelle et pronostic spontané des malformations artério-veineuses cérébrales. Neurochirurgie 39:205–211

Jungreis CA, Horton JA, Hecht ST (1989) Blood pressure changes in feeders to cerebral arteriovenous malformations during therapeutic embolization. AJNR Am J Neuroradiol 10:575–577

Kader A, Young WL, Pile-Spellman J, et al (1994) The influence of hemodynamic and anatomic factors on hemorrhage from cerebral arteriovenous malformations. Neurosurg 34:801–808

Kader A, Goodrich JT, Sonstein WJ (1996) Arteriovenous malformations after negative postoperative angiograms. J Neurosurg 85:14–18

Kaminaga T, Hayashida K, Iwama T, et al (1999) Hemodynamic changes around cerebral arteriovenous malformation before and after embolization measured with PET. J Neuroradiol 26:236–241

Kamiryo T, Nelson PK, Bose A, et al (2000) Familial arteriovenous malformations in siblings. Surg Neurol 53:255–259

Karlsson B, Lax I, Soderman M, et al (1996) Prediction of results following Gamma-Knife surgery for brain stem and other centrally located arterio-venous malformations: relation to natural course. Stereotact Funct Neurosurg 66 [Suppl 1]:260–268

Karlsson B, Kihlström L, Lindquist C, et al (1998) Gamma Knife surgery for previously irradiated arterio-venous malformations. Neurosurg 42:1–6

Kerber C (1976) Balloon catheter with a calibrated leak: a new system for superselective angiography and occlusive catheter therapy. Radiology 120:547–550

Kish KK, Rapp SM, Wilner HL, et al (1983) Histopathologic effects of transarterial bucrylate occlusion of intracerebral arteries in mongrel dogs. AJNR Am J Neuroradiol 4: 385–387

Kjeldsen AD, Vase P, Green A (1999) Hereditary haemorrhagic telangiectasia: a population-based study of prevalence and mortality in Danish patients. J Intern Med 245:31–39

Kjellberg RN (1986) Stereotactic Bragg peak proton beam radiosurgery for cerebral arteriovenous malformations. Ann Clin Res 18 [Suppl 47]:17–19

Kjellberg RN (1989) Radiosurgery. Neurosurgery 25:670–672

Kondziolka D, Humphreys RP, Hoffman HJ (1992) Arteriovenous alformations of the brain in children: a forty-year experience. Can J Neurol Sci 19:40–45

Kondziolka D, Lunsford LD, Flickinger JC (1993) Gamma Knife stereotactic radiosurgery for cerebral vascular malformations. In: Alexander E III, Loeffler JS, Lunsford LD (eds) Stereotactic radiosurgery. McGraw Hill, New York, pp 136–146

Kondziolka D, Lunsford LD, Kanal E, et al (1994) Stereotactic magnetic resonance angiography for targeting in arteriovenous malformations radiosurgery. Neurosurgery 35: 585–591

Krapf H, Siekmann R, Freudenstein D, et al (2001) Spontaneous occlusion of a cerebral arteriovenous malformation: angiography and MR imaging: follow-up and review of the literature. AJNR Am J Neuroradiol 22:1556–1560

Krayenbuhl HA (1977) Angiographic contribution to the problem of enlargement of cerebral arteriovenous malformations. Acta Neurochir (Wien) 36:215–242

Kricheff II, Madayag M, Braunstein P (1972) Transfemoral catheter embolization of cerebral and posterior fossa arteriovenous malformations. Radiology 120:457–550

Kvam DA, Michelsen J, Quest DO (1980) Intracerebral hemorrhage as a complication of artificial embolization. Neurosurgery 7:491–494

Kwon OK, Han DH, Han MH, et al (2000) Palliatively treated cerebral arterio-venous malformations: follow-up results. J Clin Neurosci 7:69–72

Kwon Y, Ryong S, Hoon J, et al (2000) Analysis of the causes of treatment failure in gamma knife radiosurgery for intracranial arteriovenous malformations. J Neurosurg 93:104–106

Lamy B, Jourdan R, Deschamps J, et al (1990) Hematome intracerebral par rupture d'une arteriovenous malformations cerebral. Analyse et pronostic d'une serie de 35 patients comateux admis en reanimation. Agressologie 31:299–302

Lanzino G, Fergus AH, Jensen ME, et al (1997) Long-time outcome after surgical excision of parenchymla arteriovenous malformations in patients over 60 years of age. Surg Neurol 47:258–263

Lasjaunias P, Berensteins A (1993a) Surgical neuroangiography, vol 2. Springer, Berlin Heidelberg New York, pp 379–383

Lasjaunias P, Berensteins A (1993b) Surgical angiography, vol 4. Springer, Berlin Heidelberg New York, pp 268–317

Lasjaunias P, Piske R, TerBrugge K, et al (1988) Cerebral arteriovenous malformations (CVM) and associated arterial aneurysms(AA): analysis of 101 CAVM cases, with 37 AA in 23 patients. Acta Neurochir (Wien) 91:29–36

Latchaw RE, Hu X, Ugurbil K, et al (1995) Functional magnetic resonance imaging as a management tool for cerebral arteriovenous malformations. Neurosurgery 37:619–626

Lawton MT, Hamilton MG, Spetzler RF (1995)Multimodality treatment of deep arteriovenous malformations: thalamus, basal ganglia, and brain stem. Neurosurgery 37:29–36

Lazar RM, Marshall RS, Pile-Spellman J, et al (2000) Interhemispheric transfer of language in patients with left frontal cerebral arteriovenous malformation. Neuropsychologia 38:1325–1332

Lindquist M, Karlsson B, Guo WY, et al (2000) Angiographic long-term follow-up data for arteriovenous malformation previously proven to be obliterated after Gamma Knife radiosurgery. Neurosurgery 46:803–810

Liu K, Rutt BK (1998) Sliding interleaved kY (SLINKY) acquisition: A novel 3D MRA technique with suppressed slab boundary artifact. J Magn Reson Imaging 8:903–911

Lombardi D, Scheithauer BW, Piepgras D, Meyer FB, Forbes GS (1991) "Angioglioma" and the arteriovenous malformation-glioma association. J Neurosurg 75:589–596

Luessenhop AJ, Spence WT (1960) Artificial embolization of cerebral arteries:report of use in a case of arteriovenous malformation. JAMA 172:1153–1155

Lunsford LD (1993) The role of stereotactic radiosurgery in the management of brain vascular malformations. In: Alexander E III, Loeffler JS, Lunsford LD (eds) Stereotactic radiosurgery. McGraw-Hill, New York, pp 111–121

Lunsford LD, Kondziolka D, Flickinger JC, et al (1991) Stereotactic radiosurgery for arteriovenous malformations of the brain. J Neurosurg 75:512–524

Maisonpierre PC, Suri C, Jones PF, Bartunkova S, et al (1997) Angiopoietin-2, a natural antagonist for Tie2 that disrupts in vivo angiogenesis. Science 277:55–60

Manchola IF, De Salles AA, Foo TK, Ackerman TH, et al (1993) Arteriovenous malformation hemodynamics: a transcranial Doppler study. Neurosurgery 33:556–562

Maldjian J, Atlas SW, Howard RS, et al (1996) Functional magnetic resonance imaging of regional brain activity in patients with intracranial arteriovenous malformations before surgical or endovascular therapy. J Neurosurg 84: 477–483

Mandybur TI, Nazek M (1990) Cerebral arteriovenous malformations. A detailed morphological and dimmunohistochemical study using actin. Arch Pathol Lab Med 114: 970–973

Mansmann U, Meisel J, Brock M, et al (2000) Factors associated with intracranial hemorrhage in cases of cerebral arteriovenous malformation. Neurosurg 46:272–281

Marchal G, Bosmans H, Van Fraeyenhoven L, et al (1990) Intracranial vascular lesions: optimization and clinical evaluation of three-dimensional time-of-flight MR angiography. Radiology 175:443–448

Marks MP, Lane B, Steinberg GK, et al (1990) Hemorrhage in intracerebral arteriovenous malformations: angiographic determinants. Radiology 176:807–813

Marks MP, Lane B, Steinberg GK, Chang P (1991) Vascular characteristics of intracerebral arteriovenous malformations in patients with clinical steal. AJNR Am J Neuroradiol 12:489–496

Marks MP, Lane B, Steinberg GK, et al (1992) Intranidal aneurysms in cerebral arteriovenous malformations: evaluation and endovascular treatment. Radiology 183:355–360

Massoud TF, Hademenos GJ, Young WL, et al (2000) Can induction of systemic hypotension help prevent nidus rupture commplicating cerebral arteriovenous malformation embolization? Analysis underlying mechanisms achieved using a theoretical model. AJNR Am J Neuroradiol 21:1255–1267

Mast H, Mohr JP, Osipov A, et al (1995) „Steal“ is an unestablished mechanism for the clinical presentation of cerebral arteriovenous malformations. Stroke 26:1215–1220

Mast H, Youg WL, Koennecke HC, et al (1997) Risk of spontaneous haemorrhage after diagnosis of cerebral arteriovenous malformation. Lancet 350:1065–1068

Matsubara S, Manzia JL, Terbrugge K, et al (2000) Angiographic and clinical characteristics of patients with cerebral arteriovenous malformations associated with hereditary hemorrhagic telangiectasia. AJNR Am J Neuroradiol 21:1016–1020

Mawad ME, Hilal SK, Michelsen WJ, Stein B, et al (1984) Occlusive vascular disease associated with cerebral arteriovenous malformations. Radiology 153:401–408

McAllister KA, Grogg KM, Johnson DW, et al (1994) Endoglin, a TGF-beta binding protein of endothelial cells, is the gene for hereditary haemorrhagic telangiectasis type 1. Nat Genet 8:345–351

McCormick WF (1966) The pathology of vascular (arteriovenous) malformations. J Neurosurg 24:807–816

Meisel HJ, Mansmann U, Alvarez H, et al (2000) Cerebral arteriovenous malformations and associated aneurysms: analysis of 305 cases from a series of 662 patients. Neurosurgery 46:793–800

Mendelow AD, Erefurth A, Grossart K, et al (1987) Do cerebral arteriovenous malformations increase in size? J Neurol 50: 980–987

Merland JJ, Rufenacht D, Laurent A, et al (1986) Endovascular treatment with isobutyl cyanoacrylate in patients with arteriovenous malformation of the brain: indications, results and complications. Acta Radiol 369:621–622

Minakawa T, Tanaka R, Koike T, et al (1989) Angiographic follow-up study of cerebral arteriovenous malformations with reference to their enlargement and regression. Neurosurgery 24:68–74

Miyasaka Y, Yada K, Ohwada T, Kitahara T (1992) An analysis of the venous drainage system as a factor in hemorrhage from arteriovenous malformations. J Neurosurg 76:239–243

Miyasaka Y, Kurata A, Tanaka, et al (1997) Mass effect caused by clinically unruptured cerebral arteriovenous malformations. Neurosurgery 41:1060–1064

Mobin F, De Salles AA, Abdelaziz O, et al (1999) Stereotactic radiosurgery for arteriovenous malformations: appearance of perinidal T2 hyperintensity signal as a predictor of favorable treatment response. Stereotact Funct Neurosurg 73:50–59

Moret J, Cognard C, Weill A, Castaings L, Rey A (1997) The "remodelling technique" in the treatment of wide-neck intracranial aneurysms. Angiographic results and clinical follow-up in 56 cases. Intervent Neuroradiol 3:21–35

Morgan MK, Johnston IH, Hallinan JM, et al (1993) Complications of surgery for arteriovenous malformations of the brain. J Neurosurgery 78:176–182

Muacevic A, Steiger HJ (1999) Computer-assisted resection of cerebral arteriovenous malformations. Neurosurgery 45: 1164–1170

Munshi I, Macdonald RL, Weir BK (1999) Intraoperative angiography of brain arteriovenous malformations. Neurosurgery 45:491–497

Murayama Y, Vinuela F, Ulhoa A, et al (1998) Nonadhesive liquid embolic agent for cerebral arteriovenous malformations: preliminary histopathological studies in swine rete mirabile. Neurosurgery 43:1164–1175

Murayama Y, Vinuela F, Duckwiler G, et al (1999) Non-adhesive liquid embolic agent for the treatment of cerebral AVM: clinical results at UCLA. Intervent Neuroradiol 5:78

Nakahara I, Taki W, Kikuchi H, et al (1999) Endovascular treatment of aneurysms on the feeding arteries of intracranial arteriovenous malformations. Neuroradiology 41:60–66

Nakstad PH, Nornes H (1994) Superselective angiography, embolisation and surgery in treatment of arteriovenous malformations of the brain. Neuroradiology 36:410–413

Nakstad PH, Bakke SJ, Hald JK (1992) Embolization of intracranial arteriovenous malformations and fistulas with polyvinyl alcohol particles and platinum fibre coils. Neuroradiology 34:348–351

Nataf F, Meder JF, Roux FX, et al (1997) Angioarchitecture associated with haemorrhage in cerebral arteriovenous malformations: a prognostic statistical model. Neuroradiol 39:52–58

Nataf F, Meder JF, Merienne L, et al (1998) Stratégie thérapeutique des malformations artérioveineuses cérébrales. Neurochirurgie 44:83–93

Nataf F, Merienne L, Sclienger M, et al (2001a) Résultats de la série de 705 malformations artério-veineuses cérébrales traitées par radiochirurgie. Neurochirurgie 47:268–282

Nataf F, Merienne L, Schlienger M (2001b) La radiochirurgie des malformations artério-veineuses de grande taille. Neurochirurgie 47:298–303

Nataf F, Ghossoub M, Missir O, et al (2001c) Parenchymal changes after radiosurgery of cerebral arteriovenous malformations. Clinical and MRI data. Neurochirurgie 47:355–368

Nataf F, Meder JF, Oppenheim C, et al (2001d) Radiochirurgie des malformations artério-veineuses cérébrales choroïdiennes et cisternales. Neurochirurgie 47:283–290

Nazek M, Mandybur TI, Kashiwagi S (1988) Oligodendroglial proliferative abnormality associated with arteriovenous malformation: report of three cases with review of the literature. Neurosurgery 23:781–785

Norbash AM, Marks MP, Lane B (1994) Correlation of pressure measurements with angiographic characteristics predisposing to hemorrhage and steal in cerebral arteriovenous malformations. AJNR Am J Neuroradiol 15:809–813

Nornes H,Grip A (1980) Hemodynamic aspects of cerebral arteriovenous malformations. J Neurosurg 53:456–464

Nüssel F, Wegmüller H, Huber P (1991) Comparison of magnetic resonance, angiography magnetic resonance imaging and conventional angiography in cerebral arteriovenous malformation. Neuroradiology 33:56–61

Ogilvy CS, Stieg PE, Awad I, et al (2001) Recommendation for the management of intracranial arteriovenous malformations: a statement for health-care professionals from a special writing group of the Stroke Council, American Stroke Association. Stroke 32:1458–1471

Ondra SL, Troupp H, George ED, et al (1990) The natural history of symptomatic arteriovenous malformations of the brain: a 24-year follow-up assessment. J Neurosurg 73: 387–391

Oppenheim C, Meder JF, Trystram D, et al (1999) Radiosurgery of cerebral arteriovenous malformations: is an early angiogram needed? AJNR Am J Neuroradiol 20:475–481

Osipov A, Koennecke HC, Hartmann A, et al (1997) Seizures in cerebral arteriovenous malformations: type, clinical, course, and medical management. Intervent Neuroradiol 3:37–41

Pan DH, Guo WY, Chung WY, et al (2000) Gamma knife radiosurgery as a single treatment modality for arteriovenous malformations. J Neurosurg 12:113–119

Patan S (1998) TIE1 and TIE2 receptor tyrosine kinases inversely regulate embryonic angiogenesis by the mechanism of intussusceptive microvascular growth. Microvasc Res 56:1–26

Patel V, Gupta SC (1990) Wyburn-Mason syndrome. A case report and review of the literature. Neuroradiology 31: 544–546

Patil A (1997) Recurrent AVMs after negative angiography. J Neurosurg 86:170

Pelz DM, Fox AJ, Vinuela F, Drake CC, Ferguson GG (1988) Preoperative embolization of brain AVMs with isobutyl-2 cyanoacrylate. AJNR Am J Neuroradiol 9:757–764

Pevsner PH (1977)Micro-balloon catheter for superselective angiography and therapeutic occlusion. AJR Am J Roentgenol 128:225–230

Picard L, Moret J, Lepoire J, et al (1984) Endovascular treatment of intracerebral arteriovenous angiomas. Technique, indications and results. J Neuroradiol 11:9–28

Picard L, Bracard S, Anxionnat R, Macho J (1999) Long-term anatomic and clinical outcomes in embolized brain AVMs. World Federation of Interventional and Therapeutic Neuroradiology, Algarve (Portugal)

Picard L, Costa EDA, Anxionnat R, et al (2001) Acute spontaneous hemorrhage after embolization of cerebral arteriovenous malformations with n-butyl cyanoacrylate. J Neuroradiol 28:147–165

Pietila TA, Stendel R, Jansons J, et al (1998) The value of intraoperative angiography for surgical treatment of cerebral arteriovenous malformations in eloquent brain areas. Acta Neurochir (Wien) 140:1161–1165

Pik JHT, Margan MK (2000) Microsurgery for small arteriovenous malformations of the brain: results in 110 consecutive patients. Neurosurgery 47:571–577

Pile-Spellman J, Young WL, Joshi S, et al (1999) Adenosine-induced cardiac pause for endovascular embolization of cerebral arteriovenous malformations: technical case report. Neurosurgery 44:881–887

Piotin M, Ross IB, Weill A, et al (2001) Intracranial arterial aneurysms associated with arteriovenous malformations: endovascular treatment. Radiology 220:506–513

Pollock BE, Lunsford LD, Kondziolka D, et al (1994) Patients' outcome after radiosurgery for "operable" arterio-venous malformations. Neurosurgery 35:1–7

Pollock BE, Flickinger JC, Lunsford LD, et al (1996a) Factors that predict the bleeding risk of cerebral arteriovenous maformations. Stroke 27:1–6

Pollock BE, Kondziolka D, Lunsford LD, et al (1996b) Repeat stereotactic radiosurgery of arteriovenous malformations: factors associated with incomplete obliteration. Neurosurg 38:318–324

Pollock BE, Flickinger JC, Lunsford LD, et al (1998) Factors associated with successful arteriovenous malformation radiosurgery. Radiosurgery 42:1239–1247

Porteous ME, Brun J, Proctor SJ (1992) Hereditary haemorrhagic telangiectasia: a clinical analysis. J Med Genet 29:527–530

Purdy PD, Samson D, Batjer HH, et al (1990) Preoperative embolization of cerebral arteriovenous malformations with polyvinyl alcohol particles: experience in 51 adults. AJNR Am J Neuroradiol 11:501–510

Purdy PD, Batjer HH, Samson D (1991a) Management of hemorrhagic complication from preoperative embolization of arteriovenous malformation. J Neurosurgery 74:205–211

Purdy PD, Batjer HH, Samson D, et al (1991b) Intra-arterial sodium amytal administration to guide pre-operative embolization of cerebral arteriovenous malformations. J Neurosurg Anesth 3:103–106

Putman CM, Chaloupka JC, Fulbright RK, et al (1996) Exceptional multiplicity of cerebral arteriovenous malformations associated with hereditary hemorrhagic telangiectasia (Osler-Weber-Rendu syndrome). AJNR Am J Neuroradiol 17:1733–1742

Puzzilli F, Mastronardi L, Ruggeri A, et al (1998) Eealy surgical treatment of intracerebral hemorrhages caused by AVM: our experience in 10 cases. Reurosurg Rev 21:87–92

Ralls PW, Johnson MB, Radin R, et al (1992) Hereditary hemorrhagic telangiectasia: findings in the liver with color Doppler sonography. AJNR Am J Neuroradiol 159:59–61

Rao VR, Mandalam KR, Gupta AK, et al (1989) Dissolution of isobutyl 2-cyanoacrylate on long-term follow-up. AJNR Am J Neuroradiol 10:135–141

Rauch RA, Vinuela F, Dion J, et al (1992a) Preembolization functional evaluation in brain arteriovenous malformations: The superselective amytal test. AJNR Am J Neuroradiol 13:303–308

Rauch RA, Vinuela F, Dion J, et al (1992b) Preembolization functional evaluation in brain arteriovenous malformations: the ability of superselective Amytal test to predict neurologic dysfunction before embolization. AJNR Am J Neuroradiol 13:309–314

Redekop G, TerBrugge K, Montanera W, et al (1998) Arterial aneurysms associated with cerebral arteriovenous malformations: classification, incidence, and risk of hemorrhage. J Neurosurg 89:539–546

Regis J, Massager N, Levrier O (2001) Traitement radiochirurgical Gamma knife des malformations artério-veineuses du tronc cérébral Neurochirurgie 47:291–297

Roman G, Fisher M, Perl DP, et al (1978) Neurological manifestations of hereditary hemorrhagic telangiectasia (Rendu-Osler-Weber disease): report of two cases and review of the literature. Ann Neurol 4:130–144

Rosenblum MK, BilbaoJM, Ang LC (1996) Central nervous system. In: Rosai J (ed) Ackerman's surgical pathology. Mosby, St Louis, pp 2238–2241

Salcman M, Scholtz H, Numaguchi Y (1992) Multiple intracerebral arteriovenous malformations: report of three cases and review of the literature. Surg Neurol 38:121–128

Sampei K, Hashimoto N, Kazekawa K, et al (1996) Histological changes in brain tissue and vasculature after intracarotid infusion of organic solvents in rats. Neurordiology 38: 291–294

Samson D, Ditmore QM, Beyer CW jr (1981) Intravascular use of isobutyl 2-cyanoacrylate: 1. Treatment of intracranial arteriovenous malformations. Neurosurgery 8:43–51

Sano K, Ueda Y, Saito I (1978) Subarachnoid hemorrhage in children. Childs Brain 4:38–46

Sasaki T, Kurita H, Saito I, et al (1998) Arteriovenous malformations in the basal ganglia and thalamus: management and results in 101 cases. J Neurosurg 88:285–292

Sato TN, Tozawa Y, Deutshc U, Wolburg-Buchholz K, et al (1995) Distinct roles of the receptor tyrosine kinases Tie-1 and Tie-2 in blood vessel formation. Nature 376:70–74

Schaller C, Schramm J, Haun D (1998) Significance of factors contributing to surgical complications and to late outcome after elective surgery of cerebral arteriovenous malformations. J Neurol Neurosurg Psychiatry 65:547–554

Schlienger M, Atlan D, Lefkopoulos D, et al (2000) Linac radiosurgery for cerebral arteriovenous: results in 169 patients. Int J Radiat Biol Phys 46:1135–1142

Schlienger M, Merienne L, Lefkopoulos D, et al (2001) Réirradiation des malformations artérioveineuses cérébrales. Neurochirurgie 47:324–331

Schlosser MJ, Mc Carthy G, Fulbright RK, et al (1997) Cerebral vascular malformations adjacent to sensorimotor and visual cortex. Stroke 28:1130–1137

Schumacher M, Horton JA (1991) Treatment of cerebral arteriovenous malformations with PVA: results and analysis of complications. Neuroradiology 33:101–105

Serbinenko FA (1974) Balloon catheterization and occlusion of major cerebral vessels. J Neurosurg 41:125–145

Shalaby F, Rossant Y, Yamaguchi TP, Gertsenstein M, WU XF, et al (1995) Failure of blood-island formation and vasculogenesis in Flk-1 deficient mice. Nature 376:62–66

Shovlin CL, Hughes JM, Scott J, Seidman CE, Seidman JG (1997) Characterization of endoglin and identification of novel mutations in hereditary hemorrhagic telangiectasia. Am J Hum Genet 61:68–79

Sisit MB, Kader A, Stein BM (1993) Microsurgery for 67 intracranial arteriovenous malformations less than 3 cm in diameter. J Neurosurg 65:476–483

Smith HJ, Strother CM, Kikuchi Y, et al (1988a) MR imaging in the management of supratentorial intracranial AVMs. AJR Am J Roentgenol 150:1143–1153

Smith HJ, Strother CM, Kikuchi Y, et al (1988b) MR imaging in the management of supratentorial intracranial AVMs. AJNR Am J Neuroradiol 9:225–235

Sobel D, Norman D(1984) CNS malformations of hereditary hemorrhagic telangiectasia. AJNR Am J Neuroradiol 5: 569–573

Sorimachi T, Takeuchi S, Koike T, et al (1995) Blood pressure monitoring in feeding arteries of cerebral arteriovenous malformations during embolization: a preventive role in hemodynamic complication. Neurosurgery 37:1041–1048

Spetzler RF, Martin NA (1986) A proposed grading system for arteriovenous maformations. J Neurosur 65:476–483

Spetzler RF, Wilson CB, Weinstein P, et al (1978) Normal perfusion pressure breakthrough theory. Clin Neurosurg 25: 651–672

Spetzler RF, Martin NA, Carter LP, et al (1987) Surgical management of large AVMs by staged embolization and operative excision. J Neurosurg 67:17–28

Spetzler RF, Hargraves RW, McCormick PW, et al (1992) Relationship of perfusion pressure and size to risk of hemorrhage from arteriovenous malformations. J Neurosur 76: 918–923

Stapf C, Mohr JP (2000) New concepts in adult brain arteriovenous malformations. Curr Opin Neurol 13:63–67

Stapf C, Mohr JP, Sciacca RR, et al (2000) Incident hemorrhage risk of brain arteriovenous malformations located in the arterial border zones. Stroke 31:2365–2368

SteinbergGK, Levy RP, Marks MP, et al (1993) Charged-particle radiosurgery. In: Alexander E III, Loeffler JS, Lunsford LD (eds) Stereotactic radiosurgery. McGraw Hill, New York, pp 122–134

Steiner L (1988) Stereotactic radiosurgery with the cobalt-60 gamma unit in the surgical treatment of intracranial tumor and cerebral arteriovenous malformations. In: Schmidek HH, Sweet WH (eds) Operative neurosurgical techniques. Grune and Stratton, New York, pp 515–529

Steiner L, Lindquist C, Adler JR, et al (1992) Outcome of radiosurgery for cerebral AVM. J Neurosurg 77:823

Steiner L, Lindquist C, Cail W, et al (1993) Microsurgery and radiosurgery in brain arteriovenous malformations. J Neurosurg 79:647–652

Takano K, Utsunomiya H, Ono H, et al (1999) Dynamic contrast-enhanced subtraction MR angiography in intracranial vascular abnormalities. Eur Radiol 9:1909–1912

Takeuchi S, Kikuchi H, Karasawa J, Naruo Y, et al (1987) Cerebral hemodynamics in arteriovenous malformations: evaluation by single-photon emission CT. AJNR Am J Neuroradiol 8:193–197

Taki W, Kikuchi H, Iwata H, et al (1990) Embolization of arteriovenous malformations using EVAL mixture (a new liquid embolization material). Neuroradiology 33s:195–196

Terada T, Nakamura Y, Nakai K, Tsuura M, et al (1991) Embolization of arteriovenous malformations with peripheral aneurysms using ethylene vinyl alcohol copolymer: report of three cases. J Neurosurg 75:655–660

The Arteriovenous Malformation Study Group (1999) Arteriovenous malformations of the brain in adults. N Engl J Med 340:1812–1818

Theron J, Newton TH, Hoyt WF(1974) Unilateral retinocephalic vascular malformations. Neuroradiology 7:185–196

Thompson RC, Steinberg GK, Levy RP, et al (1998) The management of patients with arteriovenous malformations and associated intracranial aneurysms. Neurosurgery 43: 202–212

Turjman F, Massoud TF, Vinuela F, et al (1994) Aneurysms related to cerebral arteriovenous malformations: superselective andiographic assessment in 58 patients. AJNR Am J Neuroradiol 15:1601–1605

Turjman F, Massoud TF, Vinuela F, et al (1995a) Correlation of the angioarchitectural features of cerebral arteriovenous malformations with clinical presentation of hemorrhage. Neurosurgery 37:856–860

Turjman F, Massoud TF, Sayre JW, et al (1995b) Epilepsy associated with cerebral arteriovenous malformations: a multivariate analysis of angioarchitectural characteristics. AJNR Am J Neuroradiol 16:345–350

U HS, Kerber CW, Todd MM (1992) Multimodality treatment of deep periventricular cerebral arteriovenous malformations. Surg Neurol 38:192–203

Uranischi R, Baev NI, Ng PY, Kim JH, Awad IA (2001) Expression of endothelial cell angiogenesis receptors in human cerebrovascular malformations. Neurosurgery 48:359–367

Vikingstad EM, Cao Y, Thomas AJ, et al (2000) Language hemispheric dominance in patients with congenital lesions of eloquent brain. Neurosurg 47:562–570

Vinters HV, Galil KA, Lundie MJ, et al (1985) The histotoxicity of cyaoacrylates. Neuroradiology 27:279–291

Vinters HV, Lundie MJ, Kaufmann JCE (1986) Long-term pathological follow-up of cerebral arteriovenous malformation treated by embolization with bucrylate. N Engl J Med 314:477–483

Vinuela F (1992) Functional evaluation and embolization of intracranial arterio-venous malformations. In: Vinuela F, Van Halbach V, Dion J (eds) Interventional neuroradiology, endovascular therapy of the central nervous system. Raven, New York, pp 77–86

Vinuela F, Debrun GM, Fox AJ, et al (1983a) Dominant-hemisphere arteriovenous malformations: therapeutic embolization with isobutyl-2-cyanoacrymate. AJNR Am J Neuroradiol 4:959–966

Vinuela F, Fox AJ, Debrun G, et al (1983b) Progressive thrombosis of brain arteriovenous malformations after embolization with isobutyl-2 cyanoacrylate. AJNR Am J Neuroradiol 4: 1233–1238

Vinuela F, Fox AJ, Debrun G, et al (1984) Preembolization superselective angiography: role in the treatment of brain arteriovenous malformations with isobutyl-2 cyanoacrylate. AJNR Am J Neuroradiol 5:765–769

Vinuela F, Fox AJ, Pelz D, et al (1986) Angiographic follow-up of large cerebral AVMs incompletely embolized with isobutyl-2 cyanoacrylate. AJNR Am J Neuroradiol 7:919–925

Vinuela F, Dion JE, Duckwiler G, et al (1991) Combined endovascular embolization and surgery in the management of cerebral arteriovenous malformations: experience with 101 cases. J Neurosurg 75:856–864

Wada J, Rasmussen T (1960) Intracarotid injection of sodium amytal for the lateralization of cerebral speech dominance: experimental and clinical observations. J Neurosurg 17: 266–282

Wallace RC, Flom RA, Khayata MH, et al (1995) The safety and effectiveness of brain arteriovenous malformation embolization using acrylic and particles: the experiences of a single institution. Neurosurgery 37:606–618

Warren DJ, Hoggard N, Radatz MWR, et al (2001) Cerebral arteriovenous malformations: comparison of novel magnetic resonance angiographic techniques and conventional catheter angiography. Neurosurgery 48:973–983

Wikholm K, Taki W, Lwata H, et al (1995) Occlusion of cerebral arteriovenous malformations with N-butyl cyano-acrylate is permanent. AJNR Am J Neuroradiol 16:479–482

Wikholm K, Lundqvist C, Svendsen (1996) Embolization of cerebral arteriovenous malformations, part I. Technique, morphology, and complications. Neurosurgery 39:448–459

Willemse RB, Mager JJ, Westermann CJ, et al (2000) Bleeding risk of cerebrovascular malformations in hereditary hemorrhagic telangiectasia. J Neurosurg 92:799–784

Willinsky RA, Lasjaunias, Terbrugge K, et al (1988) Malformations arterio-veineuses cérébrales. J Neuroradiol 15: 225–237

Willinsky RA, Lasjaunias P, Terbrugge K (1990) Multiple cerebral arteriovenous malformations (AVMs): review of our experience from 203 patients with cerebral vascular lesions. Neuroradiology 32:207–210

Wilms G, Goffin J, Plets C, Van Calenbergh F, Van Hemelrijck J, Van Aken H, Baert AL (1993) Embolization of arteriovenous malformations of the brain: preliminary experience. J Belge Radiol 76:299–303

Wong JH, Awas IA, Kim JH (2000) Ultrastructural pathological feature of cerebrovascular malformations: a preliminary report. Neurosurgery 46:1454–1459

Yakes WF, Krauth L, Ecklund J, Swengle R, et al (1997) Ethanol endovascular management of brain arteriovenous malformations: initial results. Neurosurgery 40:1145–1154

Yamamoto M, Jimbo M, Ide M, et al (1992) Long-term follow-up of radiosurgically treated arterio-venous malformations in children. Surg Neurol 38:95–100

Yamamoto Y, Coffey RJ, Nichols DA, et al (1995) Interim report on the radiosurgical treatment of cerebral arteriovenous malformations. The influence of size, dose, time and technical factors on obliteration rate. J Neurosurg 83: 832–837

Yamashita K, Taki W, Iwata H, et al (1994) Characteristics of ethylene vinyl alcohol copolymer (EVAL) mixtures. AJNR Am J Neuroradiol 15:1103–1105

Yasargil MG (1988) Deep central AVMs. In: Yasargil MG (ed) Microneurosurgery IIIB. AVM of the brain. Clinical considerations, general and special operative techniques, surgical results, nonoperated cases, cavernous and venous angiomas, neuroanesthesia. Thieme, Stuttgart, pp 204–368

Yokoyama K, Asano Y, Murakawa T, Takada M (1991) Familial occurrence of arteriovenous malformation of the brain. J Neurosurg 74:585–589

Young WL, Kader A, Pile-Spellman J, et al (1994a) Columbia University AVM study project: Arteriovenous malformations draining vein physiology and determinants of transnidal pressure gradients. Neurosurgery 35:389–396

Young WL, Pile-Spellman J, Prohovnik I, et al (1994b) Columbia University AVM study project: evidence for adaptive autoregulatory displacement in hypotensive cortical territories adjacent to arteriovenous malformations. Neurosurgery 34:601–611

Young WL, Kader A, Ornstein E, et al (1996) Cerebral hyperemia after arteriovenous malformations resection is related to "breakthrough" complications but not to feeding artery pressure. Neurosurgery 38:1085–1095

4 Dural Arteriovenous Malformations

I. Szikora

CONTENTS

4.1 Pathology

4.1.1 Definition

Dural arteriovenous malformations (DAVMs), first described by Sachs and Tonnis (Aminoff 1973), are defined as abnormal connections ("shunts") between the arterial and the venous side of the vascular tree located on the surface of the dura mater. Arterial supply is provided by meningeal branches, and either dural sinuses or meningeal or subarachnoid veins drain the lesions. By definition, DAVMs are located within the dura, most frequently on the wall of or immediately around the venous sinuses (Fig. 4.1a). The currently used terminology is not uniform. The term malformation is used to express the frequent "spontaneous" etiology of these lesions and to describe similarities with brain or spine arteriovenous malformations (AVM). However, this term involves the developmental origin of the lesion, which is probably not the case with DAVM. While some of them are connatal, the majority seem to be acquired. To avoid confusion, many authors use the term dural arteriovenous fistula (DAVF). This may be more appropriate concerning etiology, but it implies a single type of morphology (fistula) and therefore is less adequate in this regard. As of today, both terms are used in the literature without indicating either a certain etiologic origin or a particular angioarchitecture of the lesion. In this chapter, the term DAVM will be used as the general name of the pathology.

I. Szikora, MD, PhD
National Institute of Neurosurgery, Amerikai ut 57, 1025 Budapest, Hungary

4.1.2 Etiology, Pathogenesis

Dural AVMs are relatively rare lesions, constituting approximately 10%–15% of all intracranial vascular malformations (Newton and Cronqvist 1969). Originally, these lesions were thought to be congenital (Aminoff 1973). Coincidence with other vascular anomalies, such as aneurysms (Kaech et al. 1987; Murai et al. 1999; Friedman et al. 2000; Suzuki et al. 2000), intradural arteriovenous fistulae (Ratliff and Voorhies 1999), brain arteriovenous AVM (Lasjaunias and Berenstein 1987; Yamada et al. 1993) and others (Hieshima et al. 1977; Yamada et al. 1993) has also been reported, pointing towards a congenital origin of the lesions.

However, many DAVMs have been proved to be acquired. It is hypothesized that DAVMs develop

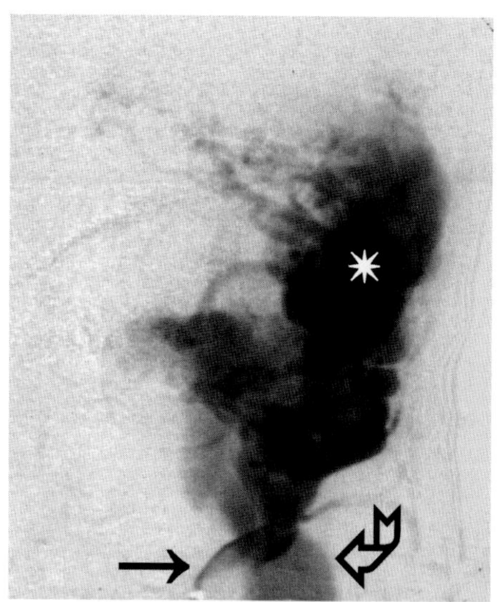

Fig. 4.1a–e. Pathomorphology of dural arteriovenous malformations. **a** Selective digital subtraction angiography (DSA) of a DAVM (*asterisk*) involving the sigmoid sinus on the left. Left occipital artery injection (*arrow*), anteroposterior (AP) view. The DAVM is drained by the ipsilateral jugular vein (*broken arrow*). **b** Macroscopic image of the same DAVM taken during autopsy. The sigmoid sinus on the left is opened (*arrow*). Spongy, fibrous material (*broken arrow*) fills the lumen of the involved segment of the sinus. **c** Lumen of the sigmoid sinus following removal of the fibrous material. **d** Microscopic section of the spongy tissue removed from the sinus, demonstrating multiple cross sections of thin-walled sinusoidal vascular structures (*arrows*) within fibrous proliferating tissue (hematoxylin-eosin stain, +40). **e** Cross section of a large vessel with irregular elastic laminae (*arrowheads*). The lumen is filled with organizing thrombus, containing cross sections of newly formed blood vessels (*arrows*) representing neovascularization

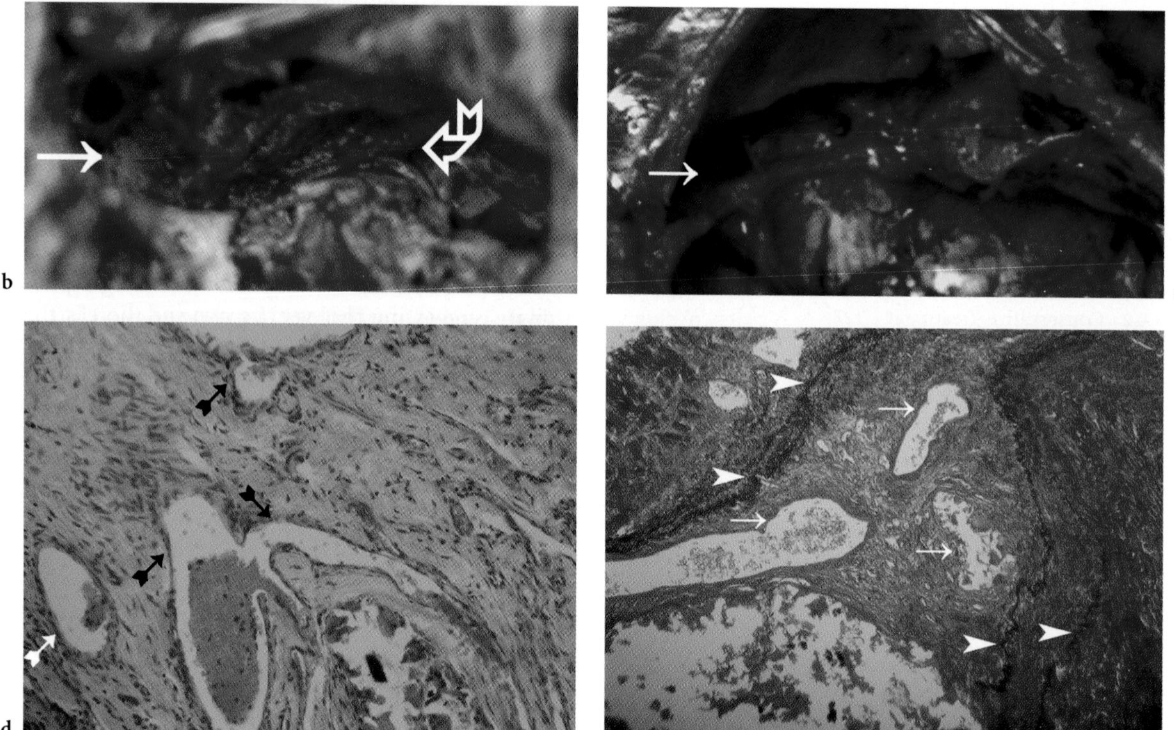

either (1) by opening of existing microshunts within the dura or (2) by angioneogenesis, leading to the development of new shunts. The triggering factor for the development of DAVM is thought to be a change of the normal arteriovenous pressure gradient within the dura. Either elevation of the arterial pressure (arterial hypertension) or increase of the venous pressure (venous obstruction) may dilate existing arteriovenous communications, leading to hemodynamically significant shunts. While the predisposing factor for the development of a permanent DAVM remains unknown, several events may increase the venous pressure and serve as a trigger. These include developmental anomalies of the venous system, venous thrombosis, head trauma, or transcranial surgery (Watanabe et al. 1984). It is presumed that head trauma caused by either surgery or injury may induce venous thrombosis or at least alteration of the venous outflow, subsequently resulting in changes of the arteriovenous pressure gradient (LASJAUNIAS and BERENSTEIN 1987). The frequent coincidence of DAVMs with previous major surgery (other than transcranial) and child delivery suggests that increased systemic thrombotic activity may serve as a trigger, too. Dural AVMs occurring in association with pregnancy and the menopausal period suggest that hormonal changes may also play a role, potentially by inducing increased angiogenesis (DJINDJAN and MERLAND 1978).

4.1.2.1
Venous Occlusive Disease

Dural AVMs are frequently associated with stenosis or occlusion of the draining dural sinuses (DJINDJAN and MERLAND 1978). In 1979, Houser reported two cases of DAVM that developed years after documented sinus thrombosis (HOUSER et al. 1979). Later, Chaudhary demonstrated the development of DAVM in patients following head trauma (CHAUDHARY et al. 1982). They proposed that sinus thrombosis might be the primary factor leading to the development of a DAVM. During the normal recanalization process, arteries within the sinus wall penetrate the intraluminal organizing thrombus, establishing a communication between mural arteries and the lumen of the sinus. A number of publications have since reported association of sinus thrombosis or sinus occlusive disease and DAVM (AL-MEFTY et al. 1986; CONVERS et al. 1986; BARNWELL et al. 1991; PIEROT et al. 1993; COGNARD et al. 1998). Significant controversy exists, however, as to whether thrombosis is the cause or the result of DAVM.

Some observations suggest that dural sinus thrombosis is the primary factor leading to the development of DAVM. This hypothesis seems to be substantiated by findings related to increased thrombotic activity in some patients. Prothrombin gene mutation was found in a patient who developed sinus thrombosis and later DAVM (SINGH et al. 2001). The most frequent cause of venous thrombotic disease, resistance to activated protein C (APCR), was detected with significantly higher prevalence in patients with DAVM as compared with normal controls. In addition, factor V Leyden was found in these patients as a result of a mutation in factor V gene (KRAUS et al. 1998, 2000).

On the other hand, several studies have reported nonthrombotic occlusion of the dural sinuses as the primary cause in the pathogenetic process. Occlusion of the sinuses due to the direct compression of tumors (ARNAUTOVIC et al. 1998) or due to the surgical sacrifice of the sinus during tumor removal may equally result in development of DAVM as late as up to 7 years following surgery (SAKAKI et al. 1996). These later findings suggest that venous congestion and hypertension, rather than sinus thrombosis, lead to dural AV shunts. To check this assumption a number of animal experiments were recently carried out. In rats, surgically induced venous hypertension by artificial carotid-jugular fistula and proximal jugular vein ligation resulted in development of arteriovenous malformations, one of them located on a dural sinus (TERADA et al. 1994). A combination of significant (three- to sixfold) increase of the venous pressure (by ligation of the draining vein of the transverse sinus) and artificially induced superior sagittal sinus thrombosis resulted in arteriovenous fistulae that developed within the dura near the thrombosed section of the sinus. However, a direct connection between the fistula and the thrombus was found in only half of the cases (HERMAN et al. 1995). In another series of experiments, superior sagittal sinus thrombosis was induced in all animals, with or without venous hypertension. Angiogenic activity of the dura mater adjacent to the thrombosed section of the sinus was tested and found to be positively correlated with venous hypertension but was not correlated with sinus thrombosis. Development of dural AV fistulae correlated positively with both venous hypertension and increased angiogenic activity, suggesting that venous hypertension is the primary etiologic factor in the development of DAVM (LAWTON et al. 1997). Evidence of increased angiogenic activity was found in association with DAVM in human beings, too. Surgically excised specimens were studied that had been removed from patients harboring DAVMs associated with sinus thrombosis. The subendothelial and medial layer of the sinus wall as well as the wall of proliferating vessels and connective tissue around the involved sinuses expressed basic fibroblast growth factor (bFGF) on immunohistochemical staining. The endothelium of the sinus expressed vascular endothelial growth factor (VEGF) (URANISHI et al. 1999).

Although this study proves the role of increased vasogenic activity in the development of human DAVM, it does not provide information regarding the cause of such increased activity. As DAVMs, particularly those involving the cavernous sinus, have a high incidence in women in the menopausal age, the potential role of hormonal changes has also been investigated, but it remains unclear. Sudden decrease of blood estradiol levels was implicated as a precipitating factor in cavernous sinus DAVM in women (KURATA et al. 1999). In contrast, ovariectomy with or without estrogen therapy did not induce an increased rate of DAVM formation in experimental rats (Terada et al. 1998).

4.1.2.2 Histopathology

Most histopathological studies demonstrate thickening of the dura and intensive vascular proliferation within and around the wall of the involved sinus. In some cases, a spongy mass of fibrous tissue can be found inside lumen of the sinus. This mass contains numerous irregular vascular spaces (Graeb and Dolman 1986) (Fig. 4.1). Increasing evidence suggests that the primary arteriovenous shunt exists within the wall of the sinus, with secondary shunting between the venous side of the proliferating vascular network and the lumen of the sinus. In several studies a mass of dilated small dural vessels was found in subendothelial location within the sinus wall. Multiple microshunts were seen connecting those dural arteries and veins with each other (Nishijima et al. 1992; Momoji et al. 1997). One study demonstrated arteriovenous connections within the sinus wall via small abnormal vessels of approximately 30 µm in diameter ("crack-like vessels"). Histologically, these vessels were proven to be veins (Hamada et al. 1997). Larger openings (approximately 200 µm) provided connection between intramural veins and the lumen of the sinus (Momoji et al. 1997). On the other hand, signs of organized thrombus and neovascularization were confirmed in only a few of the studied cases (Sakaki et al. 1996). The location of the arteriovenous shunts within the dura and the sinus wall may explain why some DAVMs drain into major dural sinuses, others into meningeal veins, yet others directly into subarachnoid veins adjacent to sinuses.

4.1.2.3 Pathogenesis

The etiology and pathogenesis of DAVM is still not fully understood. It is now generally accepted that DAVMs are acquired lesions. It has been postulated that even DAVMs presenting in infants are not congenital, but rather connatal, and develop during the fetal period in response to venous obstruction (Lasjaunias and Berenstein 1987). Increasing evidence suggests that the primary pathogenetic factor is venous hypertension related to either thrombotic or nonthrombotic reduction of venous outflow. Significant increase of venous pressure may lead to opening of existing microshunts within the dura. Such microshunts have been proposed previously by Kerber intracranially and by Manelfe intraspinally (Manelfe et al. 1972; Kerber and Newton 1973). Alternatively, venous hypertension results in cerebral hypoperfusion and ischemia. This may secondarily produce sprouting vasogenesis and the development of arteriovenous shunts within the adjacent meninges (Lawton et al. 1997). Sinus thrombosis maybe one of the primary factors leading to venous hypertension and initiating the vicious circle that leads to a DAVM. In those cases predisposing factors for venous thrombosis, such as hypercoagulopathy, trauma, or surgery, may play an etiologic role. Alternatively, sinus thrombosis may occur secondary to DAVM by several mechanisms. The growing mass of proliferating vessels within the sinus wall may gradually narrow its lumen, leading to either stenosis or occlusion of the sinus.

Fast and/or turbulent arterial flow within the sinus due to existing DAVM may result in intimal injury, secondary hyperplasia, and sinus stenosis or occlusion. In some cases the two mechanisms may be involved simultaneously. In a case reported by Wakamoto, angiographically proven sinus thrombosis resulted in venous infarction without an arteriovenous shunt. A DAVM developed 4 months later (presumably as a result of sinus thrombosis), at which time the sinus has already recanalized. The DAVM persisted and resulted in rethrombosis of the sinus within another year (Wakamoto et al. 1999).

Venous thrombosis has been proposed as the most probable pathogenetic mechanism for spinal DAVMs, although minor venous anomalies have also been recognized in such patients that may serve as predisposing factors (McCutcheon et al. 1996).

The behavior of sinus thrombosis may impact the natural history of an individual lesion. Cessation of venous hypertension by complete recanalization of the thrombosed sinus will interrupt the vicious circle and may lead to spontaneous cure of the disease. Progressive thrombosis or occlusion of the venous outflow channels may further increase venous hypertension, however, leading to an aggressive clinical course (Lawton et al. 1997).

4.1.3 Morphology

Dural AVMs consist of arterial feeders and draining venous structures with or without an intervening mesh of small vessels. Arterial supply is primarily by periosteal and meningeal arteries but in large DAVMs enlarged collaterals from cutaneous or even subarachnoid branches may also contribute. The feeding pedicles are connected with the draining venous structure via single or multiple holes between those vessels (fistulae, Fig. 4.2a) or through a tangle of small abnormal vascular channels (nidus, Fig. 4.2b). This later corresponds to the thick, fibrous sections of the dura that is rich in vascular channels, as seen on pathological specimens (Fig. 4.1d). The shunt is drained either by one of the dural sinuses, or by meningeal or subarachnoid veins, or both. Single or multiple narrowing or occlusion of the dural sinus system frequently results in rerouting of the venous outflow. In some DAVMs with meningeal or subarachnoid venous drainage enlarged varices or venous lakes are seen on the venous side. Arterial aneurysms may develop on the feeding pedicles or elsewhere on the cerebral arteries.

Concerning spinal DAVM, Kendall introduced the concept that the majority of spinal intradural AVMs are actually enlarged arterialized draining veins of dural AVMs (Kendall and Logue 1977). This has been confirmed by microangiography studies of surgically removed specimens demonstrating dural branches of the radiculomedullary arteries that feed a network of small vessels within the dura. This network is connected directly (without a capillary bed) to the draining vein, usually an enlarged intradural, perimedullary vein (McCutcheon et al. 1996). Spinal DAVMs may also drain into periosteal and epidural veins (Borden et al. 1995; McCutcheon et al. 1996).

4.1.4 Location

DAVMs may occur anywhere within the cranium or in the spinal column. Intracranial DAVMs are located either in the anterior cranial fossa on or around the ethmoid groove (Fig. 4.3, 1), in the middle cranial fossa at the cavernous sinuses (Fig. 4.3, 2), in the posterior fossa at the transverse (Fig. 4.3, 3) or the sigmoid (Fig. 4.3/4) sinuses, at the confluens sinuum (Fig. 4.3, 5), or around the foramen magnum (Fig. 4.3, 6). DAVMs are found on the base (Fig. 4.3, 7) and at the free margin of the tentorium (Fig. 4.3, 8). Lesions of the straight sinus or the vein of Galen are rare (Fig. 4.3, 9) (Halbach et al. 1989). Finally, DAVMs are found on the dura of the convexity and at the superior sagittal sinus (not demonstrated in Fig. 4.3). In a meta-analysis of 258 published cases, Lucas found 26% on the cavernous sinus, 25% on the transverse and sigmoid sinuses, 26% at the tentorial incisura, 11% on the convexity and superior sagittal sinus, 9% in the anterior fossa, and 4% in the middle fossa outside of the cavernous sinus (Lucas et al. 1997). Multiple lesions are found in 7%–8 % of all cases (Barnwell et al. 1991; Fujita et al. 2001; van Dijk et al. 2002). DAVMs of the anterior fossa may drain into frontal veins and the olfactory vein; lesions of the cavernous sinus drain either into the superior ophthalmic vein, the contralateral cavernous sinus, the inferior petrosal sinus(es) or into temporal subarachnoid veins. Venous drainage for transverse

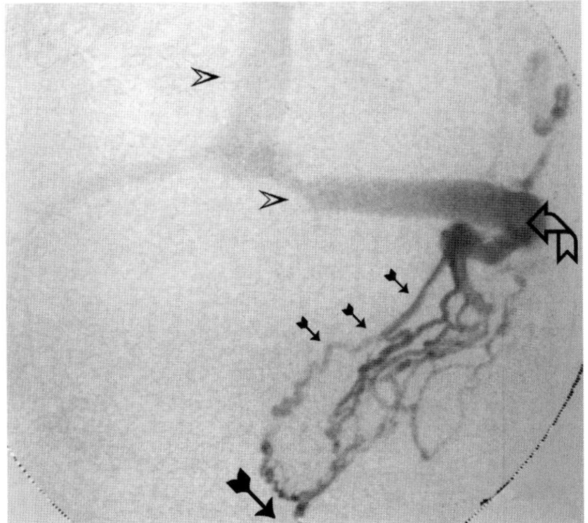

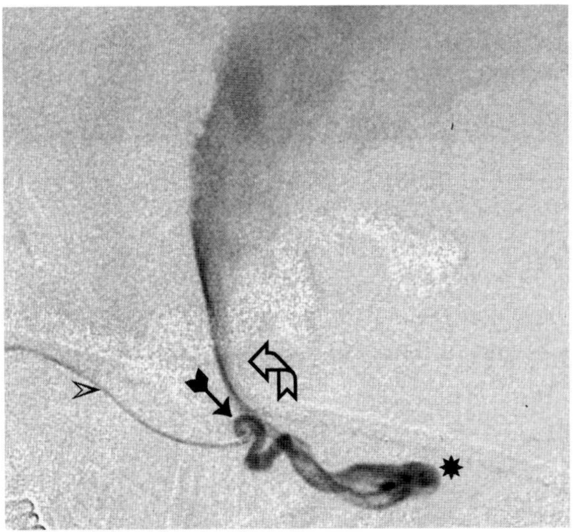

Fig. 4.2a, b. Morphological characteristics of the arteriovenous shunt within DAVMs. **a** Plexiform nidus. DSA, superselective injection of the middle meningeal artery (*arrow*) supplying a DAVM involving the left sigmoid sinus (*broken arrow*), AP view. Arteriovenous shunt is established via a meshwork of small vessels (*small arrows*). The ipsilateral sigmoid sinus is occluded. Note reflux into the transverse sinuses and the superior sagittal sinus (*arrowheads*). **b** Direct arteriovenous fistula. DSA, superselective injection of a middle meningeal artery feeder (*arrow*) draining directly (*asterisk*) into an extremely enlarged transverse sinus (*broken arrow*). Lateral view

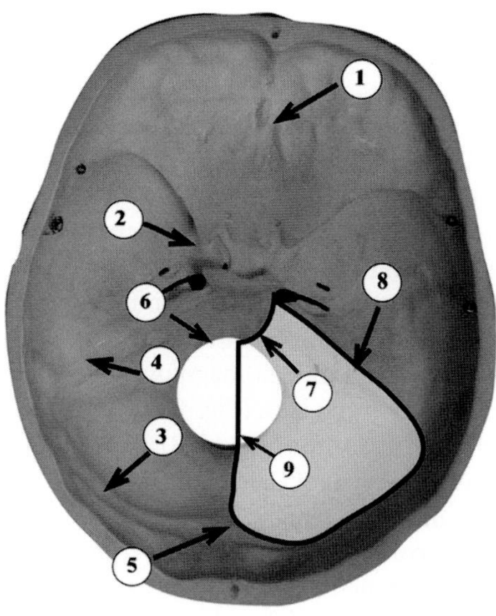

Fig. 4.3. Typical locations of intracranial DAVMs. *1* anterior fossa, *2* cavernous sinus, *3* transverse sinus, *4* sigmoid sinus, *5* confluens sinuum, *6* foramen magnum, *7* tentorial incisura, *8* base of the tentorium, *9* straight sinus and vein of Galen

Table 4.1. Venous drainage pathways of intracranial DAVM in different locations

Location	Potential venous drainage pathway
Anterior fossa	Olfactory vein, frontal veins
cavernous sinus	Contralateral cavernous sinus, ophthalmic veins, inferior petrosal sinus, temporal veins
Transverse, sigmoid sinus	Sigmoid sinus, jugular vein, straight sinus, superior sagittal sinus, temporal occipital veins
Confluens sinuum	Superior sagittal sinus, transverse sinuses, straight sinus, occipital veins, temporal veins
Tentorium	Superior petrosal sinus, petrous vein, tentorial veins, vein of Rosenthal, lateral mesencephalic vein, spinal perimedullary veins
Foramen magnum	Clival venous plexus, spinal perimedullary veins

and sigmoid sinus DAVMs may be provided by the ipsi- or contralateral or bilateral transverse-sigmoid sinus – internal jugular vein system and/or temporal subarachnoid veins, mainly the vein of Labbé. Lesions at the confluens sinuum drain into both or either one of the transverse sinuses, into the superior sagittal sinus in a retrograde fashion or into occipital or temporal subarachnoid veins. DAVMs of the tentorium are connected with either the superior petrosal sinus, the petrous vein, tentorial veins, or the basal vein of Rosenthal. Shunts located around the tentorial incisura may drain into lateral mesencephalic veins and into spinal epidural veins. Lesions located around the foramen magnum and on the clivus drain into the clival venous plexus and towards spinal epidural veins (Lasjaunias and Berenstein 1987) (Table 4.1).

Spinal DAVMs are considered the most common spinal vascular malformations, constituting 80% of all spinal AVMs (Anson and Spetzler 1992; Lee et al. 1998). The majority of these lesions are located in the thoracolumbar region.

4.1.5 Hemodynamics

The rate of flow through a DAVM is related to the size of the draining venous system. Direct fistulae on patent sinuses may have exceedingly high flow; others, particularly those with small venous channels, such as many cavernous sinus and spinal dural fistulae demonstrate slow flow. In theory, both the arterial steal phenomenon and increased venous pressure can be implicated as hemodynamic effects of DAVMs. Clinically, elevated venous pressure seems to be the single most important hemodynamic effect that is related to the venous outflow pattern and largely independent from the flow rate. Reduced regional cerebral blood flow (rCBF) and increased regional cerebral blood volume (rCBV) were demonstrated by single photon emission computerized tomography (SPECT) and positron emission tomography (PET), indicating venous congestion and impaired cerebral perfusion in cases with retrograde cortical venous drainage and sinus occlusion. These hemodynamic effects were not related to the flow rate of the fistula (Tanimoto et al. 1984; Kawaguchi et al. 2000).

4.2 Clinical Presentation

4.2.1 Signs and Symptoms

Intracranial DAVMs are rare in infancy and childhood (Boet et al. 2001; Kincaid et al. 2001). In adults they present mostly in middle-aged or elderly patients with a mean age of 50–60 years. Spinal

DAVMs commonly present after the 4th decade. Men and women are equally affected except for cavernous sinus fistulae, which have a significantly higher incidence in women (85% of all lesions) (COGNARD et al. 1995). Clinical signs and symptoms most commonly associated with DAVM include pulsatile tinnitus, objective bruit, cranial nerve palsies, ocular symptoms including proptosis and chemosis ("red eye"), optic nerve atrophy, papilledema, headaches, nausea and/or vomiting as signs of elevated intracanial pressure (ICP), epileptic seizures, focal neurological deficit, and intracranial hemorrhage. High-flow fistulae that typically present in infants and children may lead to heart failure. Hydrocephalus may also develop mostly in children with fast-flow lesions. Symptoms are strongly related to the location and hemodynamic pattern of the lesion. Table 4.2 summarizes the most typical symptoms of each DAVM location. Potential pathomechanisms include venous congestion, perfusion deficit due to venous hypertension, mass effect, and arterial steal phenomenon (LASJAUNIAS et al. 1986). As a general rule, involvement of leptomeningeal veins in venous drainage is associated with increased incidence of hemorrhagic and nonhemorrhagic neurological complications and therefore is considered an indicator of aggressive clinical course (see later). This is thought to be related to high pressure within subarachnoid veins, leading to venous rupture and subarachnoid hemorrhage (SAH), and/or venous ischemia, resulting in venous infarction and subsequent parenchymal hemorrhage.

Dural AVMs in the anterior fossa frequently present with intradural bleeding, likely caused by the obligate leptomeningeal venous drainage in this condition (Fig. 4.4).

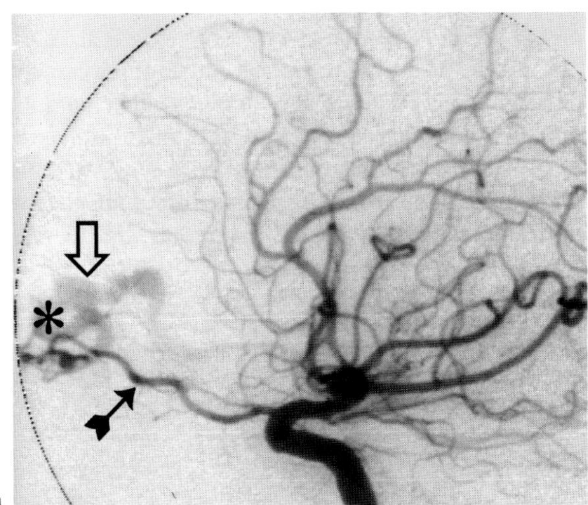

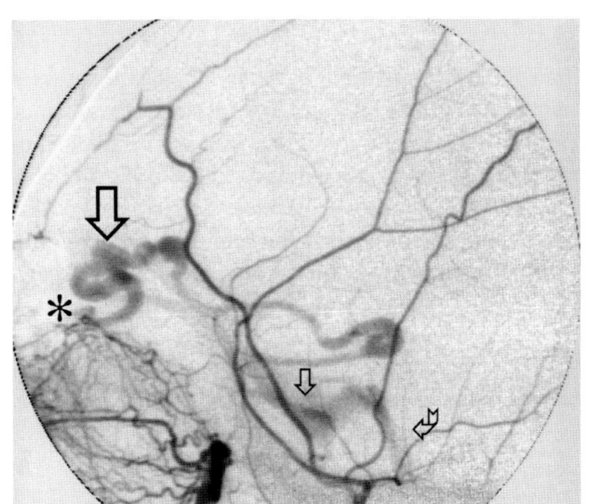

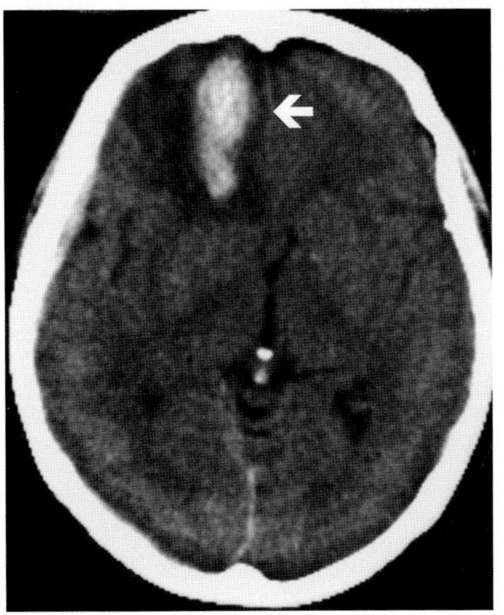

Fig. 4.4a–c. DAVM located in the anterior fossa. **a** Right internal carotid artery injection. DSA, lateral view, demonstrating DAVM fed by an ethmoidal branch of the ophthalmic artery (*arrow*) and drained by a frontal vein (*open arrow*). **b** Right external carotid artery injection of the same DAVM demonstrating arterial supply from ethmoidal branches of the distal internal maxillary artery and venous drainage via the cavernous sinus (*small open arrow*) and the inferior petrosal sinus (*small broken arrow*). **c** Computer tomography of the same patient demonstrating parenchymal hemorrhage (*arrow*) within the right frontal lobe

Table 4.2. Characteristic signs and symptoms associated with DAVMs in different locations

	ICH	Bruit	Pulsatile tinnitus	Ocular palsy	"Red eye"	Nonocular cranial nerve	Headaches	Seizures	Papilledema	Neurological deficit
Anterior fossa	+						+			
Cavernous sinus		+	+	+	+		+			+
Transverse-sigmoid sinuses	+	+	+				+	+	+	
Confluens sinuum	+	+	+				+	+	+	
Tentorium	+		+			+	+		+	
Straight sinus and vein of Galen			+				+	+	+	+
Foramen magnum	+		+			+	+		+	+
Convexity	+						+	+		+
Superior sagittal sinus							+	+	+	+
Spinal										+

Cavernous sinus DAVMs have a characteristic clinical presentation including proptosis, chemosis (Fig. 4.5a,b), ocular movement disorder due to sixth and/or third nerve palsy, leading to double vision, retinal hemorrhages, reduced vision, pulsatile tinnitus, and bruit. Most of those symptoms are related to venous overload of the primary draining veins, namely the superior ophthalmic vein (SOV) and the inferior petrosal sinus (Fig. 4.5c, d). Congestion in the SOV results in chemosis, proptosis, and retinal hemorrhage and is probably involved in visual loss due to hypoperfusion of the optic nerve and the retina. Fast arterialized flow within the SOV leads to bruit that can be detected over the eye. Involvement of the inferior petrosal sinus, if present, produces pulsatile tinnitus. Cranial nerve paresis leading to ocular movement disorder can be explained by mass effect within the cavernous sinus and the orbit, although arterial steal phenomenon has also been mentioned as a potential cause (Lasjaunias et al. 1986). Thrombosis of the major venous outlets of the cavernous sinus may occur, further aggravating symptoms. Rerouting of the venous flow toward the contralateral cavernous sinus results in contralateral eye symptoms (Fig. 4.5e). Venous drainage via temporal veins maybe associated with neurological symptoms and in rare cases with hemorrhage (Fig. 4.5f, i).

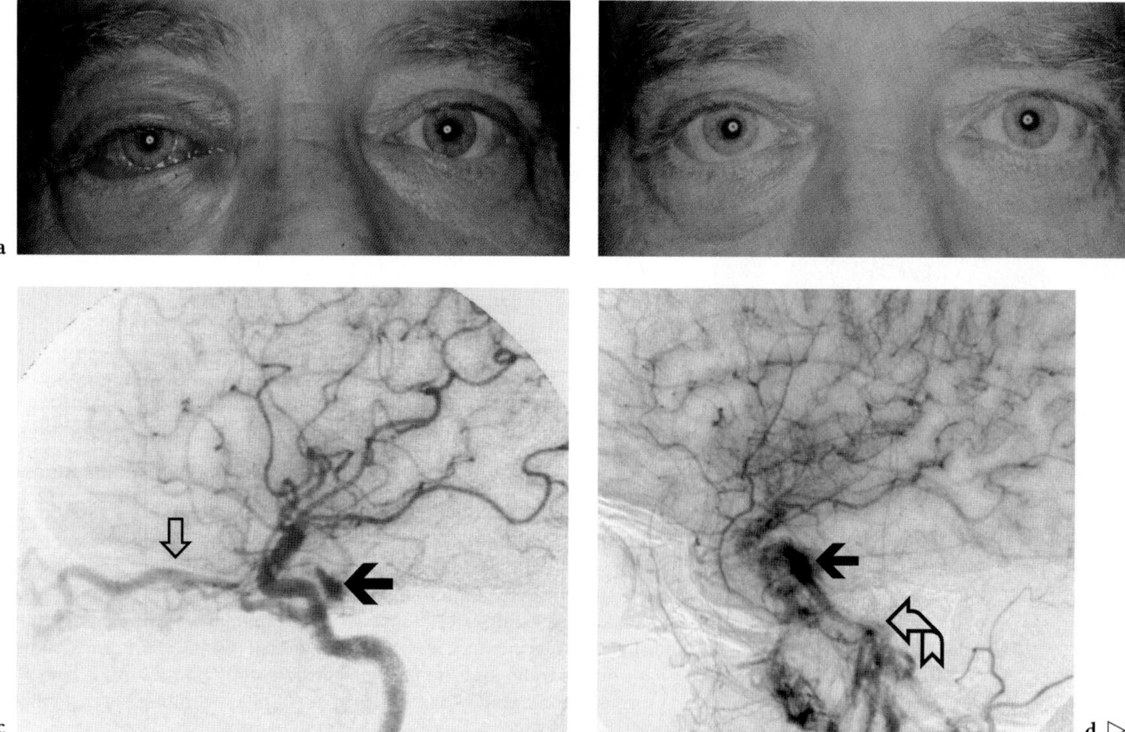

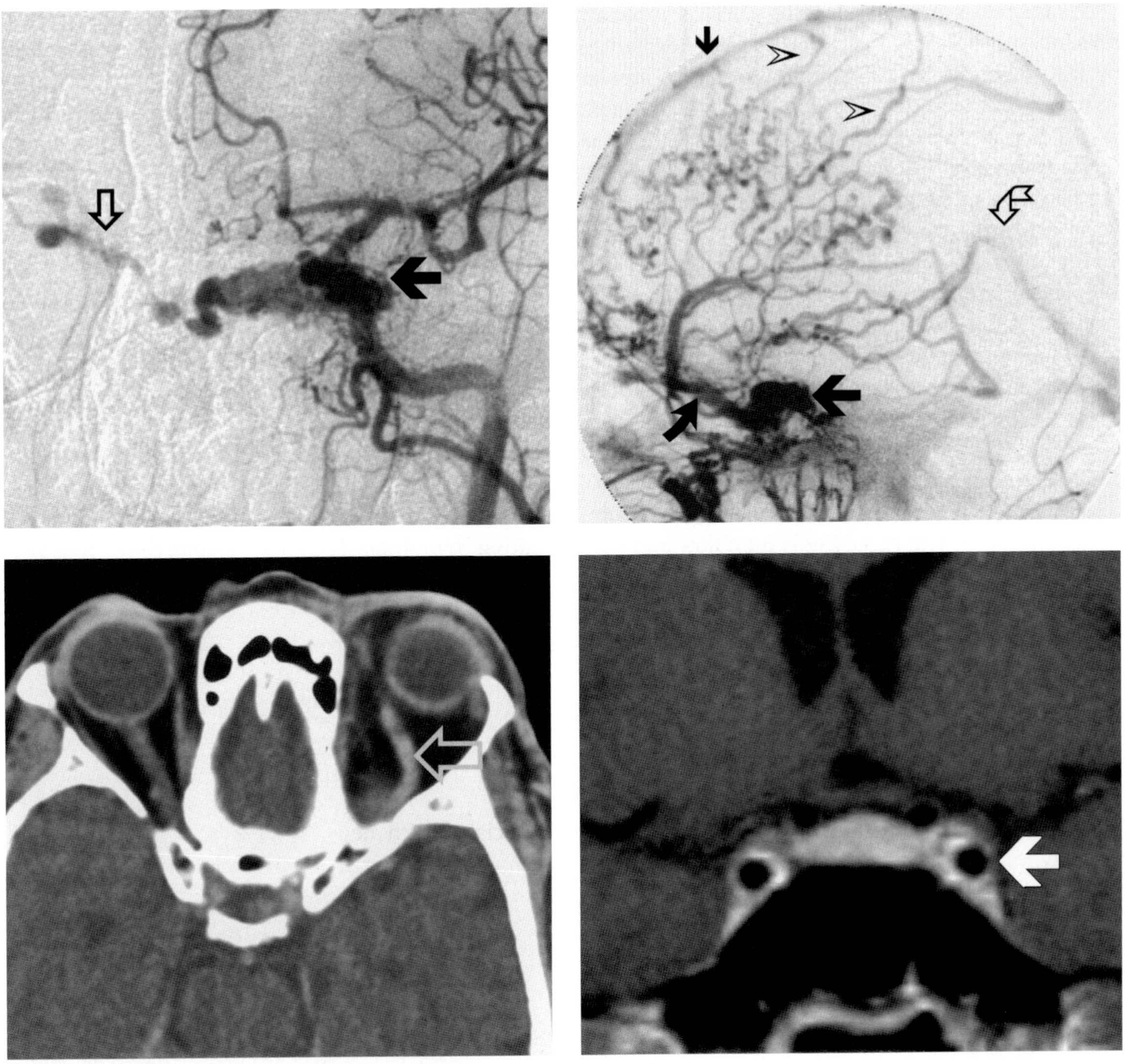

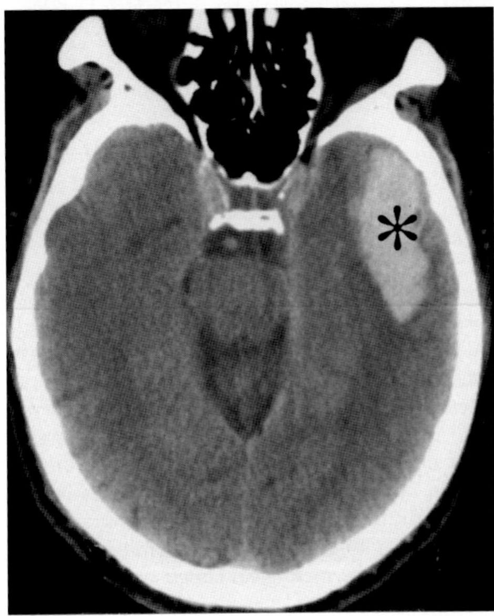

Fig. 4.5a–i. Clinical and radiomorphological characteristics of cavernous sinus (CS) DAVM. **a** Typical ocular signs of CS DAVM on the right, including moderate exophthalmos, chemosis, and conjunctival hyperemia ("red eye"). **b** Resolution of the ocular signs following successful treatment of the lesion. **c** Typical angiographic appearance of CS DAVM (*arrow*) with exclusive venous drainage via the superior ophthalmic vein (SOV) (*open arrow*). DSA, internal carotid artery (ICA) injection, lateral view. **d** Venous drainage of a CS (*arrow*) DAVM via the inferior petrosal sinus (*broken arrow*). Note that the SOV is not opacified. DSA, ICA injection, lateral view. **e** Cavernous sinus DAVM drained via the intercavernous sinus and the contralateral SOV (*open arrow*). DSA, common carotid artery (CCA) injection, AP view. **f** Cortical venous drainage of a CS DAVM (*arrow*) via the sylvian vein (*curved arrow*) and multiple frontal cortical veins (*arrowheads*) towards the superior sagittal sinus (*small arrow*) and the vein of Labbé (*broken arrow*). **g** Contrast-enhanced CT scan of the patient demonstrated in **c**, exhibiting an enlarged SOV that intensely enhances with contrast material (*open arrow*). **h** Magnetic resonance image (MRI) of the same patient: T_1-weighted (T_1-W) coronal section following contrast administration demonstrates an enlarged CS (*arrow*). **i** Noncontrast CT scan of the patient demonstrated in **f** depicting left temporal lobe hemorrhage (*asterisk*)

Transverse and sigmoid sinus DAVMs typically present with pulsatile bruit that is easily explained by fast flow within the sigmoid sinus and jugular vein close to the middle ear (Fig. 4.6a). The frequent association of either contra- or ipsilateral occlusion of the transverse or sigmoid sinuses leads to rerouting of venous flow towards the contralateral transverse sinus, the superior sagittal sinus and/or into leptomeningeal veins. This may result in elevated venous and intracranial pressure and subsequent papilledema, neurological symptoms, seizures, and optic nerve atrophy (Fig. 4.6b). High-flow fistulae typically involve this region in infants and children. The resulting extreme enlargement of the sinus may cause mass effect, chronic venous hypertension, and communicating hydrocephalus (Fig. 4.6c).

Similarly, DAVMs involving the confluens sinuum tend to be large, with exceedingly high flow and with reflux into the straight and superior sagittal sinuses, producing frequent hemorrhagic and nonhemorrhagic neurological complications (Fig. 4.7).

DAVMs located on the tentorium frequently bleed; this is thought to be related to the typical leptomeningeal venous drainage of this region (Fig. 4.8).

Lesions in the posterior fossa, and particularly that of the clivus and the foramen magnum, may have a very special clinical presentation. As some of them tend to drain into spinal perimedullary veins, they typically produce spinal venous hypertension. The resulting hypoperfusion of the spinal cord results in myelopathy and subsequent neurological deficit (Woimant et al. 1982; Cognard et al. 1995; Brunereau et al. 1996; Ricolfi et al. 1999; Slaba et al. 2000; Reinges et al. 2001). Most patients present with a long history of slowly progressing and fluctuating symptoms (Fig. 4.9). Hemorrhage has also

a

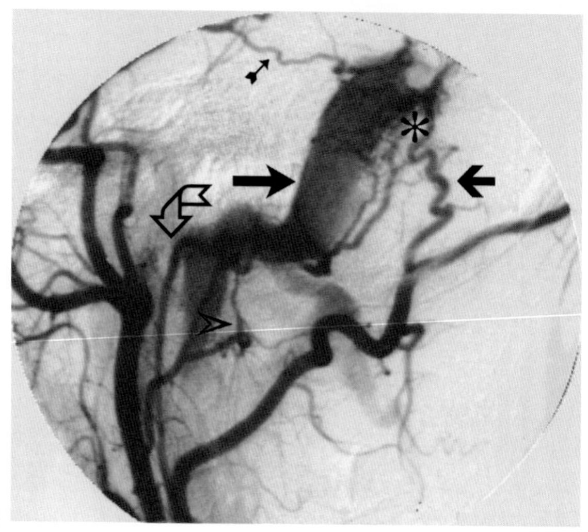

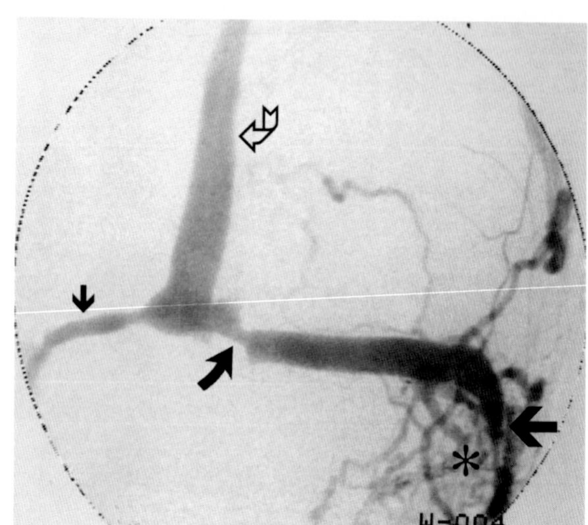

b

c

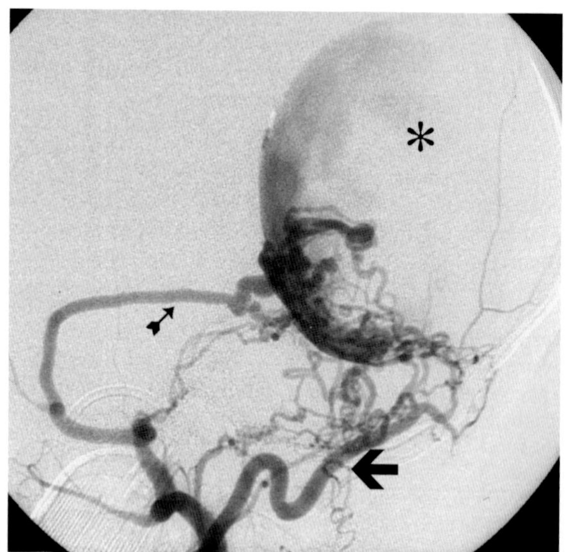

Fig. 4.6a–c. Angiographic features of DAVMs involving the transverse and sigmoid sinuses. **a** DSA, external carotid artery (ECA) injection, lateral view, demonstrating a sigmoid sinus (SS) DAVM (*asterisk*). Venous drainage is antegrade via SS (*large arrow*). Multiple feeding pedicles of the middle meningeal (*small arrow*), the occipital (*arrow*), the ascending pharyngeal (*broken arrow*), and the retroauricular (*arrowhead*) arteries are delineated. **b** DSA of an SS DAVM (*asterisk*) with ECA injection in AP view. The SS is occluded (*arrow*). Venous drainage is retrograde. Note severe stenosis of the ipsi- (*curved arrow*) and contralateral (*small arrow*) transverse sinuses (TS) and reflux into the superior sagittal sinus (SSS) (*broken arrow*). **c** DSA in lateral view, ECA injection delineating an extensive DAVM draining into an ectatic transverse sinus (*asterisk*). Patient is a 10-month-old baby. Prominent feeders arise from the middle meningeal (*small arrow*) and the occipital (*arrow*) arteries

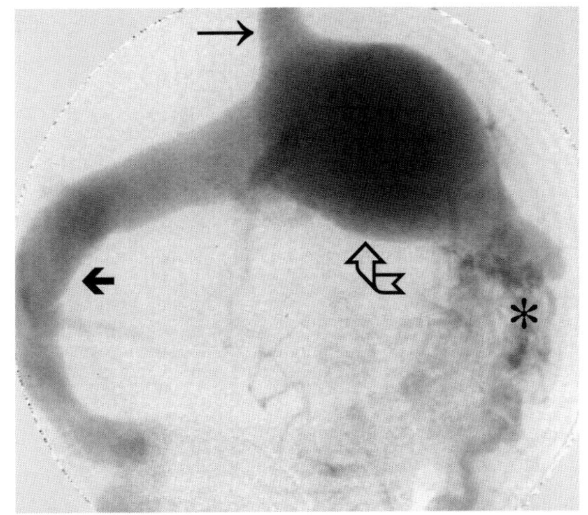

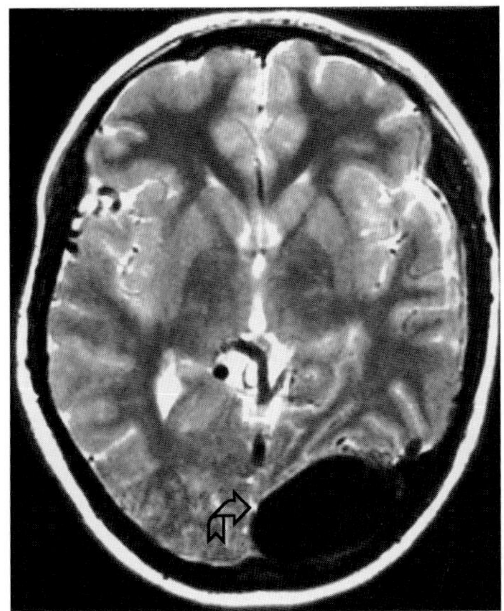

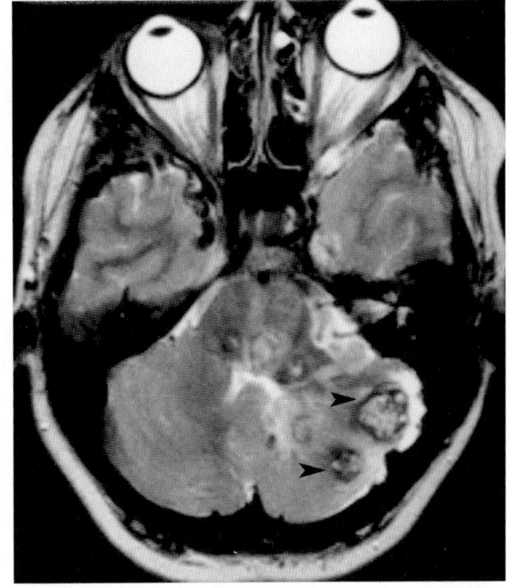

Fig. 4.7a–c. Dural arteriovenous malformation involving the confluens sinuum. **a** The medial segment of the transverse sinus is extremely enlarged (*broken arrow*). The sinus ectasia involves the confluens sinuum. The sigmoid sinus on the left is occluded (*asterisk*). Note reflux into the SSS (*arrow*) and retrograde flow within the contralateral transverse sinus (*small arrow*). **b** T_2-W MRI demonstrates dilatation of the TS with mass effect. **c** T_2-W MRI depicting multiple areas of mixed signal intensity within the cerebellum (*arrowheads*) corresponding to repeated small hemorrhages due to significant venous hypertension and perfusion deficit

been reported in cases of spinal epidural drainage (Cognard et al. 1995).

Arteriovenous malformations of the superior sagittal sinus produce a complex neurological picture. These lesions tend to be morphologically complex with multiple arterial feeders and high flow. Subsequently, the venous overload is significant, resulting in highly elevated intracranial pressure, headaches, papilledema, visual disturbances, progressive dementia, neurological deficits, and seizures. Sinus thrombosis is frequently associated, leading to bizarre venous flow patterns. Occlusion of the superior sagittal sinus itself leads to retrograde venous drainage via subependymal veins. These patients typically present with headaches and progressive dementia (Jaillard et al. 1999). Occlusion of the transverse sinuses will reroute venous flow into cortical veins and into the straight sinus. Blood may eventually exit the cranium via the superior ophthalmic vein (producing exophthalmos and bruit) and via perimesencephalic veins towards the spinal perimedullary venous system. Ectatic draining veins may produce a mass effect on the brain stem or the spinal cord, further complicating the neurological course (Fig. 4.10).

Arteriovenous shunts on the dura of the convexity commonly present with hemorrhage due to the obligate leptomeningeal venous drainage (Fig. 4.11).

Spinal DAVMs are rare. These lesions produce slowly progressing symptoms of spinal myelopathy, including weakness, gait disturbances, sensory deficit of the lower extremities, and sphincter dysfunction, thought to be a result of the venous hypertension and resulting hypoperfusion. Symptoms typically develop in a slow and fluctuating fashion, frequently delaying the diagnosis significantly (Stecker et al. 1996; Kataoka et al. 2001) (Fig. 4.12).

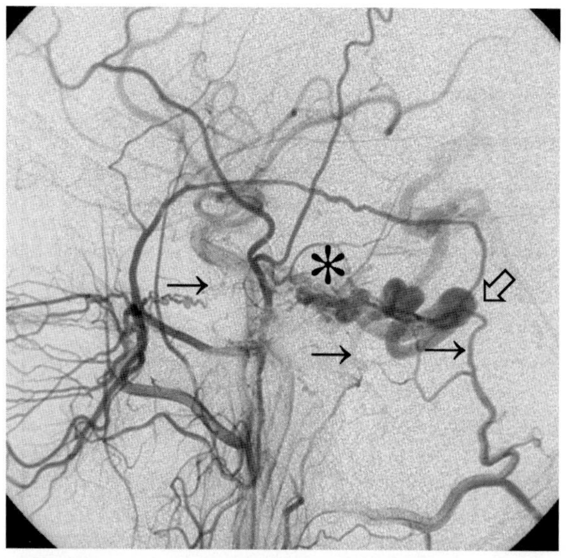

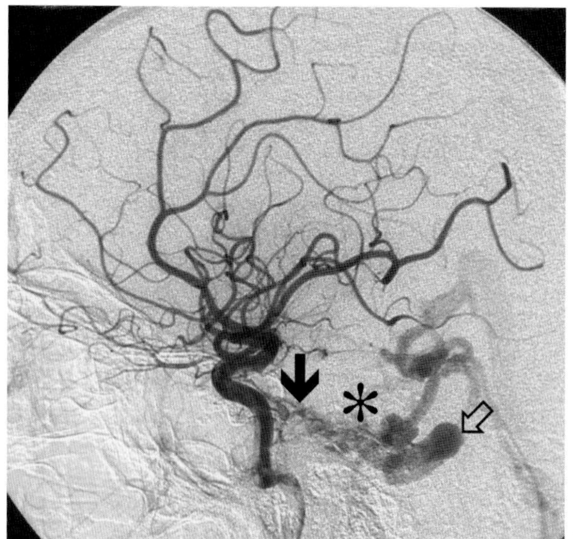

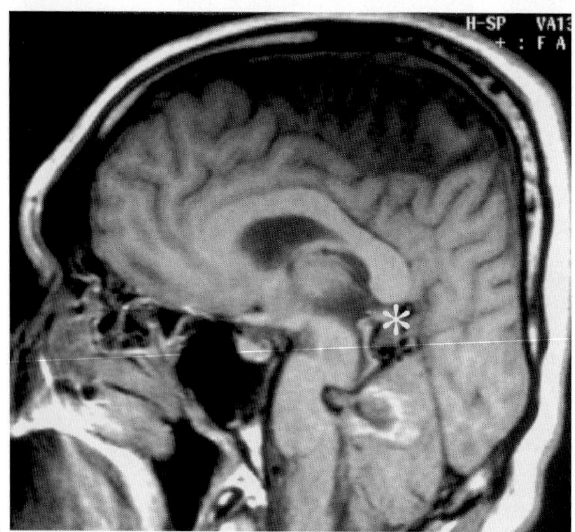

Fig. 4.8a–e. Radiomorphological characteristics of DAVMs involving the tentorium. **a** and **b** DSA, ECA (**a**) and ICA (**b**) injection, lateral view. The DAVM (*asterisk*) is located in the tentorial incisura and drains directly into an enlarged leptomeningeal vein (*open arrow*) towards the straight sinus. Arterial supply is provided by multiple ECA branches (*small arrows*) and the tentorial marginal branch of the ICA (*arrow*). **c** and **d** demonstrate location of the DAVM (*asterisk*), the draining vein, and its dilated segment (*open arrow*) within the tentorial incisura with mass effect on the cerebellum. **e** Noncontrast CT scan of the same patient demonstrates perifocal hemorrhage around the dilated draining vein (*broken arrow*)

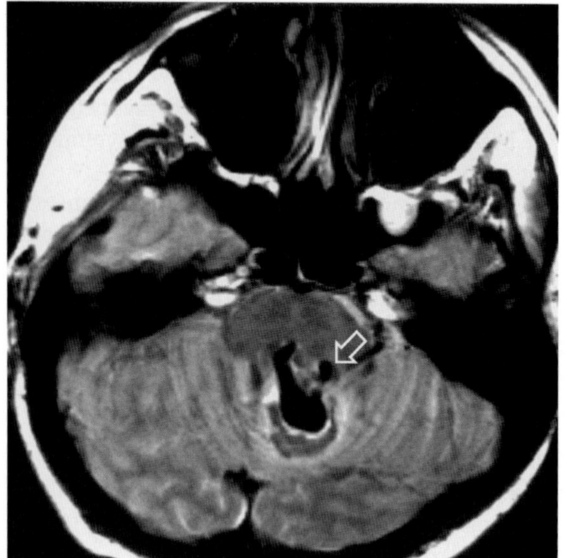

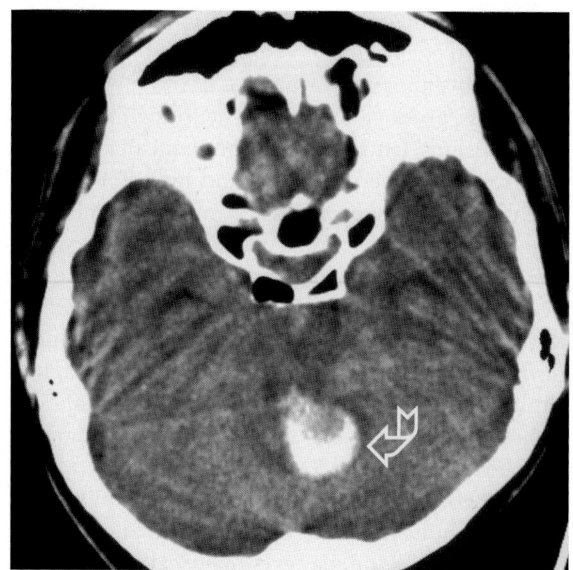

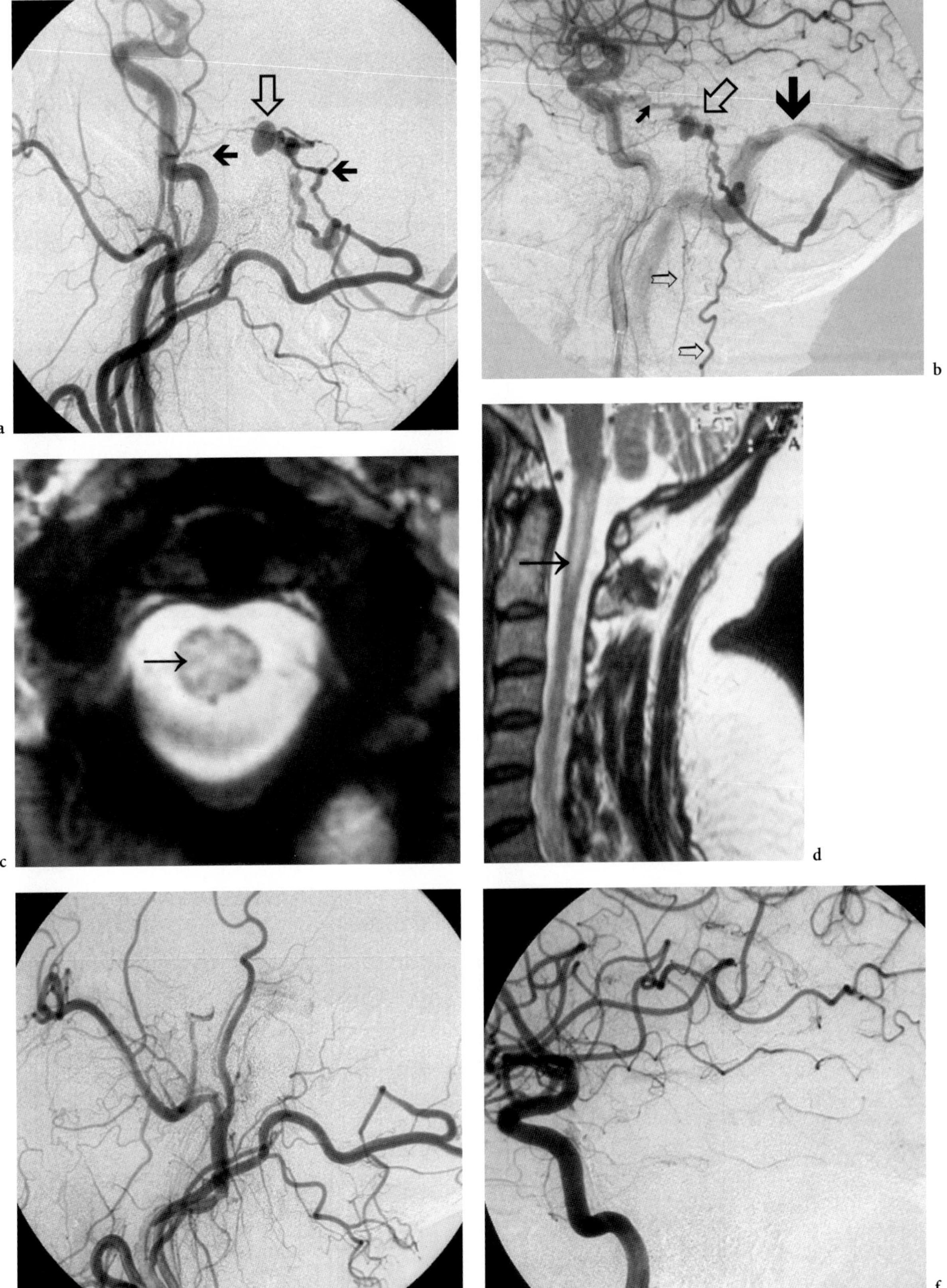

Fig. 4.9a–f. Dural AVM of the posterior fossa with spinal perimedullary drainage. **a** and **b** Common carotid injection, lateral view. Multiple ECA branches (*arrows*) and the tentorial marginal branch of the ICA (*small curved arrow*) feed an arteriovenous connection with a venous varix (*open arrow*). Narrow, irregular vein drains the DAVM towards the transverse sinus (*large arrow*) and pontomesencephalic veins into anterior and posterior intradural spinal veins (*small open arrows*). **c** and **d** Noncontrast, T_2-W axial (**c**) and sagittal (**d**) MRI images demonstrating hyperintense signal within the medulla, representing venous ischemia (*arrow*). **e** and **f** Post-treatment ECA (**e**) and ICA (**f**) angiograms demonstrating complete occlusion of the malformation following embolization from all feeders with diluted cyanoacrylate glue (Histoacryl)

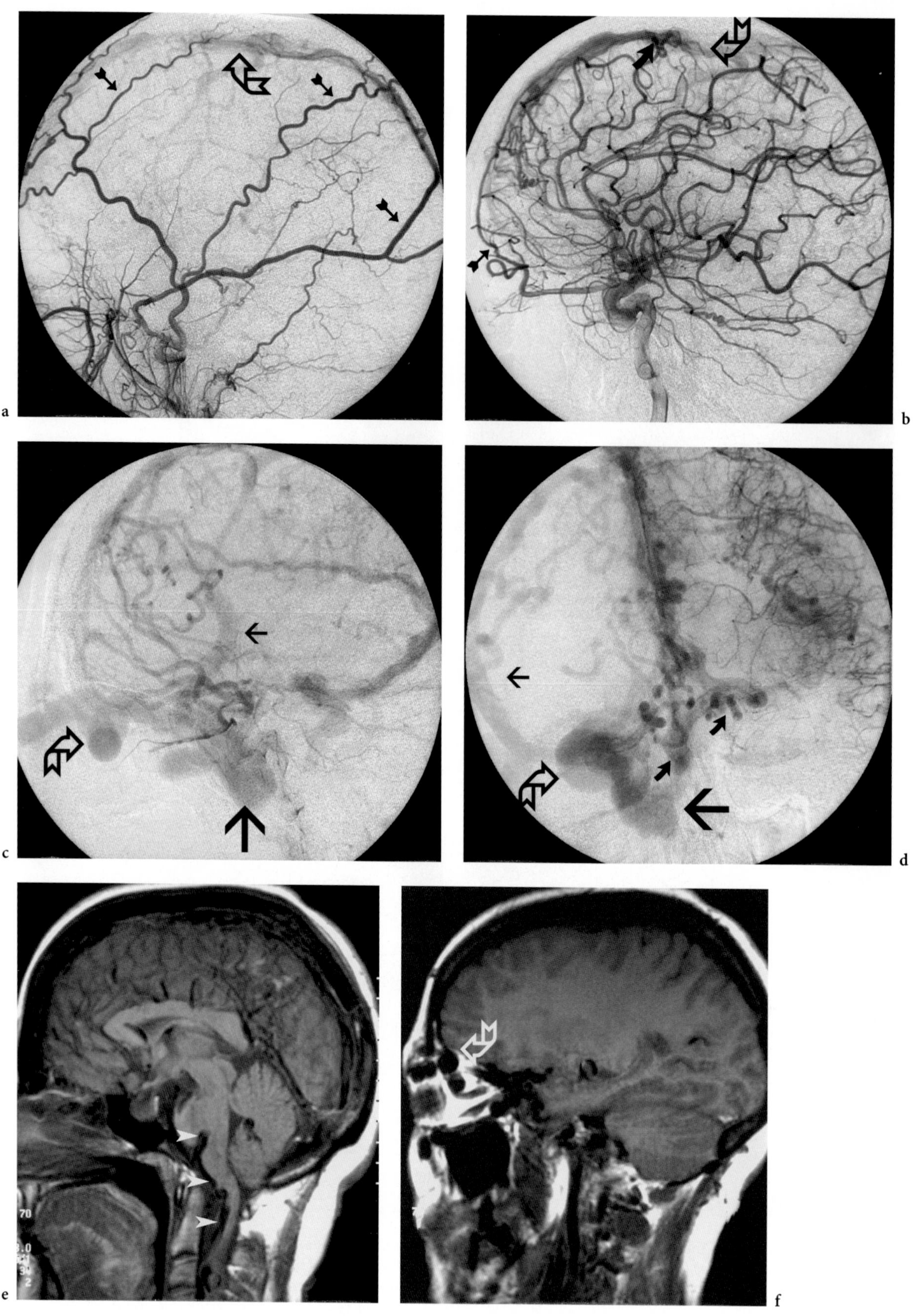

Fig. 4.10a–f. Dural arteriovenous malformation of the superior sagittal sinus with significant venous occlusive disease. **a** and **b** DSA with selective ECA and ICA injections in lateral view demonstrates intense filling of the SSS (*broken arrow*) in the arterial phase from multiple ECA feeders including transosseal branches of the superficial temporal and branches of the middle meningeal artery (*small arrows* in **a**), from the anterior meningeal artery (*small arrow* in **b**) and from subarachnoid branches of the anterior cerebral artery (*small curved arrow*). **c** and **d** Left ICA injection, late venous phase, lateral (**c**) and AP (**d**) views. Both transverse sinuses are occluded. Anteriorly, venous drainage is provided by a large frontal cortical vein (*small arrow*) and the sylvian vein into cavernous sinus. An extremely dilated SOV (*broken arrow*) drains the CS. Posteriorly, retrograde flow is seen within the straight sinus and the vein of Labbé draining into a large pontomesencephalic vein (*small curved arrows*) and spinal perimedullary veins. **e** and **f** MRI study, T_1-W sagittal sections depicting the giant SOV (*broken arrow*) producing exophthalmos and the large pontomesencephalic vein with severe mass effect on the brain stem and the spinal cord (*arrowheads*)

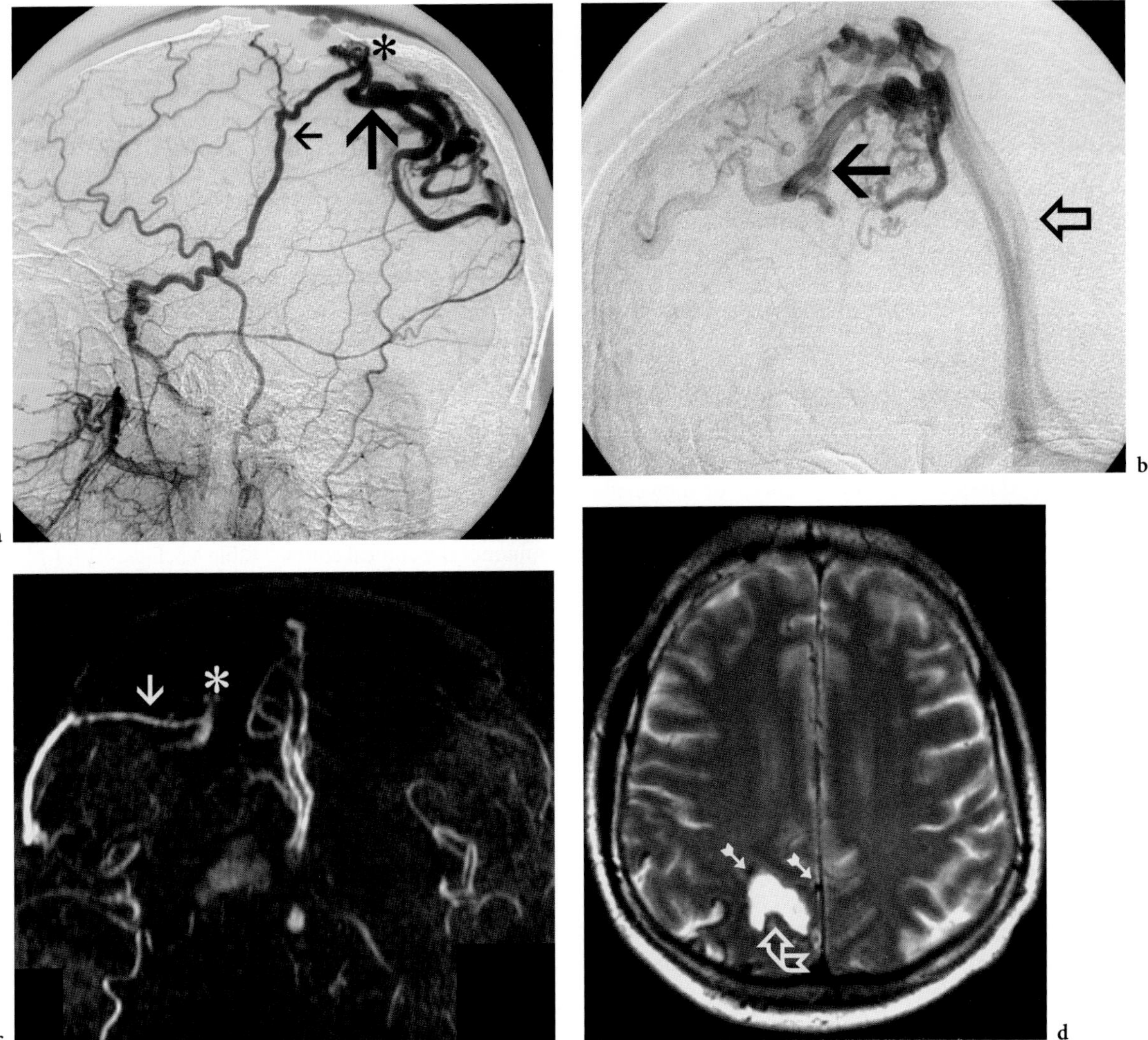

Fig. 4.11a–d. Dural AVM of the convexity. **a** and **b** Direct communication (*asterisk*) between the middle meningeal artery (*arrow*) and a tortuous leptomeningeal vein of the frontal convexity (*large arrow*) close to the superior sagittal sinus (*open arrow*). **c** Time of flight (TOF) magnetic resonance angiography (MRA), maximum intensity projection (MIP), delineates the feeding pedicle (*small arrow*) and arteriovenous shunt (*asterisk*). **d** T_2-W MRI demonstrates cross sections of multiple large vessels by signal void within the subarachnoid space corresponding to enlarged veins (*small arrows*). A small intraparenchymal hemorrhage is seen within the frontal parasagittal parenchyma (*broken arrow*)

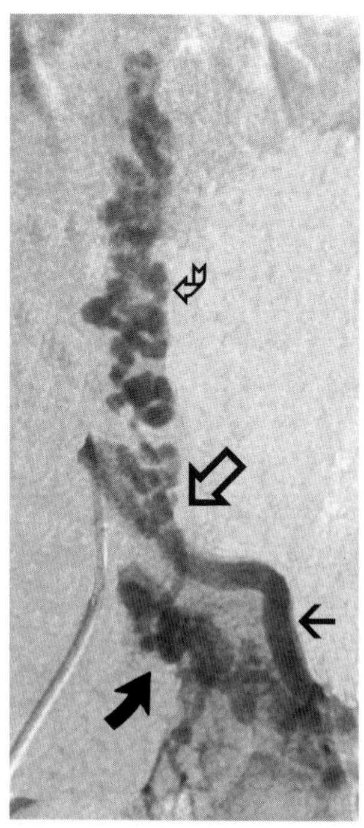

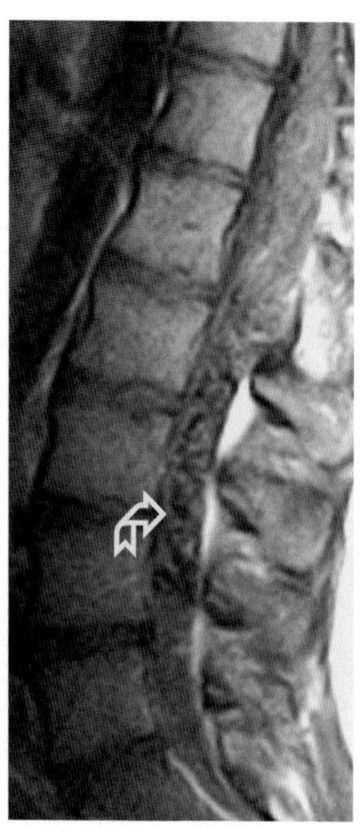

Fig. 4.12a, b. Spinal dural arteriovenous malformation. **a** DSA, selective injection of an L.IV segmental artery on the left (*arrow*) demonstrates a DAVM involving the nerve root sheath (*curved arrow*), draining into a perimedullary vein (*open arrow*) and into dilated spinal intradural veins (*broken arrow*). **b** Sagittal T_1-W MRI study demonstrates large intradural vessels within the L.I–IV segments (*broken arrow*), typical of spinal DAVM. Contrast enhancement at the lower thoracic level is due to previous surgery

4.2.2 Natural History and Classification

DAVMs are dynamic lesions with a highly variable clinical course that extends from spontaneous cure to fatal hemorrhage. The clinical presentation of DAVMs has been classified as either benign or aggressive. Lesions producing ocular symptoms, pulsatile tinnitus, bruit, and/or local cranial nerve deficits only are considered benign. Those associated with intracranial hemorrhage or nonhemorrhagic neurological deficit are classified as aggressive. While symptomatology is influenced by location, the natural history is dominated by the venous flow pattern. Growing evidence suggests that retrograde venous drainage and venous drainage into leptomeningeal veins is associated with more severe clinical presentation and a more aggressive natural history. Careful analysis of the hemodynamics as demonstrated by angiography is therefore prerequisite to proper therapeutic decision-making. During the past several decades, several classification systems have been developed based on the venous flow pattern.

Djindjan recognized the significance of retrograde venous drainage early on and created a classification system as demonstrated in Table 4.3 and Figs. 4.13, 4.14 (Djindjan and Merland 1978). In this system, grade 1 lesions drain into the involved sinus in either an ante- or a retrograde fashion Fig. 4.13a–c). Grade 2 lesions drain into sinuses, too, but have reflux into cerebral veins (Fig. 4.13d, e). Grade 3 lesions are characterized by exclusive drainage into cortical veins (Fig. 4.13e–g, j), and grade 4 DAVMs drain into or towards large venous lakes (Fig. 4.13h).

Cognard retrospectively analyzed a series of 205 patients with DAVMs (Cognard et al. 1995) and modified Djindjan's classification based on further details of the venous pathway that he found to significantly influence the clinical course (Table 4.3, Figs. 4.13, 4.14). In his system, type I. lesions drain into dural sinuses in an antegrade direction only (Fig. 4.13a). Type II. is characterized by disproportionately high arterial load and insufficient antegrade venous drainage, resulting in retrograde flow. This category is further divided into three subgroups, including II/a, with retrograde flow within the sinuses only (Fig. 4.13b, c), II/b, with antegrade flow within the sinus and reflux into cortical veins (Fig. 4.13d), and II/a+b, with retrograde flow within both the sinus and cortical veins (Fig. 4.13e). Type III lesions drain exclusively into cortical veins (Fig. 4.13f). Type IV Lesions drain into cortical veins with venous ectasia (Fig. 4.13h). Finally, Cognard added another entity, lesions that drain into spinal perimedullary veins, classified as type V. (Fig. 4.13j). In his analysis of 205 patients, Cognard found an aggressive clinical course in one of 84 patients with type I fistulae, 45% in type II, 76% in type III, 96% in type IV, and in 100% in type V. In addition, hemorrhage, as the most severe complication, was related strictly to cortical venous drainage. No hemorrhage was found

Table 4.3. Classification of intracranial DAVM-s in relation to venous drainage pattern

Venous drainage pattern: intracranial DAVM		Fig. 4.2	Classification		
Site of shunt	Venous outflow		Djindjan	Cognard	Borden
Dural sinus/meningeal vein	Sinus, antegrade	A	1	1	1
Dural sinus/meningeal vein	Sinus, ante/retrograde	B	1	2/A	1
Dural sinus/meningeal vein with sinus occlusion	Sinus, retrograde	C	1	2/A	1
Dural sinus/meningeal vein	Sinus antegrade + reflux into subarachnoid vein	D	2	2/B	2
Dural sinus/meningeal vein	Sinus ante/retrograde + reflux into subarachnoid vein	E	2	2/A+B	2
Subarachnoid vein	Subarachnoid vein	F	3	3	3
Isolated sinus with reflux into subarachnoid vein	Subarachnoid vein	G	3	3	3
Venous lake	Subarachnoid vein	H	4	4	3
Spinal perimedullary vein	Subarachnoid vein	J	3	5	3

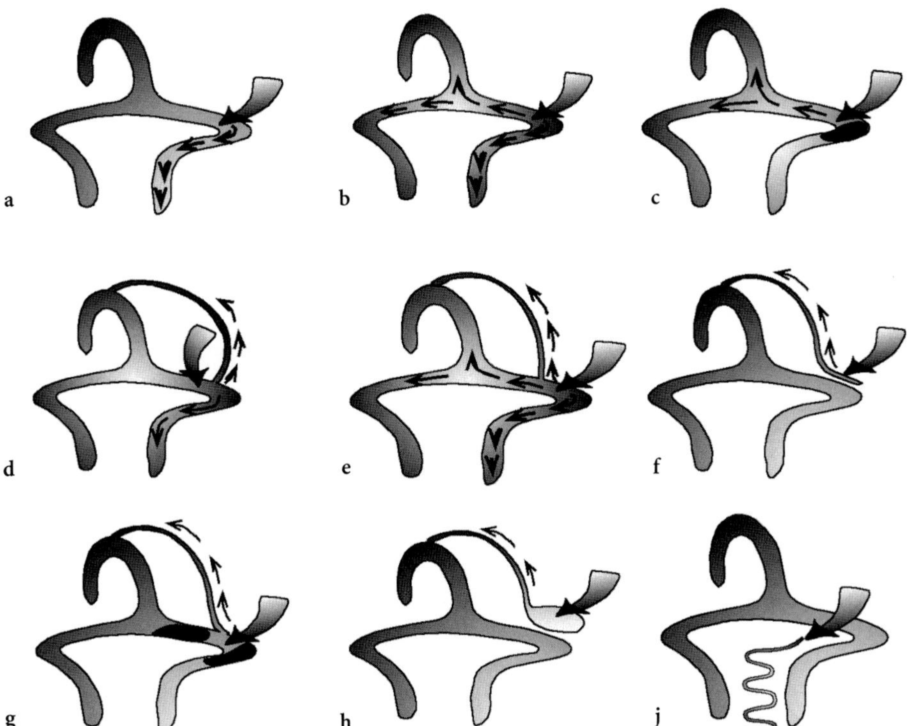

Fig. 4.13a–j. Schematic representation of venous drainage patterns of intracranial DAVMs. **a–c** DAVM shunting into a dural sinus with antegrade (**a**), ante- and retrograde (**b**), and exclusively retrograde flow (due to sinus occlusion, **c**) within the sinus system. **d** and **e** DAVM shunting into a dural sinus with retrograde flow in leptomeningeal veins due to venous overload of the sinus, with (**e**) or without (**d**) retrograde flow inside the sinus itself. **f** DAVM shunting directly into a leptomeningeal vein. **g** Isolated sinus due to sinus occlusion with retrograde leptomeningeal venous drainage. **h** DAVM draining into venous ectasia. **j** Intracranial DAVM draining into spinal perimedullary veins

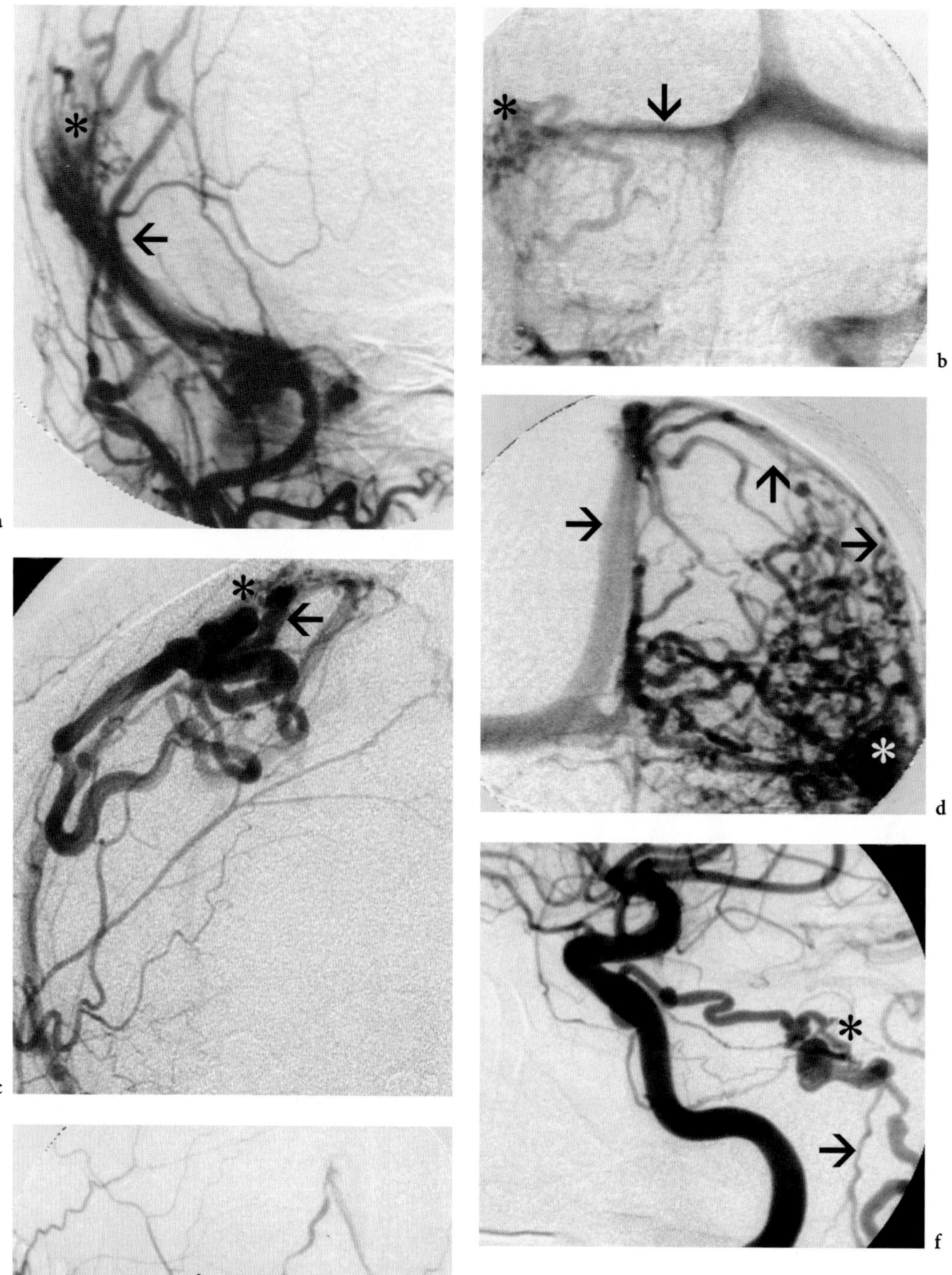

Fig. 4.14a–f. Examples of intracranial DAVMs with different venous drainage patterns. **a** DAVM (*asterisk*) of the SS, shunting into the sinus (*arrow*) with antegrade flow only. DSA, ECA injection, AP view. **b** DAVM (*asterisk*) of the sigmoid-transverse sinus with retrograde flow (*arrow*) and reflux into the SSS. DSA, ECA injection, AP view. **c** DAVM of the SS (*asterisk*) on the left with retrograde flow within multiple cortical veins (*arrows*) draining into the SSS (*arrow*). DSA, left ECA injection, AP view. **d** DAVM of the frontal convexity (*asterisk*) draining into a dilated cortical vein (*arrow*). DSA, Right ECA injection, AP view. **e** DAVM at the tentorial incisura (*asterisk*) draining into a venous varix (*arrow*). DSA with ECA injection, lateral view. **f** DAVM on the clivus draining into spinal perimedullary veins (*arrow*). DSA, ICA injection, lateral view

in types I and II/a, 20% in type II/b, 6% in type II/a+b, 40% in type III, and 66% in type IV. Five of 12 patients with spinal venous drainage had hemorrhage, and in all of them the spinal drainage was directed into the epidural space in the cervical region. The significant difference between type III and IV demonstrates that venous ectasia is associated with a particularly high likelihood of hemorrhage. Histopathological signs of venous wall degeneration have been found in such venous pouches (Hamada et al. 2000). This classification system, although somewhat complicated, has a high predictive value regarding aggressive clinical course and particularly concerning hemorrhage.

Finally, Borden created a simplified system by combining the previous two and including spinal DAVMs in the same classification (Tables 4.3 and 4.4, Figs. 4.13–4.15) (Borden et al. 1995). This system is dominated by an aggressive clinical course, hemorrhagic or not, that requires treatment. All malformations draining into dural sinuses or meningeal or spinal epidural veins with normal (antegrade) flow within the subarachnoid/leptomeningeal veins are considered type I (Fig. 4.13a–c). Those that drain into sinuses or meningeal or epidural veins resulting in reversed flow within normal veins draining into those sinuses are classified as type II (Fig. 4.13d, e, g). Lesions draining directly into subarachnoid veins (brain or spine) belong to type III (Fig. 4.13f, j). Type I lesions in an intracranial location have a benign course, but those located spinally may present with medullopathy or epidural hemorrhage. Type II lesions, either spinal or cranial, present with hemorrhage or neurological symptoms due to venous hypertension. Type III lesions typically present with hemorrhage intracranially and with medullopathy spinally.

In an attempt to validate the classifications described above, Davies et al. applied both systems retrospectively to 102 patients harboring DAVMs (Davies et al. 1996). By definition, Cognard types I and II/a were considered as Borden type I, Cognard II/b and II/a+b as Borden II. and Cognard III, IV, and V as Borden III (Table 4.3.). Of the 102 patients, 31 (30%) had an aggressive presentation: 16 had hemorrhage and 15 had nonhemorrhagic neurological symptoms. Aggressive presentation correlated well with both Borden and Cognard grades: Either hemorrhagic or nonhemorrhagic aggressive symptoms were found in 2% of Borden I, 39% of Borden II, and 79% of Borden III cases. In the Borden I group Cognard type II/a patients had more nonhemorrhagic

Table 4.4. Classification of spinal DAVMs in relation to venous drainage pattern

Venous drainage pattern: spinal DAVM		Classification
Site of shunt	Venous outflow	Borden
Nerve root sleeve, dura	Periosteal, epidural veins	1
Nerve root sleeve, dura	Epidural veins with reflux into perimedullary veins	2
Nerve root sleeve, dura	Perimedullary veins	3

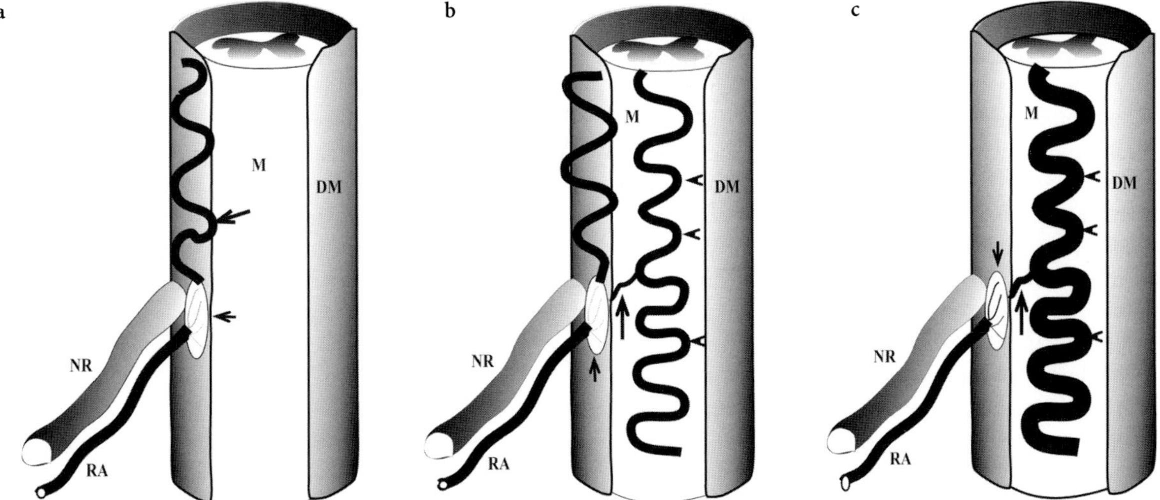

Fig. 4.15a–c. Schematic representation of venous drainage patterns of spinal DAVMs. (*NR* nerve root, *RA* radicular artery, *DM* dura mater, *M* medulla). Meningeal branch of the radicular artery feeds arteriovenous shunt located on the dura (*small arrow*). **a** Venous drainage by epidural veins (*arrow*). **b** Venous drainage via epidural veins and a perimedullary vein (arrow) into the coronal venous plexus (*arrowheads*). **c** Exclusive venous drainage by perimedullary vein (*arrow*) and the coronal venous plexus (*arrowheads*)

symptoms (7%) than those with Cognard type I. lesions (0%). In the Borden III group, the incidence of hemorrhagic presentation correlated positively with Cognard grades, demonstrating 38% incidence in type III., 50% in type IV, and 75% in type V. While the Borden classification reliably predicts aggressive clinical presentation, the Cognard system provides more precise correlation between hemorrhage and venous drainage.

In addition, the clinical presentation was analyzed in relation to location of the lesions by several authors. In a meta-analysis of 100 benign and 277 aggressive DAVM cases, Awad and colleagues found no correlation between aggressive presentation and flow rate. Although the lowest rate of aggressive behavior was found in transverse and cavernous sinus locations and the highest in tentorial DAVMs, no location was immune to an aggressive neurological course. Leptomeningeal venous drainage, venous dilatations, and galenic drainage were found to significantly correlate with aggressive symptoms (Awad et al. 1990). No aggressive symptoms were found in association with lesions involving the cavernous sinus, while there were aggressive symptoms in 27% of transverse sinus DAVMs, in 100% of those at the confluens sinuum, in 65% at the superior sagittal sinus, in 92% at the tentorium, and in 88% in the anterior fossa (Cognard et al. 1995). Analysis of the venous drainage pattern demonstrated that high incidence of aggressive symptoms in certain locations was related to the typical venous anatomy in each location rather than to the location itself. Only Borden type III lesions were found in the anterior cranial fossa: 78% of them on the tentorium, 13% on the transverse sinus, and none on the cavernous sinus (Davies et al. 1996). Multiple DAVM location was found to correlate significantly with leptomeningeal venous drainage (84%) and subsequently with aggressive presentation. These patients had a three times higher incidence of hemorrhage than those with single a DAVM (van Dijk et al. 2002). In general, location has a significant impact on the venous drainage pattern but the clinical presentation is determined by the venous drainage itself, and not by the location.

While the above-cited studies provide good correlation between venous morphology and clinical symptomatology at the time of the initial presentation, this is of limited value regarding the natural history and the prognosis of the disease. Some DAVMs may disappear without treatment (Bitoh and Sakaki 1979; Chaudhary et al. 1982; Lasjaunias et al. 1984; Meder et al. 1995; Luciani et al. 2001); others may lead to death. As treatment is complicated and carries certain risks, proper selection of patients requiring treatment necessitates reliable prognosis of each particular case. Davies and colleagues analyzed the clinical course of 55 Borden grade I (benign) and 46 Borden grade II–III intracranial DAVM patients for 133 patient years and for 344 patient months, respectively, following presentation. Twenty-one of 26 Borden I patients improved and five remained stable without treatment. In contrast, four of the 29 Borden III patients treated conservatively died within the follow-up period. This group had a 19%/year incidence of hemorrhaging, 11%/year of nonhemorrhagic complications, and a 19%/year mortality (Davies et al. 1997a,b). Although the number of observed cases is small, this study supports the concept that the type of venous drainage not only determines the first clinical presentation but also reliably predicts the natural history, and therefore may serve as a basis for therapeutic decision-making.

4.3 Diagnostic Imaging

Although plain X-ray films may occasionally demonstrate prominent vascular impressions on the skull, the contribution of conventional radiography to the imaging diagnosis of DAVM is limited. Although myelography depicts enlarged intradural vessels by negative contrast, this does not justify using this technique for the demonstration of spinal DAVM (Chen et al. 1995). Cross-sectional imaging techniques such as computed tomography (CT) and magnetic resonance imaging (MRI) demonstrate consequences of the dural arteriovenous shunt on the brain and the cerebrospinal fluid (CSF) spaces. Less invasive or noninvasive angiographic techniques such as CT angiography (CTA) or MR angiography (MRA) are capable of depicting the vascular pathology itself. Catheter angiography is required for the accurate localization of the shunt and evaluation of the hemodynamic pattern.

4.3.1 Computer Tomography

Computer tomography (CT) scan without contrast demonstrates changes secondary to DAVMs. These include hydrocephalus, cortical atrophy, and hemorrhage (Figs. 4.4, 4.5, 4.8, 4.16.) that can be either subarachnoid (Kagawa et al. 2001), subdural,

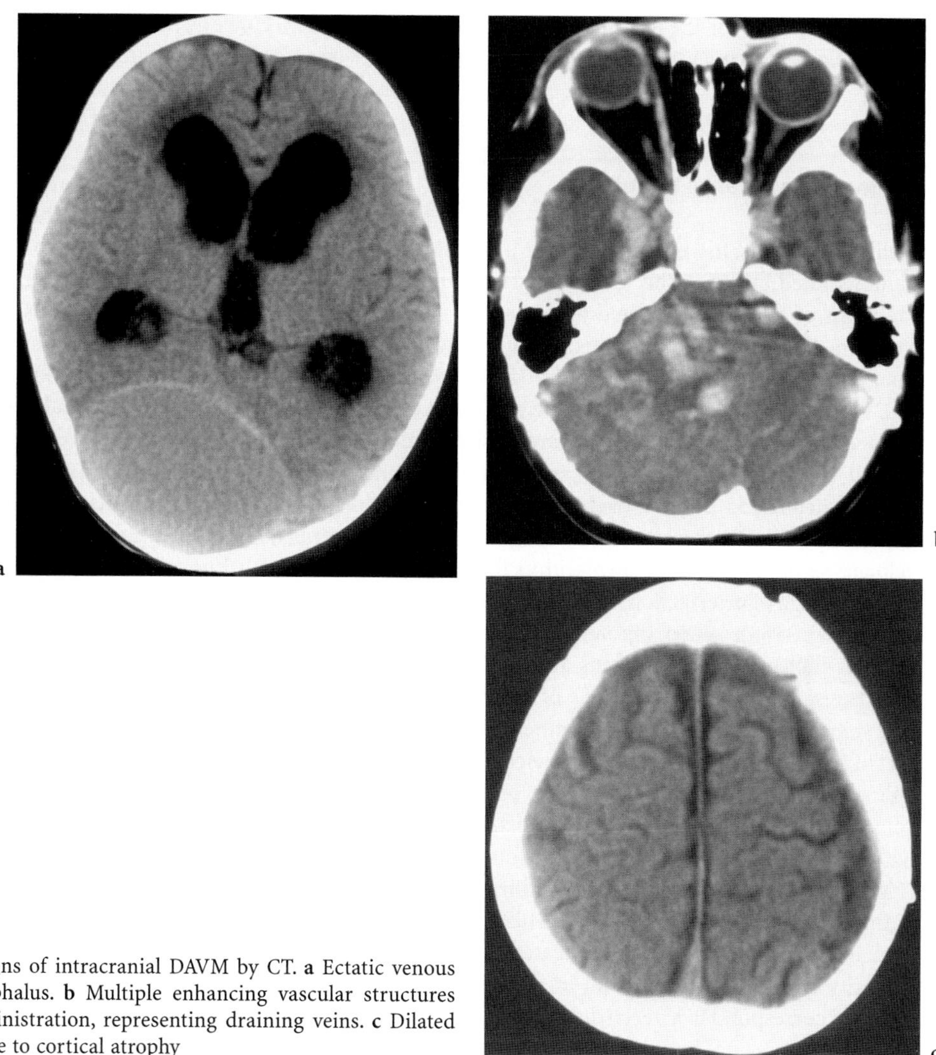

Fig. 4.16a–c. Typical signs of intracranial DAVM by CT. **a** Ectatic venous structure and hydrocephalus. **b** Multiple enhancing vascular structures following contrast administration, representing draining veins. **c** Dilated subarachnoid spaces due to cortical atrophy

parenchymal (Solis et al. 1977), or intraventricular (Kawaguchi et al. 1999). Noncontrast CT scan may raise the suspicion of sinus thrombosis by hyperdensity within the involved sinus. Contrast-enhanced CT delineates enlarged draining veins as serpentine enhancing structures. This is particularly characteristic in cavernous sinus DAVM with superior ophthalmic vein (SOV) drainage in which the enlarged SOV is well demonstrated as tubular enhancement within the orbit that also exhibits signs of associated exophthalmos (Fig. 4.5g). If coupled with typical clinical symptoms, these signs on CT may provide the diagnosis of a cavernous sinus arteriovenous shunt; however, differentiation between direct carotid cavernous fistula and a cavernous sinus DAVM is not possible based on CT scan. Enlarged draining veins are delineated in cases of DAVM in other locations with either direct leptomeningeal venous drainage or reflux into leptomeningeal veins due to venous overload of the sinuses. Mass effect from venous varices is well depicted (Fig. 4.16a, b). In cases of DAVM with antegrade sinus drainage, CT scan is usually normal (Chiras et al. 1982). The use of multislice CT (Klingebiel et al. 2001) and CT angiography (CTA) (Alberico et al. 1999) has been proposed for the less invasive evaluation of cerebral vascular malformation. DAVMs, particularly those with large and complex nidi, are likely to be detected by CTA. However, the dynamic evaluation of the lesion necessary for making a therapeutic decision may not be possible by CT/CTA techniques. Computer tomography with contrast is useful in demonstrating sinus thrombosis as lack of contrast enhancement within the involved sinus(es) in association with DAVM. CT scanning has been applied to evaluate the results following embolization of spinal DAVM, but it cannot be successfully used for the initial diagnostic imaging of such lesions (Cognard et al. 1996).

4.3.2 Magnetic Resonance Imaging

Unlike pial AVMs, the nidus of a DAVM is usually not demonstrated by spin echo (SE) MRI. This is because the nidus of a DAVM is located within a thin sheet of the dura that is difficult to detect by cross-sectional imaging. MRI depicts indirect signs of DAVM. Similar to CT, hydrocephalus, cortical atrophy, and mass effect from enlarged venous structures are easily demonstrated (Figs. 4.7b, 4.8d, 4.10e). Large draining veins are well delineated by flow void on spin echo images either intraorbitally or intracranially (Fig. 4.10e, f). High velocity signal loss can be seen within the cavernous sinus as a sign of arterial flow, indicating DAVM (Hirabuki et al. 1988). When the venous flow is diverted towards the subependymal veins and midline venous structures, multiple cross sections of enlarged medullary veins may be seen within the white matter as small foci of flow void. Although the nidus itself is usually not delineated, the presence of dilated pial vessels (draining veins) without an AVM nidus is suggestive of DAVM with venous occlusive disease and venous congestion (Fig. 4.11d). This is found in over two thirds of patients with venous reflux (De Marco et al. 1990; Willinsky et al. 1994). Venous ischemia is indicated by high signal intensity on T_2-weighted (T_2-W) images that typically does not correspond to arterial distribution (Figs. 4.19c, d, 4.17f). High signal intensity areas may enhance with gadolinium, indicating disruption of the blood-brain barrier due to venous hypoperfusion (Willinsky et al. 1994; Kawaguchi et al. 2001). Bithalamic T_2 hyperintensities have been described as a result of reversible venous ischemia (Greenough et al. 1999). Intradural hemorrhage, either subdural or parenchymal, due to DAVM is easily detected by MRI as mixed signal intensity on SE images (Figs. 4.7c, 4.8c, 4.11/d). Dural sinus thrombosis that is frequently associated with DAVM might be demonstrated as lack of signal loss within the involved segment of the sinus on SE images. This can be confirmed by the lack of contrast enhancement and lack of visualization of the occluded sinus by venous MRA. However, correct assessment of venous occlusive disease by MRI might be difficult. Parenchymal hemorrhage is commonly associated with venous infarction. SE MRI in cases of DAVM with antegrade sinus drainage might be normal (De Marco et al. 1990).

Magnetic resonance angiography improves the delineation of the site of the shunt and feeding and draining pedicles. Either two- and three-dimensional phase contrast (PC) or time of flight (TOF) MRA may demonstrate the nidus. Phase-contrast MRA may demonstrate flow reversal in sinuses or draining veins (Cellerini et al. 1999). Stenosis or occlusion of sinuses and dilated cortical veins, however, might be missed by either PC or TOF MRA (Chen et al. 1992; Cellerini et al. 1999). (Figs. 4.11c, 4.17d). First-pass, gadolinium-enhanced fast MRA significantly improves delineation of the nidus, feeding pedicle, and draining veins (Farb et al. 2001).

An intracranial DAVM draining into the spinal venous system produces spinal venous ischemia, indicated by enlargement and increased T_2 signal intensity of the cervical spinal cord (Fig. 4.9c, d). Diffuse gadolinium contrast enhancement of the cervical medulla has also been reported (Bousson et al. 1999). Enlarged intradural draining veins may or may not be depicted by MRI of the cervical spine. Clinical evidence of myelopathy with cervical spinal cord signal changes should raise the suspicion of such DAVM and prompt intracranial vascular studies (MRA, DSA) (Ernst et al. 1997; Chen et al. 1998; Bousson et al. 1999).

Most spinal DAVMs generate spinal venous hypertension leading to myelopathy that, if untreated, results in permanent disabling neurological deficit. Symptoms commonly develop in a slow and fluctuating manner, making the clinical diagnosis extremely difficult. Proper imaging is of the utmost importance to establish the diagnosis before permanent damage to the spinal cord occurs. Yet the average time from the onset of symptoms until diagnosis was found to be 27 months in a large study of 66 patients with spinal DAVM (Gilbertson et al. 1995). As localization of the lesion by clinical signs is often difficult or impossible and spinal catheter angiography is highly invasive, MRI and MRA play an outstanding role as noninvasive tools in the diagnosis of spinal DAVM.

Fig. 4.17a–f. Typical signs of intracranial DAVM by MRI. **a–d** DAVM of the tentorial incisura. DSA with left ECA injection (**a**) demonstrates the DAVM draining into a venous lake (*arrow*). The dilated draining vein is demonstrated by flow void on T_2-W MRI (*arrow* in **b**) and by flow enhancement on the source image of TOF MRA (*arrow* in **c**). MIP reconstructed MRA delineates the draining vein (*arrow* in **d**). **e–f** DAVM of the superior sagittal sinus with occlusion of both transverse sinuses. Sinus occlusion is demonstrated be DSA (*arrow*) in **e**. Am ischemic area of increased T_2 signal intensity (*arrow* in **f**) is seen as a result of venous hypertension. Figure 4.10 demonstrates further details of the case

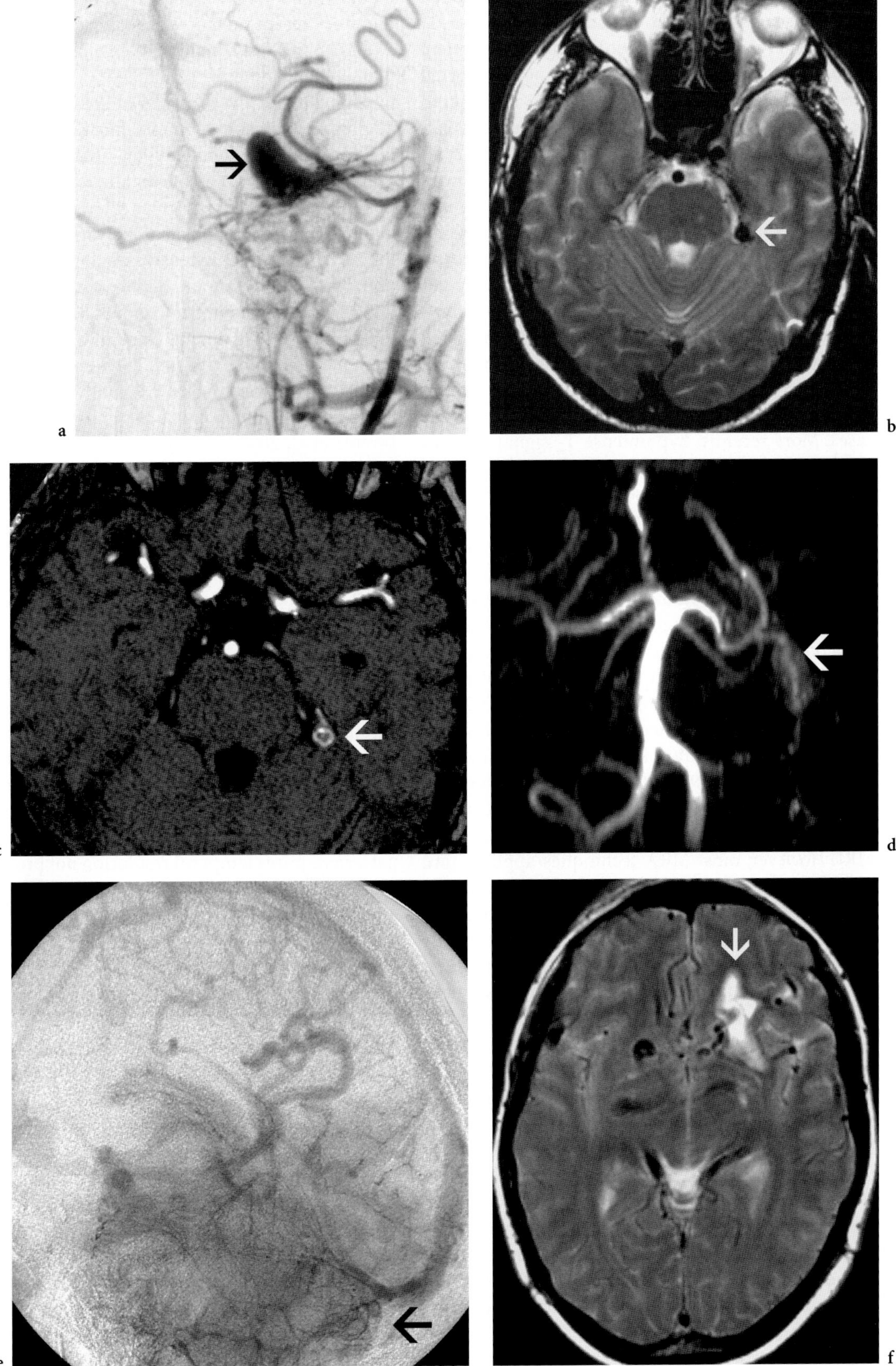
a
b
c
d
e
f

The most common signs of spinal DAVM are related to venous ischemia and include hyperintense T_2 signal, enlargement, and gadolinium enhancement of the spinal cord. These signs have been reported in 94%–100%, 45%–65% and 60%–88% of patients, respectively. Intradural, serpentine structures visualized by flow void and contrast enhancement are typical direct signs of the vascular dural arteriovenous shunts, representing enlarged veins of the coronal venous plexus that drains the lesion (Fig. 4.12). These vessel-like linear areas, located mostly on the dorsal surface of the cord, are present in 45%–82% of cases (TERWEY et al. 1989; GILBERTSON et al. 1995; WILLINSKY et al. 1995). Changes most commonly associated with spinal DAVM are therefore nonspecific, and enlarged vessels lead the diagnosis in the correct direction in only one half to three quarter of the cases. More recently, hypointense T_2 signal changes were found on the periphery of the medulla in a consecutive series of 11 cases of spinal DAVM. This is thought to be a sign of venous myelopathy, specific to venous hypertension and arteriovenous shunt. These findings and their explanation need to be confirmed in larger studies (HURST and GROSSMAN 2000). Presently, magnetic resonance angiography is increasingly being used to confirm the diagnosis of DAVM based on direct signs and to localize the fistula prior to selective angiography. Both TOF and PC MRA were tested in demonstrating spinal DAVM (GELBERT et al. 1992; BOWEN et al. 1995; MASCALCHI et al. 1995, 1997, 1999, 2001; BOWEN and PATTANY 1997, 1998, 2000; BINKERT et al. 1999; SHIGEMATSU et al. 2000) and were found to improve the specificity of MRI. However, most MRA techniques applied until recently demonstrate enlarged intradural vessels but are not capable of delineating the feeding pedicle and draining vein, and therefore do not contribute to the localization of the fistula itself. Contrast-enhanced TOF and PC sequences (BOWEN and PATTANY 1997, 1998) and phase display of 2D PC MRA (MASCALCHI et al. 1999) have been found useful in some cases in delineating the fistula site. Rapidly repeated 3D angiographic sequences immediately following administration of gadolinium contrast agent and detection of the first pass of gadolinium improved visualization of the draining vein within the neural foramen (BINKERT et al. 1999; SHIGEMATSU et al. 2000). Most recently, Farb and colleagues applied automatic triggering of a fast, three-dimensional MR angiographic sequence by detection of the first pass of gadolinium within the aorta. This technique allowed accurate delineation of the feeding pedicle, and the draining vein and determination of the foraminal level of the fistula in all of their nine cases (FARB et al. 2002). With the most recent advances in MRA technology, MRI and MRA studies should be the primary tools in the diagnostic workup for spinal DAVM with an attempt to delineate the level and site of the fistula. Selective angiography is still required, focusing on the level previously determined by MRA. The goal of catheter angiography is to evaluate small anatomical details, such as the origin of radicular arteries supplying the anterior spinal artery, and to perform endovascular therapy if possible. Extensive angiographic workup of the entire spine should be avoided.

Magnetic resonance techniques are also used for follow-up after treatment. Gradual disappearance of intramedullary high signal, cord enlargement, and contrast enhancement by MRI within 1–23 months following treatment (WILLINSKY et al. 1995; HORIKOSHI et al. 2000), as well as lack of enlarged perimedullary vessels by MRA (MASCALCHI et al. 2001), confirms the result of either surgical or endovascular disconnection of the arteriovenous shunt.

4.3.3 Angiography

Noninvasive or minimally invasive imaging techniques including CT, MRI, and MRA, coupled with careful analysis of the clinical history, allow for establishing the diagnosis of a DAVM with relatively high confidence in many cases. Borden type I. lesions, however, may not produce any pathological changes on CT and MRI. Moreover, analysis of the hemodynamic pattern requires temporal resolution not provided by MRA. Details of the venous circulation and associated venous occlusive disease may not be properly visualized by MR/CT techniques (CHEN et al. 1992; KALLMES et al. 1998; CELLERINI et al. 1999). As these details are critical in evaluating the risks associated with the individual pathology, selective angiography remains necessary for therapeutic decision-making.

Proper angiographic evaluation of patients with intracranial DAVM requires analysis of all potential sources of arterial supply as well as draining veins and venous structures. The reach vascular supply of the dura provides anastomotic connections between different territories, and even the falx or the tentorium does not provide a barrier between the two hemispheres or the infra- and supratentorial compartments (LASJAUNIAS and BERENSTEIN 1987). Selective injections of all arteries that potentially supply a certain anatomical location are therefore indispensable for proper angiographic evaluation (Table 4.5) (DJINDJAN and MERLAND 1978). While analysis of the arterial supply is important in disclosing the diagnosis, thorough study and understanding of the venous outlet is critical in order to establish the proper prognosis. This will allow appropriate indication of treatment and selection of the adequate therapeutic modality.

Anterior fossa DAVMs are fed by branches of either ophthalmic artery (OphA), distal branches of the internal maxillary artery (IMA), and the middle meningeal artery (MMA) (Fig. 4.4a, b). In cavernous sinus DAVM, the most common arterial supply arises from cavernous branches of the ipsi- and contralateral internal carotid arteries (ICA), distal branches of the IMA, cavernous branches of the (MMA), and the anterior division of the ascending pharyngeal artery (APA) (Figs. 4.5, 4.19). Transverse, sigmoid sinus, and confluens sinuum DAVMs receive blood from the tentorial branch of the ipsi- and sometimes contralateral ICA, the MMA, the posterior auricular (PA), the occipital (OA), and the posterior meningeal branches of the vertebral (VA) arteries. High-flow DAVMs in these locations may recruit a blood supply from large branches

Table 4.5. Expected feeding pedicles, recommended selective injections, and projections for intracranial DAVMs in different locations

Location of DAVM	Expected arterial supply			Selective injections recommended				
	Branches	Ipsilateral	Contralateral	Arteries projection	Ipsilateral		Contralateral	
					AP	Lateral	AP	Lateral
Anterior fossa	OphA	+	+	ICA	+	+	+	
	IMA	+	+	ECA	+	+	+	
	MMA	+		VA				
Cavernous sinus	ICA	+	+	ICA	+	+	+	
	IMA	+	+	ECA	+	+	+	
	MMA	+	+	VA				
	APA	+	+					
Transverse and sigmoid sinuses	ICA	+		ICA		+		
	MMA	+		ECA	+	+	+	
	APA	+		VA	+	+	+	+
	PA	+						
	OA	+	+					
	VA	+	+					
Confluens sinuum	ICA	+	+	ICA		+		+
	MMA	+	+	ECA	+	+	+	+
	APA	+	+	VA	+	+	+	+
	PA	+	+					
	OA	+	+					
	VA	+	+					
Tentorium	ICA	+	+	ICA	+	+		+
	MMA	+		ECA	+	+	+	
	APA	+	+	VA	+	+	+	
	OA	+						
	VA	+	+					
Foramen magnum	ICA	+		ICA	+	+		
	MMA	+		ECA	+	+	+	
	APA	+	+	VA	+	+	+	
	OA	+	+					
	VA	+	+					
Convexity	OphA	+	+	ICA	+	+	+	
	MMA	+		ECA	+	+	+	
	OA	+	+	VA	+	+	+	
	VA	+	+					
Superior sagittal sinus	ICA	+	+	ICA	+	+	+	+
	OphA	+	+	ECA	+	+	+	+
	IMA	+	+	VA	+	+		+
	MMA	+	+					
	APA	+	+					
	OA	+	+					
	VA	+	+					

of the subclavian artery such as the ascending cervical artery (Fig. 4.6). Lesions involving the tentorium are supplied by tentorial branches of the ICA bilaterally, by the neuromeningeal trunk of the APA on either side, and by the posterior division of the MMA, OA, and meningeal branches of the VA (Fig. 4.8). The blood supply to DAVMs around the foramen magnum may be recruited from tentorial branches of the ICA, posterior division of the MMA, neuromeningeal trunk of the APA, OA, and VA (Fig. 4.9). Superior sagittal sinus DAVMs have complex supply involving branches of the anterior (from OphA), middle, and posterior (from VA) meningeal arteries, and meningeal branches of the OAs. These usually high-flow lesions recruit arterial feeders from transosseal and subcutaneous sources such the superficial temporal arteries (STA) and from pial arteries, such as branches of the anterior cerebral arteries. Blood supply is typically bilateral (Fig. 4.10). Dural shunts located on the convexity in the middle cranial fossa are supplied mostly by MMA branches (Fig. 4.11). The differential diagnosis of slowly progressing myelopathy should include spinal DAVM that leads to spinal venous hypertension and hypoperfusion. Usually, MRI discloses spinal cord ischemia and enlarged intradural vessels. Spinal angiography is used to demonstrate the feeding pedicle and the draining vein of the fistula. Unless MRA provides accurate information on the foraminal level, selective injections of all segmental arteries potentially providing blood supply to the involved region of the spinal column must be studied, until the fistula is found. Spinal cord ischemia might be remote from the fistula site, which may make angiographic evaluation of the entire spine necessary, particularly if venous stasis is seen in spinal veins (Willinsky et al. 1990). If arteriovenous shunt within the spine cannot be demonstrated, a DAVM within the posterior fossa must be suspected that drains into spinal perimedullary veins, and appropriate injections must be performed (Fig. 4.9).

Expected feeding pedicles and recommended injections and projections are listed in Table 4.5. Because of the many anatomical variants and the dynamic nature of the disease, however, strict rules cannot be established and the angiographer should use the best individual judgment to explore all potential feeders. Long series with delayed images are necessary to study the venous drainage of the lesion. In addition to studying the venous outlet of the fistula itself, the venous drainage of the brain parenchyma must be demonstrated. All major dural sinuses should be studied to disclose venous occlusive disease and to demonstrate patency and direction of flow within the major venous channels draining the brain.

4.4 Therapy

4.4.1 Indications

Currently available therapeutic options include no treatment, conservative treatment, palliative or definitive endovascular treatment, surgery, a combination of endovascular treatment and surgery, and radiosurgery. As detailed in Sects. 4.2.2 and 4.2.3, the natural history of DAVM may vary from spontaneous cure (Magidson and Weinberg 1976; Bitoh and Sakaki 1979; Endo et al. 1979; Luciani et al. 2001) (Fig. 4.18) to fatal hemorrhage (Awad et al. 1990). With this large spectrum, not the diagnosis, but rather the expected prognosis of the disease should indicate treatment. This makes proper classification of patients by angiography mandatory.

In a recent study by Davies et al., 21 of 26 patients with Borden type I. DAVMs experienced resolution or improvement of their symptoms without any treatment, and the other five remained unchanged. Owing to the low risk implied by the natural history of this type, and considering that malignant transformation following incomplete treatment may occur (Watanabe et al. 1984, 2000), this group of patients should be observed or treated conservatively until symptoms are tolerated. Palliative or (if possible without high risk) definitive endovascular treatment should be offered for those whose symptoms (for instance pulsatile tinnitus) result in significant impairment of their quality of life. Similarly, progressive decrease of visual acuity or imminent loss of vision may prompt endovascular intervention in cases of cavernous sinus DAVM.

Spontaneous transformation of a benign (Borden I) DAVM to a malignant (Borden II–III) one has been reported (Cognard et al. 1997). Patients with high-flow Borden I DAVM, particularly those in the subgroup of Cognard II/a, may develop malignant elevation of ICP. Subsequently, patients with conservative or incomplete treatment should be closely observed and treated if necessary (Cognard et al. 1995; Davies et al. 1997).

On the other hand, the high risk of DAVM with leptomeningeal venous drainage (Borden I–II) has been well documented (Awad et al. 1990; Borden et al. 1995; Cognard et al. 1995; Davies et al. 1996). Four of 14 such patients died, representing a 19% yearly mortality (Davies et al. 1997). The malignant course of the disease in this group requires aggressive therapy leading to permanent elimination of factors

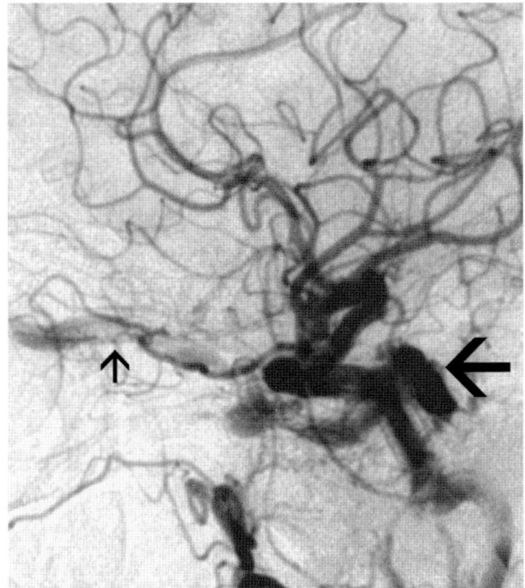
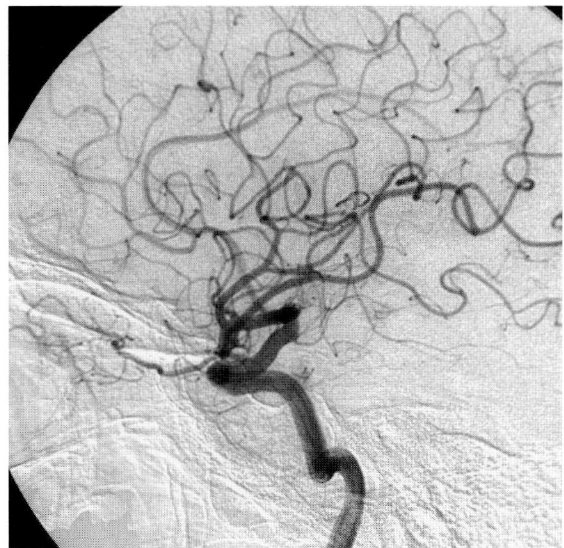

Fig. 4.18a, b. Spontaneous cure of DAVM. **a** Common carotid artery DSA in lateral view demonstrates CS DAVM (*arrow*) that drains into the SOV (*small arrow*). **b** Follow-up angiography 2 months later demonstrates complete obliteration of the DAVM. No treatment was performed

posing a high risk. The treatment modality should be chosen by a team of experienced neurointerventionists and neurosurgeons based on the individual pathology.

4.4.2 Conservative Treatment

Conservative treatment is offered to patients with Borden I fistula, who most often have their lesion on the cavernous sinus or on the transverse/sigmoid sinuses. These two are the most benign and the most common location of intracranial DAVMs. In a retrospective study by Cognard et al., 69% of transverse sinus and 87% of cavernous sinus lesions had no leptomeningeal venous drainage (Borden I) and these two locations corresponded to 66% of all DAVMs studied (Cognard et al. 1995).

Conservative treatment has two components. Manual vascular compression is utilized to facilitate spontaneous closure of the fistula. Medical treatment is used to control ocular symptoms if present.

In case of benign transverse sinus fistulae, the pulsating occipital artery can be compressed over the mastoid by the patient for up to 30 min per treatment. This may reduce flow and induce spontaneous thrombosis with a reported frequency of 27% (Halbach et al. 1987). Patients harboring DAVMs on the cavernous sinus might be treated similarly. In these cases, the common carotid artery–jugular vein complex is compressed (Matas maneuver) on the side of the fistula. As this manipulation carries some risks, patients with atherosclerotic carotid disease should not be treated. Patients in this group are instructed to compress their carotid bifurcation with their contralateral hand, so that if cerebral ischemia occurs the resulting motor weakness will automatically interrupt the procedure. The suspected mechanism is simultaneous decrease of the arterial and increase of the venous pressure, promoting thrombosis of the arteriovenous connection. Halbach reported a 33% rate of success with manual compressions of 10–30 s four to six times in each hour while awake for up to 6 weeks (Valavanis 1993). As the incidence of spontaneous thrombosis (Fig. 4.18) is unknown, the efficacy of the treatment cannot be established.

In cavernous sinus DAVM the ocular symptoms require ophthalmological and medical therapy, including control of the (frequently elevated) intraocular pressure and protective treatment of the conjunctiva in cases of extensive chemosis. Mild diuresis utilizing furosemide (Lasix), 5–10 mg/day usually provides significant relief of the external ocular symptoms. Visual acuity, fundus, and intraocular pressure should be periodically checked in patients under conservative treatment.

In our practice we initially propose observation only to patients with benign DAVM (regardless of location). Compression therapy is offered to patients presenting with significant ocular symptoms and those complaining of poorly tolerated tinnitus.

Additional medical and ophthalmological therapy is applied if necessary. Patients are followed in cooperation with the ophthalmologist. Spontaneous closure of cavernous sinus DAVM is frequently preceded by transient worsening of the symptoms, including retinal hemorrhages and reduced vision. Central retinal vein thrombosis has been implicated as the underlying pathomechanism (Miki et al. 1988; Suzuki et al. 1989). If the ocular symptoms progress to an imminent loss of vision we consider repeat angiography and embolization. Significant change of the symptoms, including improvement such as cessation of tinnitus, may indicate spontaneous closure. However, this should raise the suspicion of a change in the venous drainage pattern and prompt repeat studies before the patient is considered cured.

4.4.3 Endovascular Treatment

The goal of aggressive treatment of a DAVM can be (a) cure of the lesion, (b) conversion of a high-risk fistula to a low-risk one, and (c) palliation of symptoms caused by a low-risk lesion. As previously shown, the pathological entity of DAVM seems to be located within the wall of dural sinuses, veins, or leptomeningeal veins. The pathophysiological effect of the shunt is exercised on the venous system. Complete and permanent cure can be achieved only by closing all pathological connections between the arterial and venous side of the lesion. Theoretically, this can be obtained (a) by approaching the site of shunt through the feeding arteries and plugging the arteriovenous communication with an embolic material, or (b) by sealing the lumen of the draining venous structure off from the arteriovenous shunt (that exists inside its wall) by packing the entire section of that venous structure with an embolic material.

4.4.3.1 Transarterial Embolization

Considering the multiplicity of the arterial feeders that drain into a single venous channel and the multiple microshunts that exist inside the wall of the vein between arteriolae and venulae (Nishijima et al. 1992; Hamada et al. 1997; Momoji et al. 1997), complete closure is difficult or impossible to achieve from the arterial side. Embolic material injected from the feeding arteries is very likely to get wedged proximal to the shunt. Transarterial embolization therefore rarely results in complete cure of DAVMs and should be reserved for those cases in which the fistula cannot be reached via the transvenous route (goal *a*), for the palliation of symptoms in case of low-risk DAVMs (goal *c*), or as a preoperative measure to facilitate surgery (goal *a*).

Technically, solid – i.e., polyvinyl alcohol particles (PVA), platinum coils – and liquid embolics are used that are delivered through microcatheters coaxially introduced into a distal superselective position within the feeding pedicles. Dangerous anastomoses should always be considered prior to transarterial embolization. Potential connections between the IMA and the OphA, the MMA and the OphA and ICA, between the anterior division of the APA and the ICA, the posterior division of the APA and the VA, the OA and the VA must always be kept in mind, even if not visualized by superselective injection. The blood supply to cranial nerves should be considered when embolizing from the MMA and APA (Lasjaunias and Berenstein 1987). Inadvertent injection of the embolic material into cerebral arteries via dangerous anastomotic channels will result in stroke. Application of particles as an embolic agent carries little risk of stroke, as these particles are unlikely to reach intracerebral vessels via small-caliber anastomoses. Intra-arterially delivered microcoils will stay at the site of delivery and therefore carry no risk of intracerebral embolization (Nakstad et al. 1992). This material will, however, produce proximal occlusion of the feeding pedicles, which will result in collateral blood supply to the shunt.

In our experience, using transarterial embolization with particles in cavernous sinus DAVM may facilitate spontaneous occlusion of the fistula by decreasing the arterial load towards the draining vein. We apply this technique in cases where treatment is necessitated by progressive symptoms and the lesion is not reachable via the venous route. Transient worsening of the ocular symptoms may occur after partial transarterial embolization and can be attributed to progressive thrombosis of the superior ophthalmic vein (Sergott et al. 1987; Nagy et al. 1995) or the central retinal vein (Hashimoto et al. 1989). This requires aggressive dehydration including the administration of furosemide, mannitol, and steroids. In most cases this is followed by gradual improvement and (probably spontaneous) cure (Sergott et al. 1987). During this period, patients need to be carefully followed, their ocular status and visual acuity regularly checked. In case of progressive loss of vision a more effective treatment modality must be considered.

Multiple ECA feeders can be embolized with small PVA particles (50–250 μm). Generally, the smaller the particles, the better the result that can be expected.

In the presence of dangerous anastomoses, larger particles should be selected to avoid complications. Catheterization of small cavernous branches of the ICA is usually difficult, frequently impossible. Embolization with small particles from a narrow, short meningeal branch might be dangerous even if technically feasible (HALBACH et al. 1989). In such cases microcoils can be placed to reduce flow via ICA branches followed by extensive embolization through ECA feeders (Fig. 4.19).

Particulate embolization can also be applied preoperatively for lesions requiring extensive surgery. As fast recanalization is expected, surgery should follow embolization with little delay (Fig. 4.20).

In case of high-risk (Borden I–II) DAVMs, particulate embolization as a sole treatment does not provide safe and permanent prevention from subsequent bleeding. If transarterial embolization is considered in such cases because neither surgery nor transvenous embolization is feasible or recommended,

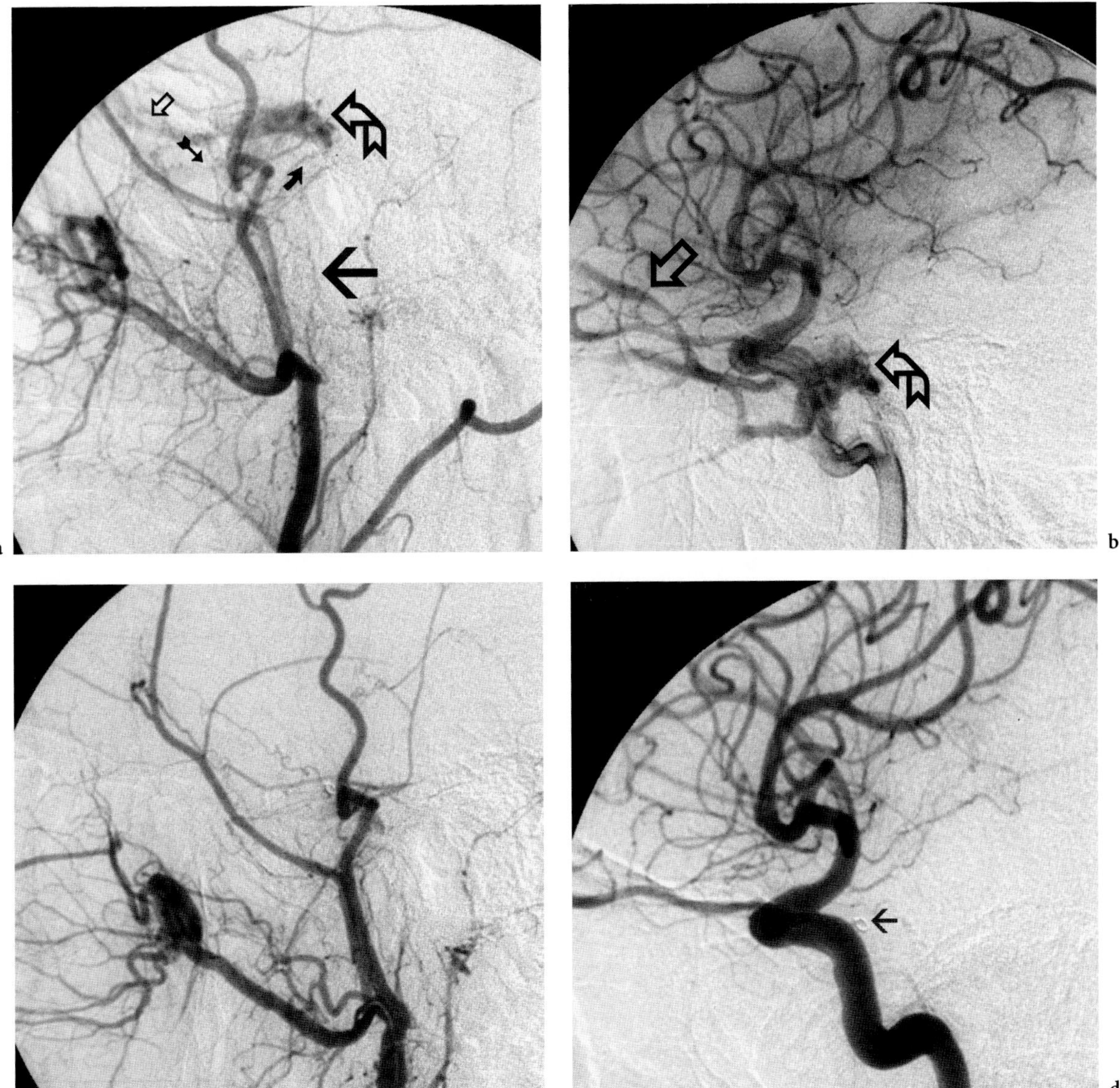

Fig. 4.19a–d. Endovascular treatment of DAVM by transarterial embolization. **a** and **b** DSA with Selective ECA (**a**) and ICA (**b**) injections demonstrates CS DAVM (*broken arrow*) draining into the SOV (*open arrow*), fed by distal internal maxillary (*small arrow*), middle meningeal (*small curved arrow*), ascending pharyngeal (*arrow*) branches and a prominent dural pedicle of the meningohypophyseal branch of the ICA. **c** and **d** Complete obliteration of the DAVM following transarterial embolization of the ECA branches using PVA and occlusion of the meningohypophyseal pedicle by deposition of a small detachable microcoil within its lumen (*arrow*)

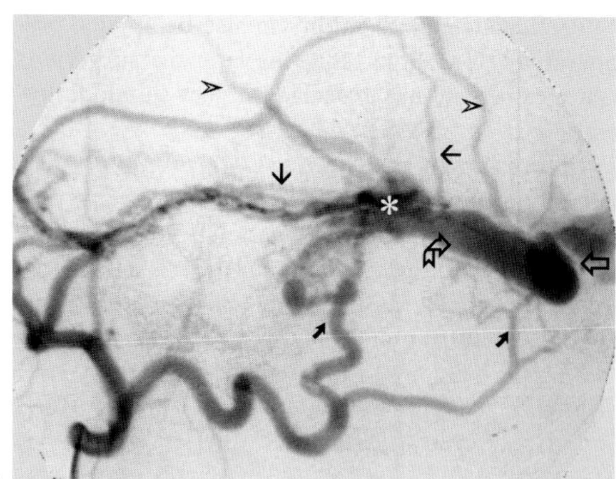

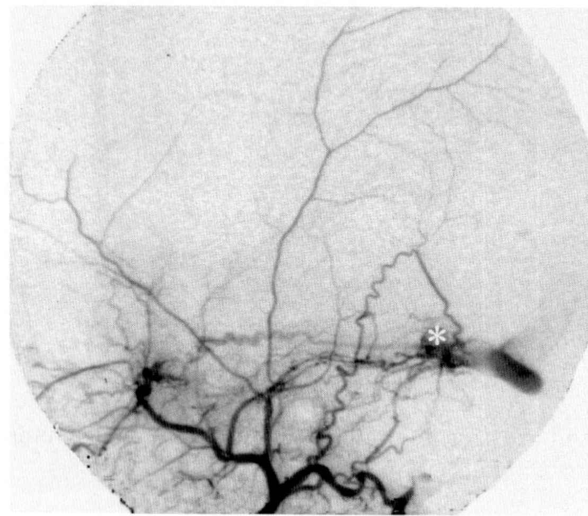

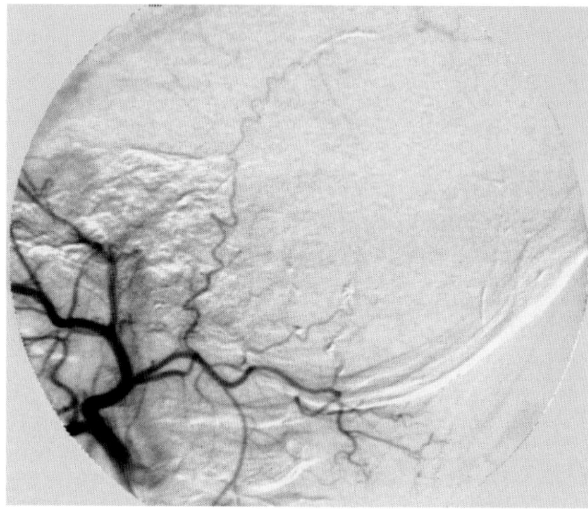

Fig. 4.20a–c. Combined treatment of DAVMs involving preoperative embolization and surgical excision. DSA images with selective ECA injections in lateral view. **a** DAVM of the sigmoid sinus (*asterisk*) with ipsilateral sigmoid sinus occlusion, severe stenosis of the ipsilateral transverse sinus and retrograde flow (*broken arrow*) towards the contralateral transverse sinus and into subarachnoid veins (*arrowheads*). Arterial feeders include branches of the middle meningeal artery (*small arrows*) and of the occipital artery (*small curved arrows*). **b** Persistent DAVM with significant reduction of flow following multiple sessions of transarterial embolization utilizing cyanoacrylate glue. Retrograde venous drainage is not seen. **c** Complete obliteration of the fistula and normal arterial flow following surgical resection

liquid embolics should be chosen. Cyanoacrylate glue mixed with Lipiodol is most commonly employed as a liquid embolic agent. The glue, N-butyl-cyanoacrylate, polymerizes quickly in an ionic environment such as blood. Lipiodol, a radiopaque oil, is added to provide radiopacity and to regulate solidification time (Cromwell and Kerber 1979; Kerber et al. 1979; Bank et al. 1981). Most DAVMs have relatively small-caliber feeders and a meshwork of fine arteries within the nidus. For effective embolization, the microcatheter must be placed in a very distal position and the glue needs to be highly diluted with Lipiodol (Liu et al. 2000; Iizuka et al. 2001). Depending on the arteriovenous transit time, a glue-to-oil ratio of 1:3–1:7 is frequently used. The best result of transarterial embolization with glue is achieved if the radiopaque glue reaches the venous site of the lesion without producing occlusion of major draining veins (Fig. 4.9). In case of direct arteriovenous communication, much lower dilution or even undiluted glue needs to be applied to avoid undesired venous occlusion or pulmonary embolism. Both potential dangerous anastomoses and the cranial nerve blood supply must be seriously considered if diluted glue is used, since the risk of stroke or cranial nerve ischemia is significantly higher than if particles are used. Reflux of glue proximal to the microcatheter tip may also lead to inadvertent embolization of normal arteries.

Because transvenous embolization is not feasible for spinal lesions, transarterial embolization with glue is the treatment of choice for a spinal DAVM with an arterial feeder that allows safe and distal catheterization and does not supply the anterior spinal artery. Glue should be pushed until it reaches the draining vein (Cognard et al. 1996; Song et al. 2001).

4.4.3.2 Transvenous Embolization

While it is difficult to obliterate multiple arteriovenous connections via the feeding arteries, this can be easily achieved by packing the lumen of the single venous channel of the lesion. Although this might induce transient pressure elevation inside the nidus, rupture and bleeding does not occur, as the nidus is located within the dura and is surrounded by thick walls, reinforced by connective tissue proliferation (HOUDART et al. 1993). In contrast to brain AVMs, venous occlusion is feasible and highly effective for DAVMs (HALBACH et al. 1989). Permanent and complete sacrifice of a dural sinus is feasible without causing venous infarction if the involved section does not drain the brain tissue. Venous embolization therefore requires thorough study of the venous circulation. Venous drainage of both the anterior and posterior circulation needs to be investigated on both sides. Long angiographic series must be obtained. Drainage of the malformation is seen in the late arterial phase. Venous drainage of the brain tissue can be observed on late venous phase images, frequently with long delay representing venous congestion. Visualization of the same venous structure (sinus or cortical vein) in both the early and late phases demonstrates participation of the involved segment in normal venous flow. Occlusion of a venous segment draining brain tissue may result in venous infarction and should not be performed. If the venous flow cannot be properly clarified, the normal venous routes can be studied during temporary test occlusion of the involved sinus using detachable balloons (URTASUN et al. 1996; ROY and RAYMOND 1997).

The venous approach to intracranial DAVMs is variable. A simultaneous transfemoral arterial catheterization of one of the main feeding arteries is necessary. This will provide the possibility of generating a road map of the venous system using the late phase of the arterial injection. It will also allow for control arterial injections during the procedure. The transfemoral approach via the femoral vein provides the most convenient access to the intracranial sinuses. Usually 5- or 6-French (F) guiding catheters are used, except if balloon test occlusion or permanent balloon occlusion is entertained that requires 8-F guides. Catheter navigation into the internal jugular veins, however, might be difficult or impossible. In such cases, direct retrograde puncture of the internal jugular vein should be considered (URTASUN et al. 1996). If even this maneuver does not allow access to the involved segment of the dural sinuses, a more distal direct venous puncture can be obtained, depending on the individual anatomy as demonstrated by angiography. As an example, microcatheters can be introduced into the superior ophthalmic vein and the cavernous sinus via the facial vein on some occasions. Finally, direct puncture of the superior sagittal sinus and transverse/sigmoid sinuses can be obtained via surgically created burr holes (URTASUN et al. 1996) or intraoperatively, through a small craniotomy (ENDO et al. 1998).

Occlusion or thrombosis of the major sinuses that frequently complicates DAVM may make transvenous access challenging. However, distal catheterization of the internal jugular vein generally makes introduction of microcatheters possible through occluded segments of the sigmoid or transverse sinus (GOBIN et al. 1993; NAITO et al. 2001). Alternately, access can be gained via the contralateral transverse sinus and the confluens sinuum. The ipsilateral inferior petrosal sinus provides the most convenient access to the cavernous sinus (Fig. 4.21). Even if not visualized on arteriograms, its entrance can usually be found with some manipulation of the guidewire within the jugular vein (HALBACH et al. 1989). With the help of micro-guidewires, hydrophilic microcatheters can than be easily navigated into the cavernous sinus. A phlebogram using a large volume of contrast medium may help in identifying a remnant of the inferior petrosal sinus (BENNDORF et al. 2000). If the ipsilateral inferior petrosal sinus is not found, the cavernous sinus might be catheterized with microcatheters introduced via the contralateral inferior petrosal sinus into the contralateral cavernous sinus and crossing the midline via intercavernous veins (HALBACH et al. 1989).

In none of the above avenues are feasible, for cavernous sinus DAVM the superior ophthalmic vein offers an excellent approach (LABBE et al. 1987; HANNEKEN et al. 1989; MILLER et al. 1995; QUINONES et al. 1997; KLINK et al. 2001). Through a small incision in the upper sulcus of the superior eyelid the orbital septum is opened and the superior ophthalmic vein is exposed within the retroseptal orbital fat. Once identified, the superior ophthalmic vein is incised between ligatures and a microcatheter is introduced under fluoroscopy into the cavernous sinus. Either microballoons or microcoils can be used to occlude the fistula. In case of normal drainage of the sylvian vein into the same cavernous sinus, the compartment receiving the shunt should be selectively occluded (NAKAMURA et al. 1998). Either the superior ophthalmic vein is permanently ligated or the incision is closed with microsutures at the end of the procedure (MILLER et al. 1995). Direct puncture of the superior ophthalmic vein has also been reported (BENNDORF et al. 2001). In case of DAVM involving subarachnoid veins that drain into sinuses, selective transvenous retrograde catheterization of the vein itself can be attempted. If successful, the vein itself can be occluded

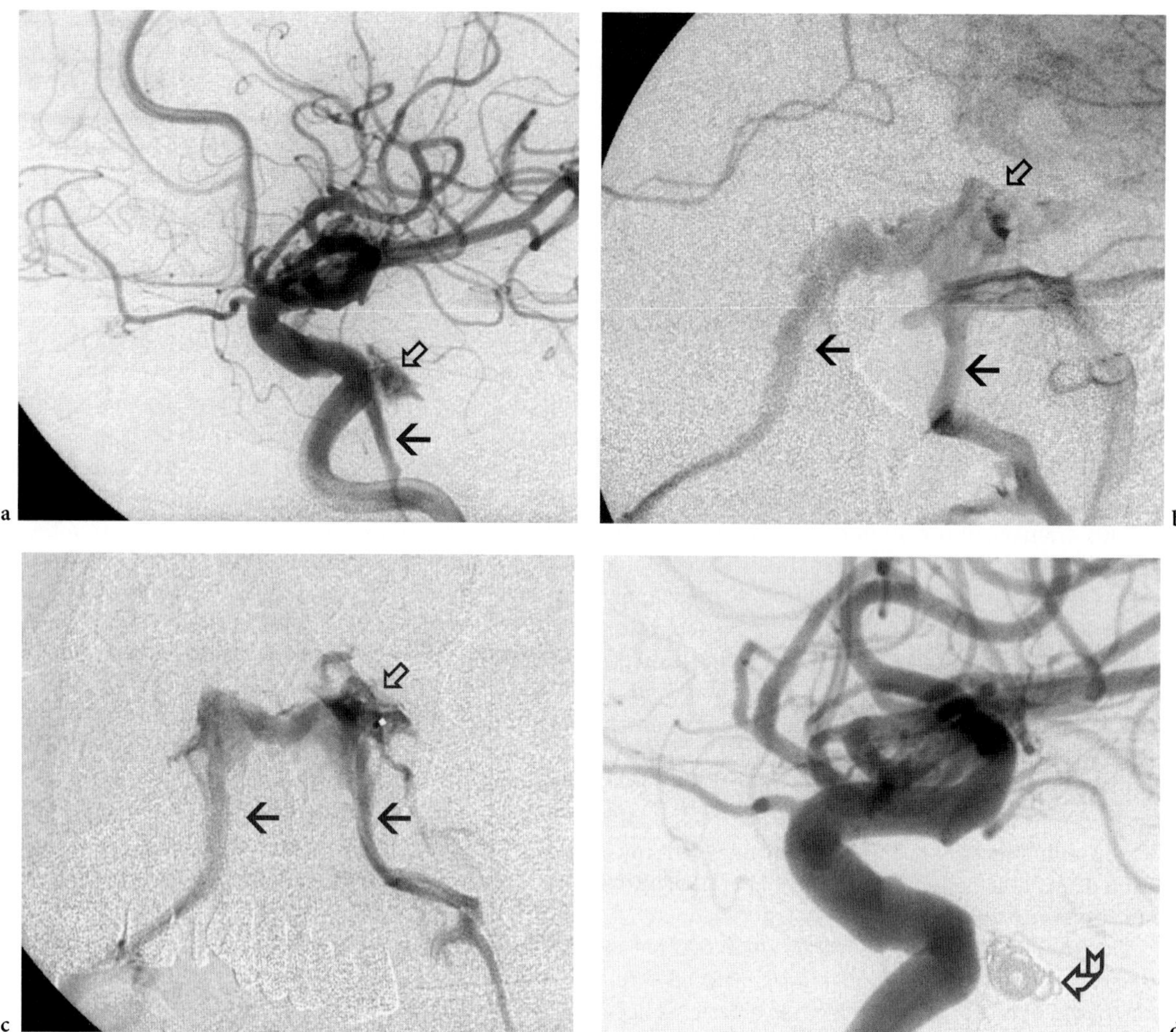

Fig. 4.21a–d. Endovascular treatment of cavernous sinus DAVM with transvenous embolization. **a** DSA with ICA injection, lateral view demonstrates DAVM of the posterior CS (*open arrow*) draining via the inferior petrosal sinus (IPS) (*arrow*). **b** Late venous phase of a ICA injection in an oblique view demonstrates bilateral SPS drainage (arrows). **c** Superselective injection of the ipsilateral CS (*open arrow*) following transfemoral catheterization of the ipsilateral internal jugular vein and introduction of a microcatheter via the IPS. Bilateral IPS drainage is well seen. **d** Complete obliteration of the DAVM is demonstrated by ICA injection in lateral view following the deposition of several detachable microcoils within the posterior CS (*broken arrow*)

with microcoils, and patency of the sinus (which in this case is normal) can be spared (Mironov 1998). The draining vein can be occluded from a transarterial approach, too, if enlarged arterial feeders and the arteriovenous connection allow the microcatheter to pass the fistula (Fukai et al. 2001).

Once transvenous access to the fistula site has been secured, the involved venous segment can be occluded using detachable balloons, microcoils, detachable microcoils, or glue. The segment that carries the malformation and any cortical veins that drain into the same sinus must be identified with extreme care. The entire section with fistulous connections must be tightly packed. Failure to occlude all arteriovenous connections may convert an originally benign venous pattern to a more aggressive one by blocking its antegrade outlet and forcing high-pressure arterial blood into the retrograde direction or, more malignantly (Davies et al. 1997), into cortical veins. On the other hand, closure of the entrance of normal subarachnoid veins may lead to venous infarction and hemorrhage. The use of detachable microballoons allows precise analysis of the venous circulation by temporary test occlusion prior to permanent closure (Urtasun et al. 1996; Roy and Raymond 1997). The disadvantage of using balloons is that they require a large (8-F) guiding catheter. Furthermore, any space remaining unpacked between balloons within the sinus will become an isolated sinus. If that segment carries residual arterial feeders as well as cortical veins, a high-grade fistula (Borden III) has been created. Alternatively, detachable and free pushable microcoils are being used to pack dural sinuses. Detachable coils can be delivered with more accuracy, in relation to any vascular structure (normal veins) that needs to be spared. One or more detachable coils can be placed at the end of the involved segment that is distal in relation to the tip of the guiding catheter. Once the distal edge of the occlusion is secured, the rest of the sinus is packed with free pushable coils, proceeding proximally. The disadvantage of using coils is that usually a large number of expensive microcoils and a lengthy procedure are required to achieve complete occlusion (Fig. 4.22). To reduce the number of coils, glue can be injected in combination with coils once the flow has been significantly reduced, or flow can be diminished by manual compression of the eyeball in case of cavernous sinus DAVM (Roy and Raymond 1997). To facilitate transvenous occlusion of DAVM, transarterial embolization may be obtained prior to venous occlusion to reduce arterial load.

In studies analyzing results of transvenous embolization in series of 20–24 patients with nonselected DAVM, anatomical cure of 71%–88%, significant flow reduction of 12%, clinical cure in 83%–96%, and clinical improvement of 13% are reported (Urtasun et al. 1996; Roy and Raymond 1997). Patients in series of 10–13 with cavernous sinus DAVM treated via the superior ophthalmic vein approach experienced a 92%–100% clinical and anatomical cure rate and 15% transient worsening of the ocular symptoms (Miller et al. 1995; Quinones et al. 1997).

Other transient complications including cranial nerve palsies and hearing loss (Roy and Raymond 1997; Oishi et al. 1999), as well as subdural hematoma associated with direct sinus puncture through a burr hole and perforation of sinus wall (Urtasun et al. 1996), are reported with low incidence (Irie et al. 2001). Recurrence of DAVM at another location following transvenous obliteration of cavernous sinus lesions occurs (Nakagawa et al. 1992; Kawaguchi et al. 1999; Kubota et al. 1999). It is unclear whether this is related to a permanent elevation of venous pressure, increased release of angiogenetic factors, or increased thrombogenic activity.

Combined surgical-endovascular approaches for sinus occlusion have been reported by several authors. Sections of sinuses isolated by complete sinus thrombosis can be packed with coils through a small craniotomy (Endo et al. 1998). During such procedures, direct measurements demonstrated 30%–60% of systemic blood pressure and purely arterial blood gas levels within the involved sinuses prior to treatment. If surgically exposed, the involved segment of the sinus can be isolated by surgical clamping, the subarachnoid veins draining into this segment ligated, and the sinus injected with glue (Halbach et al. 1989). The disadvantage of these combinations are that they require intraoperative angiographic facilities that are not always available, and even if they are, the quality may not be that of a dedicated endovascular laboratory. With currently used techniques endovascular access to intracranial sinuses can be gained with a high success rate. If this is not feasible, surgical treatment of the disease (with preoperative embolization if necessary) seems more reasonable than endovascular techniques applied in a surgical environment. This latter combination should be reserved for cases where neither embolization nor surgery can be safely employed.

4.4.3.3 Sinus Recanalization

Although the relationship between sinus thrombosis and DAVM is not yet fully understood, the etiologic role of thrombosis has been raised. If the occlusion or thrombosis of a dural sinus is the primary cause of a DAVM, then recanalization of that sinus would be a highly reasonable approach to treatment. Revascularization of thrombosed sinuses using local fibrinolysis with selective infusion of urokinase has been employed in cases of DAVM associated with symptomatic sinus thrombosis (Barnwell et al. 1991; Smith et al. 1994). More recently, mechanical recanalization of an occluded sigmoid sinus has been attempted using balloon angioplasty and stent placement. Balloon angioplasty resulted in conversion of the fistula from Borden II to Borden I by reestablishing antegrade venous drainage through the sigmoid sinus. Rethrombosis of the sinus occurred and a second procedure was performed, resulting in complete obliteration of the DAVM, normal antegrade flow within the sinus, and clinical improvement of the patient (Murphy et al. 2000). The implication of this report is controversial. Reopening of an occluded venous channel seems more physiological than what has been widely practiced: artificial occlusion of what was not yet (completely) occluded. On the other hand, the recanalization procedure applying selective infusion of fibrinolytics and systematic use of antiaggre-

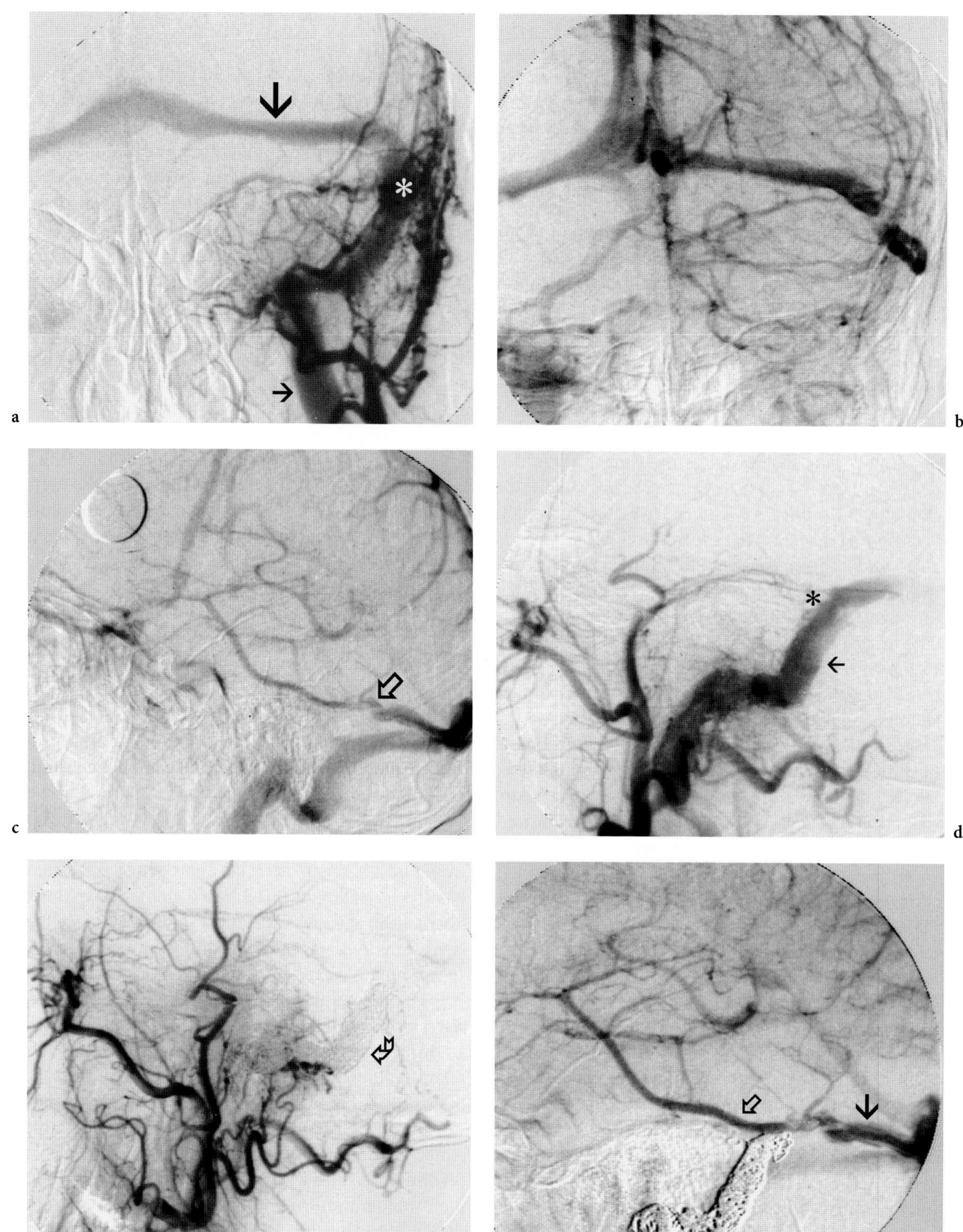

Fig. 4.22a–f. Endovascular treatment of sigmoid sinus DAVM with transvenous embolization. **a** DSA with Left ECA injection demonstrates DAVM involving the SS (*asterisk*) on the left with antegrade (*small arrow*) and retrograde (*arrow*) flow within the sinus. **b** Left ICA injection, AP view, late phase demonstrates "functional occlusion" of the sigmoid sinus on the left: arterial pressure from the DAVM prevents venous drainage of the brain parenchyma. **c** Lateral view of the ICA injection in the late phase demonstrates a prominent ipsilateral vein of Labbé (*open arrow*) that drains into the sinus in a retrograde fashion. **d** DSA, ECA injection following extensive transarterial embolization reduction of shunt flow and antegrade venous drainage only. The patient continued complaining of intolerable pulsatile tinnitus. **e** Complete occlusion of the DAVM following endovascular packing of the sigmoid sinus with several microcoils (*broken arrow*). DSA, left ECA injection, lateral view. **f** ICA injection confirms patency of the vein of Labbé (*arrow*) following sinus and DAVM occlusion

gants in association with stent placement may significantly increase the risks of bleeding that may occur as a result of a high-grade DAVM. Further research needs to be done to clarify current controversies.

4.4.4 Surgical Treatment

The goal of surgical treatment is permanent cure of the DAVM (goal *a*). For DAVMs that drain directly into leptomeningeal veins, simple interruption of that vein at the level of the dural entry results in complete elimination of the DAVM (Thompson et al. 1994; Hoh et al. 1998; Collice et al. 2000). For spinal DAVMs surgical disconnection of the draining vein at the dural level is the obligate treatment.

Lesions draining into sinuses are more complex are require extended surgery. The surrounding dura that contains the multiple arteriovenous shunts needs to be cut off the sinus ("skeletonization") and/or the diseased segment of the sinus needs to be removed or occluded (Sundt and Piepgras 1983). With proper preoperative angiographic analysis, the most appropriate surgical technique can be selected (Collice et al. 2000).

Skeletonization, or removal of the sinus, requires extensive exploration of the dura and may be associated with significant blood loss and morbidity. Preoperative transarterial embolization is therefore recommended if that type of surgery is required. Such a combination is usually associated with excellent results: an anatomical cure rate of 100%, with 0% permanent procedure-related morbidity and no mortality, is reported by several studies in series consisting of 17–34 patients with high-risk intracranial DAVM (Goto et al. 1999; Collice et al. 2000).

Preoperative embolization should concentrate on reduction of blood flow towards the nidus of the lesion. This is best achieved using liquid embolics; however, temporary results can be obtained with particles, too, which is associated with fewer risks. It should be kept in mind that superficial arterial feeders, such as those arising from the occipital artery, can be relatively easily handled during surgery, while blood supply from the tentorial branch of the ICA creates more difficulties for the surgeon. Transosseous blood supply and venous drainage results in significant blood loss that is difficult to control surgically. Surgery should follow preoperative embolization within a few days to avoid recanalization (Fig. 4.20).

The treatment of spinal DAVM by surgery is easy, safe, and effective and requires interruption of the draining vein at its dural entrance only (Anson and Spetzler 1992). Therefore, embolization of spinal DAVM should be offered only if the feeding pedicle provides a safe approach to a position close to the fistula site and it does not give rise to radiculomedullary branches supplying the anterior spinal artery. If there is a risk of reflux into the anterior spinal artery, surgery is significantly safer and should be selected.

4.4.5 Stereotactic Irradiation (Radiosurgery)

Several authors investigated stereotactic irradiation as a treatment modality for intracranial DAVM. Targeting of the lesions may require stereotactic angiography and image fusion with MRI (Guo et al. 1998). Maximum target doses of 22–30 Gy are used, delivered by gamma knife. In some series, preoperative embolization was applied either to alleviate symptoms or in an attempt to block leptomeningeal venous drainage and subsequently reduce the risk of hemorrhage during the latency period of gamma knife radiosurgery (Link et al. 1996; Pollock et al. 1999). In series of 18–29 patients treated, 72%–86% rates of angiographically complete occlusion and recurrence of symptoms in 15% are reported within a follow up of 12–36 months, without significant complication and no bleeding after irradiation (Link et al. 1996; Guo et al. 1998; Pollock et al. 1999). While these numbers are promising, considering the benign nature and propensity for spontaneous resolution of many DAVMs, it is difficult to draw a conclusion regarding the efficacy of this treatment modality. Radiosurgery is reported in a number of cavernous sinus DAVMs. Many cavernous sinus lesions do not necessitate treatment, and those that do require fast resolution of ocular symptoms that cannot be achieved by irradiation. In view of the natural history of DAVM (as presently known), we believe that radiosurgery should be reserved for cases in which treatment is necessary and no other alternative is feasible.

4.4.6 Management Strategy and Choice of Treatment

Indication for treatment should be based primarily on angiographic assessment of venous drainage and secondarily on clinical presentation. Patients without leptomeningeal drainage (Borden I) do not need to be treated if symptoms are well tolerated and do not cause an imminent visual loss. Medical and ophthalmological treatment should be applied as needed. If symptoms are not tolerated, treatment should be offered. Although complete closure of the shunt is desirable, palliative therapy is acceptable considering the low risk of the disease in this group. Within the Borden I category, Cognard type II/a lesions require closer follow-up. If signs of elevated ICP are detected aggressive treatment is recommended to avoid complications. All Borden type II and III patients require definitive closure of the arteriovenous shunt because of the high risk of bleeding or neurological deterioration in these cases (Fig. 4.23).

If treatment is decided on, medical conditions, location, arterial and venous anatomy need to be taken into consideration in order to select the best operative technique. In a recent meta-analysis of 258 reported cases, results of endovascular, surgical, and combined endovascular and surgical procedures, as well as surgical feeding artery ligation, were compared. Treatment was considered successful if complete angiographic occlusion was achieved. Not surprisingly, proximal occlusion of the feeding artery was found highly ineffective. For transverse-sigmoid sinus DAVMs, combined endovascular-surgical treatment (including all potential endovascular and surgical techniques) was more effective than all the other techniques together, demonstrating a success rate of 68%. Embolization alone was effective in 41% only. Similarly, DAVMs of the tentorial incisura were obliterated by the combined approach in 89%, while surgery alone demonstrated 78% and embolization alone 31% success. All cavernous sinus DAVMs were treated endovascularly. The venous approach was effective in 78%, arterial embolization in 62% only. Anterior fossa DAVMs were treated by surgery only, with a success rate of 95%. The number of cases located on the superior sagittal sinus or on the convexity was too low to draw a statistical conclusion (Lucas et al. 1997).

As shown by this report, cavernous sinus DAVM is primarily an endovascular disease, while anterior fossa lesions are generally better treated by surgery. Selection of the most appropriate technique for all other locations requires careful individual analysis of the anatomy in close cooperation between the neurosurgeon and the neurointerventionist. Not only the decision-making but also the operation itself may require collaboration of the two parties. The personal experience of both surgeon and endovascular therapist will greatly influence the choice of technique. If an endovascular procedure is selected, the benefits and disadvantages of both the venous and the arte-

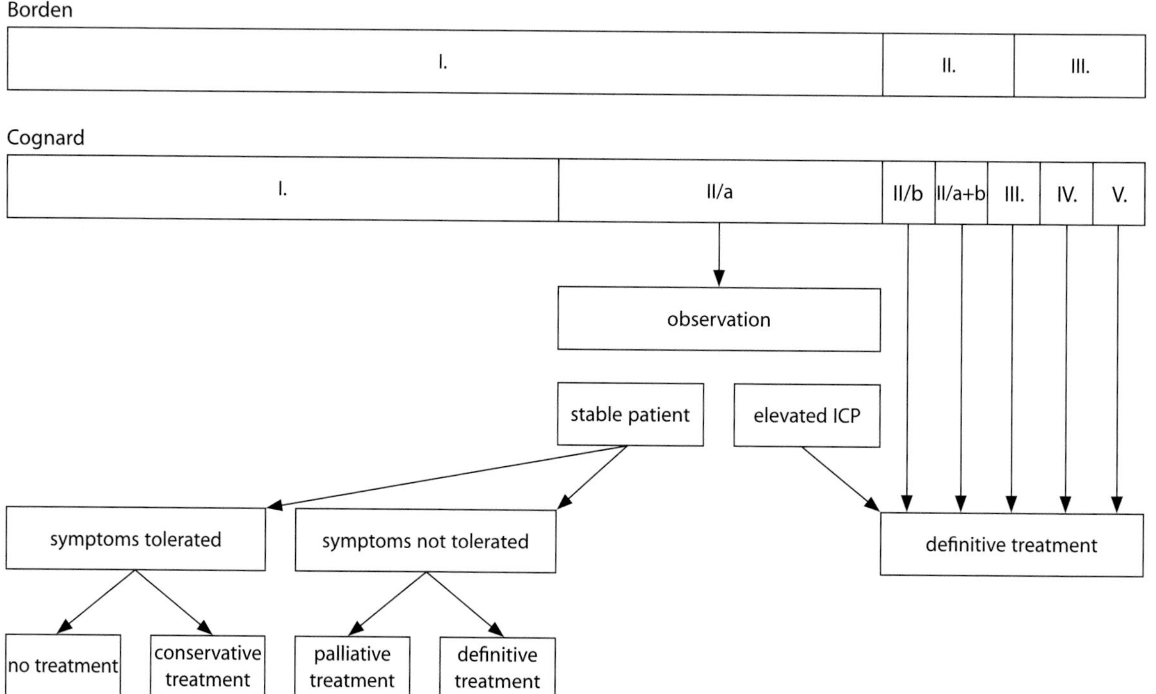

Fig. 4.23. Management strategy and indications for treatment

rial approach should be carefully analyzed. For cavernous sinus DAVM, transarterial embolization may be applied as a palliative treatment that in some case may also facilitate spontaneous cure. In case of complex arterial supply involving meningeal branches of the ICAs, the venous approach is preferred. For other locations, venous occlusion should be considered first, with or without previous arterial embolization. For permanent arterial occlusion a liquid embolic material must be employed. If complete occlusion of the sinus or meningeal vein is not feasible, surgery always needs to be taken into consideration. Preoperative transarterial embolization provides effective help for the surgical treatment while preoperative venous embolization may not be necessary. Stereotactic radiosurgery should be offered to those patients who need to be treated and are not candidates for either embolization or surgery. Although DAVMs present one of the most challenging groups of cerebrovascular disease for surgeons and radiologists, with state-of-the-art imaging techniques, thorough analysis, and understanding of the pathology, and with the common effort of an experienced neurosurgical–neuroendovascular team, most patients can be successfully managed, either conservatively or aggressively.

References

Al-Mefty O, Jinkins JR, Fox JL (1986) Extensive dural arteriovenous malformation. Case report. J Neurosurg 65: 417–420

Alberico RA, Barnes P, Robertson RL, et al (1999) Helical CT angiography: dynamic cerebrovascular imaging in children. AJNR Am J Neuroradiol 20:328–334

Aminoff MJ (1973) Vascular anomalies in the intracranial dura mater. Brain 96:601–612

Anson J, Spetzler R (1992) Classification of spinal arteriovenous malformations and implication for treatment. BNIQ 8:2–10

Arnautovic KI, Al-Mefty O, Angtuaco E, et al (1998) Dural arteriovenous malformations of the transverse/sigmoid sinus acquired from dominant sinus occlusion by a tumor: report of two cases. Neurosurgery 42:383–388

Awad IA, Little JR, Akarawi WP, et al (1990) Intracranial dural arteriovenous malformations: factors predisposing to an aggressive neurological course. J Neurosurg 72:839–850

Bank WO, Kerber CW, Cromwell LD (1981) Treatment of intracerebral arteriovenous malformations with isobutyl 2-cyanoacrylate: initial clinical experience. Radiology 139:609–616

Barnwell SL, Halbach VV, Dowd CF, et al (1991a) Multiple dural arteriovenous fistulas of the cranium and spine. AJNR Am J Neuroradiol 12:441–445

Barnwell SL, Higashida RT, Halbach VV, et al (1991b) Direct endovascular thrombolytic therapy for dural sinus thrombosis. Neurosurgery 28:135–142

Benndorf G, Bender A, Lehmann R, et al (2000) Transvenous occlusion of dural cavernous sinus fistulas through the thrombosed inferior petrosal sinus: report of four cases and review of the literature. Surg Neurol 54:42–54

Benndorf G, Bender A, Campi A, et al (2001) Treatment of a cavernous sinus dural arteriovenous fistula by deep orbital puncture of the superior ophthalmic vein. Neuroradiology 43:499–502

Binkert CA, Kollias SS, Valavanis A (1999) Spinal cord vascular disease: characterization with fast three-dimensional contrast-enhanced MR angiography. AJNR Am J Neuroradiol 20:1785–1793

Bitoh S, Sakaki S (1979) Spontaneous cure of dural arteriovenous malformation in the posterior fossa. Surg Neurol 12:111–114

Boet RS, Poon WS, Chan MY, et al (2001) Childhood posterior fossa pial-dural arteriovenous fistula treated by endovascular occlusion. Childs Nerv Syst 17:681–684

Borden JA, Wu JK, Shucart WA (1995) A proposed classification for spinal and cranial dural arteriovenous fistulous malformations and implications for treatment. J Neurosurg 82:166–179

Bousson V, Brunereau L, Vahedi K, et al (1999) Intracranial dural fistula as a cause of diffuse MR enhancement of the cervical spinal cord. J Neurol Neurosurg Psychiatry 67: 227–230

Bowen BC, Pattany PM (1997) Spine MR angiography. Clin Neurosci 4:165–173

Bowen BC, Pattany PM (1998) MR angiography of the spine. Magn Reson Imaging Clin North Am 6:165–178

Bowen BC, Pattany PM (2000) Contrast-enhanced MR angiography of spinal vessels. Magn Reson Imaging Clin North Am 8:597–614

Bowen BC, Fraser K, Kochan JP, et al (1995) Spinal dural arteriovenous fistulas: evaluation with MR angiography. AJNR Am J Neuroradiol 16:2029–2043

Brunereau L, Gobin YP, Meder JF, et al (1996) Intracranial dural arteriovenous fistulas with spinal venous drainage: relation between clinical presentation and angiographic findings. AJNR Am J Neuroradiol 17:1549–1554

Cellerini M, Mascalchi M, Mangiafico S, et al (1999) Phase-contrast MR angiography of intracranial dural arteriovenous fistulae. Neuroradiology 41:487–492

Chaudhary MY, Sachdev VP, Cho SH, et al (1982) Dural arteriovenous malformation of the major venous sinuses: an acquired lesion. AJNR Am J Neuroradiol 3:13–19

Chen CJ, Ro LS, Cheng WC, et al (1995) MRI/myelographic localization of fistulous tract in spinal dural arteriovenous malformations prior to arteriography. J Comput Assist Tomogr 19:893–896

Chen CJ, Chen CM, Lin TK (1998) Enhanced cervical MRI in identifying intracranial dural arteriovenous fistulae with spinal perimedullary venous drainage. Neuroradiology 40: 393–397

Chen JC, Tsuruda JS, Halbach VV (1992) Suspected dural arteriovenous fistula: results with screening MR angiography in seven patients. Radiology 183:265–271

Chiras J, Bories J, Leger JM, et al (1982) CT scan of dural arteriovenous fistulas. Neuroradiology 23:185–194

Cognard C, Gobin YP, Pierot L, et al (1995) Cerebral dural arteriovenous fistulas: clinical and angiographic correlation with a revised classification of venous drainage. Radiology 194:671–680

Cognard C, Miaux Y, Pierot L, et al (1996) The role of CT in evaluation of the effectiveness of embolisation of spinal dural arteriovenous fistulae with N-butyl cyanoacrylate. Neuroradiology 38:603–608

Cognard C, Houdart E, Casasco A, et al (1997) Long-term changes in intracranial dural arteriovenous fistulae leading to worsening in the type of venous drainage. Neuroradiology 39:59–66

Cognard C, Casasco A, Toevi M, et al (1998) Dural arteriovenous fistulas as a cause of intracranial hypertension due to impairment of cranial venous outflow. J Neurol Neurosurg Psychiatry 65:308–316

Collice M, D'Aliberti G, Arena O, et al (2000) Surgical treatment of intracranial dural arteriovenous fistulae: role of venous drainage. Neurosurgery 47:56–66; discussion 66–57

Convers P, Michel D, Brunon J, et al (1986) Dural arteriovenous fistulas of the posterior cerebral fossa and thrombosis of the lateral sinus. Discussion of their relations and treatment apropos of 2 cases. Neurochirurgie 32:495–500

Cromwell LD, Kerber CW (1979) Modification of cyanoacrylate for therapeutic embolization: preliminary experience. AJR Am J Roentgenol 132:799–801

Davies MA, Ter Brugge K, Willinsky R, et al (1996) The validity of classification for the clinical presentation of intracranial dural arteriovenous fistulas. J Neurosurg 85:830–837

Davies M, Saleh J, Ter Brugge K, et al (1997a) The natural history and management of dural arteriovenous fistulae, part 1. Bening lesions. Intervent Neuroradiol 3:295–302

Davies M, Ter Brugge K, Willinsky R, et al (1997b) The natural history and management of intracranial dural arteriovenous fistuilae, part 2. Aggressive lesions. Intervent Neuroradiol 3:303–311

De Marco JK, Dillon WP, Halback VV, et al (1990) Dural arteriovenous fistulas: evaluation with MR imaging. Radiology 175:193–199

Djindjan R, Merland J (1978) Superselective angiography of the external carotid artery. Springer, Berlin Heidelberg New York

Endo S, Koshu K, Kodama N, et al (1979) Spontaneous regression of a posterior fossa dural arteriovenous malformation (author's translation). No Shinkei Geka 7:1001–1004

Endo S, Kuwayama N, Takaku A, et al (1998) Direct packing of the isolated sinus in patients with dural arteriovenous fistulas of the transverse-sigmoid sinus. J Neurosurg 88: 449–456

Ernst RJ, Gaskill-Shipley M, Tomsick TA, et al (1997) Cervical myelopathy associated with intracranial dural arteriovenous fistula: MR findings before and after treatment. AJNR Am J Neuroradiol 18:1330–1334

Farb RI, McGregor C, Kim JK, et al (2001) Intracranial arteriovenous malformations: real-time auto-triggered elliptic centric-ordered 3D gadolinium-enhanced MR angiography – initial assessment. Radiology 220:244–251

Farb RI, Kim JK, Willinsky RA, et al (2002) Spinal dural arteriovenous fistula localization with a technique of first-pass gadolinium-enhanced MR angiography: initial experience. Radiology 222:843–850

Friedman JA, Pollock BE, Nichols DA (2000) Development of a cerebral arteriovenous malformation documented in an adult by serial angiography. Case report. J Neurosurg 93: 1058–1061

Fujita A, Nakamura M, Tamaki N (2001) Multiple dural arteriovenous fistulas involving both the cavernous sinus and the posterior fossa: report of two cases and review of the literature. No Shinkei Geka 29:1065–1072

Fukai J, Terada T, Kuwata T, et al (2001) Transarterial intravenous coil embolization of dural arteriovenous fistula involving the superior sagittal sinus. Surg Neurol 55: 353–358

Gelbert F, Guichard JP, Mourier KL, et al (1992) Phase-contrast MR angiography of vascular malformations of the spinal cord at 0.5 T. J Magn Reson Imaging 2:631–636

Gilbertson JR, Miller GM, Goldman MS, et al (1995) Spinal dural arteriovenous fistulas: MR and myelographic findings. AJNR Am J Neuroradiol 16:2049–2057

Gobin YP, Houdart E, Rogopoulos A, et al (1993) Percutaneous transvenous embolization through the thrombosed sinus in transverse sinus dural fistula. AJNR Am J Neuroradiol 14:1102–1105

Goto K, Sidipratomo P, Ogata N, et al (1999) Combining endovascular and neurosurgical treatments of high-risk dural arteriovenous fistulas in the lateral sinus and the confluence of the sinuses. J Neurosurg 90:289–299

Graeb DA, Dolman CL (1986) Radiological and pathological aspects of dural arteriovenous fistulas. Case report. J Neurosurg 64:962–967

Greenough GP, Mamourian A, Harbaugh RE (1999) Venous hypertension associated with a posterior fossa dural arteriovenous fistula: another cause of bithalamic lesions on MR images. AJNR Am J Neuroradiol 20:145–147

Guo WY, Pan DH, Wu HM, et al (1998) Radiosurgery as a treatment alternative for dural arteriovenous fistulas of the cavernous sinus. AJNR Am J Neuroradiol 19:1081–1087

Halbach VV, Higashida RT, Hieshima GB, et al (1987) Dural fistulas involving the transverse and sigmoid sinuses: results of treatment in 28 patients. Radiology 163:443–447

Halbach VV, Higashida RT, Hieshima GB, et al (1989a) Embolization of branches arising from the cavernous portion of the internal carotid artery. AJNR Am J Neuroradiol 10:143–150

Halbach VV, Higashida RT, Hieshima GB, et al (1989b) Transvenous embolization of dural fistulas involving the cavernous sinus. AJNR Am J Neuroradiol 10:377–383

Halbach VV, Higashida RT, Hieshima GB, et al (1989c) Transvenous embolization of dural fistulas involving the transverse and sigmoid sinuses. AJNR Am J Neuroradiol 10:385–392

Halbach VV, Higashida RT, Hieshima GB, et al (1989d) Treatment of dural fistulas involving the deep cerebral venous system. AJNR Am J Neuroradiol 10:393–399

Hamada J, Yano S, Kai Y, et al (2000) Histopathological study of venous aneurysms in patients with dural arteriovenous fistulas. J Neurosurg 92:1023–1027

Hamada Y, Goto K, Inoue T, et al (1997) Histopathological aspects of dural arteriovenous fistulas in the transverse-sigmoid sinus region in nine patients. Neurosurgery 40: 452–456; discussion 456–458

Hanneken AM, Miller NR, Debrun GM, et al (1989) Treatment of carotid-cavernous sinus fistulas using a detachable balloon catheter through the superior ophthalmic vein. Arch Ophthalmol 107:87–92

Hashimoto M, Yokota A, Matsuoka S, et al (1989) Central retinal vein occlusion after treatment of cavernous dural arteriovenous malformation. AJNR Am J Neuroradiol 10 [Suppl 5]:S30–S31

Herman JM, Spetzler RF, Bederson JB, et al (1995) Genesis of a dural arteriovenous malformation in a rat model. J Neurosurg 83:539–545

Hieshima GB, Cahan LD, Berlin MS, et al (1977) Calvarial, orbital and dural vascular anomalies in hereditary hemorrhagic telangiectasia. Surg Neurol 8:263–267

Hirabuki N, Miura T, Mitomo M, et al (1988) MR imaging of dural arteriovenous malformations with ocular signs. Neuroradiology 30:390–394

Hoh BL, Choudhri TF, Connolly ES Jr, et al (1998) Surgical management of high-grade intracranial dural arteriovenous fistulas: leptomeningeal venous disruption without nidus excision. Neurosurgery 42:796–804; discussion 804–795

Horikoshi T, Hida K, Iwasaki Y, et al (2000) Chronological changes in MRI findings of spinal dural arteriovenous fistula. Surg Neurol 53: 243–249

Houdart E, Gobin YP, Casasco A, et al (1993) A proposed angiographic classification of intracranial arteriovenous fistulae and malformations. Neuroradiology 35:381–385

Houser OW, Campbell JK, Campbell RJ, et al (1979) Arteriovenous malformation affecting the transverse dural venous sinus - an acquired lesion. Mayo Clin Proc 54:651–661

Hurst RW, Grossman RI (2000) Peripheral spinal cord hypointensity on T2-weighted MR images: a reliable imaging sign of venous hypertensive myelopathy. AJNR Am J Neuroradiol 21:781–786

Iizuka Y, Maehara T, Hishii M, et al (2001) Successful transarterial glue embolisation by wedged technique for a tentorial dural arteriovenous fistula presenting with a conjunctival injection. Neuroradiology 43:677–679

Irie K, Kawanishi M, Kunishio K, et al (2001) The efficacy and safety of transvenous embolisation in the treatment of intracranial dural arteriovenous fistulas. J Clin Neurosci 8 [Suppl 1]:92–96

Jaillard AS, Peres B, Hommel M (1999) Neuropsychological features of dementia due to dural arteriovenous malformation. Cerebrovasc Dis 9:91–97

Kaech D, de Tribolet N,Lasjaunias P (1987) Anterior inferior cerebellar artery aneurysm, carotid bifurcation aneurysm, and dural arteriovenous malformation of the tentorium in the same patient. Neurosurgery 21:575–582

Kagawa K, Nishimura S, Seki K (2001) Cavernous sinus dural arteriovenous shunt presenting with subarachnoid hemorrhage and acute subdural hematoma: a case report. No Shinkei Geka 29:457–463

Kallmes DF, Cloft HJ, Jensen ME, et al (1998) Dural arteriovenous fistula: a pitfall of time-of-flight MR venography for the diagnosis of sinus thrombosis. Neuroradiology 40:242–244

Kataoka H, Miyamoto S, Nagata I, et al (2001) Venous congestion is a major cause of neurological deterioration in spinal arteriovenous malformations. Neurosurgery 48:1224–1229; discussion 1229–1230

Kawaguchi T, Kawano T, Kaneko Y, et al (1999a) Dural arteriovenous fistula of the transverse sigmoid sinus after transvenous embolization of the carotid cavernous fistula. No To Shinkei 51:1065–1069

Kawaguchi T, Kawano T, Kaneko Y, et al (1999b) Dural arteriovenous fistula of the transverse-sigmoid sinus with intraventricular hemorrhage: a case report. No Shinkei Geka 27:1133–1138

Kawaguchi T, Kawano T, Kaneko Y, et al (2000) rCBF study with 123I-IMP SPECT of dural arteriovenous fistula. No To Shinkei 52:991–996

Kawaguchi T, Kawano T, Kaneko Y, et al (2001) Classification of venous ischaemia with MRI. J Clin Neurosci 8 [Suppl 1]: 82–88

Kendall BE, Logue V (1977) Spinal epidural angiomatous malformations draining into intrathecal veins. Neuroradiology 13:181–189

Kerber CW, Newton TH (1973) The macro and microvasculature of the dura mater. Neuroradiology 6:175–179

Kerber CW, Bank WO,Cromwell LD (1979) Cyanoacrylate occlusion of carotid-cavernous fistula with preservation of carotid artery flow. Neurosurgery 4:210–215

Kincaid PK, Duckwiler GR, Gobin YP, et al (2001) Dural arteriovenous fistula in children: endovascular treatment and outcomes in seven cases. AJNR Am J Neuroradiol 22: 1217–1225

Klingebiel R, Zimmer C, Rogalla P, et al (2001) Assessment of the arteriovenous cerebrovascular system by multi-slice CT. A single-bolus, monophasic protocol. Acta Radiol 42: 560–562

Klink T, Hofmann E, Lieb W (2001) Transvenous embolization of carotid cavernous fistulas via the superior ophthalmic vein. Graefes Arch Clin Exp Ophthalmol 239:583–588

Kraus JA, Stuper BK, Berlit P (1998) Association of resistance to activated protein C and dural arteriovenous fistulas. J Neurol 245:731–733

Kraus JA, Stuper BK, Nahser HC, et al (2000) Significantly increased prevalence of factor V Leiden in patients with dural arteriovenous fistulas. J Neurol 247:521–523

Kubota Y, Ueda T, Kaku Y, et al (1999) Development of a dural arteriovenous fistula around the jugular valve after transvenous embolization of cavernous dural arteriovenous fistula. Surg Neurol 51:174–176

Kurata A, Miyasaka Y, Oka H, et al (1999) Spontaneous carotid cavernous fistulas with special reference to the influence of estradiol decrease. Neurol Res 21:631–639

Labbe D, Courtheoux P, Rigot-Jolivet M, et al (1987) Bilateral dural carotid-cavernous fistula. Its treatment by way of the superior ophthalmic vein. Rev Stomatol Chir Maxillofac 88: 120–124

Lasjaunias P, Berenstein A (1987) Surgical neuroangiography, 1st edn, vol 2. Springer, Berlin Heidelberg New York

Lasjaunias P, Halimi P, Lopez-Ibor L, et al (1984) Endovascular treatment of pure spontaneous dural vascular malformations. Review of 23 cases studied and treated between May 1980 and October 1983. Neurochirurgie 30:207–223

Lasjaunias P, Chiu M, Ter Brugge K, et al (1986) Neurological manifestations of intracranial dural arteriovenous malformations. J Neurosurg 64:724–730

Lawton MT, Jacobowitz R, Spetzler RF (1997) Redefined role of angiogenesis in the pathogenesis of dural arteriovenous malformations. J Neurosurg 87:267–274

Lee TT, Gromelski EB, Bowen BC, et al (1998) Diagnostic and surgical management of spinal dural arteriovenous fistulas. Neurosurgery 43:242–246; discussion 246–247

Link MJ, Coffey RJ, Nichols DA, et al (1996) The role of radiosurgery and particulate embolization in the treatment of dural arteriovenous fistulas. J Neurosurg 84:804–809

Liu HM, Huang YC, Wang YH, et al (2000) Transarterial embolisation of complex cavernous sinus dural arteriovenous fistulae with low-concentration cyanoacrylate. Neuroradiology 42:766–770

Lucas CP, Zabramski JM, Spetzler RF, et al (1997) Treatment for intracranial dural arteriovenous malformations: a meta-analysis from the English language literature. Neurosurgery 40:1119–1130; discussion 1130–1112

Luciani A, Houdart E, Mounayer C, et al (2001) Spontaneous

closure of dural arteriovenous fistulas: report of three cases and review of the literature. AJNR Am J Neuroradiol 22: 992–996

Magidson MA, Weinberg PE (1976) Spontaneous closure of a dural arteriovenous malformation. Surg Neurol 6:107–110

Manelfe C, Lazorthes G, Roulleau J (1972) Artères de la duremère rachidienne chez l'homme. Acta Radiol 13:829–841

Mascalchi M, Bianchi MC, Quilici N, et al (1995) MR angiography of spinal vascular malformations. AJNR Am J Neuroradiol 16:289–297

Mascalchi M, Quilici N, Ferrito G, et al (1997) Identification of the feeding arteries of spinal vascular lesions via phase-contrast MR angiography with three-dimensional acquisition and phase display. AJNR Am J Neuroradiol 18: 351–358

Mascalchi M, Cosottini M, Ferrito G, et al (1999) Contrast-enhanced time-resolved MR angiography of spinal vascular malformations. J Comput Assist Tomogr 23:341–345

Mascalchi M, Ferrito G, Quilici N, et al (2001) Spinal vascular malformations: MR angiography after treatment. Radiology 219:346–353

McCutcheon IE, Doppman JL, Oldfield EH (1996) Microvascular anatomy of dural arteriovenous abnormalities of the spine: a microangiographic study. J Neurosurg 84:215–220

Meder JF, Devaux B, Merland JJ, et al (1995) Spontaneous disappearance of a spinal dural arteriovenous fistula. AJNR Am J Neuroradiol 16:2058–2062

Miki T, Nagai K, Saitoh Y, et al (1988) Matas procedure in the treatment of spontaneous carotid cavernous sinus fistula: a complication of retinal hemorrhage. No Shinkei Geka 16: 971–976

Miller NR, Monsein LH, Debrun GM, et al (1995) Treatment of carotid-cavernous sinus fistulas using a superior ophthalmic vein approach. J Neurosurg 83:838–842

Mironov A (1998) Selective transvenous embolization of dural fistulas without occlusion of the dural sinus. AJNR Am J Neuroradiol 19:389–391

Momoji J, Mukawa J, Yamashiro K, et al (1997) Histopathological examinations of dural arteriovenous malformations of posterior fossa. No Shinkei Geka 25:137–142

Murai Y, Yamashita Y, Ikeda Y, et al (1999) Ruptured aneurysm of the orbitofrontal artery associated with dural arteriovenous malformation in the anterior cranial fossa – case report. Neurol Med Chir (Tokyo) 39:157–160

Murphy KJ, Gailloud P, Venbrux A, et al (2000) Endovascular treatment of a grade IV transverse sinus dural arteriovenous fistula by sinus recanalization, angioplasty, and stent placement: technical case report. Neurosurgery 46: 497–500; discussion 500–491

Nagy ZZ, Nemeth J, Suveges I, et al (1995) A case of paradoxical worsening of dural-sinus arteriovenous malformation syndrome after neurosurgery. Eur J Ophthalmol 5:265–270

Naito I, Iwai T, Shimaguchi H, et al (2001) Percutaneous transvenous embolisation through the occluded sinus for transverse-sigmoid dural arteriovenous fistulas with sinus occlusion. Neuroradiology 43:672–676

Nakagawa H, Kubo S, Nakajima Y, et al (1992) Shifting of dural arteriovenous malformation from the cavernous sinus to the sigmoid sinus to the transverse sinus after transvenous embolization. A case of left spontaneous carotid-cavernous sinus fistula. Surg Neurol 37:30–38

Nakamura M, Tamaki N, Kawaguchi T, et al (1998) Selective transvenous embolization of dural carotid-cavernous sinus fistulas with preservation of sylvian venous outflow. Report of three cases. J Neurosurg 89:825–829

Nakstad PH, Bakke SJ, Hald JK (1992) Embolization of intracranial arteriovenous malformations and fistulas with polyvinyl alcohol particles and platinum fibre coils. Neuroradiology 34:348–351

Newton TH,Cronqvist S (1969) Involvement of dural arteries in intracranial arteriovenous malformations. Radiology 93: 1071–1078

Nishijima M, Takaku A, Endo S, et al (1992) Etiological evaluation of dural arteriovenous malformations of the lateral and sigmoid sinuses based on histopathological examinations. J Neurosurg 76:600–606

Oishi H, Arai H, Sato K, et al (1999) Complications associated with transvenous embolisation of cavernous dural arteriovenous fistula. Acta Neurochir (Wien) 141:1265–1271

Pierot L, Chiras J, Duyckaerts C, et al (1993) Intracranial dural arteriovenous fistulas and sinus thrombosis. Report of five cases. J Neuroradiol 20:9–18

Pollock BE, Nichols DA, Garrity JA, et al (1999) Stereotactic radiosurgery and particulate embolization for cavernous sinus dural arteriovenous fistulae. Neurosurgery 45: 459–466; discussion 466–457

Quinones D, Duckwiler G, Gobin PY, et al (1997) Embolization of dural cavernous fistulas via superior ophthalmic vein approach. AJNR Am J Neuroradiol 18:921–928

Ratliff J, Voorhies RM (1999) Arteriovenous fistula with associated aneurysms coexisting with dural arteriovenous malformation of the anterior inferior falx. Case report and review of the literature. J Neurosurg 91:303–307

Reinges MH, Thron A, Mull M, et al (2001) Dural arteriovenous fistulae at the foramen magnum. J Neurol 248:197–203

Ricolfi F, Manelfe C, Meder JF, et al (1999) Intracranial dural arteriovenous fistulae with perimedullary venous drainage. Anatomical, clinical and therapeutic considerations. Neuroradiology 41:803–812

Roy D, Raymond J (1997) The role of transvenous embolization in the treatment of intracranial dural arteriovenous fistulas. Neurosurgery 40:1133–1141; discussion 1141–1134

Sakaki T, Morimoto T, Nakase H, et al (1996) Dural arteriovenous fistula of the posterior fossa developing after surgical occlusion of the sigmoid sinus. Report of five cases. J Neurosurg 84:113–118

Sergott RC, Grossman RI, Savino PJ, et al (1987) The syndrome of paradoxical worsening of dural-cavernous sinus arteriovenous malformations. Ophthalmology 94:205–212

Shigematsu Y, Korogi Y, Yoshizumi K, et al (2000) Three cases of spinal dural AVF: evaluation with first-pass, gadolinium-enhanced, three-dimensional MR angiography. J Magn Reson Imaging 12:949–952

Singh V, Meyers PM, Halbach VH, et al (2001) Dural arteriovenous fistula associated with prothrombin gene mutation. J Neuroimaging 11:319–321

Slaba S, Smayra T, Hage P, et al (2000) An unusual cause of acute myelopathy: a dural arteriovenous fistula at the craniocervical junction. J Med Liban 48:168–172

Smith TP, Higashida RT, Barnwell SL, et al (1994) Treatment of dural sinus thrombosis by urokinase infusion. AJNR Am J Neuroradiol 15:801–807

Solis OJ, Davis KR, Ellis GT (1977) Dural arteriovenous malformation associated with subdural and intracerebral hematoma: a CT scan and angiographic correlation. Comput Tomogr 1:145–150

Song JK, Gobin YP, Duckwiler GR, et al (2001) N-butyl 2-cyanoacrylate embolization of spinal dural arteriovenous fistulae. AJNR Am J Neuroradiol 22:40–47

Stecker MM, Marcotte P, Hurst R, et al (1996) Spinal dural arteriovenous malformations. Intraoperative evoked potential evidence for pathophysiology. A case report. Spine 21: 512–515

Sundt TM Jr, Piepgras DG (1983) The surgical approach to arteriovenous malformations of the lateral and sigmoid dural sinuses. J Neurosurg 59:32–39

Suzuki S, Tanaka R, Miyasaka Y, et al (2000) Dural arteriovenous malformations associated with cerebral aneurysms. J Clin Neurosci 7 [Suppl 1]:36–38

Suzuki Y, Kase M, Yokoi M, et al (1989) Development of central retinal vein occlusion in dural carotid-cavernous fistula. Ophthalmologica 199:28–33

Tanimoto M, Tamaki N, Kuwamura K, et al (1984) Hemodynamic study of cerebral arteriovenous malformation by using 133Xe inhalation method. No Shinkei Geka 12: 1513–1520

Terada T, Higashida RT, Halbach VV, et al (1994) Development of acquired arteriovenous fistulas in rats due to venous hypertension. J Neurosurg 80:884–889

Terada T, Higashida RT, Halbach VV, et al (1998) The effect of oestrogen on the development of arteriovenous fistulae induced by venous hypertension in rats. Acta Neurochir (Wien) 140:82–86

Terwey B, Becker H, Thron AK, et al (1989) Gadolinium-DTPA enhanced MR imaging of spinal dural arteriovenous fistulas. J Comput Assist Tomogr 13:30–37

Thompson BG, Doppman JL,Oldfield EH (1994) Treatment of cranial dural arteriovenous fistulae by interruption of leptomeningeal venous drainage. J Neurosurg 80:617–623

Uranishi R, Nakase H, Sakaki T (1999) Expression of angiogenic growth factors in dural arteriovenous fistula. J Neurosurg 91:781–786

Urtasun F, Biondi A, Casaco A, et al (1996) Cerebral dural arteriovenous fistulas: percutaneous transvenous embolization. Radiology 199:209–217

Valavanis A (ed) (1993) Interventional neuroradiology. Medical radiology. Springer, Berlin Heidelberg New York

Van Dijk JM, TerBrugge KG, Willinsky RA, et al (2002) Multiplicity of dural arteriovenous fistulas. J Neurosurg 96: 76–78

Wakamoto H, Miyazaki H, Shinoda A, et al (1999) The natural history of a dural arteriovenous fistula associated with sinus thrombosis: a case report. No Shinkei Geka 27: 563–568

Watanabe A, Takahara Y, Ibuchi Y, et al (1984) Two cases of dural arteriovenous malformation occurring after intracranial surgery. Neuroradiology 26:375–380

Watanabe T, Matsumaru Y, Sonobe M, et al (2000) Multiple dural arteriovenous fistulae involving the cavernous and sphenoparietal sinuses. Neuroradiology 42:771–774

Willinsky R, Lasjaunias P, Terbrugge K, et al (1990) Angiography in the investigation of spinal dural arteriovenous fistula. A protocol with application of the venous phase. Neuroradiology 32:114–116

Willinsky R, Terbrugge K, Montanera W, et al (1994) Venous congestion: an MR finding in dural arteriovenous malformations with cortical venous drainage. AJNR Am J Neuroradiol 15:1501–1507

Willinsky RA, Ter Brugge K, Montanera W, et al (1995) Posttreatment MR findings in spinal dural arteriovenous malformations. AJNR Am J Neuroradiol 16:2063–2071

Woimant F, Merland JJ, Riche MC, et al (1982) Bulbospinal syndrome related to a meningeal arteriovenous fistula of the lateral sinus draining into spinal cord veins. Rev Neurol (Paris) 138:559–566

Yamada T, Okuchi K, Tuji H, et al (1993) A case of intracerebral AVM fed by the anterior ethmoidal artery. No Shinkei Geka 21:459–462

5 Intracranial Aneurysms

I. WANKE, A. DÖRFLER, M. FORSTING

CONTENTS

I. WANKE, MD; A. DÖRFLER, MD; M. FORSTING, MD, PhD
Institute of Diagnostic and Interventional Radiology, Department of Neuroradiology, University of Essen, Hufelandstrasse 55, 45122 Essen, Germany

Intracranial aneurysms do not fall precisely into the category of true vascular malformations; they are usually acquired. However, we included them because any neuroradiologist with an interest in vascular malformations and/or endovascular therapy clearly expects this entity to be covered extensively in a book such as this. Instead of using the modern way of communicating data (coloured boxes and tables), we have used the traditional form of writing with reiteration, mixing facts with opinions and illustrating as much as possible with radiological images. It is our hope that many people will read the chapter from beginning to end, and that redundancy and images will help to memorize new information.

5.1 Pathology

5.1.1 Classification

Classification of intracranial aneuryms may be based on morphology, size, location and etiology. The majority of intracranial aneurysms are true aneurysms containing all layers or components of the normal vessel wall. In contrast, in false aneurysms or pseudoaneurysms the vascular lumen does not enlarge, although the external diameter of the abnormal segment may be increased. These aneurysms are rare within the skull.

Usually, intracranial aneurysms are divided into three basic types: saccular, fusiform and dissecting. They can arise as solitary (70%–75%) or multiple (25%–30%) vascular lesions, usually located at the Circle of Willis. While traumatic, infectious or tumor-associated aneurysms are rare, most of them develop spontaneously. However, the pathogenetic criteria for the development of spontaneous aneurysms are only partially understood. Endogenous factors like elevated arterial blood pressure, special anatomical relationships given by the Circle of Willis, altered flow conditions, and exogenous factors like cigarette smoking, heavy alcohol consumption and anticoagulant or contraceptive medications have all been found to be associated with the occurrence of cerebral aneurysms (Juvela et al. 2001; Longstreth et al. 1985; Stehbens 1989; Teunissen et al. 1996; Weir et al. 1998). The most common causes for the development of an aneurysm are hemodynamically induced vascular injuries, atherosclerosis, underlying vasculopathy and high flow states. More uncommon etiologies are trauma, infection, drug abuse and neoplasms.

5.1.2 Saccular Aneurysms

Saccular aneurysms are berry-like vessel outpouchings mostly arising from arterial bifurcations and account for 66%–98% of intracranial aneurysms (Yong-Zhong and van Alphen 1990). The vast majority of aneurysms (85%) are located in the anterior and only 15% are located in the posterior circulation (Kassell and Torner 1983).

The majority of saccular aneurysms are not considered to be congenital, but develop during life. Cerebral aneurysms are rare in children and almost never occur in neonates (Heiskanen 1989). If a neonate or young baby suffers from an aneurysmal hemorrhage, usually a connective tissue disease is the underlying cause.

In adults the role of acquired changes in the arterial wall is likely because there are general risk factors for subarachnoid hemorrhage (SAH) and presumably for the development of aneurysms like hypertension, smoking and alcohol abuse (Teunissen et al. 1996). These factors might contribute to general thickening of the intimal layer in the arterial wall, distal and proximal to branching sites. These "intimal pads" are probably the earliest stages of aneurysm formation. Within these pads, the intimal layer is inelastic and therefore causes increased strain of the more elastic portions of the vessel wall (Crompton 1966). Abnormalities in structural proteins of the extracellular matrix additionally contribute to aneurysm formation (Chyatte et al. 1990). However, it is not known why only some adults develop aneurysms at arterial bifurcations and most do not. The popular theory of a congenital defect in the tunica media of the muscle layer as a weak spot through which the inner layer of the arterial wall would bulge has had doubt cast upon it by a number of contradicting observations. Gaps in the muscle layer are equally present in patients with and without aneurysms (Stehbens 1989). If the aneurysm has formed, any defect in the muscle layer is not located at the neck, but somewhere in the aneurysmal wall of the sac (Stehbens 1989).

The most plausible pathogenetic theory is that they are acquired due to hemodynamic stress on the relatively unsupported bifurcations of cerebral arteries (Timperman et al. 1995). This is supported by the

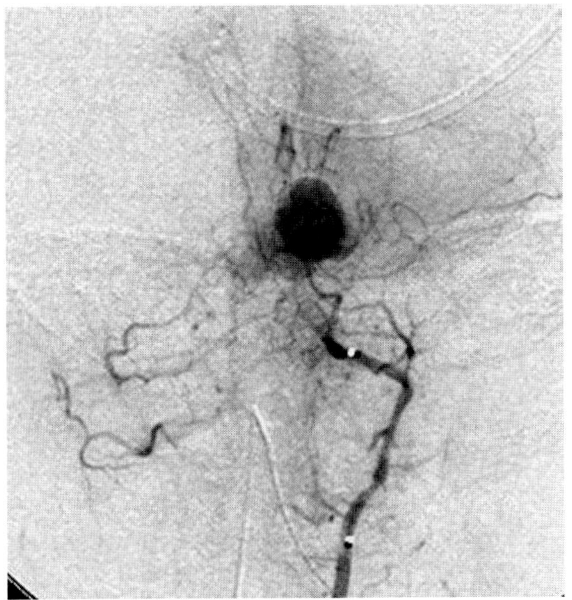

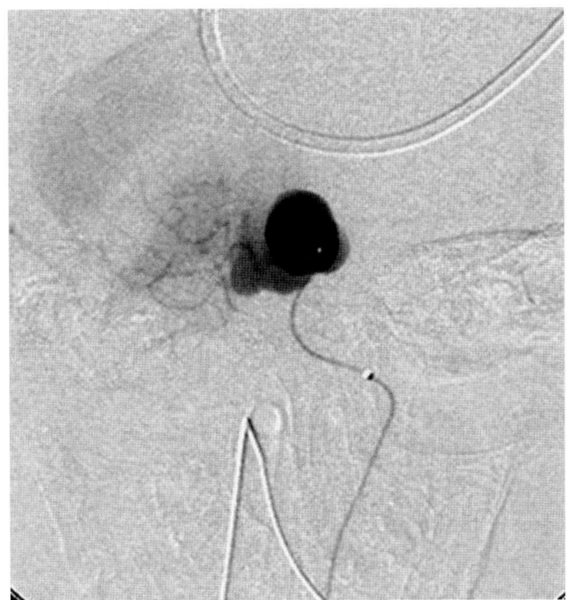

Fig. 5.1.1. a Aneurysm of the basilar artery in a newborn (ap view). **b** Aneurysmography revealed a large bilobulated aneurysm (ap view)

clinical observation that many patients with an anterior communicating artery (Acom) aneurysm do have one hypoplastic or absent A1 segment and thus an increased hemodynamic stress on the AcomA. Other factors than hemodynamics and structural alterations of the vessel wall contributing to the development of saccular aneurysms may be genetic, infection, trauma, neoplasms, radiation or idiopathic.

5.1.3 Dissecting Aneurysms

Spontaneous arterial dissection has been well recognized at the cervical portion of the carotid artery and extracranial vertebral artery as an important cause of ischemic stroke in young adults. In contrast, intracranial or intradural dissections more often cause subarachnoid hemorrhage instead of stroke. The true prevalence of intracranial dissections is unknown. SASAKI et al. (1991) described dissecting aneurysms accounting for 4.5% of the autopsy cases of SAH. In contrast to saccular aneurysms dissecting aneurysms occur much more often in the vertebrobasilar system and more often in man than in woman (YAMAURA et al. 2000).

Dissecting aneurysms of the extracranial carotid and vertebral arteries are often traumatic in origin. However, they may also be caused by fibromuscular dysplasia, atherosclerosis, infection, arthritis, heritable connective tissue disorders and chiropractic manoeuvres, or may occur spontaneously. Dissecting aneurysms are usually false aneurysms consisting of a false lumen within an injured arterial wall. An intimal tear is followed by an intramural hemorrhage between the media and adventitia (SCHIEVINK 2001). The majority of dissecting aneurysms in supraaortal vessels are found at extracranial segments. However, if dissections occur intracranially, e.g. at the intradural portion of the vertebral or carotid artery, these can clearly cause subarachnoid hemorrhage. In our experience these dissecting aneurysms may be the most often overlooked cause of the so-called non-perimesencephalic form of non-aneurysmal SAH.

Magnetic resonance imaging is the diagnostic modality of choice, since the intramural hematoma can be directly visualized. Angiography may reveal luminal dilatation followed by tapering of the vessel (string sign). The major clinical concern of extracranial dissections are distal embolization or subsequent arterial occlusion. Rupture of an extracranial dissecting aneurysm is rare (SCHIEVINK 2001). The therapeutic gold standard is anticoagulation and this usually leads to a good outcome. Surgical or endovascular therapy is generally reserved for those patients who do not respond to medical therapy or those with enlarging lesions.

The major clinical feature of intracranial arterial dissection is SAH due to rupture (58%). Ischemic infarction due to stenosis or occlusion by the intramural hematoma or by remote embolism occurs in around 42% of patients (Yamaura et al. 2000). Intracranially, there is some difficulty in differentiating dissection from stenotic lesions. Isolated unusual locations of arterial stenosis as well as the presence of smooth rather than irregular narrowing should help to differentiate dissection from vasospasm due to SAH. The optimal treatment of intracranial dissection has not been determined. Dissections that result in a complete stroke are beyond treatment; however, those within a certain time window might be candidates for recanalization therapy.

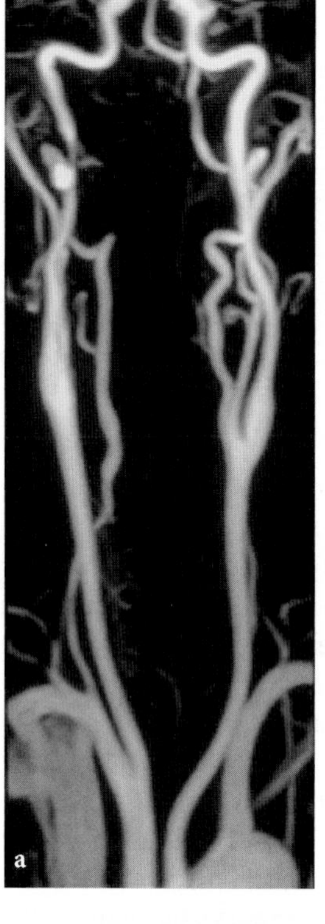

Fig. 5.1.2. Dissection of the right internal carotid artery with extracranial enlarging pseudoaneurysm. **a** Contrast-enhanced MR angiography demonstrating the aneurysm at the extracranial ICA. **b** Conventional DSA, oblique view. **c** CT angiography, sagittal reformation reveals the small aneurysm neck. **d** Conventional DSA before and (**e, f**) after endovascular coil embolization demonstrating aneurysm occlusion with preservation of the internal carotid artery

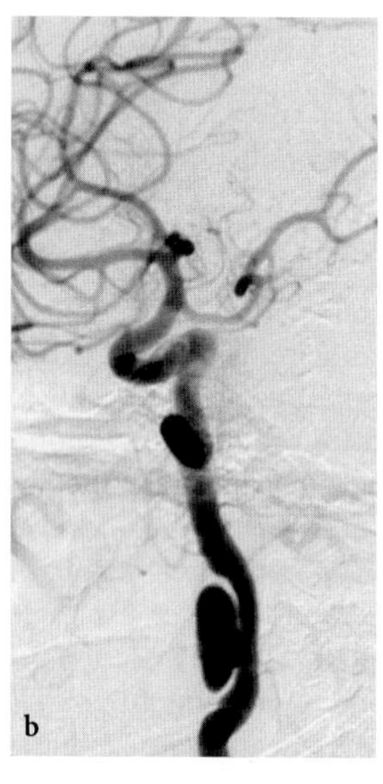

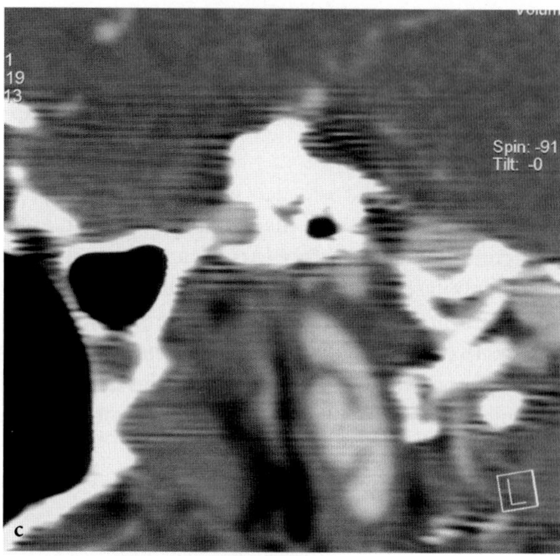

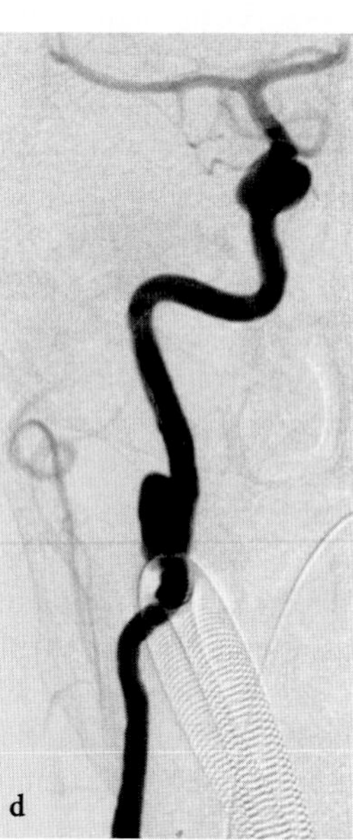

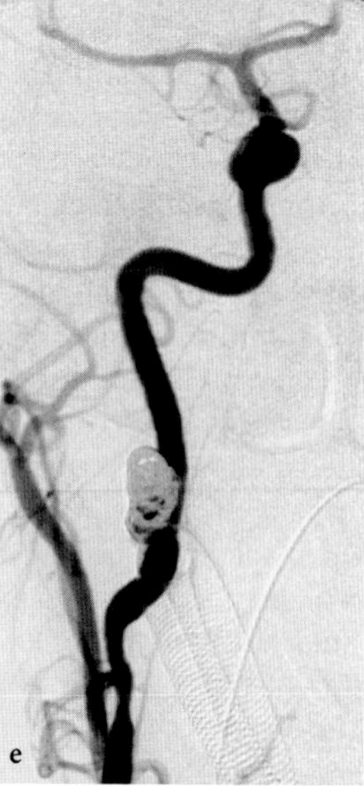

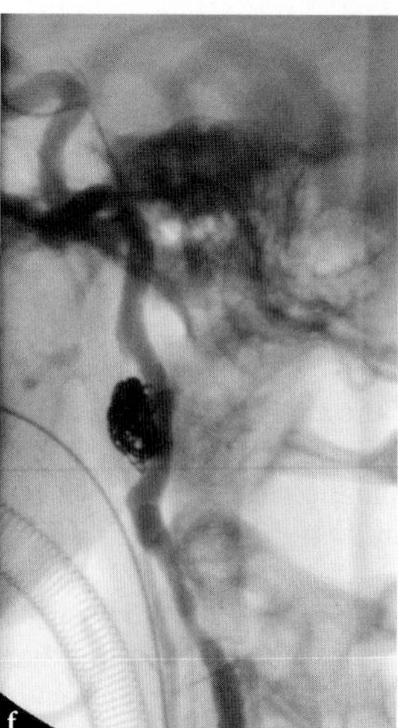

In patients with SAH due to dissecting aneurysms endovascular therapy with stents to remodel the lumen will probably be the future type of therapy.

In contrast to extracranial dissections, the intramural hematoma in most intracranial dissections forms between the internal elastic lamina and the media (Endo et al. 1993). Intracranial dissections may not be explained solely by a defect in the media. Rather, they originate at intimal alterations due to defects of the elastic tissue. The absence of external elastica may allow rupture into the subarachnoid space. Aneurysmal dilatation might occur if the underlying media is also abnormal (Endo et al. 1993).

5.1.4 Fusiform Aneurysms

Fusiform aneurysms are dilated, tortuous and elongated arterial segments. The term dolichoectasia describes a giant ectatic vessel of this type of aneurysms. Fusiform aneurysms are characterized by the absence of a defined neck, circumferential involvement of the parent artery and a longish course. The aneurysm can be partially thrombosed.

The spectrum of fusiform aneurysms may arise from congenital, acquired, or iatrogenic defects in the vessel wall, with or without atherosclerosis, and hypertension, or may develop after intimal tear from dissection (Anson et al. 1996; Gobin et al. 1996). Fusiform aneurysms can occur in any location; however, they most frequently occur in the distal vertebral artery, basilar artery, P1 segment of the posterior cerebral artery and the supraclinoid internal carotid artery. Hemorrhage from these aneurysms is unusual. Presenting symptoms such as cranial neuropathy, brain stem compression and cerebral ischemia are mainly due to mass effect and distal embolization.

A distinct subgroup of fusiform aneurysms are serpentine aneurysms: large and partially thrombosed tortuous aneurysms with a central parent channel, eccentrically located within the intraluminal clot. This channel is not endothelialized and does not contain elastic lamina or media. The clot may become organized or calcified over time. The etiology of serpentine aneurysms is still totally unclear. They may develop from a degenerative form of atherosclerosis, infection, or may be congenital (Mawad and Klucznik 1995). They occur most commonly in the internal carotid artery, the middle cerebral artery and posterior cerebral artery. Typically, they present with symptoms of mass effect. Subarachnoid or intracerebral hemorrhage is rare. MRI may reveal different stages of hemoglobin degradation within the thrombosed part of the aneurysm.

Fusiform aneurysms are usually not suitable for endovascular obliteration because they do not have a circumscribed neck. In selected cases, endovascular parent vessel occlusion may be a therapeutic option, particularly if mass effect is the leading symptom. The aneurysm may subsequently shrink in size or completely resolve (Mawad and Klucznik 1995).

5.1.5 Infectious Aneurysms

The first infectious intracranial aneurysm was probably described by Church in 1869 when he established a relationship between an intracranial aneurysm and infectious endocarditis. The term "infectious aneurysm" should be preferred, "bacterial" or "mycotic" should be used only if bacteria or fungi are demonstrated as the causative organisms. The frequently used term "mycotic" is misleading in the vast majority of patients because bacterial infection represents the most common cause for infectious cerebral aneurysms.

The pathogenesis of infectious aneurysm formation has been well characterized in animal models. After septic emboli arise, polymorphonuclear leucocytes infiltrate the vessel wall from toward the internal elastic membrane. Most of them concentrate within Virchow-Robin spaces.

Infectious intracranial aneurysms account for 2%–3% of all intracranial aneurysms. They commonly result from embolization of cardiac vegetations in endocarditis, with *Streptococcus* as the most frequent organism, followed by *Staphylococcus* and *Enterococcus*. Infected tissue debris entering the blood stream may embolize in cerebral artery walls leading to aneurysmal dilatation. The risk of aneurysm formation due to endocarditis is 5%. While there is decreasing overall incidence of infectious cerebral aneurysms, the incidence of infectious aneurysms increased in drug abusers and immunocompromised patients.

Pathologically, a loss of intima is characteristic in bacterial cerebral aneurysms. Subendothelial inflammation and necrosis of the media and internal elastic lamina results in weakening of the vessel wall, leading to aneurysm formation. Aneurysms associated with infective endocarditis are often irregularly shaped, fusiform, frequently multiple and peripheral and in the majority of patients located at distal branches of the middle cerebral artery. The time interval from septic embolism to aneurysmal dilatation can be as short as 24 h.

True mycotic aneurysms are rare. The underlying condition is often a craniofacial infection with aspergillus, phycomycetes or candida endocarditis. In contrast to bacterial etiology the time course of mycotic aneurysms is longer, sometimes taking months to develop. Mycotic aneurysms are typically proximal in location (carotid or basilar artery) and fusiform (Lau et al. 1991). Rupture of such aneurysms may lead to massive SAH in the basal cisterns, indistinguishable from SAH of saccular aneurysms. Aspergillosis is difficult to diagnose, but should be considered particularly in patients undergoing long-term treatment with steroids, immunosuppressive agents and antibiotics, or in HIV-infected patients.

The course of infectious aneurysms is unpredictable. Under antibiotic or antimycotic therapy they may shrink, or completely disappear. However, enlargement during treatment has also been reported (Brust et al. 1990). Septic aneurysms can be obliterated surgically or by endovascular treatment (Chapot et al. 2002; Phuong et al. 2002; Steinberg et al. 1992). The theoretical assumption that implantation of foreign material – like platinum coils – into an infectious lesion might worsen the problem is not true for infectious intracranial aneurysms.

Mortality due to rupture of bacterial cerebral aneurysms is reported to be up to 60% (Barrow and Prats 1990; Bohmfalk et al. 1978; Clare and Barrow 1992).

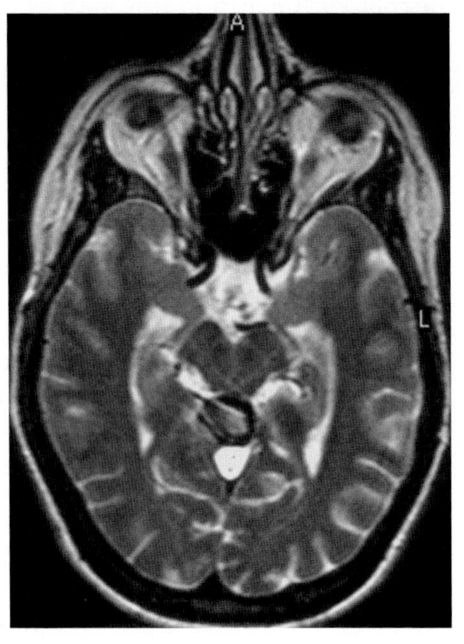

a

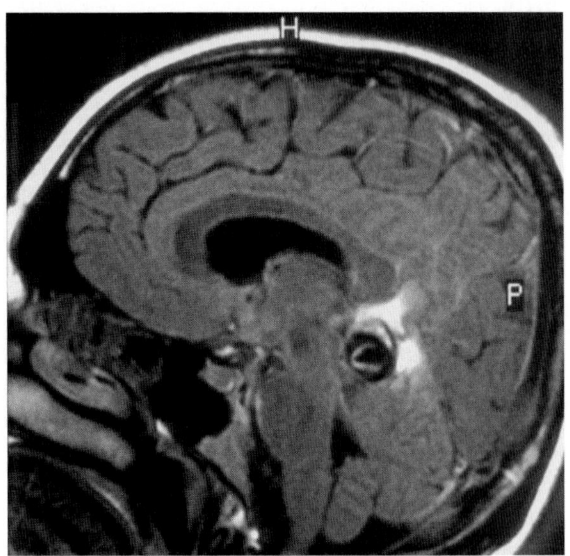

b

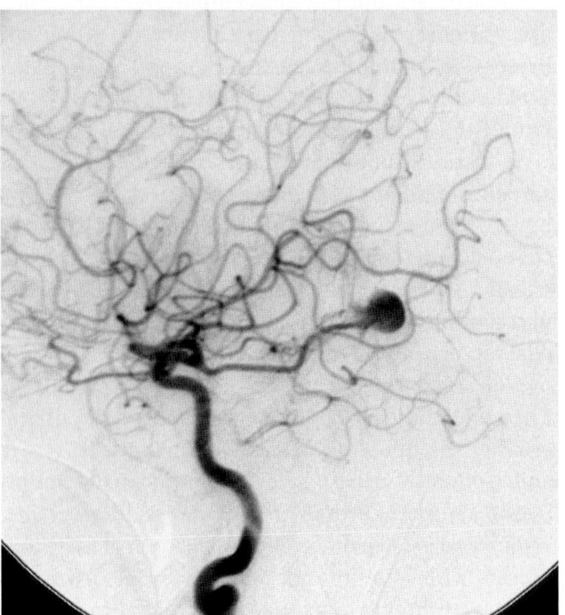

c

Fig. 5.1.3. Infectious aneurysm of the right posterior cerebral artery. T2-weighted image (**a**), FLAIR image (**b**) with subarachnoid blood around the aneurysm and DSA (**c**)

There is no scientific opinion about screening high risk patients for infectious aneurysms, e.g. those with a bacterial endocarditis. However, this may be a field of collaboration between cardiologists and neuroradiologists.

5.1.6 Traumatic Aneurysms

Traumatic aneurysms result from a direct injury to the arterial wall or to acceleration-induced shear. Cervical, cerebral or meningeal arteries can be affected. Traumatic aneurysms may develop within hours after trauma and the majority are false aneurysms. More than 50% of traumatic aneurysms are associated with a skull fracture (Holmes and Harbaugh 1993). Traumatic aneurysms tend to develop on the longitudinal aspect of the injured vessel.

The majority of intracranial traumatic aneurysms are located at the distal middle cerebral artery (MCA) or at anterior cerebral artery (ACA) branches. Angiography typically demonstrates irregular aneurysms, absence of a true neck, and a peripheral location (Amirjamshidi et al. 1996). They may regress, thrombose, enlarge or rupture. Late, often fatal subarachnoid or intraparenchymal hemorrhage may occur in up to 60% with an associated mortality of 50% (Holmes and Harbaugh 1993).

5.1.7 Inflammatory Aneurysms

Inflammatory transmural angiitis in systemic lupus erythematosus, polyarteritis nodosa, or giant cell arteritis cause focal fibrinoid necrosis and elastic tissue disruption. Subacute or chronic changes usually produce ectasia and may facilitate aneurysm formation. Aneurysms in acute arteritis tend to be multiple, peripheral and non side-wall in configuration.

5.1.8 Neoplastic and Radiation-Induced Aneurysms

Oncotic aneurysms may arise from cerebral embolization of neoplastic cells with infiltration of the vessel wall and subsequent aneurysm formation. Thus, the underlying pathomechanism is quite similar to infectious aneurysms. Subarachnoid or intraparenchymal hemorrhage may result. Neoplastic aneurysms have been reported with cardiac myxoma, choriocarcinoma, bronchogenic and undifferentiated carcinomas. Treatment consists of resection of the involved segment, if possible, and evacuation of the symptomatic lesion (Weir et al. 1978).

Formation of fusiform aneurysms following radiation and radioactive intrathecal gold therapy has been reported after treatment of germinoma and medulloblastoma. These aneurysms are located in the midline or parasellar region, and tend to enlarge and rupture (Benson and Sung 1989).

5.1.9 Aneurysms Associated with Arteriovenous Malformations

There is an increased incidence, or better, an increased amount of visible aneurysms associated with arteriovenous malformations. The incidence of these aneurysms in AVMs is up to 25% (Brown et al. 1990; Stapf et al. 2002). Approximately 50% of these aneurysms are located on a feeding artery, 25% within the nidus. Stapf and colleagues analysed their extensive AVM database and figured out that feeding artery aneurysms are an important independent determinant for an increased risk of hemorrhage in AVM.

Flow-related aneurysms probably develop due to hemodynamic stress caused by increased flow and pressure, with subsequent dilatation and pathologic changes in feeding arteries.

AVM-associated aneurysms contribute to an increased risk of hemorrhage. A 7% risk of hemor-

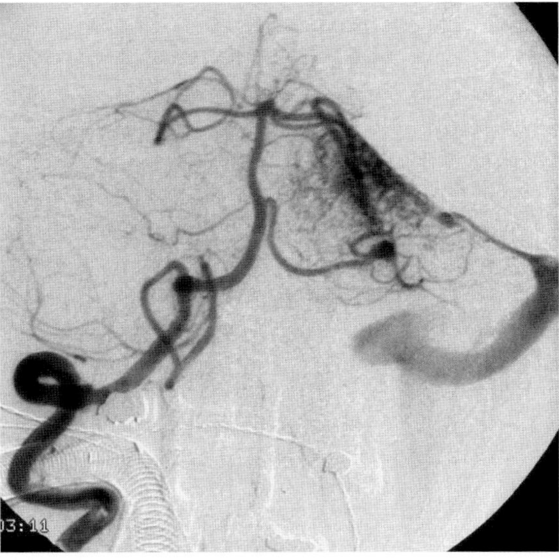

Fig. 5.1.4. Distal small aneurysm of the anterior inferior cerebellar artery (AICA) associated with a high-flow arterious-venous malformation

rhage for these combined lesions is estimated compared to a 1.7%–3% risk for AVMs without associated aneurysms (Turjman et al. 1994). In case of rupture the hemorrhage is more often located intraparenchymally than subarachnoidally (Brown et al. 1990). Management of these combined lesions is still discussed controversially. However, in our opinion these aneurysms should be treated – preferentially by the endovascular route-in order to reduce the bleeding risk of the combined lesion. In fact, elimination of the AVM with subsequent change in hemodynamics might place the aneurysm at risk. In accordance to our opinion, other authors also advocate to treat the aneurysm before eliminating the AVM (Nakahara et al. 1999; Thompson et al. 1998). On the other hand, proximal asymptomatic aneurysms may regress after removal of the AVM. If this is not the case, an interval of 3 months after AVM treatment might be justified before considering a further therapy for a proximal aneurysm. However, aneurysms located in the posterior circulation associated with an AVM are at higher risk of rupture and therefore should be treated as soon as possible even if they have not ruptured before.

5.1.10 Distribution

Most arterial aneurysms arise at the bifurcation of major arteries, and this is also true for the intracranial location. Around 85% of all intracranial aneurysms originate from the anterior circulation. The most common location (30%–35%) is the anterior communicating artery (Acom). However, many of these so-called Acom aneurysms do have their origin at the A1/A2 junction of the anterior cerebral artery and do not involve the anterior communicating artery. Internal carotid and posterior communicating artery aneurysms account for 30% and middle cerebral artery (MCA) bifurcation aneurysms for 20%. Around 15% of intracranial aneurysms arise at the vertebrobasilar circulation. Half of them develop at the basilar tip (with various degrees of involvement of the P1 segments) and the other 50% from other posterior fossa vessels. Aneurysms of the anterior inferior cerebellar artery (AICA) and vertebral artery (VA) aneurysms without involvement of the VA-PICA junction or the vertebrobasilar union are extremely rare.

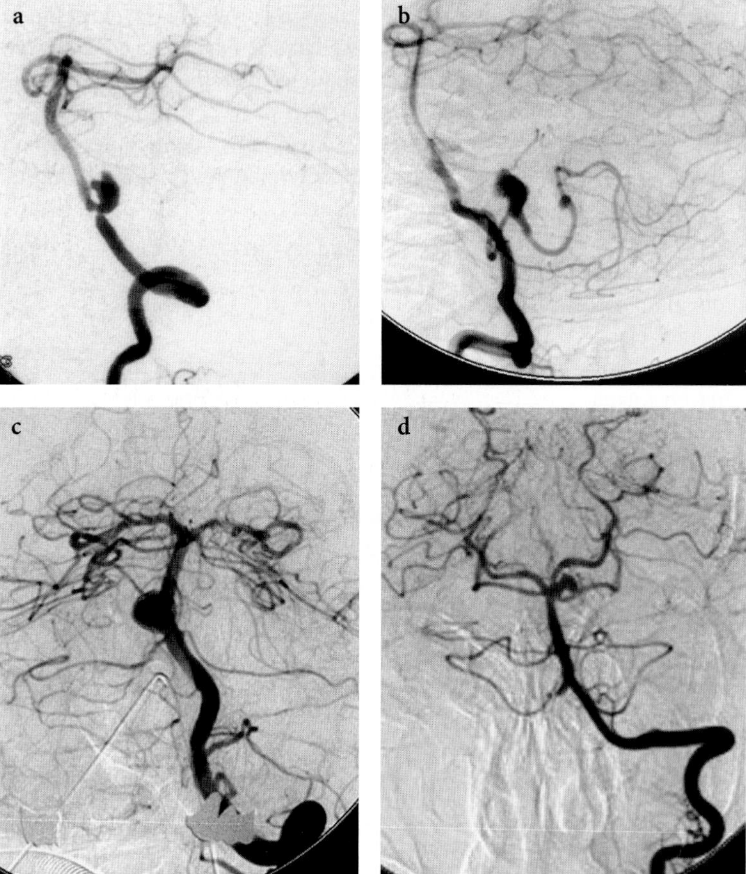

Fig. 5.1.5a–d. Various locations of aneurysms. **a** Vertebral basilar junction aneurysm. **b** True PICA aneurysms. **c** Basilar trunk aneurysm. **d** Basilar trunk aneurysm between origin of superior cerebellar artery and posterior cerebral artery, so-called superior cerebellar artery aneurysm.

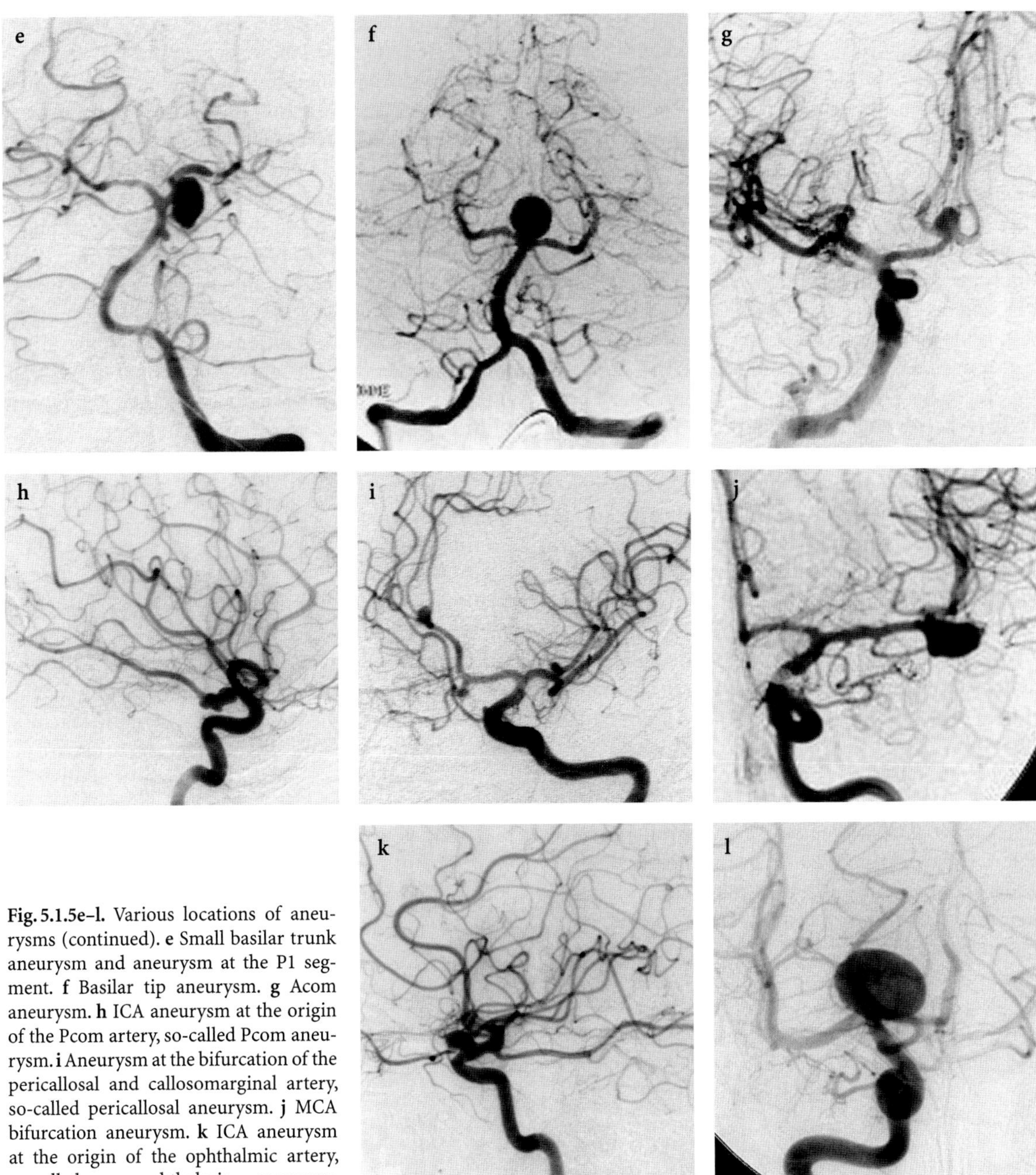

Fig. 5.1.5e–l. Various locations of aneurysms (continued). **e** Small basilar trunk aneurysm and aneurysm at the P1 segment. **f** Basilar tip aneurysm. **g** Acom aneurysm. **h** ICA aneurysm at the origin of the Pcom artery, so-called Pcom aneurysm. **i** Aneurysm at the bifurcation of the pericallosal and callosomarginal artery, so-called pericallosal aneurysm. **j** MCA bifurcation aneurysm. **k** ICA aneurysm at the origin of the ophthalmic artery, so-called paraophthalmic aneurysm. **l** Distal carotid bifurcation aneurysm

5.1.11 Familial Occurrence

The prevalence of intracranial aneurysms among first-degree relatives of patients with cerebral aneurysms is higher than in the general population. The risk for a first-degree relative harbouring an aneurysm is about three to four times higher than for someone from the general population (Raaymakers 1999, 2000; Ronkainen et al. 1997). In other words: The incidence of intracranial aneurysms is between 8% and 9% in persons with two or more relatives who have had a SAH or an aneurysm (Raaymakers et al. 1998b; Ronkainen et al. 1997).

Recently, this was confirmed by Okamoto and colleagues (2003). They found that the SAH risk was elevated when: (1) any first degree relative had a positive episode of SAH, (2) a mother or father had a relative with a positive episode of SAH (an effect much greater in magnitude in a positive maternal rather than paternal history), (3) any first-degree relative <50 had had a SAH. Kojima et al. (1998) confirmed that asymptomatic aneurysms were more likely to rupture among family members with aneurysmal SAH than among those without. According to the group around Leblanc (Leblanc 1996; Lozano and Leblanc 1987) cerebral aneurysms in patients with a positive family history might result from a mesenchymal defect affecting the cerebral vessel wall produced by a lesion of chromosome 16. Okamoto et al. (2003) found an urgent need for early prevention of SAH by screening individuals with any positive family members (first-degree relatives with an episode of SAH).

Various hereditary connective tissue disorders have been associated with formation of aneurysms, most likely as a result of the weakening of the vessel wall. Intracranial aneurysms may develop in 10%–15% of patients with polycystic kidney disease, an autosomal dominant disorder. Although Marfan syndrome was previously identified as a risk factor for aneurysms, a recent study did not find any significant relationship (Conway et al. 1999). Coarctation of the aorta, fibromuscular dysplasia and pheochromocytoma have been associated with intracranial aneurysms, most likely because of the elevated blood pressure that occurs in these conditions.

There are some presumptions on neurofibromatosis type 1 (NF1) and intracranial aneurysms. In a recent study, Conway and colleagues (2001) concluded from their own data and an extensive analysis of the literature that an association between NF1 and intracranial aneurysms has never been identified in large clinical studies of NF1 patients and that there is no evidence for any association between NF1 and intracranial aneurysms.

5.2 Clinical Presentation

Most intracranial aneurysms remain undetected until the time of rupture. SAH, a medical emergency, is by far the most common initial clinical presentation. A history of abrupt onset of a severe headache of atypical quality ("the worst headache in my life") is typical of SAH. Headache onset may or may not be associated with brief loss of consciousness, nausea and vomiting, focal neurologic deficits or meningism. Despite the characteristic history, SAH is frequently misdiagnosed. Nearly half of the patients present with milder symptoms caused by a warning leak before full rupture of the aneurysm (Ostergaard 1991). Another problem – from a clinical point of view – is the so-called thunderclap headache which is caused by a SAH in only 10%–20%. Other findings in these patients are: cerebral infarction, meningitis, intracerebral hemorrhage, cerebral edema or even nothing. From a pure clinical standpoint it sometimes can be difficult to decide whether a thunderclap headache was related to the SAH/warning leak complex or not. There is no clear evidence what to do in a situation like this; our recommendation is to perform a CSF examination and a MRI plus MRA. Landtblom and colleagues (2002) figured out that it is clearly not justified to do an invasive angiogram in these patients (Landtblom et al. 2002).

5.2.1 Epidemiology

Although the pathogenesis and etiology of cerebral aneurysms has been studied extensively, both are still poorly understood. Endogenous factors like elevated blood pressure, the special anatomy of the Circle of Willis or the effect of hemodynamic factors, particularly originating at vessel bifurcations, are all known to be involved in the growth and rupture of an aneurysm. Arteriosclerosis and inflammatory reactions, however, might also have an impact. Exogenous factors like cigarette smoking, heavy alcohol consumption or certain medications are thought to

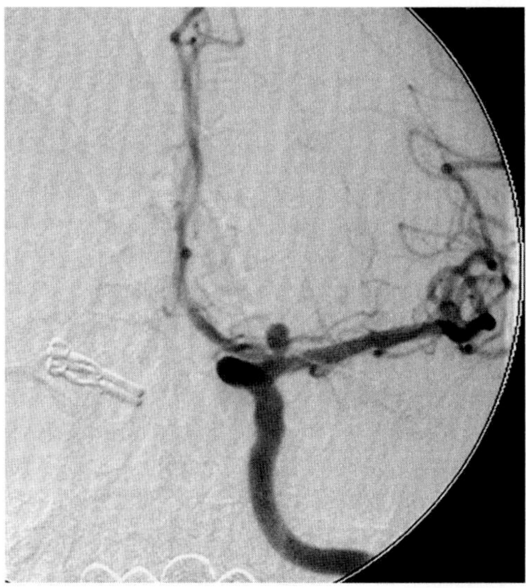

Fig. 5.2.1. Seven years after clipping an Pcom aneurysm on the right side a de novo aneurysm at the distal carotid bifurcation was found on the left side, primarily seen on MRI performed because of headache

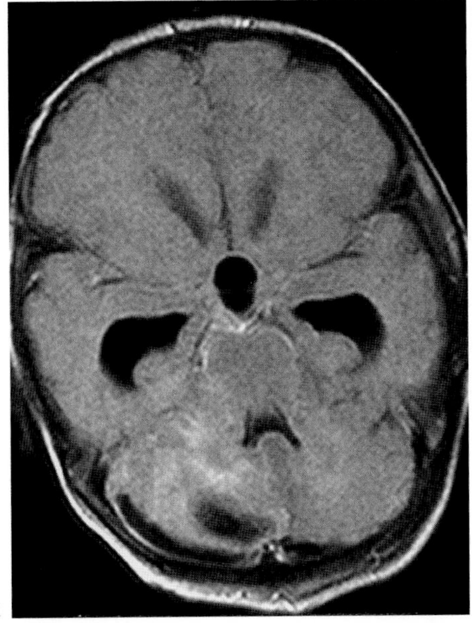

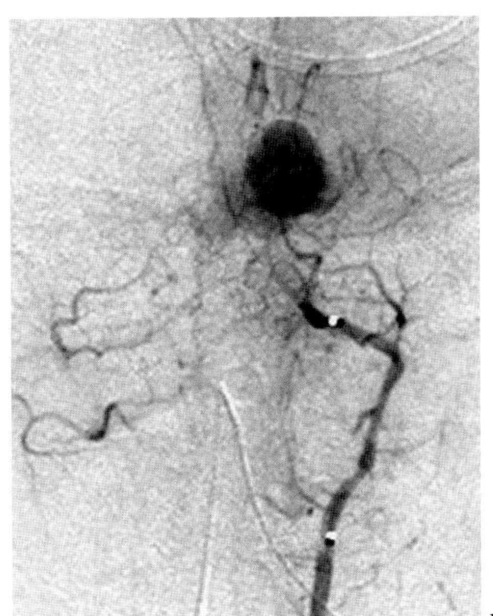

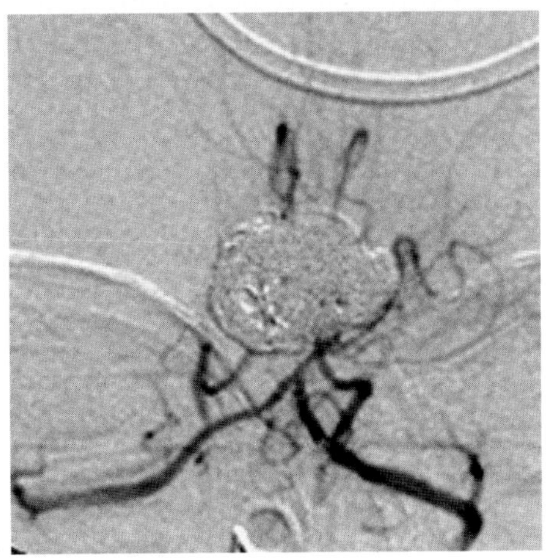

Fig. 5.2.2. Basilar trunk aneurysm in a newborn after bleeding (**a**, FLAIR) resulting in acute hydrocephalus, before (**b**) and after (**c**) endovascular treatment with selective occlusion of the aneurysm. The baby's outcome was excellent with no neurologic deficits

be risk factors in the pathogenesis of an aneurysm or at least increase the risk of rupture.

Furthermore, a genetic component is discussed. First degree relatives of patients with an aneurysmal SAH have a significant higher risk to harbour a cerebral aneurysm compared with the normal population.

5.2.2 Incidence and Risk of Rupture

Intracranial aneurysms are common. Autopsy studies have shown that the overall frequency in the general population ranges from 0.4% to 10% (Chason and Hindman 1958; Housepian and Pool 1958; Inagawa and Hirano 1990; McCormick and Acosta-Rua 1970). Rinkel et al. (1998) analysed 23 studies with 56304 patients published between 1955 and 1996 and found a prevalence of 2.3 % in adults without a risk factor for SAH and an overall annual risk of rupture of 1.9 %. They included retrospective and prospective autopsy and angiographic studies and found a higher incidence in the prospective arm of their analysis. It might be reasonable to assume that the average prevalence is around 2%. Based on this number, in the German population approximately 1.5 to 2 million people are assumed to harbour an intracranial aneurysm.

The incidence of SAH in the Western hemisphere is around 6–10 per 100,000 people per year, peaking in the sixth decade with risk for SAH increasing linearly with age. The incidence in some other countries like Finland or Japan is known to be higher – about 15/100,000 per year. SAH accounts for a quarter of cerebrovascular deaths. Aneurysms increase in frequency with age beyond the third decade, are approximately 1.6 times more common in women and are associated with a number of genetic conditions (Wardlaw and White 2000). The incidence not only of aneurysms but also of SAH is higher in Japan than in Western countries, and it has increased around three times during the past 20 years in Japan (Okamoto et al. 2003).

There are some risk factors associated with aneurysm rupture or aneurysm development beyond genetic determinants:

Elevated arterial blood pressure (hypertension) and endovascular flow conditions seem to be important for the development, growth and rupture of cerebral aneurysms. There is also a strong correlation between the presence of multiple aneurysms and hypertension: Patients with multiple aneurysms present significantly more often with hypertension than patients with solitary aneurysms or the normal population.

Other risk factors for the development of aneurysms are smoking, heavy alcohol consumption, arteriosclerosis and hyperlipidemia (for more details see Sect. 5.1.11).

5.2.3 Natural History of Ruptured Aneurysms and Patient Outcome

The peak incidence of rebleeding after the initial rupture is during the first day. Early rebleeding within hours after the onset of initial hemorrhage occurs in about 15% of patients (Fujii et al. 1996). As many as 20% of patients may rebleed within the first 2 weeks, one third in the first month, and 50% will rebleed within 6 months, if the aneurysm is not treated.

Mortality of recurrent SAH is up to 50% (Weaver and Fisher 1994). In patients surviving the first day, the risk of rebleeding is evenly distributed over the next 4 weeks with a second peak early in the third week (Hijdra et al. 1987). Between 4 weeks and 6 months after SAH, the risk of rebleeding gradually decreases from initially 1%–2% per day to a constant level of approximately 3% a year (Winn et al. 1977).

Of patients who survive the hemorrhage, approximately one third remain dependent. However, even recovery to an independent state does not necessarily mean that outcome is good. Only a small minority of patients with SAH has a truely good outcome, around 20% of them do not have a reduction of quality of life.

5.2.4 Pathophysiology of Aneurysm Rupture

There may be a small number of SAH presenting as “warning leak” or sentinel hemorrhage, usually only associated with a sudden severe headache (Hughes 1992). In general, there is a correlation between the extent of SAH and the clinical grade, incidence of vasospasm, and other complications such as cerebral ischemia, increased intracranial pressure, and hydrocephalus.

With increased severity of SAH there are increasing changes in physiologic parameters such as reduced cerebral blood flow (due to reduced cerebral autoregulation), hypovolemia, hyponatremia, hypermetabolism and cardiac arrhythmia. If intracerebral pressure is increased up to diastolic blood pressure cerebral blood flow persists during systole (Nornes 1973).

Stopping of an SAH is caused by a combination of tamponade due to reduced transmural pressure gradient across the arterial wall and coagulation.

5.2.5 Other Causes of SAH

5.2.5.1 Perimesencephalic Non-aneurysmal Hemorrhage

Perimesencephalic hemorrhage constitutes approximately 10% of all SAH. Mean age at onset is 50 years with a preponderance in male. The subarachnoid blood is confined to the perimesencephalic cisterns. The centre of the bleeding is anterior to the midbrain (Schwartz and Solomon 1996). Usually, there is no subarachnoid blood in the sylvian fissure or the anterior interhemispheric fissure. There might be some sedimented blood in the occipital horns of the lateral ventricles, but massive intraventricular hemorrhage or intracerebral hemorrhage is not a feature of this benign perimesencephalic hemorrhage.

Conventional angiography is the next step to rule out an aneurysm, although this is hardly found. In the presence of the typical CT pattern the yield of repeated angiography is low, and some investigators have abandoned it. Some of them even consider CT angiography sufficient to rule out an aneurysm. From a clinical perception, perimesencephalic non-aneurysmal hemorrhage is barely distinguishable from aneurysmal hemorrhage. The onset of headache is often more gradual than in true aneurysmal hemorrhage (Linn et al. 1998),

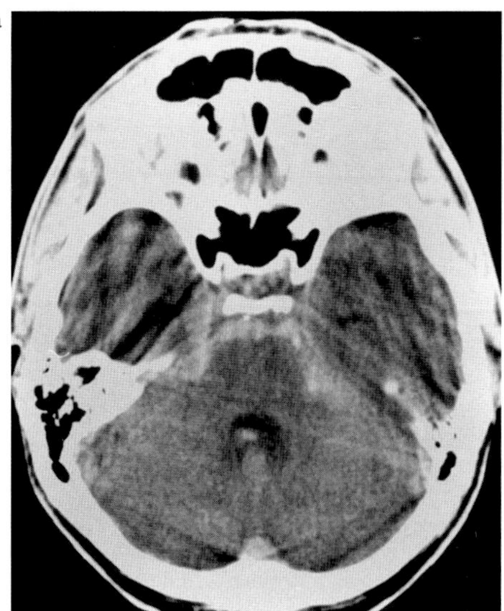

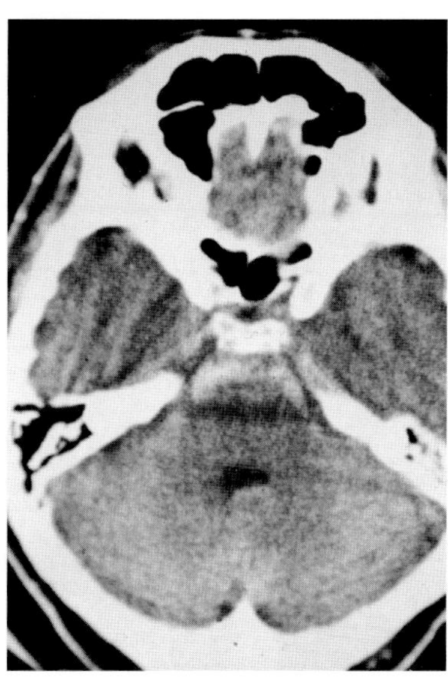

Fig. 5.2.3a,b. Typical perimesencephalic hemorrhage on CT scan

but this is a poor diagnostic hint. Focal symptoms or loss of consciousness are exceptional and do occur only transient. Usually, these patients are clinically Hunt and Hess grade I. Seizures were never reported in perimesencephalic hemorrhage. Apart from their headache the patients are in a very good clinical condition. The clinical course is typically uneventful. Rebleeding, acute hydrocephalus, or secondary cerebral ischemia due to vasospasm do not typically occur in this entity. Rebleeds after the hospital period have not been reported and the quality of life in the long-term is excellent. The time of convalescence is usually short and the outcome is good or excellent with almost all patients (94%) able to return to their previous work and activities (Brilstra et al. 1997). In summary, this is really a benign variant of SAH, but clearly requires a diagnostic work-up like a typical SAH in order not to overlook the rare aneurysmal-caused perimesencephalic SAH and other causes.

5.2.5.2 Dural Arteriovenous Fistulae

Hemorrhage from a basal dural arteriovenous fistulae might be not distinguishable from aneurysmal SAH. The risk of hemorrhage in dural arteriovenous fistulae depends on the pattern of venous drainage (Cognard et al. 1995). A cortical venous drainage is associated with a relatively high risk of hemorrhage, drainage into the main sinus is associated with a very low risk of bleeding. After a first rupture has occurred, the risk of rebleeding is very high.

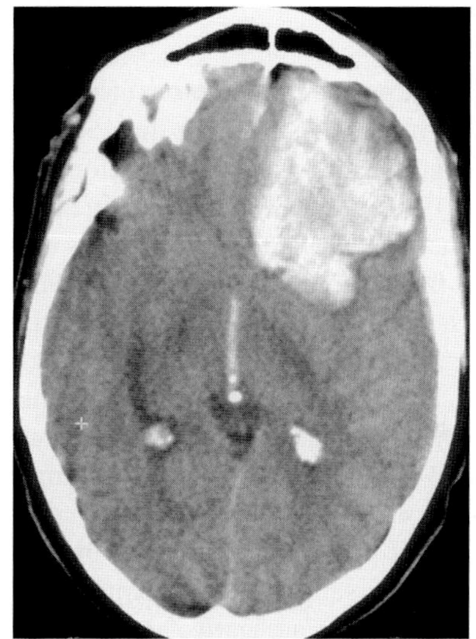

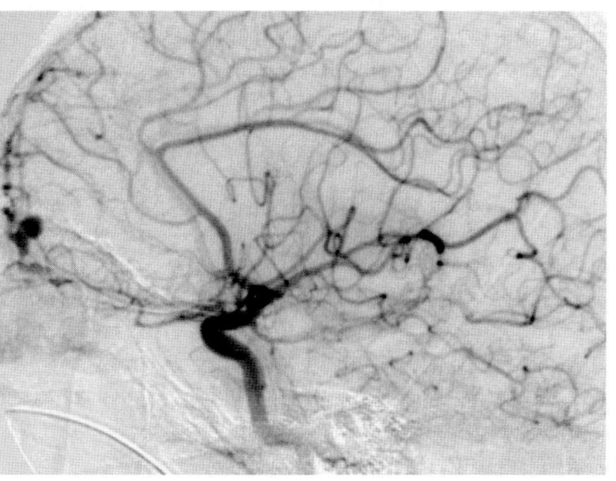

Fig.5.2.4a,b. Frontal dural AV-fistula with cortical drainage and left frontal intraparenchymal hemorrhage

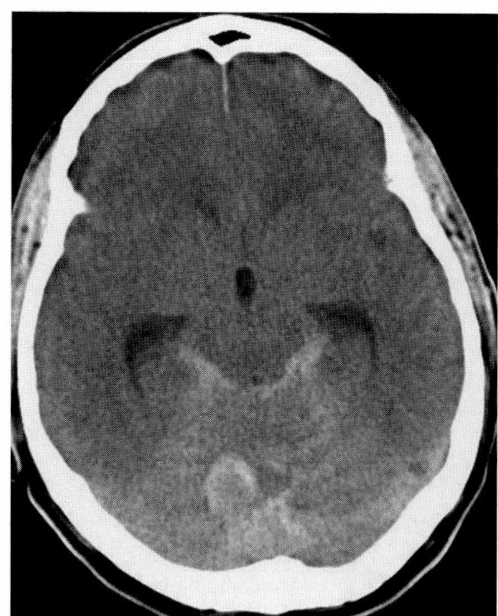

a

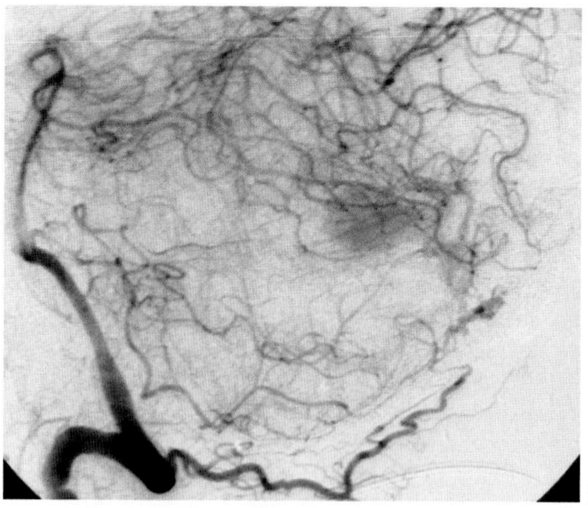

b

Fig. 5.2.5a,b. Infratentorial dural AV-fistula and subarachnoid hemorrhage

5.2.5.3
Cervical AVMs

Intracranial SAH is the presenting symptom of a spinal AVM in about 10% of patients. In more than 50% of these patients, the first hemorrhage occurs before the age of 20 (Kandel 1980). Clinically, a severe pain in the lower part of the neck radiating to the shoulders and arms may indicate the cervical source of bleeding. MRI should be the first imaging modality to localize the source of bleeding, followed by selective spinal angiography. However, it is difficult to establish the spinal source of hemorrhage. In many patients CT reveals an intracranial SAH and the four-vessel angiogram is negative. In an ideal setting cervical vessels are additionally injected, but it is clearly not routine to do a spinal angiogram in this subgroup of patients. However, in all SAH patients with a negative angiogram a cranial and spinal MR should be performed to rule out a vascular malformation.

5.2.5.4
Saccular Aneurysms of Spinal Arteries

Saccular aneurysms of spinal arteries are rare. The clinical features of spinal SAH are usually associated with those of a transverse spinal cord lesion (Mohsenipour et al. 1994).

5.2.5.5
Cardiac Myxoma

Cardiac myxoma may be a very rare cause of SAH. In exceptional cases it may metastasize into an intracranial artery, infiltrate the vessel wall and initiate aneurysm formation, even more than 1 year later after excision of the primary tumour (Furuya et al. 1995).

5.2.5.6
Sickle Cell Disease

SAH in sickle cell anemia is characterized by multiple hemorrhages, often distally and in unusual locations. CT scan demonstrates blood in the superficial cortical sulci. Angiography reveals multiple distal branch occlusions and a collateral circulation via leptomeningeal vessels. SAH is attributed to rupture of these leptomeningeal collaterals, the outcome is usually poor (Carey et al. 1990). Approximately 30% of patients with sickle cell disease and SAH are children.

5.2.5.7
Cocaine Abuse

SAH related to the abuse of cocaine is associated with an underlying aneurysm in 70% of patients using hydrochloride ("crack") versus 30%–40% of patients using the alkaloid form (Levine et al. 1990, 1991). The pattern of SAH on CT may be the same as that of a ruptured saccular aneurysm. Rebleeding frequently occurs and the outcome is often poor. The association between cocaine use and the formation and rupture of aneurysms is thought to be due to increased turbulence of blood flow and repeated, transient bouts of hypertension. Among cocaine users, aneurysms have been found in significantly younger patients and in vessels with a smaller diameter (Nanda et al. 2000).

5.2.5.8
Anticoagulants

Anticoagulant drugs are rarely the sole cause of SAH (MATTLE et al. 1989). If SAH occurs in a patient under anticoagulation therapy the outcome is poor.

5.2.5.9
Sinus-Venous Thrombosis

It is well known that sinus-venous thrombosis can cause atypical intracerebral hemorrhage. Under rare circumstances, however, thrombosis of the superior sagittal sinus can cause pure subarachnoid hemorrhage without intraaxial bleeding. Mostly, SAH is then located at the Sylvian fissure, probably due to dilated Sylvian veins, and in the parietal sulci.

5.2.6
Complications of SAH

Hydrocephalus, rebleeding from aneurysmal rerupture and cerebral vasospasm with ischemia are the three major complications following SAH.

5.2.6.1
Hydrocephalus

Acute hydrocephalus within the first 24 h of hemorrhage may develop due to blood within the basal cisterns or in the ventricular system causing CSF obstruction. Clinically, slow pupillary responses to light and deviation of the eyes is characteristic for acute hydrocephalus. If confirmed by CT, early ventricular drainage is indicated and can dramatically improve the clinical status of the patient. NOWAK and colleagues (1994) reported the use of a ventricular drainage as an early test to evaluate neurologic viability. They chose surgical candidates in whom neurologic improvement occurred after CSF drainage. Thereby, ventriculostomy might not only serve as a therapeutic device but also as an indicator which severe-grade patients should be treated more aggressively (ARNOLD et al. 1994; NOWAK et al. 1994). However, caution during placement of a ventricular drain is important, since sudden drainage may precede aneurysm rerupture, mainly because the transmural pressure along the aneurysm wall may exceed the intraventricular pressure. Large amounts of intraventricular blood are often associated with a poor clinical condition.

Hydrocephalus may also develop over days or weeks following SAH, clinically often presenting with gait disturbance, impaired intellectual function, and progressive lethargy. In these cases, ventriculo-peritoneal or ventriculo-atrial shunting is commonly indicated.

The possibility to eliminate major parts of the subarachnoid blood by intraoperative lavage and thereby decreasing the incidence of vasospasm and hydrocephalus is widely considered as an advantage of the neurosurgical approach compared to the endovascular route. However, in a retrospective study comparing 100 matched patients who had suffered SAH, the therapeutic procedure, either clipping or coil embolization, did not significantly affect the development of chronic hydrocephalus (SETHI et al. 2000).

If the initial CT already reveals early signs of hydrocephalus, the ventricular drainage should be placed before endovascular treatment starts. This schedule avoids a neurosurgical approach after having the patient on heparin and aspirin (which in many institutions is the case after coiling). In addition, a ventricular drainage is extremely helpful in the rare event of aneurysm rupture during the endovascular procedure.

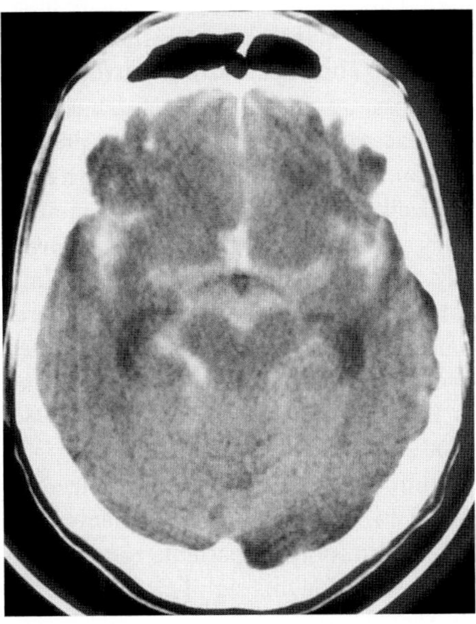

Fig. 5.2.6. CT reveals massive basal subarachnoid hemorrhage and dilated temporal horns of the lateral ventricles

5.2.6.2
Rebleeding

Rebleeding is a frequent and sometimes devastating neurologic complication of SAH and is postulated to be due to breakdown of perianeurysmal clot. Early rebleeding in the first hours after admission for the initial hemorrhage with clinical deterioration occurs in up to 18% of patients (Fujii et al. 1996). Since these early rebleedings commonly occur before the first CT scan is obtained, the true frequency of early rebleeding is definitely underestimated. As many as 20% of patients may rebleed within the first 2 weeks, one third in the first month, and 50% will rebleed within 6 months, if the aneurysm is not treated. The peak incidence of rebleeding is during the first day. There is a secondary peak 1 week after SAH. Mortality of recurrent SAH is 50% (Weaver and Fisher 1994). Between 4 weeks and 6 months after SAH, the risk of rebleeding gradually decreases from initially 1%–2% a day to a constant level of approximately 3% a year (Winn et al. 1977).

The Cooperative Aneurysm Study reported that women have a 2.2 times higher recurrence rate of hemorrhage than men. Recurrent hemorrhage was also more frequently associated with a poorer neurologic grade at presentation and increased systolic blood pressure (Torner et al. 1981). Clinically, recurrent hemorrhage may present with new neurologic deficits, increasing headache, vomiting and a depressed level of consciousness. Seizures might occur as a result, but not as the cause of bleeding.

Clot formation and tissue damage stimulate fibrinolytic activity in the CSF, increasing the potential risk of rebleeding. This observation justified the rationale for the use of antifibrinolytic drugs such as aminocaproic acid and tranexamic acid to prevent rebleeding. A randomized placebo-controlled trial, a non-randomized trial and other reports assessing the efficacy of antifibrinolytic therapy showed a significantly decreased incidence of rebleeding. However, mortality was not altered, but this therapeutic approach was associated with an increased risk of delayed cerebral ischemia, embolism, and deep venous thrombosis (Vermeulen et al. 1984; Roos et al. 2000).

The ISAT study revealed aneurysmal rebleeding before treatment in 23 neurosurgical patients – 16 of them died – and in only 14 patients randomized for coiling. The reason for this significant difference was probably that the delay between initial bleeding and surgery is longer than the interval between the bleeding and coiling (Molyneux et al. 2002). Again, this indicates strongly that early rebleeding is a significant prognostic factor and any therapeutic delay might turn into a problem for the patient. However, we are not voting for immediate angiography and subsequent endovascular therapy for all SAH patients. Usually, we provide this service during the day until 10.00 p.m.. Patients admitted later get their diagnostic angiogram and endovascular therapy early in the next morning.

5.2.6.3 Hematoma

Intracerebral hematoma (ICH) occurs in up to 30% of patients with aneurysmal rupture (van Gijn and van Dongen 1982). The outcome is clearly worse than with SAH alone. If a space-occupying hematoma compressing nerval structures is present, immediate evacuation of the hematoma is mandatory, eventually in combination with clipping of the aneurysm, if it can be identified. In this setting, CT angiography might serve as valuable and fast imaging modality to disclose the aneurysm prior to surgical intervention. Immediate surgical evacuation is also indicated in acute subdural hematoma (SDH), which is usually associated with recurrent aneurysmal rupture. However, SDH can also occur with the initial SAH or can be the only extravascular space involved after aneurysmal rupture.

There is an ongoing debate about endovascular therapy in patients with ICH due to aneurysm rupture. If the hematoma is acute life threatening, it is no question that surgical evacuation needs to be done as soon as possible. However, it is a well known clinical experience that during hematoma evacuation – due to the decrease of tissue pressure – the risk of aneurysm rerupture increases. Having this in mind it might be advantageous to coil the aneurysm first – in order to prevent rebleeding – before surgical evacuation of the hematoma in those patients with a stable clinical condition.

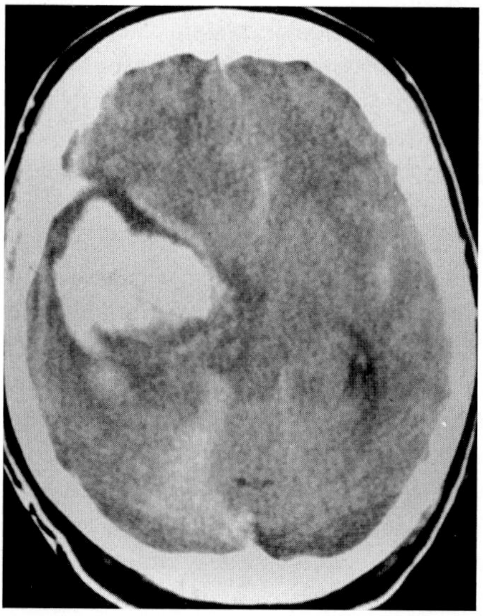

Fig. 5.2.7. Right temporal lobe intracerebral hemorrhage due to a ruptured MCA aneurysm. Beside basal subarachnoid hemorrhage CT reveals brain edema, compression of the basal cisterns and the cerebral peduncle

5.2.6.4
Vasospasm

Vasospasm is a major cause of morbidity and mortality in patients after SAH and is often associated with delayed cerebral ischemia. However, many patients are asymptomatic despite various degrees of angiographically visible vasospasm. Although vasospasm is noted angiographically in 70% after SAH, it becomes symptomatic only in about half of those patients (BILLER et al. 1988). This difference probably reflects the different collateral circulation and different degrees of vasospasm. Unlike rebleeding, the clinical presentation of vasospasm develops slowly over hours to days. Delayed cerebral ischemia occurs usually first on the third day after hemorrhage, peaks between day 4 and 12, and may persist as long as 3 weeks after SAH (BILLER et al. 1988).

Vasospasm is best detected on angiograms. However, transcranial Doppler ultrasound is the method of choice to monitor blood flow velocities in patients after SAH. The role of CTA and MRA has not been determined in this subgroup of patients.

5.2.6.5
Cerebral Ischemia and Infarction

In some patients, aneurysmal rupture leads to a prolonged period of global cerebral ischemia at the time of hemorrhage, probably as a result of increased intracranial pressure to a level above that in arterial vessels (GROTE and HASSLER 1988). Clinically, these

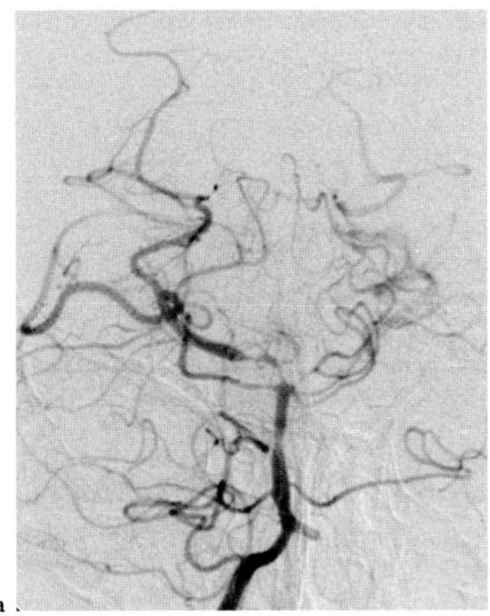
a

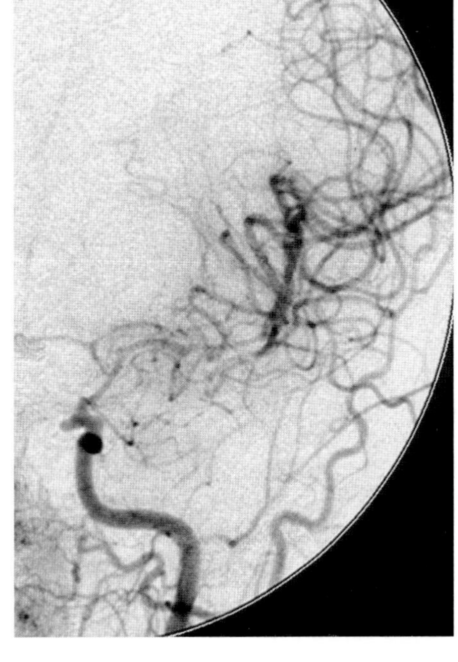
c

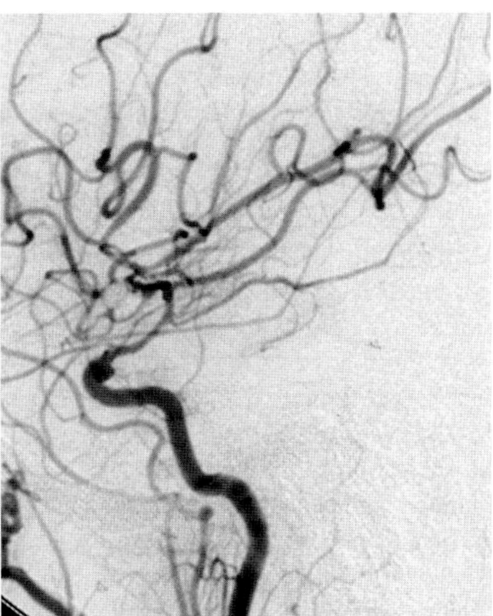
b

Fig. 5.2.8a–c. Different grades of vasospasm after SAH. **a** Moderate vasospasm of the basilar artery and severe vasospasm of both P1 segments of the posterior cerebral artery. **b,c** Severe vasospasm of the intradural ICA (sagittal view) and proximal MCA and ACA (ap view)

patients present with progressive dysfunction of the brainstem. Outcome is generally fatal. CT might reveal no other abnormality than subarachnoid blood. This entity is quite distinct from delayed cerebral ischemia, which is focal or multifocal. A major factor for this condition of global cerebral ischemia is vasospasm that in some patients occur immediately after aneurysmal rupture. From our experience aneurysm rupture during endovascular therapy has more or less no consequence in those patients without immediate severe vasospasm. Morbidity and mortality of acute aneurysm rupture is probably most strongly associated with the amount and the length of acute vasospasms.

Delayed cerebral ischemia usually occurs in the first or second week after SAH in up to one-third of patients. Despite intensive research, the pathogenesis has not been entirely elucidated. Release of yet unidentified factors into the subarachnoid space are considered to induce vasospasm and subsequent cerebral ischemia.

There is widespread postulation of a close relationship between the amount of subarachnoid blood clots and the degree of vasospasm and delayed cerebral ischemia (Fisher et al. 1980). However, there are several arguments against these assumptions. Subarachnoid blood is not a predictor of vasospasm per se, since vasospasm and delayed cerebral ischemia rarely occur in patients with SAH after rupture of an AVM or perimesencephlic SAH. Furthermore, the site of delayed cerebral ischemia does not always correspond with the distribution of subarachnoid blood (Hop et al. 1999). The fact that many patients with angiographically visible vasospasms never develop cerebral ischemia suggests additional factors determining whether and where secondary cerebral ischemia occurs. There is additional evidence that it is not simply the amount of blood that determines the severity of vasospasm. Since there is no way to remove subarachnoidal clot during coiling one would expect a lower incidence of vasospasm after clipping. But this effect has not been observed. So far, there are slight tendencies towards a lower frequency of vasospasm after coiling (Yalamanchili et al. 1998).

5.2.7 Unruptured Aneurysms

Asymptomatic aneurysms may be defined as additional aneurysms found in patients with another symptomatic aneurysm, which are not responsible for the clinical symptoms or those aneurysms found in patients investigated because they are at risk of harbouring an aneurysm. *Incidental* aneurysms may be defined as those found unexpectedly in patients undergoing investigation for any other suspected pathology. Depending on the location of an unruptured aneurysm it can be completely asymptomatic.

On the other hand, unruptured aneurysms can cause neurologic symptoms while touching cranial nerves or other cerebral structures. Symptoms can be pain, cranial nerve palsies, visual disturbances, dysesthesia, vertigo and seizures. In case of thrombembolism, mainly out of large or giant aneurysms, but also occurring in small aneurysms in any location, symptoms due to transient ischemia or permanent infarction do appear.

Ischemic events can occur distal to both small and large unruptured intracranial aneurysms (predominantly in the anterior circulation). In a series of 269 patients harbouring unruptured aneurysms ischemic strokes or transient ischemic attacks (TIAs) attributable to embolization from the aneurysmal sac were observed in 3.3% (Qureshi et al. 2000a). *Symptomatic* unruptured aneurysms are usually larger than incidental aneurysms and are often discovered near to the skull base where they are more likely to affect cranial nerves. The most frequent affected cranial nerves are the oculomotor nerve and the optic nerve.

Given the high mortality and morbidity associated with aneurysm rupture, it is crucial to determine the likelihood of rupture to decide whether to treat an aneurysm or not.

The findings of the International Study of Unruptured Intracranial Aneurysms (Wiebers 1998) were published in 1998 and in 2003. Up to now, the ISUIA is the largest evaluation of the risk of aneurysmal rupture. Examination of 2621 patient records at 53 medical centres over 7.5 years yielded an average annual rupture rates below those of previous estimates. Aneurysms less than 10 mm in diameter had an average annual rupture rate of 0.05% in patients with no history of SAH; however, the rupture rate was ten times higher for aneurysms of a similar size in patients with a history of SAH. The annual rupture rate for larger aneurysms approached 1%. However, there was a lot of criticism to that study. The authors included a large number of patients with aneurysms of the cavernous portion of the ICA. These aneurysms are usually large or giant, but due to their anatomical location they almost never cause a subarachnoid hemorrhage. Including a fairly high number of large aneurysms with almost no risk of SAH in a study cohort clearly leads to an overestimation of the critical aneurysm size. And it is a well accepted

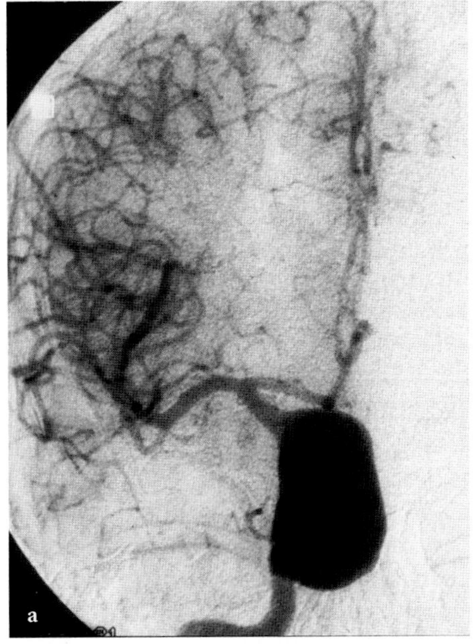

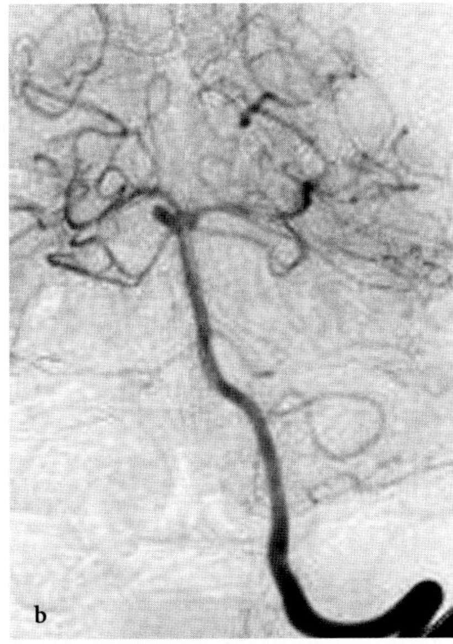

Fig. 5.2.9a–d. **a** Giant ICA aneurysm inducing optic nerve compression in a 10-year-old boy with visual deficit on the right eye. **b** Brain stem aneurysm between origin of the superior cerebellar artery and posterior cerebral artery resulting in right sided oculomotor palsy. **c, d** Pcom aneurysm (**c** DSA, lateral view) in a 46-year-old-patient with oculomotor palsy, note the close relationship of the aneurysm and the oculomotor nerve (*arrow*) but without visible contact (**d**, sagittal reconstruction of CISS sequence)

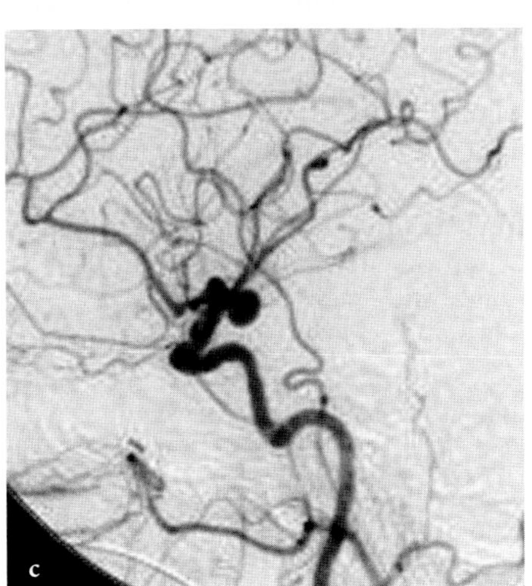

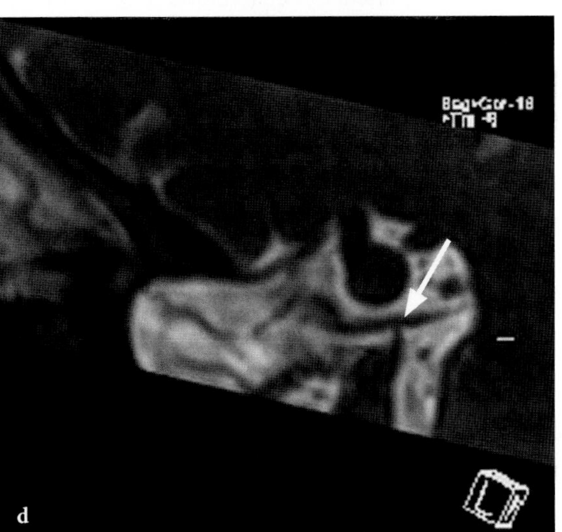

clinical experience that the majority of ruptured aneurysms are far below the ISUIA value of 10 mm; in our patient population the average aneurysms size in patients with SAH was between 4 mm and 7 mm. Very recently, the ISUIA group did redefine the critical aneurysm size from 10 mm down to 7 mm, indicating that the clinical impression and the evidence-based data are coming closer together (Wiebers et al. 2003). Nevertheless, all these results still do not explain why the majority of ruptured aneurysms are below the size of 7 mm! In our opinion there are at least two major drawbacks in the ISUIA study:

1 The criteria for or against treatment of an aneurysm remain unclear. Assuming that the majority of patients were seen and advised by experts, factors like multi-lobularity or hypoplastic vessel segments might have had a major impact on treatment decisions and thus heavily biased the results.
2 Another problem is the under-representation of Acom aneurysms and again the over-representation of those aneurysms located at the cavernous part of the ICA. Usually Acom aneurysms account for around 30% of all intracranial aneurysms, in the ISUIA study only 10% were located at that site. It may be that these aneurysms just develop, grow up to 4 mm and rupture. The cavernosal aneurysms are usually large and never – or at least rarely – do cause a SAH. This way the bias of these aneurysms is that they increase the average size of non-ruptured aneurysms.

5.3 Imaging

5.3.1 Computed Tomography

If SAH is suspected clinically, CT of the brain is the initial diagnostic imaging modality of choice and clearly the gold standard to identify, localize and quantify subarachnoid hemorrhage. Typically, the subarachnoid blood appears hyperdense on an unenhanced CT. The pattern of SAH can suggest the location of the underlying aneurysm (van Gijn and van Dongen 1982). Intraparenchymal hemorrhage occurs with aneurysms of the posterior communicating artery and middle cerebral artery more frequently than with other locations. Interhemispheric or intraventricular hemorrhage, occurring in autopsy studies in about 50% of patients, is characteristic of Acom or distal anterior cerebral artery aneurysms. Ruptured PICA aneurysms almost always coexist with hydrocephalus and intraventricular hemorrhage in the fourth ventricle, which be can also seen on CT. Intracerebral hemorrhage is also more common in patients who rebled, since the first bleeding may lead to fibrosis of the surrounding subarachnoid space and adhesion of the aneurysm to the brain. Subdural hematoma occurs in about 5% of patients, but is rarely the only location of bleeding.

Small amounts of SAH may be overlooked, CT thus should be carefully read. However, even if the CT scan is really normal (no mis-reading!), aneurysmal SAH cannot be ruled out. The sensitivity of CT for detecting SAH depends on the volume of the extravasated blood, the hematocrit, and the time elapsed after the acute event. Using modern CT scanners and performed within 24 h after the ictus CT detects SAH in up to 95%. However, due to dilution by CSF the density of the hemorrhagel decreases rapidly over time, thus after only a few days it may be impossible to demonstrate subarachnoid blood on CT (van der Wee et al. 1995). Sensitivity of CT decreases to 80% at day 3, 70% at day 5, 50% at 1 week, and 30% at 2 weeks (Adams et al. 1983).

CT may also help to distinguish aneurysmal from traumatic SAH. In traumatic SAH the subarachnoid blood is usually located on the brain convexity. In patients with basal contusions there might be a pattern of hemorrhage resembling aneurysmal SAH due to a rupture of an aneurysm at the anterior part of the Circle of Willis. The same might be the case for hemorrhage into the Sylvian fissure. In these patients, in whom it is impossible to exclude aneurysmal hemorrhage or in whom the trauma might be a consequence of the initial aneurysm rupture, conventional angiography should be performed. In patients with Sylvian fissure hemorrhages (and without angiographically visible aneurysm) any imaging modality should be used to rule out sinovenous thrombosis.

Very rarely, massive brain edema and meningitis may mimic SAH on brain CT and may lead to a false positive diagnosis of SAH.

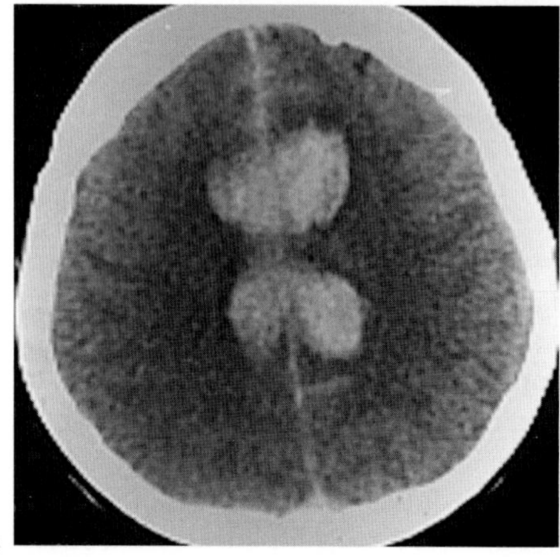
a

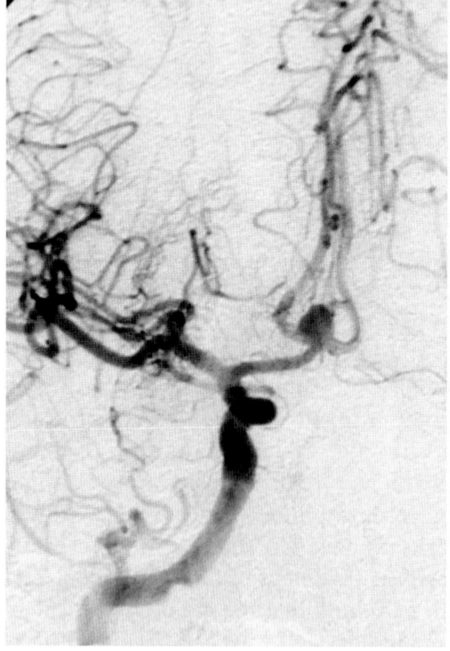
b

Fig. 5.3.1. a Massive subarachnoid and intraventricular hemorrhage. Even without any vessel visualization the pattern of hemorrhage on CT already suggests that the underlying cause will be an aneurysm of the anterior cerebral artery complex. **b** DSA reveals a typical Acom aneurysm filling from the right. The left A1 segment was hypoplastic

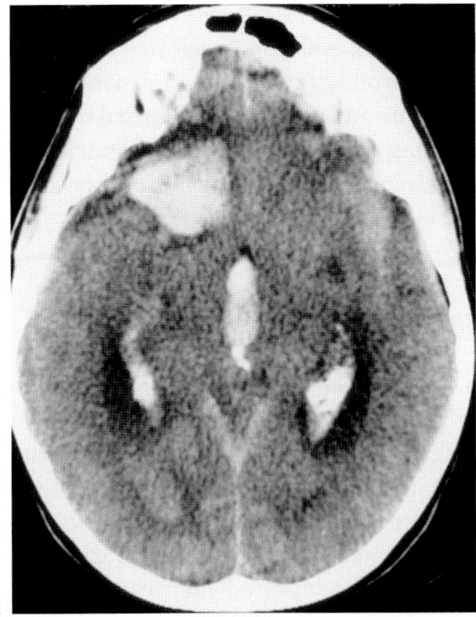

a

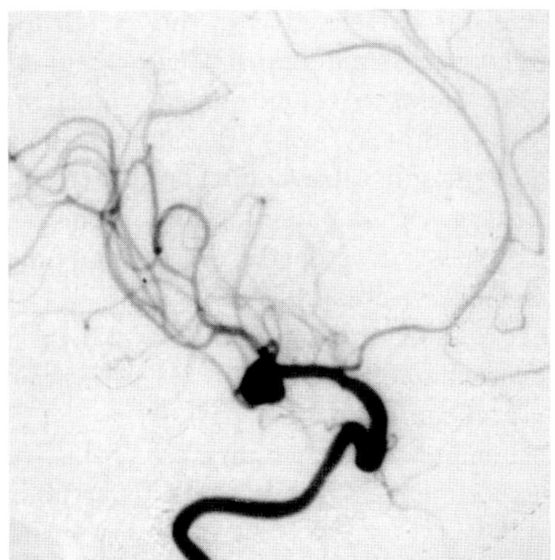

b

Fig. 5.3.2a,b. Sometimes it is more difficult to localize an aneurysm based on the bleeding pattern. **a** CT reveals frontal intracerebral hemorrhage, subarachnoid, and intraventricular hemorrhage. **b** DSA: The bleeding source in this patient was an MCA aneurysm

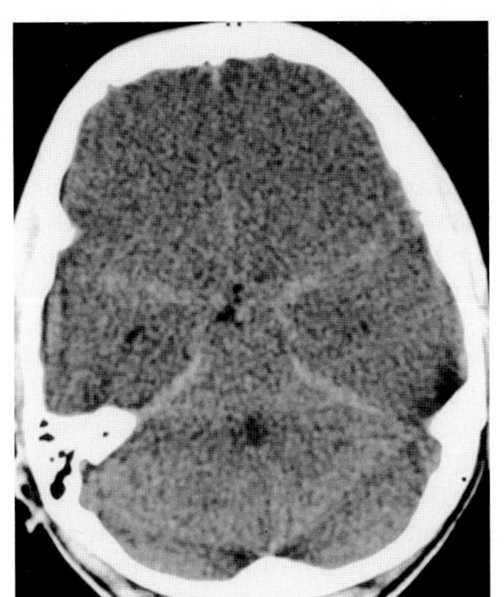

a

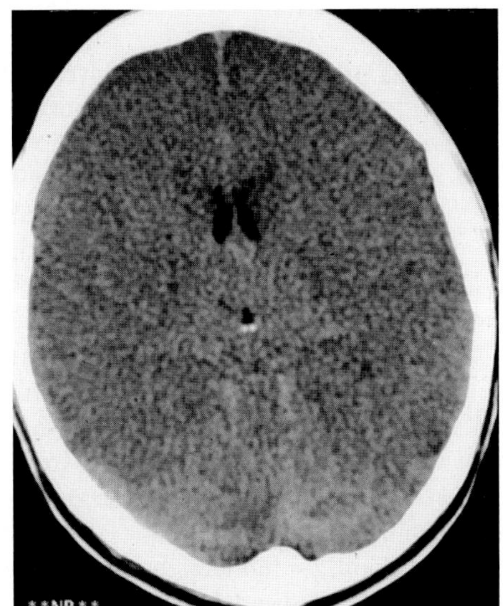

b

Fig. 5.3.3a,b. Severe hypoxia and brain edema mimicking basal SAH on CT

However, if CT is negative despite a convincing history of sudden headache, lumbar puncture is still the next diagnostic step to rule out SAH, if there is no contraindication such as bleeding disorder or space-occupying intracranial lesion (MacDonald and Mendelow 1988). Lumbar puncture should not be performed before 6 h after onset of headaches, preferably 12 h between onset of headache and spinal tap have elapsed. After this interval sufficient lysis of erythrocytes occurred to form bilirubin and oxyhemoglobin. These pigments give the CSF the "typical" xanthochrome yellowish tinge after centrifugation, an essential feature in the differentiation from traumatic SAH. This xanthochromia is invariably detectable until at least 2 weeks, usually 3 (in 70% of patients) to 7 weeks after SAH (Vermeulen et al. 1989).

Identification of factors predictive of outcome or specific complications is important in the management of SAH. The risk of a given patient to suffer from vasospasm can be estimated by the location, thickness, and density of subarachnoid blood on CT. In 1980 Fisher and colleagues provided a description of 47 patients in whom the amount and distribution of subarachnoid blood after aneurysmal rupture on the initial CT was correlated with the subsequent occurrence of vasospasm demonstrated by angiography. Two of 18 patients (11%) developed vasospasm when no or diffuse thin SAH was present on CT, whereas none did with only intraventricular or intracerebral hemorrhage. Of 24 patients with diffuse, thick SAH, 23 (96%) developed severe symptomatic vasospasm (Fisher et al. 1980). Since then, the CT-based Fisher classification of quantifying local amounts of subarachnoid blood as a powerful predictor for the occurrence of vasospasms and delayed cerebral ischemia has been confirmed by several clinical and experimental studies (Grosset et al. 1992; Findlay 1995; Jarus-Dziedzic et al. 2000; Suzuki et al. 1980). However, the predictive value of the Fisher grading system is not perfect. Never assume that a patient will not develop vasospasm just because he has a low Fisher score! All patients with SAH have to be carefully monitored during the first 2 weeks after the ictus, regardless of their initial CT score.

Table 5.3.1. Fisher's grading scale for SAH

Group	Subarachnoid blood	Risk of vasospasm
1	No blood	Low
2	Diffuse or vertical layers <1 mm	Only moderate
3	Localized clot and/or vertical layer >1 mm	High
4	Intracerebral or intraventricular clot with only diffuse or no SAH	

Hijdra et al. (1990) suggested a new grading system for the amount of subarachnoid blood estimating separately ten subarachnoid cisterns and fissures and scoring on a scale of 0 to 3, as follows: 0 = no blood, 1 = small amount of blood, 2 = moderately filled with blood, and 3 = completely filled with blood. The total SAH score is then calculated by adding the scores of the ten subarachnoid compartments (total score 0–30) (Hijdra et al. 1990). Despite the excellent idea to use a more detailed scoring system to estimate the risk of vasospasm, it was not well accepted by the clinical community and does not play a relevant role in daily practise.

Aneurysmal rupture is followed by intraventricular spread of blood in up to 50% (Le Roux and Winn 1998). Solely primary intraventricular hemorrhage is usually associated with good outcome. The outcome is particularly better than in patients with a comparable volume of subarachnoid blood, indicating that the subarachnoid blood component is by far the most important determinant for clinical outcome (Roos et al. 1995).

In a study analyzing 219 patients with ruptured aneurysms Mayfrank et al. (2001) reported increased mortality and unfavourable outcome in patients with additional moderate and severe intraventricular hemorrhage, indicating that severity of intraventricular hemorrhage is an independent predictor of mortality and functional outcome.

5.3.1.1 CT Angiography

Selective catheter angiography is still the standard method for diagnostic work-up of intracranial aneurysms (see below). Although the risk of permanent neurologic complications in patients undergoing DSA for suspected cerebral aneurysms is low, this method remains time consuming and invasive. To identify patients with unruptured aneurysms among those with thunderclap headache, an accurate non-invasive vascular imaging technique would be of considerable interest.

Sensitivity of single-slice CT angiography in the investigation of intracranial aneurysms has been reported to range from 67% to 100% (Liang et al. 1995; Vieco et al. 1995) with an accuracy of approximately 90% and an interobserver agreement ranging from 75% to 84% (White et al. 2000). Nevertheless, this technique has demonstrated a limited sensitivity for aneurysms smaller than 3 mm (25%–64% compared with 92%–100% for aneurysms > 3 mm) (Korogi et al. 1999; White et al. 2000). Moreover, CTA still has pitfalls if the aneurysm is located at a site where adjacent bone or considerable vessel overlap exist, such as the paraclinoid and terminal ICA segments or at the MCA bifurcation.

The implementation of multidetector row technology led to a major step forward in the field of CT angiography, notably for small vessels and for intracranial aneurysms. This technique offers a reduction in acquisition time despite the use of pitch values inferior to unity. The improvement of image quality and spatial resolution ends up in better diagnostic results for intracranial aneurysms. Wintermark et al. (2003) found sensitivity, specificity and accuracy values of multi-row CTA of 99%, 95.2% and 98.3%, respectively. The positive and negative predictive values on a per-patient basis were 99% and 95.2%, respectively. In aneurysms smaller than 2 mm sensitivity was 50%; in aneurysms larger than 2 mm sensitivity was 95.8%. The interobserver agreement was 98%. Multi-row CT technology will clearly make life easier at emergency departments. Patients with a first-time headache and a negative unenhanced CT scan will get a quick and reliable CTA. To optimise treatment planning and work-flow CTA may also be used to stratify patients into endovascular and surgical treatment groups. However, whether CTA really will allow us to figure out which therapeutic modality is best suited still has to be determined. In our opinion there are drawbacks when describing the anatomy of the neck and the true relationship of tiny vessels originating near to the entrance of the aneurysm or adjacent to the aneurysm dome. However, CTA clearly plays a role in the pre-therapeutic phase in large or giant aneurysms. In these patients it is often difficult to visualize the exact anatomy of the neck and the relationship to adjacent bony structures, such as in the paraophthalmic region than with conventional DSA alone. Moreover, CTA is very helpful in the pretherapeutic planning of partially calcified and thrombosed aneurysms and might help to determine the best treatment modality. In patients with large, space-occupying hematomas CTA is clearly enough to rule out an underlying aneurysm. In this specific situation DSA is probably not indicated any more.

Comparing CTA with the non-invasive competitor MRA there are pros and cons for both methods.

Patients with typical contraindications for MRA, such as ferromagnetic clips (Kluczník et al. 1993) or pacemakers, or patients on life-support devices and claustrophobia are usually candidates for CTA. CTA is more or less independent of flow rate, the images will be diagnostic even in patients with a low cardiac output, whereas in MRA this may lead to saturation effects. Flow-related artefacts seen in larger aneurysms on MRA are not seen with CTA. Additionally, CTA may depict aneurysm wall calcifications, for example at the neck, which might cause difficulties during clipping (Schwartz et al. 1994). CTA is more likely to be useful in patients after aneurysm clipping: there are reconstruction algorithms available allowing to reduce clip-related artefacts to a minimum and thus enabling us to decide whether the aneurysm is completely clipped or not (Brown et al. 1999; Vieco et al. 1996). On MRA, however, even the standard non-magnetic clips do cause severe field disturbances. Therefore, MRA is not a diagnostic tool for these patients. However, technical developments are on-going. Gonner and colleagues (2002) recently described a MRA technique with ultrashort echo times reducing clip artefacts significantly. The images are still not diagnostic, but progress is still going on.

Patients treated with endovascular methods need angiographic follow-up. But coil artefacts preclude the use of CTA in these patients. MRA is clearly an excellent tool for patients with previously coiled aneurysms. In this patient group we think time-of-flight MRA (TOF-MRA) is the method of choice (Brunereau et al. 1999; Kahara et al. 1999; Weber et al. 2001). And there are limitations of CT due to artefacts at the skull base. Furthermore, CTA requires iodine contrast agent and is associated with radiation exposure, which is a significant drawback in using CTA for community screening, particularly if this needs to be performed several times during a patient's lifetime.

5.3.2 Magnetic Resonance Imaging

Magnetic resonance imaging and MR angiography are increasingly used in the diagnostic work-up of patients with cerebral aneurysms. However, MRI is less suitable than CT in patients with acute SAH because they are often restless and need extensive monitoring. It is used in patients with a negative angiogram to detect other causes of SAH, such as a thrombosed aneurysm or spinal vascular malformation and it will increasingly be used in screening programs and as a follow-up tool after endovascular therapy.

Conventional MRI sequences are less sensitive to SAH than CT scanning. Since SAH is mostly arterial in origin, the predominant form of hemoglobin is oxy-Hb. Immediately after the extravasation of blood into the subarachnoid space, there is a shortening in T1 due to the increase in hydration layer water owing to the higher protein content of CSF. This results in an increased signal on T1-weighted and proton-density images. Fluid-attenuation inversion recovery (FLAIR) sequences are highly sensitive. The signal from CSF is almost completely reduced while producing a heavy T2-weighting. On FLAIR images SAH appears hyperintense compared to CSF and the surrounding brain (Noguchi et al. 1995). Currently, it is widely accepted that even subtle amounts of subarachnoid blood can be detected by MR when using FLAIR or proton-density weighted MR sequences (Wiesmann et al. 2002). False-positive FLAIR results which may be caused by flow-related enhancement within the CSF may occur. However, this problem could be overcome with the interpretation of protondensity weighted sequences. Even hyperacute SAH can be detected with MR. Compared with CSF the hyperacute blood has a slightly lower signal intensity on T2*-weighted gradient-echo images and increased signal intensity on T2-weighted spin-echo images (Rumboldt et al. 2003).

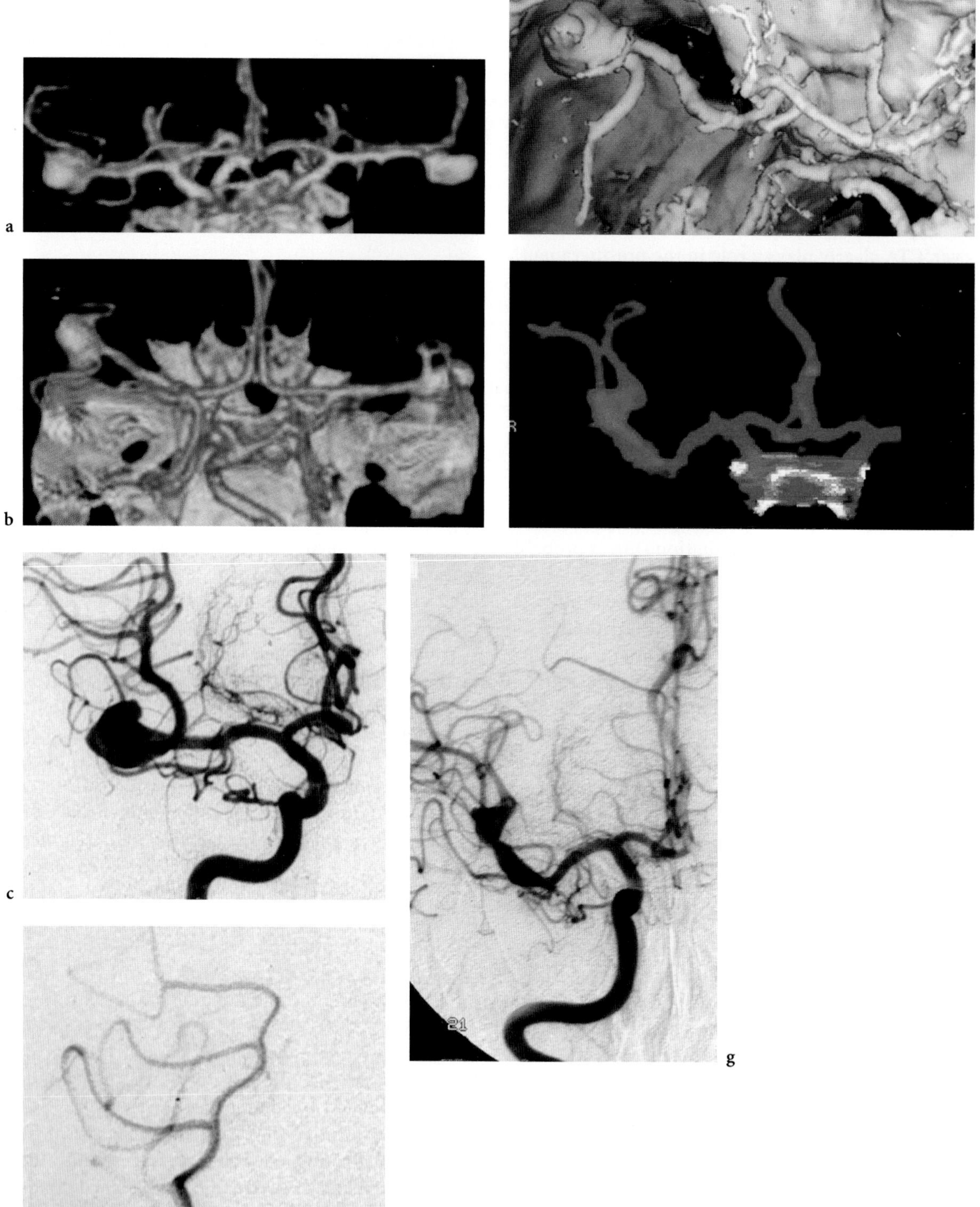

Fig. 5.3.4. a, b 3D CTA of bilateral MCA aneurysm and a small vertebral aneurysm. **c–e** DSA (ap view), aneurysmography and 3D CTA of a large MCA aneurysm demonstrating that one major MCA branch is originating very close to the neck of the aneurysm. **f, g** Fusiform MCA aneurysm: 3D CTA and DSA match perfectly. **h–j** Broad-based basilar artery aneurysm encroaching both P1 segments demonstrated on 3D CTA as well as on DSA. **k–m** Ruptured Pcom aneurysm (*arrow*)

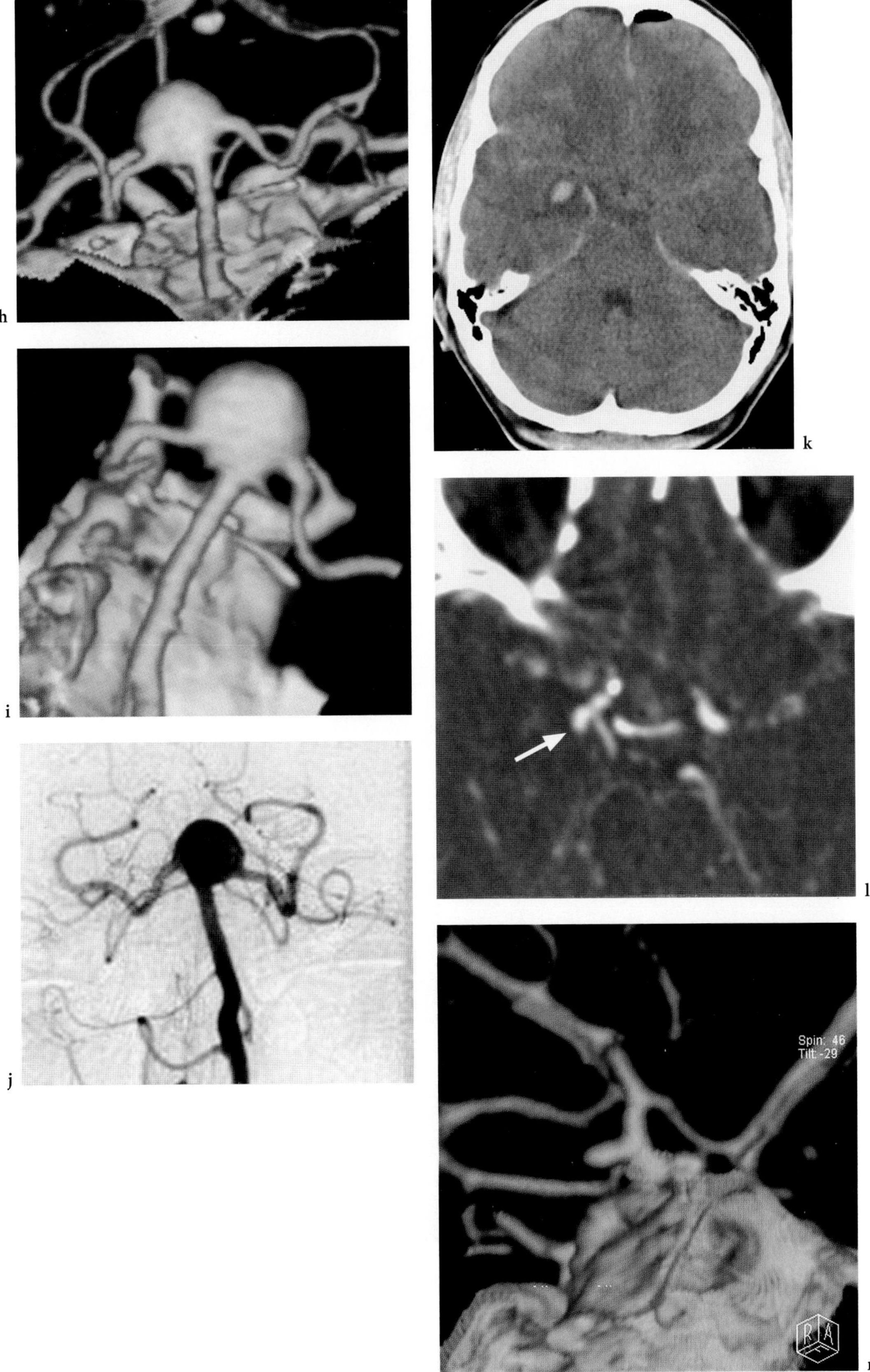
h
i
j
k
l
m
Spin: 46
Tilt: -29

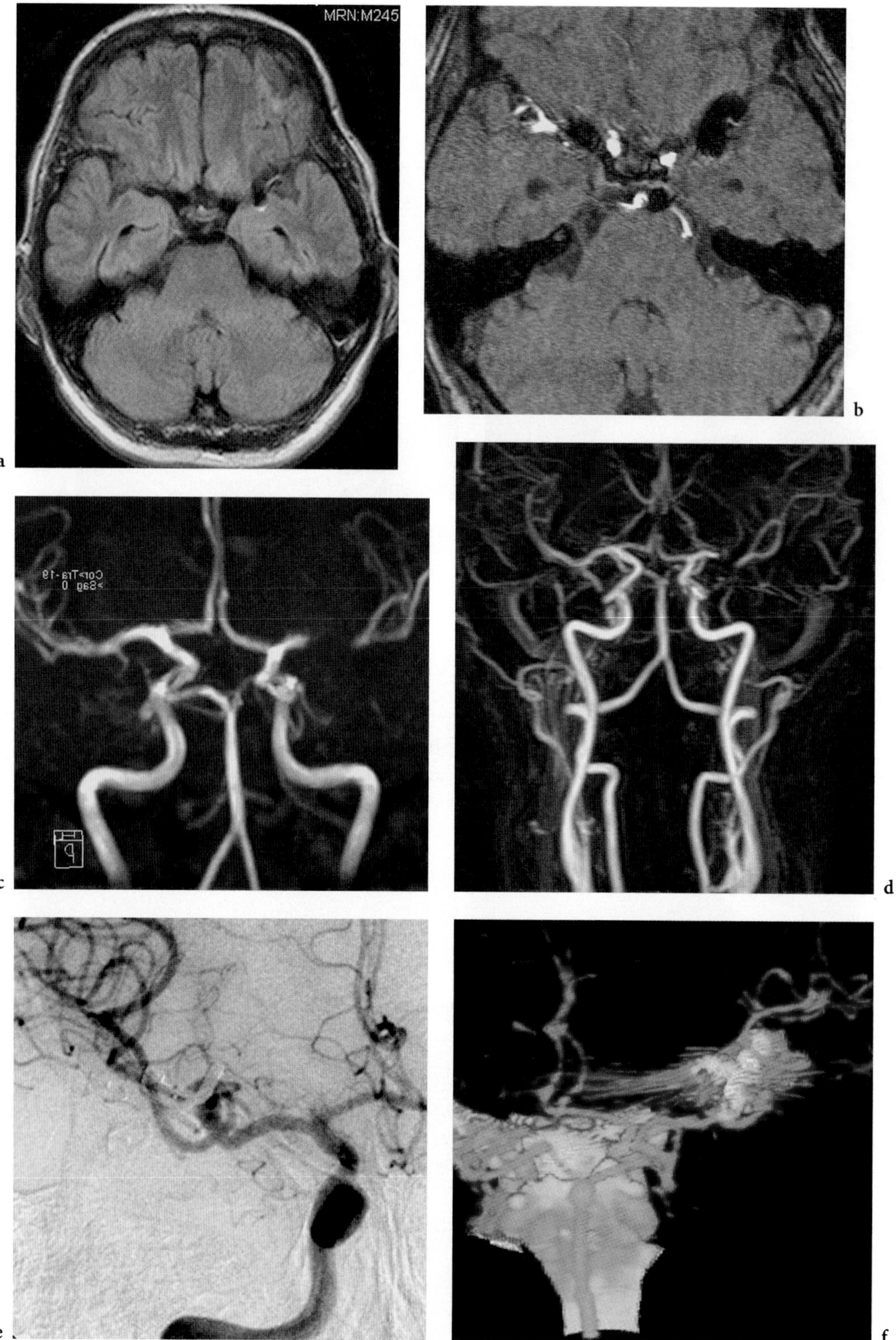

Fig. 5.3.5. **a** Flair sequence with some artefact after clipping of a MCA aneurysm on the left side. **b** Axial source image of the TOF-MRA reveals signal loss at the course of the MCA and next to the basilar artery after coiling of a left superior cerebellar artery aneurysm. **c** There is no flow signal on the 3D reconstruction images of the TOF-MRA as well as of the contrast-enhanced MRA. **d** DSA of an incompletely clipped MCA aneurysm. **e** Due to the artefacts caused by the clip 3D CTA is not useful in evaluating residual aneurysm after clipping

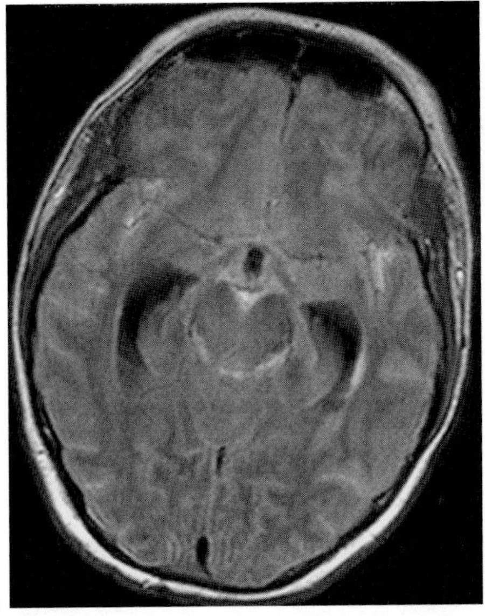
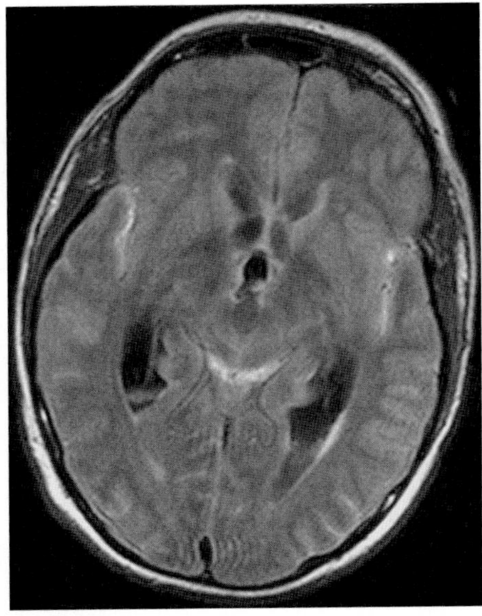

a b

Fig. 5.3.6. Flair Sequence demonstrating blood in the subarachnoid space around the brain stem and predominantly on the occipital surface and in the ventricles as well as acute hydrocephalus after rupture of a left vertebral aneurysm

5.3.2.1 Magnetic Resonance Angiography

MR angiography provides a fast, accurate and non-invasive evaluation of intracranial aneurysms without the risk of conventional angiography. The TOF-MRA technique has an excellent spatial resolution and sufficient field of view, covering all relevant intradural arteries and can be performed within a reasonable acquisition time.

However, MRA has not replaced catheter angiography yet. The accuracy of MRA depends on how the images are processed and reviewed. Using maximum intensity projection alone sensitivity for identification of at least one aneurysm per patient was 75%, increasing to 95% when axial source and spin-echo images were reviewed as well (Ross et al. 1990).

Aneurysm size is a crucial factor for sensitivity. MRA studies consistently indicate sensitivity rates of more than 95% for aneurysms larger than 6 mm, but much less for smaller aneurysms (Atlas et al. 1997). For aneurysms smaller than 5 mm, which constitute as many as a third of aneurysms in asymptomatic patients (Kojima et al. 1998) detection rates of 56% and less have been reported (Korogi et al. 1996). However, these aneurysms should not be ignored even if their rupture risk seems to be low (Wiebers et al. 2003). In our experience, in most patients MRA can detect aneurysms as small as 3 mm, the problem to detect lesions below this size is well known. The results of Atlas et al. (1997) and Korogi et al. (1996) reported problems in the identification of untreated aneurysms smaller than 3 mm in size. Therefore, TOF-MRA might not be reliable in patients with an aneurysm initially smaller than or equal to 3 mm. This should be taken into account for all screening programs, but also for those follow-up examinations (after coiling), when the initial size of the aneurysm was around 3 mm.

In a study comparing 3D TOF-MRA with intra-arterial DSA, Adams et al. examined 29 patients harbouring 42 intracerebral aneurysms. MR data were examined in different forms, i.e. axial source data, maximum intensity projection images, multi-planar reconstructions, and 3D isosurface images. Three aneurysms were not detected by MRA. These aneurysms were either smaller than 3 mm or in anatomically difficult locations (MCA bifurcation) or obscured by an adjacent hematoma. Time-of-flight techniques may obscure some anatomical details due to flow disturbances. The authors conclude that MRA is inferior to intraarterial DSA for pre-treatment assessment of intracranial aneurysms; however, MRA can provide complementary information to DSA such as intramural thrombus. If MRA is used analysis of both axial source data and reconstructed images is mandatory (Adams et al. 2000).

The study by Ronkainen et al. (1997) illustrates the current problems of non-invasive aneurysm imaging. Screening 85 families of patients with SAH using MRA, Ronkainen (1997) and colleagues found 58 aneurysms in 45 of 438 screened patients. Conventional angiogra-

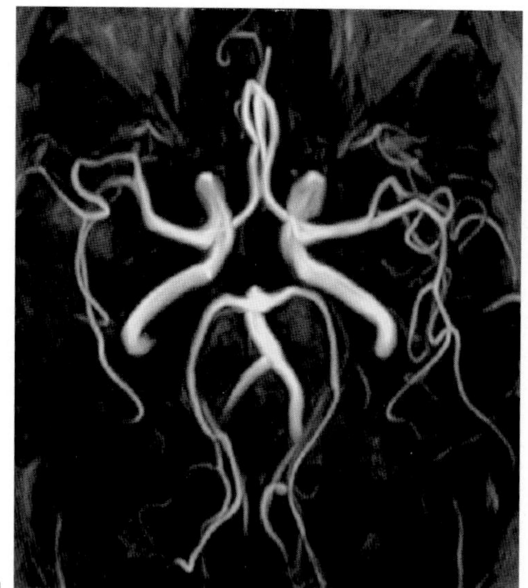

a

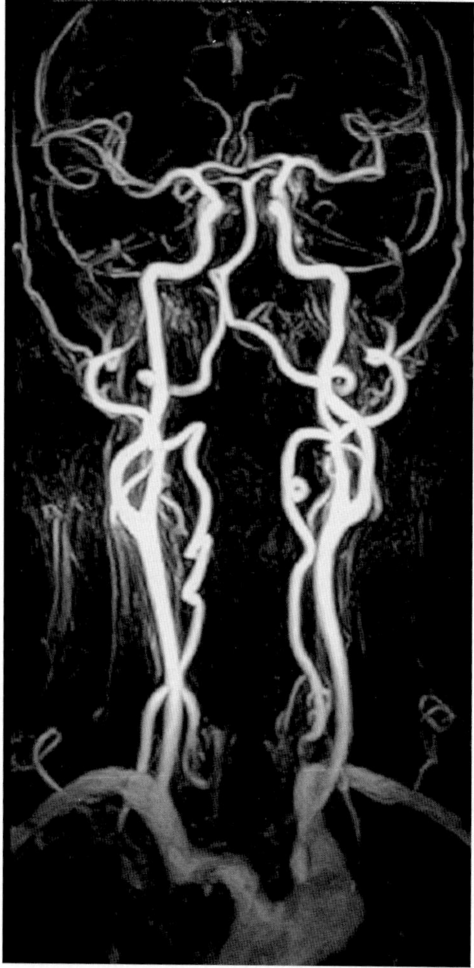

b

Fig. 5.3.7. a Time-of-flight MR angiography of normal intracranial vessels and (**b**) contrast-enhanced MRA technique with a large field-of-view covering all vessels from the aortic arch to the circle of Willis

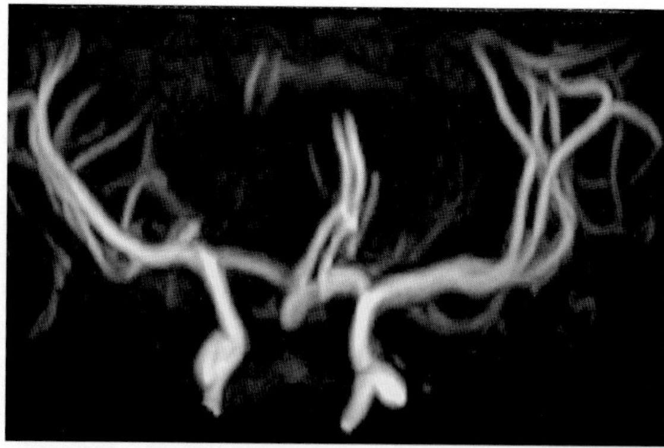

Fig. 5.3.8. TOF-MRA of a small Acom aneurysm

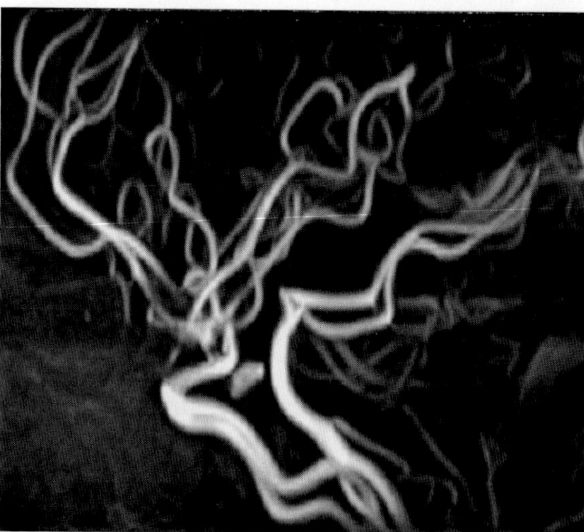

Fig. 5.3.9. TOF-MRA of an ICA/Pcom aneurysm. MRA even reveals that the aneurysm has a small neck and is suitable for endovascular therapy

phy was performed in 43 of these 45 patients, revealing that seven of these 43 did not have an aneurysm (MRA false positive), and the remaining 36 actually had 60 aneurysms (13 of which had been missed on MRA false negative). The true positive rate for MRA was 78%, the false positive rate was 15% and the false negative rate was 22%. Positive predictive value was 87%, but since 395 subjects did not undergo conventional angiography, the true negative rate and negative predictive value cannot be calculated for the whole study. Okahara et al. (2002) compared MRA with DSA in 133 patients with aneurysms. This study is of particular interest because the authors mainly focussed on evaluation of the images by a neuroradiologists, a neurosurgeon, a general radiologist and a resident in neuroradiology.

This study clearly has more clinical impact than many others done before. The diagnosis is not made by the technique – not surprising, but never mentioned with such evidence – but is dependent on the skills of the reader. The results were as follows: 79% of aneurysms were detected by the neuroradiologist, 73% by the neurosurgeon, 63% by the general radiologist and 60% by the resident in neuroradiology. Again, 3 mm was a crucial size of aneurysms: below that size, it seems to be very difficult to get reliable results.

Despite all these mentioned limitations – and we have given details about these studies, because the scientific community is still discussing this problem without an evidence based solution – MRA is increasingly used for screening of aneurysms (Kojima et al. 1998), especially in families of SAH patients.

However, another excellent indication for MRA is clearly follow-up in patients who had endovascular aneurysm treatment before. It is increasingly accepted that MRA techniques in this patient subgroup are sufficient enough to detect those aneurysm recanalizations that require retreatment. In addition to TOF techniques contrast-enhanced MR angiography is a complementary tool to visualize supraaortal and intracranial arteries. The spatial resolution is still lower than with TOF, acquisition time is much shorter (down to 12 s for a 3D data set) and the FOV covers the whole area from the aortic arch to the circle of Willis. However, up to now we do not have exact data about sensitivity and specificity of this technique in aneurysm patients.

Present indications for MRA in the evaluation of cerebral aneurysms include:

- Incidental findings on CT or MRI suspicious for an aneurysm
- Evaluation of specific clinical symptoms (i.e., third cranial nerve palsy) or non-specific symptoms in whom an aneurysm might explain the clinical presentation (thunderclap headache)
- Contraindications for conventional angiography
- Non-invasive follow-up of patients with known aneurysms or endovascular treated aneurysms
- Screening in "high risk" patients (first degree relatives of patients with SAH or multiple aneurysms, patients with polycystic kidney disease or with connective tissue disease)

5.3.4 Cerebral Angiography

Owing to its excellent spatial resolution conventional cerebral angiography is still the gold standard for the detection of a cerebral aneurysm. Currently, this is performed during the first available moment after presentation of the patient at the hospital after SAH. Considering that the risk of rehemorrhage is highest in the first 24 h (4%), an early angiogram is crucial for any therapeutic decision and for the patient‘s outcome.

Cerebral angiography can localize the lesion, reveal aneurysm shape and geometry, determine the presence of multiple aneurysms, define vascular anatomy and collateral situation, and assess the presence and degree of vasospasm. Due to the frequency of multiple aneurysms a complete four-vessel angiography is essential. However, in the case of a space occupying hematoma angiography of the most likely affected vessel is sufficient. Anteroposterior, lateral, and oblique views are systematically performed with cross-compression to demonstrate the Acom, if necessary. Additional views may be necessary to optimize demonstration of the aneurysm neck. If no aneurysm is found, selective catheterization of both external carotid arteries is performed to exclude a dural arteriovenous fistula. The potential for collateral circulation from the vertebrobasilar system may be evaluated when the vertebral artery is injected during carotid artery compression (Allcock test) demonstrating patency, size and collateral potential of the P1 segment of the PCA and the posterior communicating artery ipsilateral to the carotid artery compressed.

As a prerequisite to angiography, survey of renal function and coagulation factors is required in all patients. Digital subtraction angiography technique is necessary, biplane angiography facilitates the diagnostic workup and is useful for safe and fast therapeutic interventions. It shortens examination time and increases the safety during aneurysm obliteration. High-quality fluoroscopy and roadmapping are essential to perform intracranial interventions.

5.3.4.1 3D Rotational Angiography

The precise visualization of the aneurysm neck, the shape and the size of the aneurysm, and its relationship to parent vessels are important factors for endovascular therapy. Rotational angiography in a 2D or 3D mode is available on most new generation neurointerventional angio suites and represents a valuable supplement to standard biplane DSA. Using rotational angiography multiple oblique views are obtained as source for 3D reconstruction. Data acquisition consists of a rotational mask followed by a second run during contrast injection. During data acquisition the C-arm rotates in a continuous 200°

arc around the patients‘s head placed in the isocenter (Fahrig et al. 1997). Rotational angiography helps to define the aneurysm neck, find the appropriate working position and perform accurate measurements. 3D angiography thereby improves planning of surgical and interventional procedures, especially in complex aneurysms (Anxionnat et al. 2001). However, even the highest standard 3D DSA techniques cannot always precisely describe the exact anatomy of the neck and the exact relationship of tiny adjacent vessels to the aneurysm dome and neck. As an interventionalist you still have to rely on your experience and – sometimes – on superselective catheterization of the aneurysm itself. And sometimes you have to combine it with temporary coil placement without subsequent detachment.

Stroke complication rate for diagnostic angiography at our institution is less than 0.5%, comparable to other major interventional centres across Europe and the US (Heiserman et al. 1994). Thus the risk: benefit ratio still justifies conventional angiography in the diagnostic management of aneurysms. Other complications may include allergic reaction to contrast agent, renal failure, bleeding at the puncture site. In fact, incidence of allergic reaction seems to be very low (we did not see a single instance during the last 6 years) and bleeding complications will probably further decrease with the availability of specific devices allowing a "surgical" closure of the puncture site. Aneurysm rupture during angiography is reported in less than 3% of patients investigated with SAH. "Less than 3%" is correct, but for us it

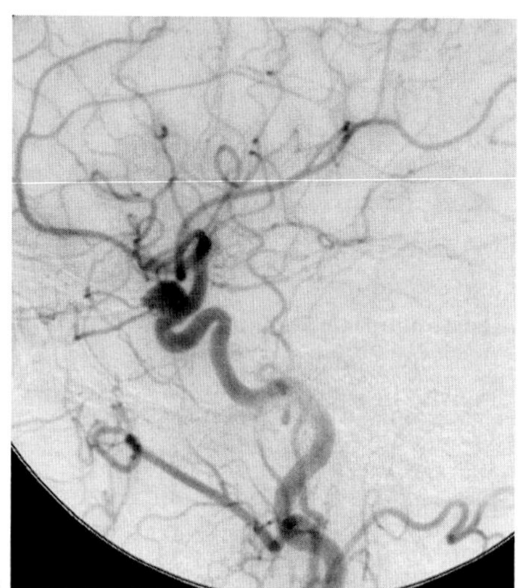

a

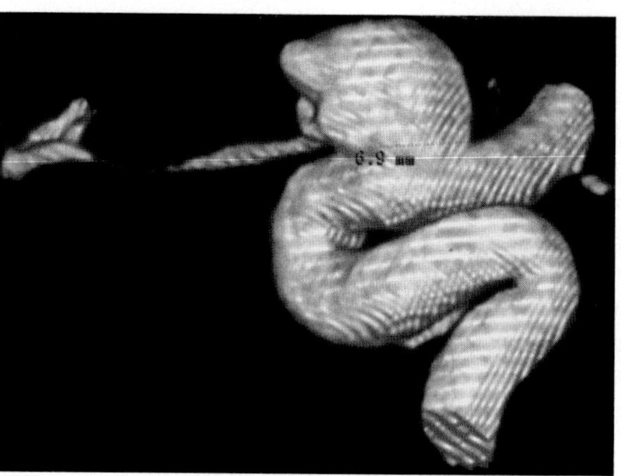

b

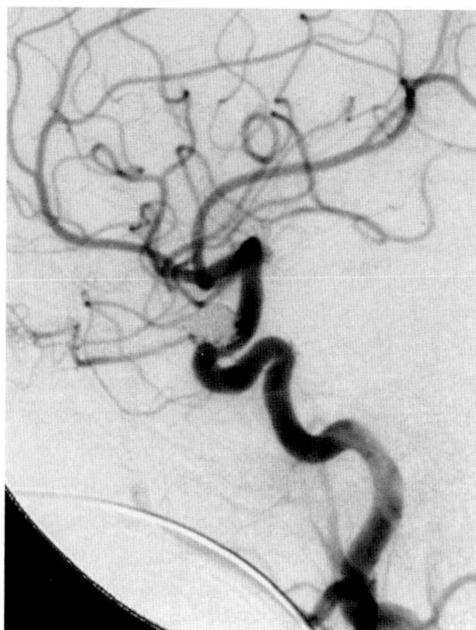

c

Fig. 5.3.10. **a** Paraophthalmic aneurysm. **b** On 3D rotational DSA the ophthalmic artery is assumed to originate from the aneurysm, but after complete occlusion of the aneurysm this vessel remained patent (**c**)

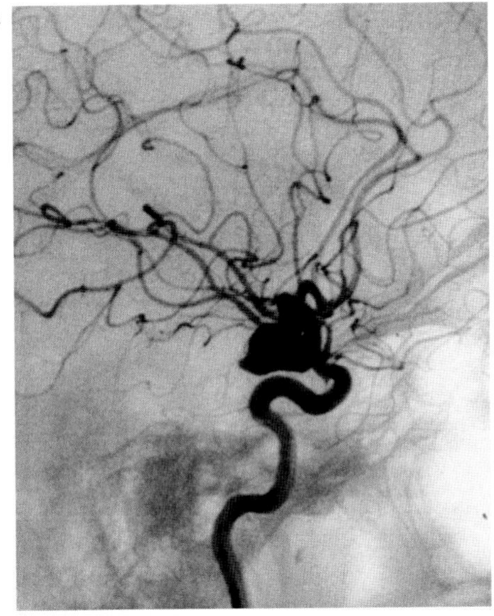

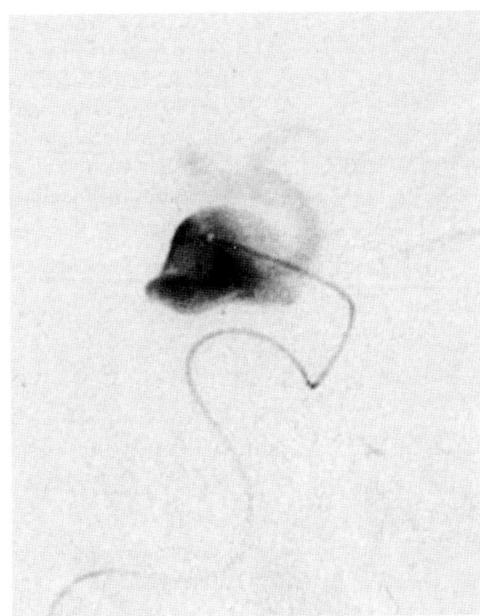

Fig.5.3.11. a ICA aneurysm. **b** Aneurysmography: selective angiography with the tip of the microcatheter placed within the aneurysm

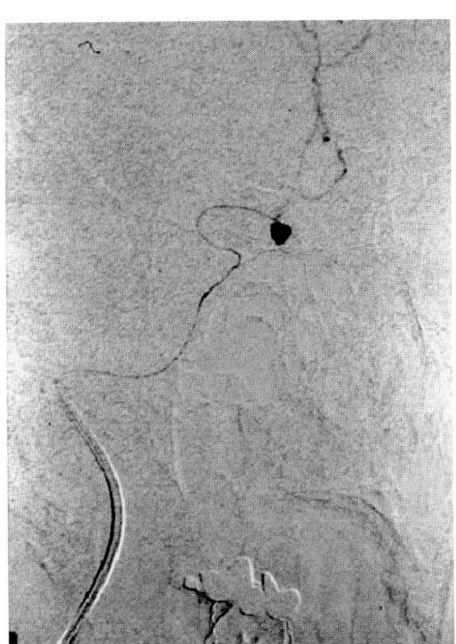

Fig. 5.3.12. Aneurysmography of a small Acom aneurysm

sounds higher than reality shows. In our institution, and now studying about 200 patients per year with intracranial aneurysms, we have not seen an aneurysm rupture during diagnostic angiography in the last 6 years.

The risk of aneurysm rupture, however, may be increased during superselective aneurysmography. Superselective angiography with the tip of the microcatheter placed within the aneurysm and gentle injection of contrast may be helpful in demonstrating morphological details of the entire aneurysm, especially concerning the identification of vessels arising from the aneurysm. GAILLOUD et al. (1997) reported a posterior perforating artery originating from the dome of a basilar tip aneurysm identified only by selective aneurysmography.

5.3.5 Patients with SAH of Unidentifiable Cause

If the initial angiography is negative despite aneurysmal pattern of hemorrhage, repeated angiography within 2–3 weeks is clearly indicated. Cranial or spinal MRI may be indicated to exclude other sources of hemorrhage. The risk of rebleeding is up to 10% (CANHAO et al. 1995). There might be several explanations for the missing radiological detection of an aneurysm: apart from technical limitations such as insufficient projections, vasospasm, aneurysm thrombosis or obliteration of the aneurysm by pressure of adjacent hematoma might contribute to the failing radiological demonstration. If a second angiogram also fails to reveal the suspected aneurysm a third angiography might be indicated after an interval of several months and may then demonstrate the aneurysm (RINKEL et al. 1991).

If cerebral angiography is negative in a pattern of perimesencephalic hemorrhage the diagnosis of non-aneurysmal hemorrhage should be established and no repeat studies are needed.

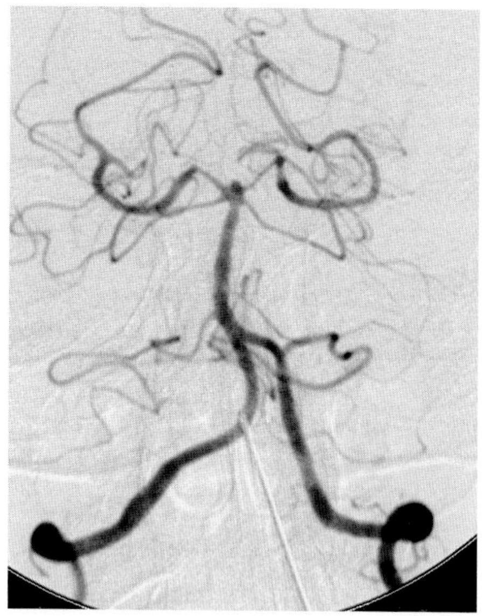

a

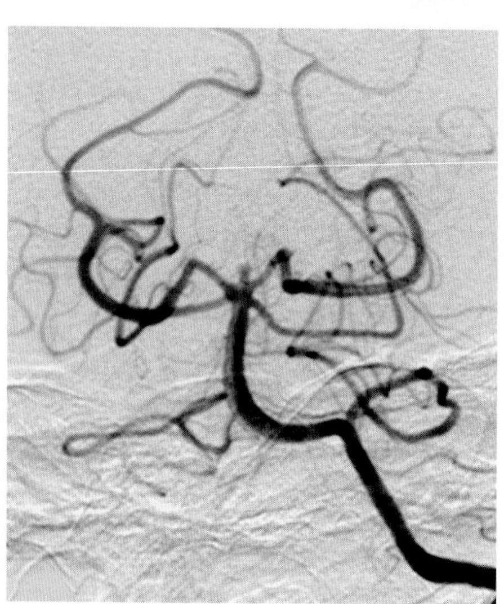

b

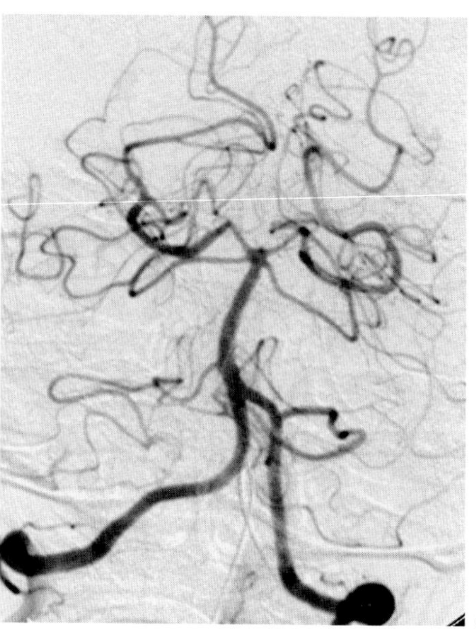

c

Fig. 5.3.13. Patient after SAH with a basilar tip aneurysm seen on CTA in an outside hospital. **a** Initial DSA did show vasospasm of the P1 segment and the superior cerebellar artery on both sides. In addition, some irregularity at the tip of the basilar artery was noted but no real aneurysm. **b** Repeated DSA 2 months later showed a small basilar tip aneurysm suitable for endovascular treatment. **c** The patient was scheduled for embolization 10 days later but the aneurysm again was not visible. The patient was referred to surgery

5.3.5.1
Screening

Screening for a cerebral aneurysm is indicated in patients in whom the risk of investigations to detect and treat the aneurysm is less than the risk of the natural history of the aneurysm. The natural history, however, is not clearly defined. Screening has been recommended for first-degree relatives of a family member with two or more aneurysms and for patients with autosomal dominant polycystic kidney disease (Schievink 1997; Schievink et al. 1997). In identical twins with one suffering SAH, the risk of harbouring an aneurysm is increased in the other and screening is also indicated.

5.3.6
Transcranial Ultrasound

Transcranial Doppler sonography (TCD) has proved to be a suitable non-invasive technique for measuring cerebral blood flow velocity in large cerebral arteries. The technique of TCD can be combined with duplex imaging and with colour coding. Colour TCD ultrasound became available in the early 1990s, with some success at identification of aneurysms (Becker et al. 1992). A recently developed technology of colour coded Doppler, i.e. colour Doppler energy or power Doppler, showed a significant greater sensitivity to flowing blood than standard colour flow imaging (Wardlaw and Cannon 1996).

However, in the detection of cerebral aneurysms power TCD is less sensitive than other non-invasive techniques such as CTA and MRA. Especially in small aneurysms of less than 6 mm sensitivity is very poor (0.35), the internal carotid artery is the most difficult segment to interpret on ultrasound (Griewing et al. 1998; White et al. 2001). Additionally, insonation of the MCA is inadequate or even not possible in 5%–20% of all patients because of insufficient ultrasound transmission through the skull (White et al. 2001). Although the technique is quick, safe, inexpensive and non invasive, it is highly dependent on the skills of the operator. At the moment, TCD for the detection of cerebral aneurysms is only of scientific interest and cannot be recommended for routine use. In fact, it does not play any role in the diagnostic work-up of SAH patients nor in screening.

5.4 Therapy

5.4.1 General Considerations

The primary treatment goal of cerebral aneurysms is prevention of rupture. Surgical clipping has been the treatment modality of choice for both ruptured and unruptured cerebral aneurysms since decades. Just over 20 years ago endovascular treatment was mainly restricted to those patients with aneurysms unsuitable for clipping due to the size or location, or in whom surgical clipping was contraindicated because of the general medical condition. Since the introduction of controlled detachable coils for packing of aneurysms (Guglielmi et al. 1991ab), endovascular embolization is increasingly used. Numerous observational studies have published complications rates, occlusion rates and short-term follow-up results. These have been summarized up to March 1997 in a systematic review of 48 eligible studies of 1383 patients with ruptured and unruptured aneurysms (Brilstra et al. 1999). Permanent procedural complications occurred in 3.7% of 1256 patients. More than 90% occlusion of the aneurysm was achieved in around 90% of patients. The most frequent procedural complication was cerebral ischemia, the second most frequent complication was aneurysm perforation, which occurred in about 2% of patients. Rerupture of angiographically successful coiled aneurysms may occur, long-term rates of rebleeding after endovascular coiling still need to be established. In 2002 the results of the ISAT study were published; the clear benefit of the endovascular treated patients will definitely change treatment strategies for patients with intracranial aneurysms (Molyneux et al. 2002). The endovascular approach will become the first line treatment option, whenever this option is available. ISAT represents a landmark in the evolution of aneurysm treatment and, therefore, a more detailed discussion of these results seems justified.

5.4.2 The ISAT Study

ISAT was a randomised, prospective, international, controlled trial of endovascular coiling versus surgical clipping for a selected group of patients with ruptured intracranial aneurysms deemed suitable for both types of therapy. Most patients were treated at high-volume centres in the United Kingdom, with the remainders from other European countries, Australia, Canada, and the United States. The primary endpoint was patient outcome, defined as a modified Rankin scale of 3–6 (dependent or deceased) at 1 year. The primary hypothesis was that endovascular treatment would reduce the proportion of patients dependent or deceased by 25% at 1 year. A total of 9559 patients with SAH were screened and around one quarter (n = 2143) were randomly assigned to both treatment groups. Those patients who were screened but not randomized were treated surgically in 39%, endovascularly in 29% or by an unrecorded therapy (11%). Most randomized patients had aneurysms located at the AcomA or intracranial ICA. A total of 94% of randomised patients were in good condition (WFNS grades I–III). The study was prematurely stopped after the results of a planned interim analysis were available: at 1 year, 23.7% of the patients allocated to endovascular treatment were dependent or dead, as compared with 30.6% of patients in the surgical group. Later on, the study group reported the revised outcome results with an even greater absolute risk reduction of 8.7% and a relative risk reduction of 26.8% for coiling over clipping (Kerr and Molyneux 2003). The results of the ISAT study were not readily accepted, particularly not in the neurosurgical community. We strongly recommend reading the statement written by the Executive Committee of the American Society of Interventional and Therapeutic Neuroradiology and the American Society of Neuroradiology (Derdeyn et al. 2003). The authors answer a lot of frequently asked questions about ISAT.

A major issue is the durability of aneurysm occlusion after coiling. It is true that long-term durability of endovascular therapy remains to be determined.

The present data, however, suggest that it is very unlikely that late aneurysm rebleeding will occur at a rate that would significantly affect the difference in outcome between surgery and coiling. The ISAT data indicate a risk of rebleeding after 1 year of 0.16% patient-years of follow-up. Thus it would take more than 40 years to overcome the benefit seen at 1 year with endovascular treatment.

Another major issue was the doubt about the competence of British neurosurgeons. However, they were very experienced – just looking at the numbers of patients they treated – and their results pretty much matched the results of the tirilazad study, a prospective multicenter study, mainly involving US neurosurgeons (HALEY et al. 1997; LANZINO and KASSELL 1999). In this study, in the 3-month follow-up, 9.2% of the grades I–III patients had died. In ISAT 8.3% of the surgically randomised patients were dead at 2 months, increasing to 10.1% at 1 year. Incidentally, similar data were reported from the European and Australasian arm of the tirilazad study (LANZINO et al. 1999a).

The low randomization rate is another point of criticism: randomization rates were less than 40% in NASCET and less than 4% in ACAS. ISAT is within the range of randomization rates given by other large studies. There is absolutely no indication that the randomisation rate could affect the final result.

Beside these frequently asked questions there are a number of important implications of ISAT: ISAT will significantly change our policy for patients with unruptured aneurysm. We look ahead for those meta-analyses based on the treatment results of ISAT.

Since ISAT it is mandatory that all patients should be seen by a neurointerventionalist to decide whether the aneurysm is suitable for coiling or not. If one treatment is recommended over another, the reasons for this decision should be documented as in accordance with the usual standards for informed consent. Furthermore, the ISAT data add support for the treatment of patients with aneurysmal SAH in high-volume centres that offer both surgery and endovascular therapy.

5.4.3 Treatment of Unruptured Aneurysms

This is still a controversial topic and up to now there is still no total agreement about indications. First of all, the easiest parts: There are two groups of unruptured aneurysms, asymptomatic aneurysms detected incidentally and those causing clinical symptoms due to compression of nerval structures or emboli arising from the non-ruptured sac. The former group also includes those aneurysms detected during angiography in patients with SAH with an aneurysm in another location.

The management of unruptured aneurysms remains controversial and depends on a full understanding of their natural history balanced against the risks of treatment and long-term protection afforded.

a 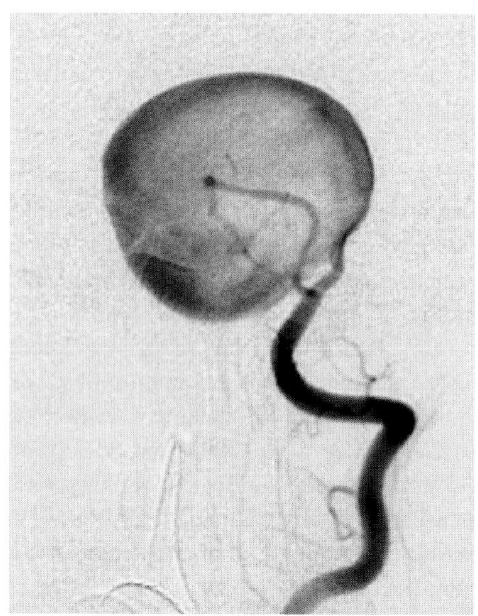

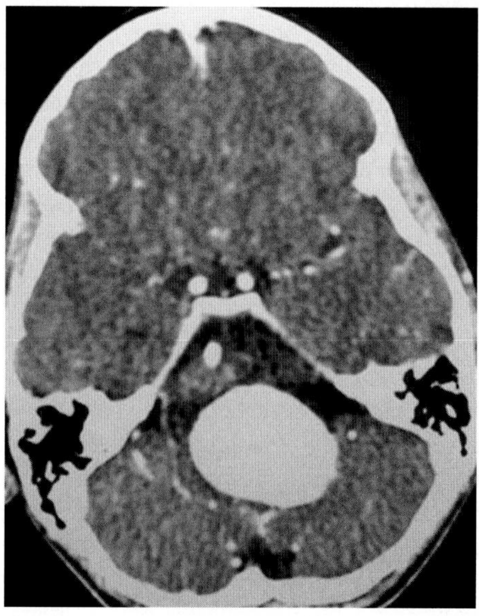 b

Fig. 5.4.1. Giant vertebral aneurysm in a 9-year-old boy with nausea and vomiting due to brain stem compression (**a**, DSA ap view; **b**, axial contrast-enhanced CCT)

Aneurysm prevalence in the general population shows wide variation. However, in those with a family history of SAH, the prevalence of unruptured aneurysms has been reported from 10% to 13% (Kojima et al. 1998). And, detection of aneurysms during life is increasing due to increased use of accurate imaging methods and due to screening programs introduced, e.g. in Japan. In summary, unruptured aneurysms will be identified with regularity in most units involved in neuroimaging and the management of these patients is a universal problem.

Unfortunately, unruptured aneurysms are a heterogeneous entity, both in terms of morphology and behaviour, e.g. tendency to rupture. This is in part reflected in the extreme variation in reported rupture risk in the literature between 0.05% and 5% a year (Wiebers 1998; Wiebers et al. 1981).

Aneurysm size seems to be an important factor to predict the risk of rupture: ISUIA part one tried to teach us that 10 mm is a critical size. Smaller aneurysms (without a history of SAH from another aneurysm) had a rupture risk of 0.05% per year. There was a lot of criticism about this study, mainly because the daily experience of nearly all physicians treating aneurysmal SAH patients is, that the vast majority of ruptured aneurysms are less than 7 mm in size. The second part of the ISUIA study – published in July 2003 – came out with a slightly different result: the critical size of the aneurysm was downsized to 7 mm and there were certain locations with an increased risk of rupture per se: Posterior circulation aneurysms and those aneurysms arising from the posterior communicating artery (Wiebers et al. 2003).

Table 5.4.1. 5-Year cumulative rupture rates of intracranial aneurysms (Wiebers et al. 2003)

Size/location	<7 mm	7–12 mm	13–24 mm	>25
ICA/AcomA/ ACA/MCA	0%	2.6%	14.5%	40%
PcomA/Posterior circulation	2.5%	14.5%	18.4%	50%

Other studies found the incidence of rupture of all coincidental aneurysms to be between 1% and 3.2% per year, with hypertension and aneurysm multiplicity being specific risk factors (Winn et al. 1983; Yasui et al. 1997). Other factors for a higher probability of rupture include: multilobular aneurysm morphology (Hademenos et al. 1998), posterior location (Hademenos et al. 1998; Rinkel et al. 1998; Wiebers et al. 2003), symptoms related to mass effect, and female sex, smoking and hypertension.

A striking observation in many studies on unruptured aneurysms is that Acom aneurysms are generally underrepresented. One possible explanation is that these aneurysms have a different natural history; they may form and subsequently rupture rapidly so that the opportunity to detect these as unruptured lesions is limited. If this explanation is true, the ISUIA findings (see Table 5.4.1) have to be interpreted with much more care than previously.

The early and late outcome after surgery of unruptured aneurysms is well documented in the literature. A meta-analysis by Raaymakers et al. (1998) of 61 studies on 2460 patients with 2568 clipped aneurysms showed a permanent morbidity of 10.9% and mortality of 2.6% with the best results in small and anterior circulation aneurysms. A study by Johnston et al. (1999a) compared the clinical outcomes of patients who had unruptured aneurysms treated by surgery and endovascular therapy. Morbidity was significantly higher in the surgical group (18.5%) than in the endovascular group (10.6%). Mortality was 2.3% after surgery and 0.4% after coiling. A further study by the same authors showed improved clinical outcomes, shorter hospital stay, shorter recovery period, reduced costs and reduced long term symptoms in those patients treated with coil embolization (Johnston et al. 2000). Technical feasibility in over 90% in our patient group and in those of other authors with a high occlusion rate justify comparison with neurosurgical data on unruptured aneurysms (Murayama et al. 1999; Wanke et al. 2002). We had a morbidity of 4.8%, mortality was zero (Wanke et al. 2002). Murayama et al. (1999) reported a morbidity of 4.3% in a total of 109 patients after endovascular treatment of unruptured aneurysms, with no morbidity in the last 65 patients. Comparisons between surgical and endovascular treatment of unruptured aneurysms demonstrated that the costs treating an unruptured aneurysm are significantly lower than treating patients with SAH regarding length of hospital stay and sequelae of morbidity (Johnston et al. 1999a,b, 2000; Murayama et al. 1999; Wardlaw and White 2000; Wiebers et al. 1992). By comparing the results of surgical clipping and coil embolization of 60 university hospitals, Johnston et al. (1999) reported significant higher costs ($43.000 vs. $30.000) and significant longer hospital stay (9.6 days vs. 4.6 days) for the surgical cases. All these facts encourage us to use the endovascular route instead of clipping in the vast majority of patients with unruptured aneurysms.

In cases of a ruptured aneurysm in another location the relative risk of rupture of an additional nonruptured aneurysm is higher than without a history of SAH (Wiebers 1998) and, therefore treatment is indicated. However, in this specific subgroup there are different opinions about the best strategy (Inagawa et al. 1992; Mizoi et al. 1995; Raaymakers et al. 1998; Wiebers 1998; Wiebers et al. 2003). The MARS group analyzed risk and benefit of screening for intracranial aneurysms in first-degree relatives of patients with SAH (626 first-degree relatives). 18 out of 25 patients with aneurysms had neurosurgical clipping of their unruptured aneurysm, none of them had endovascular therapy. They conclude that screening is not warranted at this time since the slight increase in life expectancy does not offset the risk of postoperative sequelae (Raaymakers 2000). Wardlaw and White (2000) concluded that the indication and cost-effectiveness of screening for aneurysms is totally unclear because prevalence varies, rupture rate is still unclear and non-invasive imaging modalities are not yet accurate enough to exclude aneurysms smaller than 5 mm. The major drawback of all these studies is that the results of endovascular treatment in unruptured aneurysms were not taken into account. More recently, Hoh et al. (2003) established that endovascular treatment of unruptured aneurysms has an average mortality of 1.7% and morbidity of 7.6%. However, mortality rate was lower at high-volume hospitals (1% versus 3.7%), morbidity at hospitals with high referral rates was 5.2% versus 17.6% for hospitals treating less than four unruptured aneurysms per year. In addition,

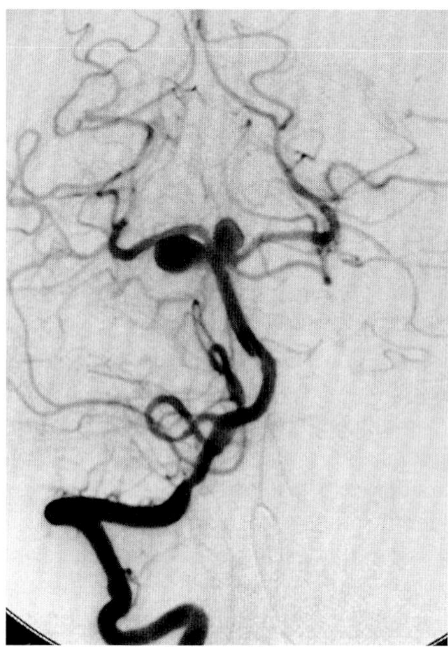

Fig. 5.4.2. Distal basilar artery aneurysms in a patient with right-sided oculomotor palsy

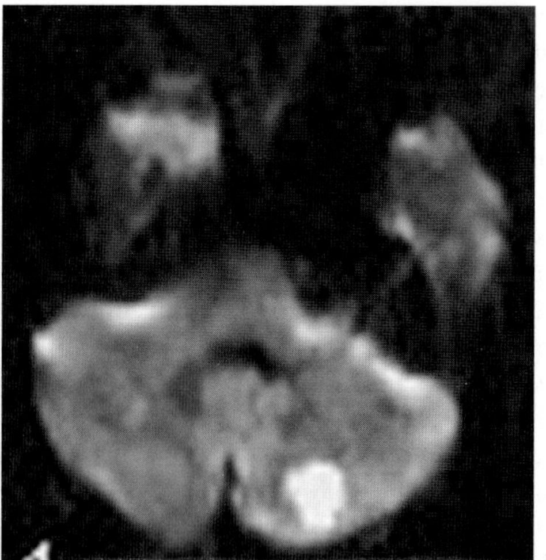

a

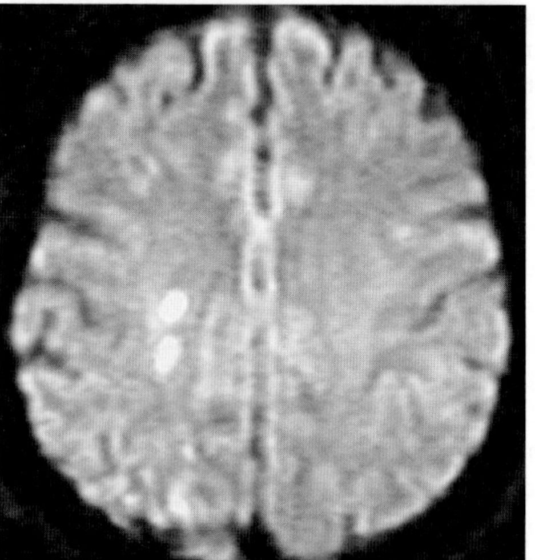

b

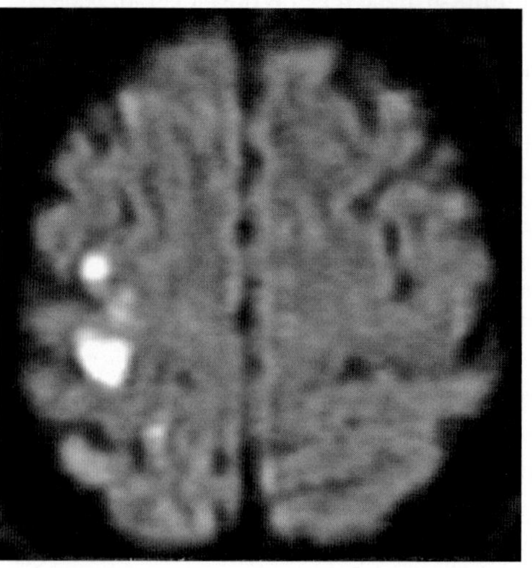

c

Fig. 5.4.3a–c. a DWI with silent small infarct of the PICA after embolization of a left vertebral aneurysm. **b, c** DWI showing small acute cerebral infarctions in the territory of the MCA after embolization of an unruptured right paraophthalmic aneurysm; the patient had no neurological symptoms

at high volume hospitals length of stay was shorter and total hospital charges were significantly lower. In conclusion, their recommendation to patients with unruptured aneurysms is to look for high-volume hospitals and physicians treating a high number of patients (Hoh et al. 2003).

Currently, healthcare is undergoing a major reorganization to meet growing economic pressure and the aspect of preventive therapy becomes more and more important. Therefore, aneurysm treatment has to be considered in several respects: what is the risk of aneurysm rupture and what are the costs to treat a subarachnoid hemorrhage? What are the costs of treating an unruptured aneurysm either neurosurgically or via an endovascular approach to avoid SAH with possibly fatal complications? Costs arising treating an aneurysmal hemorrhage have to be weighted against the risk of rupture of an incidentally detected aneurysm.

It is necessary to provide the patient all treatment options. Regarding the cost-effectiveness and the fact that endovascular treatment has a lower morbidity and mortality than neurosurgically treated patients, in our opinion, unruptured cerebral aneurysms in any location should be considered first for endovascular treatment.

5.4.4 Treatment of Ruptured Aneurysms

SAH is the most common sequelae in patients with a ruptured intracranial aneurysm. The first clinical symptom is usually an acute onset of headache. In most patients, such headache was not experienced ever before in life ("the worst headache of my life"). In patients with known migraine or other types of headache SAH can be overlooked, but usually patients themselves can clearly distinguish between these different types of headache. Aspirin should be avoided at all cost in these patients. A warning leak, defined as a sudden episode of headache, vomiting, nuchal pain, dizziness or drowsiness, might precede this event in a considerable number (Hauerberg et al. 1991). The first symptom could also be due to an intraparenchymal bleeding preceded by a minor SAH. These patients typically suffer from a frontobasal bleeding and might be referred to a psychiatric department because of a sudden onset of a psychotic episode. Therefore, cross sectional imaging is indicated in patients with sudden change of behaviour.

Very few patients do not experience the onset of SAH as an acute onset of headache, but realize the symptoms of infarction due to subsequent vasospasm.

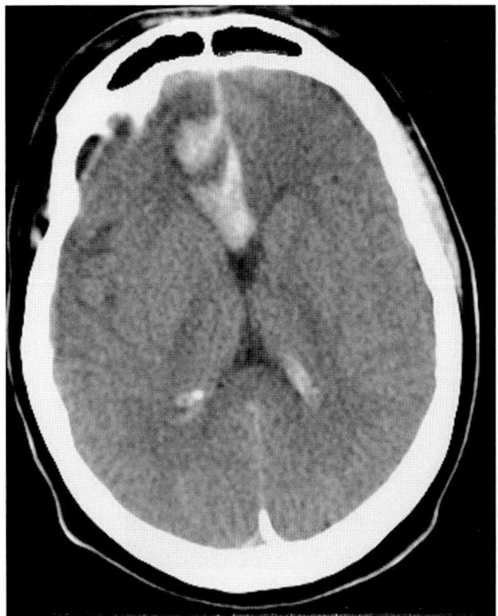
a

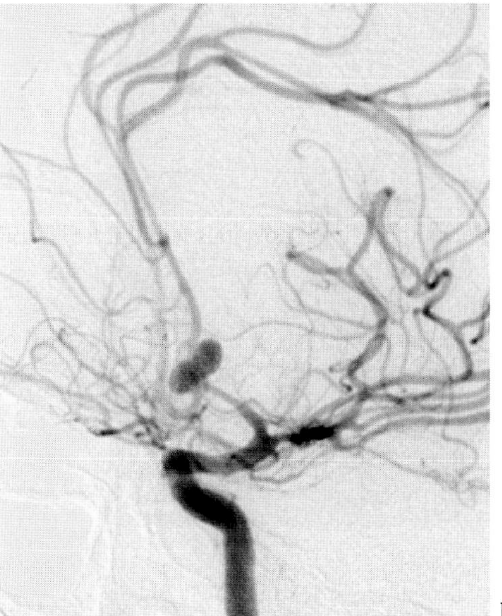
b

Fig. 5.4.4. Frontal intraparenchymal hemorrhage without SAH due to a ruptured Acom aneurysm in a patient with sudden onset of a psychotic episode

In these patients, Doppler sonography and lumbar puncture should reveal the cause of the disease.

Since the rebleeding rate of a ruptured aneurysm depending on the location is as high as 50% the urge to treat a ruptured aneurysm is obvious.

The clinical categorization of patient's symptoms was summarized by Hunt and Hess. This classification is internationally accepted and widely used to describe the patient's condition at admission after SAH.

a

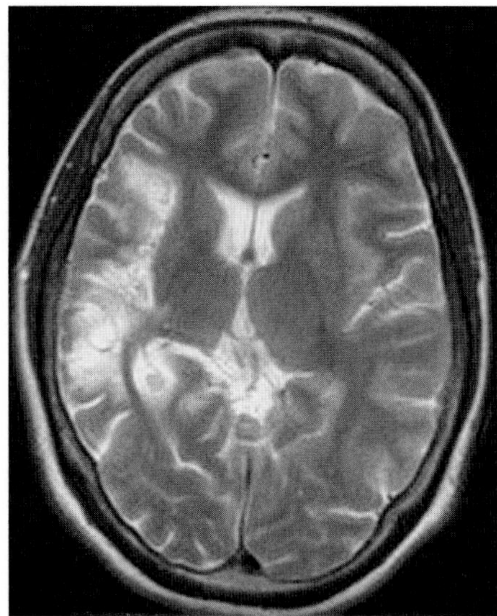

b

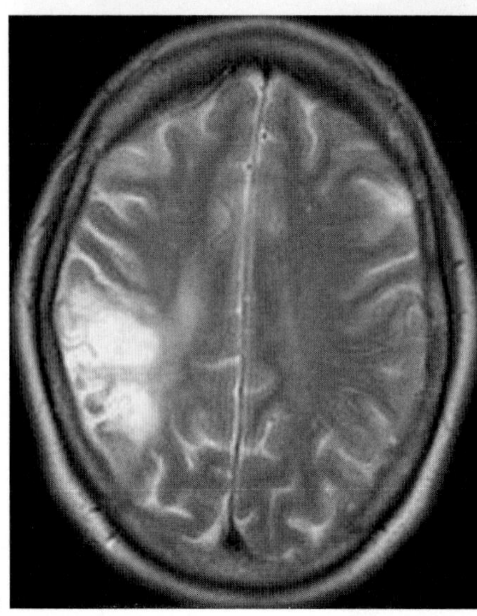

Fig. 5.4.5a,b. Right MCA infarct in a patient who was administered with mild left sided hemiparesis. Doppler sonography revealed slightly increased velocity of the ICA and MCA and lumbar puncture showed hemosiderin. The patient did not report a typical sudden onset of headache. DSA revealed a small Pcom aneurysm but no visible vasospasms

Table 5.4.2. Hunt and Hess classification of SAH

I	Asymptomatic, or minimal headache and slight nuchal rigidity
II	Moderate or severe headache, nuchal rigidity, no neurological deficit (except cranial nerve palsy)
III	Drowsiness, confusion, or mild focal deficit
IV	Stupor, moderate or severe hemiparesis, possible early decerebrate rigidity and vegetative disturbance
V	Deep coma, decerebrate rigidity, moribund

5.4.5 Endovascular Therapy

5.4.5.1 *History*

Attempts to induce thrombosis of systemic aneurysms either by introducing foreign bodies or application of electrical or thermic injury date back to the first half of the 19th century. Velpeu (1831) and Phillips (1832) independently described a method of introducing arterial thrombosis by inserting a needle into the aneurysmal lumen and withdrawing it after thrombus have formed. In 1941 Werner et al. reported successful electrothermic thrombosis of an acute ruptured intracranial aneurysm. Through a transorbital approach, a silver wire was introduced and heated, causing arrest of the aneurysmal bleeding. In 1963 Gallagher proposed a technique of inducing thrombosis of intracranial aneurysms by high-speed delivery of dog or horse hairs into the aneurysm using a pneumatic gun ("pilojection") (Gallagher 1963, 1964; Gallagher and Baiz 1964). However, despite encouraging early results this method did not gain acceptance.

Further improvements in endovascular devices, balloon techniques, and arterial catheterization, rapidly led to the idea of endovascular navigation and occlusion of the aneurysmal sac. The first successful balloon embolization was performed by Serbinenko in 1973 (Serbinenko 1974a,b), establishing the way for modern endovascular treatment of cerebral aneurysms. However, several drawbacks of latex balloons, i.e. deflation, aneurysm rupture, protrusion into the parent vessel, distal embolization, and frequent rebleedings, prompted the search for better materials for aneurysm occlusion. Although balloon occlusion of parent vessels is still a therapeutic option for large, giant, or fusiform aneurysms, this technique has been mainly abandoned in favour of coil embolization. In 1991, the Italian neurosurgeon Guido Guglielmi published his preliminary experience with electrolytically detachable platinum coils (Guglielmi Detachable Coils, GDC), opening a new era in aneurysm treatment (Guglielmi et al. 1991a,b, 1992). The GDC technique represents the current "gold standard" in endovascular aneurysm therapy with more than 80,000 patients having been treated world-wide to date. And there is still ongoing progress in the field of endovascular therapy for intracranial aneurysms with development of new coil designs or other endovascular devices. The next step is supposed to replace the simply filling techniques with materials that promote real endothelialization of the aneurysm neck.

5.4.5.2
Basic Assumptions for Endovascular Aneurysm Therapy

5.4.5.2.1
Contraindications to Endovascular Aneurysm Therapy

True contraindications to endovascular aneurysm therapy (EVT) are very rare including not manageable coagulopathies and known adverse reactions to heparin or contrast agents. Renal failure restricting the use of contrast material might be a relative contraindication.

5.4.5.2.2
General Considerations About Surgery or Endovascular Aneurysm Therapy

Initially, endovascular therapy was restricted to surgical "difficult" or inaccessible lesions, predominantly in the posterior circulation. Nowadays, the increasing experience and development of appropriate devices has widened the indications, and EVT has become a true alternative to surgical treatment (Molyneux et al. 2002).

However, the current state of the art in endovascular therapy has still some limitations such as the anatomic situation of the aneurysm, aneurysm size or unfavourable or invisible geometry (neck/fundus ratio). For aneurysms with a wide neck or difficult geometry surgery is still the preferred treatment. Relative limitations correspond to the expertise and experience of a given team. With increasing experience even wide neck or multilobulated aneurysms can be successfully treated via the endovascular approach.

The decision to treat an aneurysm endovascularly rather than surgically is not easy and requires a multidisciplinary input. It is important to jointly discuss the cases, preferentially in daily conferences and rounds. This collaboration requires both the neurosurgeon and the interventionalist to be extremely honest about what they think they can achieve with each approach. Neurosurgery and interventional neuroradiology are not competitive facilities, but the complementary nature of techniques offers the best chance for reducing treatment morbidity and improving long-term outcome in difficult aneurysms. However, currently more and more aneu-

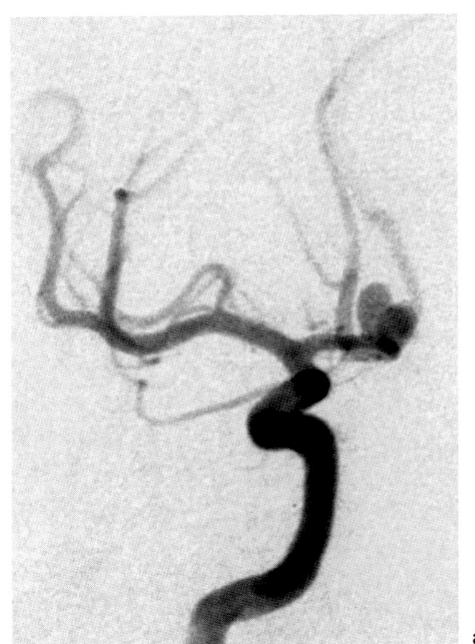
a

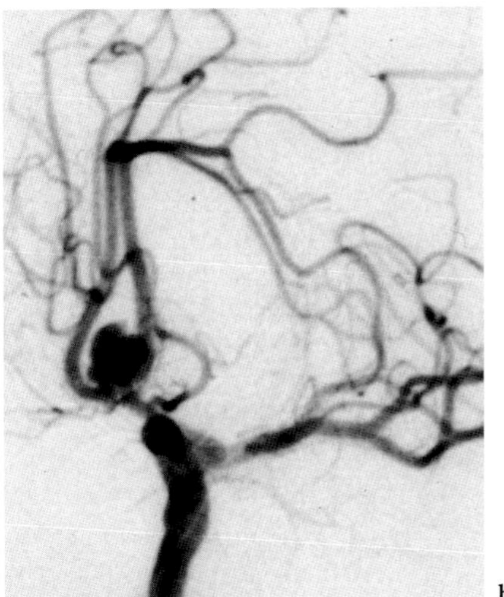
b

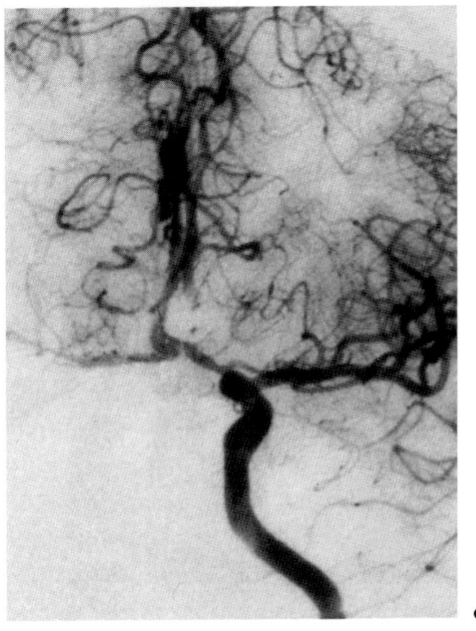
c

Fig. 5.4.6a–c. Multilobulated Acom aneurysm before (**a, b**) and after embolization (**c**)

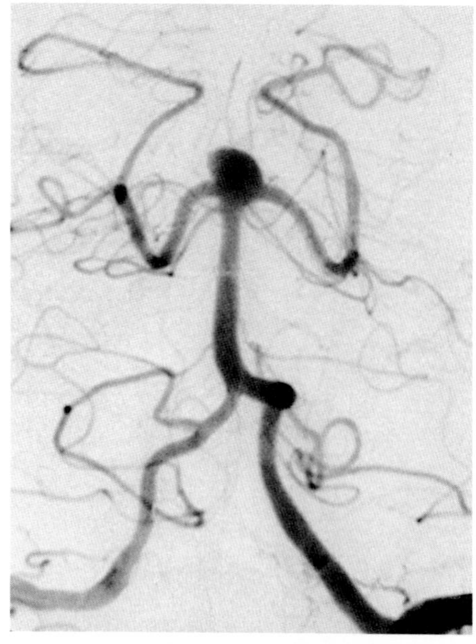
a

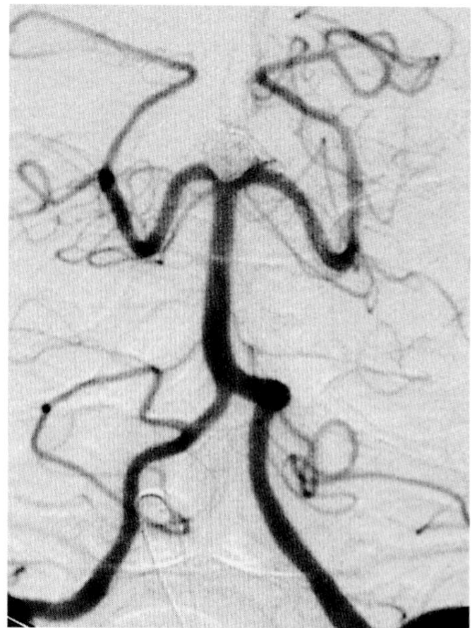
b

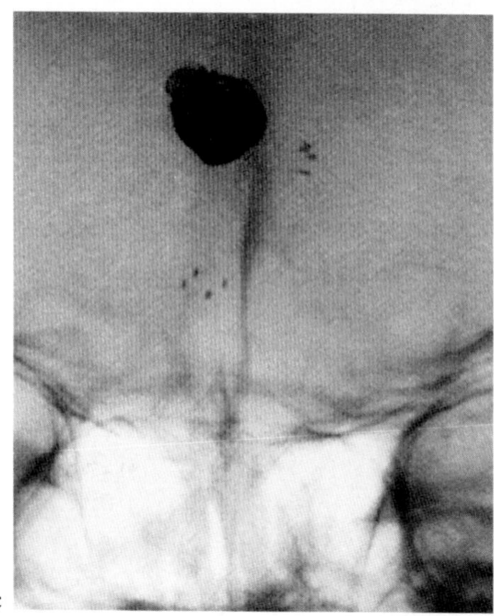
c

Fig. 5.4.7. a Broad based basilar tip aneurysm. **b, c** Endovascular treatment was performed with a stent and platinum coils. The stent was deployed with the distal end in the P1 segment left and the proximal end in the mid basilar artery (*markers*). Coiling was done through the mesh of the stent

rysms are treated via the endovascular approach and – in complete contrast to the situation of two decades ago – surgery is increasingly indicated in difficult endovascularly inaccessible aneurysms.

In our institution, the way to decide who treats the patient has changed somewhat over time. During the first 2 years each individual aneurysm was discussed between neurointerventionalists and the vascular neurosurgeons. Over time it turned out – promoted by scientific data and by the institutional experience – that the endovascular route should be preferred, if technically possible, e.g. if the geometry and anatomy of the aneurysm makes it suitable for embolization. We have reached a point where most of the aneurysms are treated by an endovascular technique (up to 75%).

Due to this circumstance the question of how to maintain the neurosurgeon's expertise is becoming increasingly important.

Timing: In recent years, the strategy of overall management has changed, focussing now on early referral and immediate therapeutic intervention to minimize the risk of rebleeding and enhance the possibilities of aggressive neurointensive care to prevent vasospasm and secondary ischemic complications. One benefit for the endovascular arm in ISAT was the earlier time of treatment compared to the surgical group.

5.4.5.2.3
Standards for Endovascular Aneurysm Therapy

The neurointerventionalist performing the procedure should have appropriate training and experience in neuroangiography and cerebral interventions, a full understanding of the disease process and alternative methods of treatment, and should fully appreciate the risks and benefits of the procedure. A thorough understanding of vascular neuroanatomy, angiographic equipment, radiation safety considerations, and physiologic monitoring equipment is taken for granted, as well as access to an adequate supply of catheters, guidewires, embolic devices, equipment for intraarterial thrombolysis or treatment of vasospasm. The neurointerventionalist should be familiar with anticoagulation regimens and the management of neuroangiographic complications, such as intraarterial thrombolysis and the treatment of vasospasm.

Endovascular treatment should be performed within an environment in which appropriate neurosurgical care can be instituted promptly. A readily available neurosurgeon should be aware of the endovascular procedure prior its start and available to back up if necessary. A CT scanner should be readily available in the facility.

5.4.5.2.4
Radiographic Equipment Standards for Endovascular Aneurysm Therapy

The availability of a biplane angiography with digital subtraction technique, a high resolution image intensifier and road-mapping fluoroscopy capability is desirable for endovascular aneurysm therapy. Specifically in difficult anatomic locations the capability of 3D angiographic techniques (either CTA or DSA) can be extremely helpful.

5.4.5.2.5
Peri- and Postprocedural Care

The role of anaesthesia in interventional neuroradiology consists in providing patient comfort by analgesia and sedation, adequate monitoring, maintenance of vital functions and (if required) the management of systemic heparinization. The patient's underlying condition, the duration and the kind of intervention have to be considered to decide on the anaesthetic management (Luginbuhl and Remonda 1999).

Embolization of intracranial aneurysms is performed with the patient in general anaesthesia at most centres. Although such an approach does not allow intraprocedural evaluation of the patient's neurological status and carries additional risks associated with general anaesthesia and mechanical ventilation (Phuong et al. 2002) we clearly prefer it during all endovascular procedures occluding intracranial aneurysms.

A British group recently published that GDC occlusion of an intracranial aneurysm can be performed in a safe manner with the patient awake (Qureshi et al. 2001). However, if aneurysm rupture occurs during treatment it is quite difficult to continue embolization if the patient is under local anaesthesia alone.

In order to minimize thromboembolic complications we recommend the administration of heparin, which we routinely start in ruptured aneurysms after insertion of the first coil. In unruptured aneurysms heparinization is started after insertion of the femoral sheath. The value of the activated clotting time (ACT) should be between 250 and 300 s and this level should be maintained for about 24–48 h postprocedure. Every patient receives aspirin (100 mg/d) for at least 3 months. If the patient was in good condition before the treatment or had an unruptured aneurysm he should be extubated in the angiosuite. This is specifically important after treatment of MCA and basilar tip aneurysms: these are usually more difficult to treat and carry a higher risk of thrombotic complications.

After the procedure the patient should be supervised on an intensive care unit and must be monitored by an experienced neurovascular team in order to detect symptomatic vasospasms before occurrence of infarction. Monitoring (clinical status including transcranial Doppler sonography, heart rate, blood pressure, pO2, puncture site) should be done at least for 24 h in all patients with an unruptured aneurysms, in case of a recent bleeding monitoring is depending upon the clinical status and on the interval of the bleeding, but should at least continue for 7 days. The patient then could be transferred to a neurosurgical step-down unit, where continuous surveillance of vital parameters and a periodically examination by experienced nurses is performed.

No endovascular procedure should be performed without an appropriate follow-up imaging protocol. In our institution, every patient gets a MR scan (MRI and MRA: TOF and contrast enhanced technique) within 3 days after the procedure. In cases of satisfied occlusion rate (total or subtotal occlusion) the patient should be scheduled for a control DSA and MRA 6 months after the procedure. If there is a good correlation between DSA and MRA at this time point follow-up could be done solely with MRA. We try to get follow-up imaging for at least 3 years.

5.4.6 Devices for Endovascular Aneurysm Therapy

5.4.6.1 Catheters and Delivery Systems

Since 1960, when LUESSENHOPP et al. reported the first intravascular cerebral embolization of an AVM by injecting silastic beads into the arteries of the neck, endovascular treatment of brain diseases has been considerably refined. There has been improvement in fluoroscopic equipment, angiographic techniques and progressive miniaturization of endovascular devices to permit increasingly more distal, so to say "superselective", catheterization. The following section tries to give an overview of the different materials to be used in endovascular therapy of intracranial aneurysms. However, it is a subjective choice. We did not want to give a complete overview, this can be done by the companies. In addition, products change so fast that a book like this cannot be up-to-date. We simply picked a few examples and give some general comments. We were not paid by any company to either mention or not mention any particular products. In general, it depends on individual experiences what type of catheter, wire or coil you use. Having the latter in mind we decided to mention our first and second choice materials. A book is written by individuals and we do have individual opinions. Every reader, however, is welcome to comment on our recommendations.

5.4.6.1.1 Guiding catheters

Distal placement of the guiding catheter in the internal carotid or vertebral artery facilitates stable navigation of the microcatheter and subsequent coil placement. A soft tip with hydrophilic coating allows atraumatic distal catheterisation. A large inner lumen enables continuous flushing and road mapping or angiograms during the procedure without a second guiding catheter in place. Continuous flushing with heparinized saline through a hemostatic valve is essential to prevent retrograde flow and clotting.

In general, this is possible with 5- or 6-F guiding catheters, such as Envoy (Cordis), or FasGuide (Boston Scientific). In our institution, we prefer the Guider XF Soft Tip (Boston Scientific) because of its soft tip and the lower risk to damage the vessel wall.

5.4.6.1.2 Microcatheters

In general, there are two types of microcatheters available: wire-directed microcatheters of 0.010- to 0.016-in. calibre, and flow-guided microcatheters usually close to 0.010-in. Flow-guided microcatheters are mainly used for the treatment of AVMs to deliver liquid embolic agents or small particles. For endovascular aneurysm therapy wire-directed microcatheters are mandatory. Their hydrophilic coating facilitates distal catheterizations. Microcatheters for aneurysm therapy usually have two markers at the distal end to allow alignment of the detachment zone of coils regardless of the type of detachment.

We prefer to use a Tracker-Excel 14 (Boston Scientific) but a Tracker-18 and Tracker-10 are also suitable to treat aneurysms.

Steam shaping of the distal tip, individually formed according the neck, direction and size of the aneurysm to be catheterized might be helpful. Microcatheters already preshaped (Prowler; Cordis Corp.) are also available, but do not have a major advantage per se. Shaping of a microcatheter should be part of the training of all neurointerventionalists.

5.4.6.1.3 Microwires

The ideal microwire is flexible, soft, shapeable, with an atraumatic tip, easy to navigate, and has no or minimal friction. These qualities are difficult to combine in one device. Neurointerventional microwires are of 0.014–0.016 in. caliber. Most of the available microwires have a hydrophilic coating. In our institution, we prefer the Transend 0.014 (Boston Scientific) combining most of these qualities. The Terumo wire 0.016 and 0.010 are of excellent torqueability, but have a very stiff preformed tip, that can easily injure the vessel wall or rupture the aneurysm sac. Therefore, we do not use them for aneurysm therapy any more.

And – surprisingly enough – it is still possible to improve the quality of these simple wires. In those situations where we are really struggling with anatomy and do not get access to the aneurysm, we switch to a wire called Synchro; this wire has a marvellous one-to-one torque and usually we can overcome the problem.

For intracranial stenting long exchange microwires (>300 cm) may be helpful. They vary considerably in stiffness. Most of the wires from cardiology are too stiff and therefore can not be recommended for intracranial use. Softer wires, like the ACS High Torque Traverse (Guidant), or the ChoICE (Boston Scientific) are better, but they still have the potential to perforate distal vessels. Recently, the Transend became available with a length of 300 cm and is now the standard wire at our institution for intracranial stent procedures. However, we are convinced that even the delay between writing the manuscript and availability of the book will give the companies enough time to further improve their products.

5.4.7 Embolic Materials for Endovascular Aneurysm Therapy

In general, there are four different types of embolic materials available: balloons, particles, coils and liquids.

5.4.7.1 Detachable Balloons

Detachable balloons, initially developed by Serbinenko for the selective treatment of aneurysms, now are mainly used for major vessel occlusion, such as the internal carotid or vertebral artery. The balloon is mounted at the distal end of a microcatheter, then navigated in the targeted position and after filling with contrast material or a solidifying agent it is detached from the microcatheter. Balloons are available with self-sealing valves ensuring that the balloon remains inflated when the microcatheter is withdrawn. There are two types of balloons available: latex balloons and silicone balloons.

Latex balloons: While latex is an essentially impermeable membrane, silicone is semipermeable. They have a tendency to undergo spontaneous deflation within days or weeks.

Silicone balloons: These have to be inflated with isomolar solutions. Silicone balloons have a higher expansion coefficient and are softer and less rigid than latex balloons. Under normal circumstances they do not deflate, unlike latex balloons, and do not induce a surrounding inflammatory reaction in adjacent tissue. Silicone balloons have a propensity for forward movement. Unfortunately, the so-called detachable silicone balloons (DSB) are not available any more. At this time it seems to be unlikely that they will be back on the market soon.

5.4.7.2 Nondetachable Balloons

Various nondetachable balloons are available for temporary vessel occlusion, angioplasty for vasospasm therapy or remodelling techniques for broad based aneurysms. Larger vessels like the carotid or vertebral artery can be occluded with a double lumen balloon catheter, i.e. Meditech (Cook). For intracranial angioplasty smaller, more flexible balloons, like the wire-directed Equinox (MTI) and Hyperglide (MTI), Commodore (Cordis), or Sentry (Boston Scientific), or the non-wire-directed Endaevor (Boston Scientific) are required. Additionally to these balloons the Hyperform (MTI) can be used for the remodelling technique.

5.4.7.3 Coils

There is a great variety of different coils currently available. Stainless steel coils have been used for a long time for peripheral embolizations. Due to an attached Dacron fibre they are extremely thrombogenic, facilitating even parent vessel occlusion. They might be increasingly used for this indication, if detachable balloons are really not available any more. However, for cerebral embolizations they are too stiff. Platinum coils are much softer than stainless steel coils. Meanwhile, there exist different types of CE marked detachable platinum coils provided from different companies. All of those are retrievable and are similar in the compound of the alloy, but they mainly differ in their technique to detach. The newest generation of coils have a coated surface in order to facilitate endothelial growth and real healing of the aneurysm entrance.

Over the last several years, the number of coil sizes has been increased, multidimensional coils have become available, and, more recently, softer coils allowing safer initial coil placement have been introduced.

They are available in different shapes, lengths and diameter for neurointerventional procedures.

5.4.7.4 Electrolytically Detachable Coils

Guglielmi et al. (1991a,b) developed electrolytically detachable platinum coils (GDC) for endovascular occlusion of aneurysms. The coil is attached to a stainless steel delivery wire. This allows repositioning and selective placement of the coil within the aneurysm. The coil can be delivered through a microcatheter and is detached electrolytically by applying a 9V positive electric current to the patient. The current dissolves the non-insulated stainless steel junction located between the GDC and the insulated delivery wire. Using the new generation GDC detachment takes about 20–30 s. GDC has to be delivered through special microcatheters, which have a radiopaque marker located 3 cm from the distal tip of the microcatheter. For detachment of the GDC the radiopaque marker of the delivery wire of the coil has to be aligned to the proximal marker of the microcatheter. The GDC design combines the advantage of very soft, compliant platinum and retrievability resulting in markedly improved safety and efficacy. An improperly fitting coil can be removed, repositioned or replaced with another coil of different size, length or shape. There are several sizes of GDCs, ranging from 2–20 mm in coil diameter and 2–30 cm in length to fit the needs

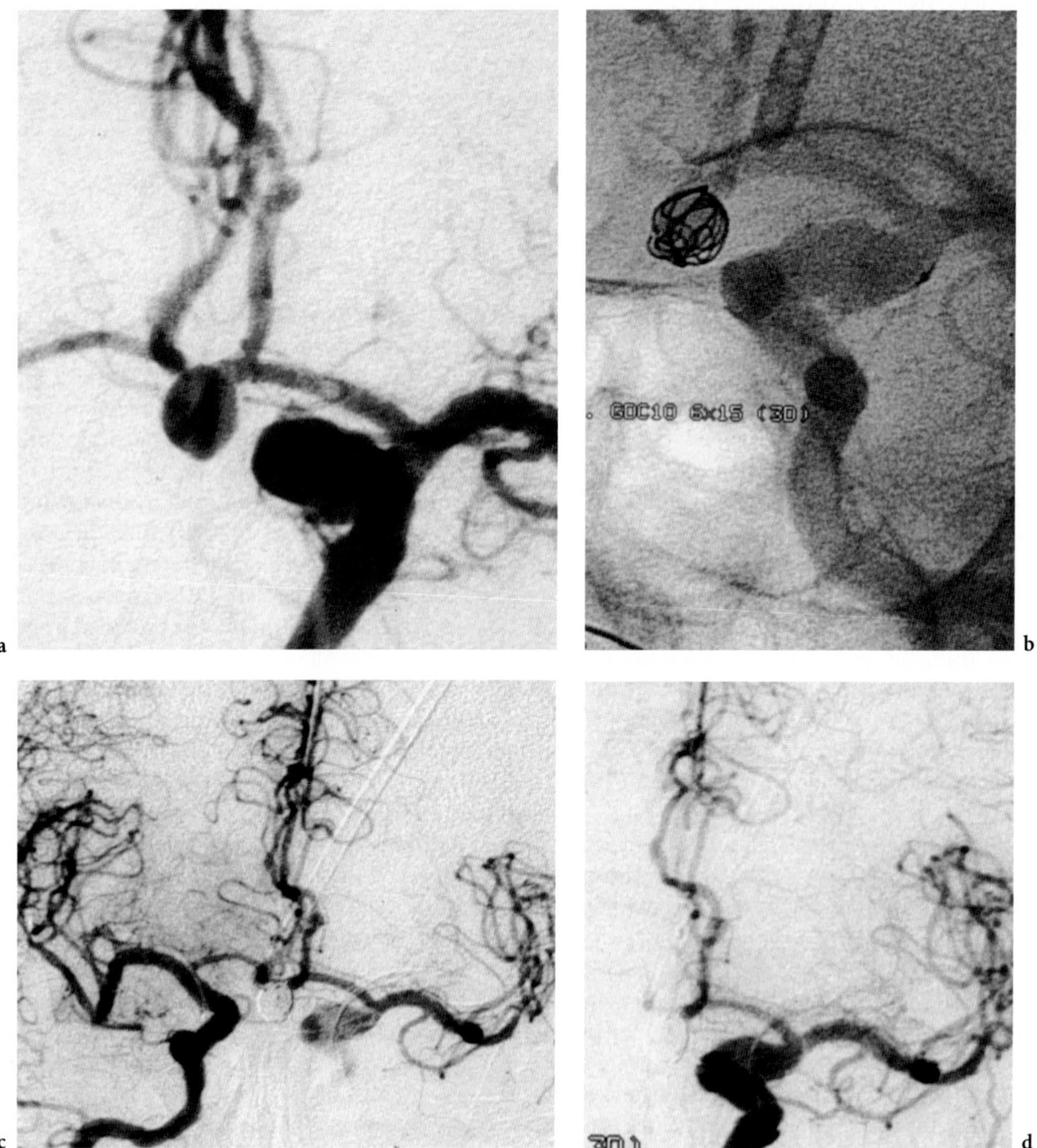

Fig. 5.4.8a–d. Acom aneurysm: angiogram before endovascular therapy, after placement of the first GDC (GDC 10: 6×15 3D) and after complete coil occlusion

of embolizing different aneurysms. GDCs exist in two thicknesses, 0.010 rather for small and acutely ruptured aneurysms and 0.015 for large and giant aneurysms.

Recently, many new designs in coil configuration, shape, and material have become available by numerous vendors and have significantly increased the versatility of this device for aneurysm therapy. Bi-dimensional GDC (2D GDC), in which the first 1.5 coil loop is of 75% smaller helical diameter, helps the following loops to stay within the aneurysm and avoids protruding into the parent artery. A three dimensional (3D)-shape GDC configuration has been developed in which the secondary structure consists of a series of omega-like loops. Due to its spherical shaped memory this 3D coil spontaneously forms a complex cage after deployment thereby serving as basket for subsequent coils. To be honest, we very rarely use this 3D type of coil. In the vast majority of patients, conventional 2D coils allow a complete and dense packing of an aneurysms. But again, this is our personal view and experience.

5.4.7.5 Hydrogel-Coils

Hydrogel-coils (MicroVention, Inc., Aliso Viejo, CA) consist of a carrier platinum coil coupled to an expandable hydrogel material, which undergoes a tremendous increase in volume when placed into a physiological environment with a certain pH value, e.g. blood. Compared to a non coated platinum coil 10, a fully expanded hydrogel coil 14 of the same length will have seven times the volume. The hydrogel coils were designed to offer an enhanced ability to fill aneurysm cavities. Distinct from previous devices aimed at speeding the organization of thrombus, the new device has been designed to entirely fill the aneurysm cavity, with complete or near-complete exclusion of thrombus. Unlike thrombus, the hydrogel material is stable and unaffected by natural thrombolytic processes and thus may reduce observed rates of aneurysm recanalization (Kallmes and Fujiwara 2002). In our own small series aneurysm treatment with hydrogel coils was extremely promising. Complication rate was not higher than usual, but so far no published data exist in patients treated with hydrogel coils. Long-term observations need to reveal if there is a real benefit over bare platinum coils. Additionally, the detachment mechanism is different; it is not based on electrolysis, but mainly on hydraulic forces.

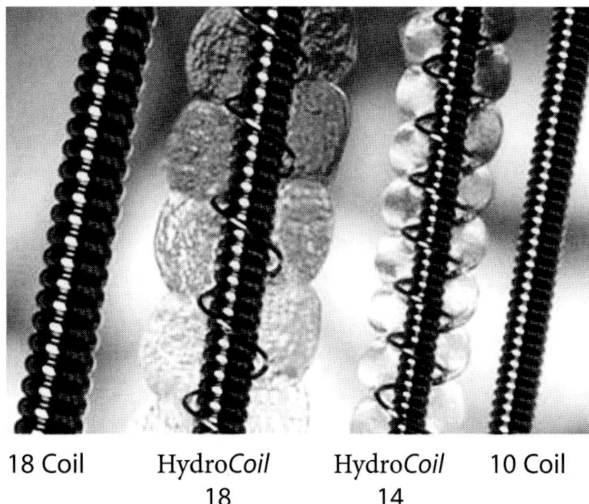

Fig. 5.4.9. Different size of Hydrogel-coated coils in comparison with bare coils

5.4.7.6 Three-Dimensional Coils: TriSpan

To support coil deposition of wide-necked aneurysms a new detachable device, the TriSpan (Boston Scientific, Fremont, USA) was designed and recently approved for clinical use in Europe. The TriSpan can be placed at the base of the aneurysm prior to coil embolization which is delivered through a second microcatheter. The TriSpan acts as a supporting structure and bridges the neck for subsequent coils. However, experience with this new device is limited mainly to broad-based basilar tip aneurysms. Further evaluation and especially long-term results are necessary to assess this new method.

5.4.7.7 Other Devices

Stretch-resistant (SR) coils have a polypropylene thread through the primary helix, associated with greater strength of the coil. It provides more safety against damage if it needs to be withdrawn from the aneurysm. We strongly recommend using the stretch-resistant-type coils whenever possible or available. This technology really helps to protect patients and reduces the stress factor for the interventionalist.

Recently there has been growing interest in modifying platinum coils by coating the surface with extracellular matrix proteins, non-biodegradable polymers, fibroblasts, and vascular endothelial growth factors. Experimental studies indicate that these modifications might promote endothelializa-

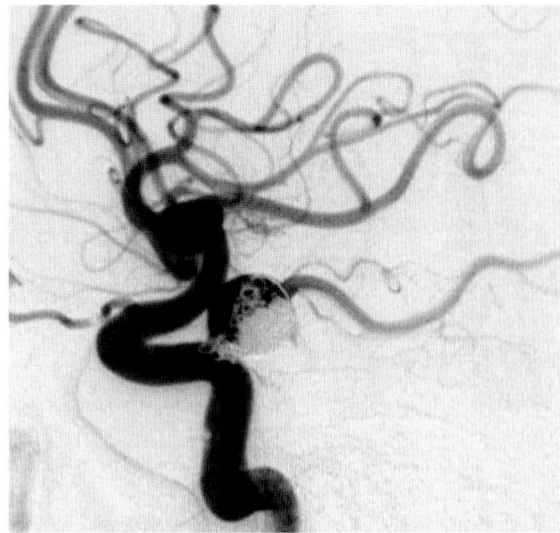
a

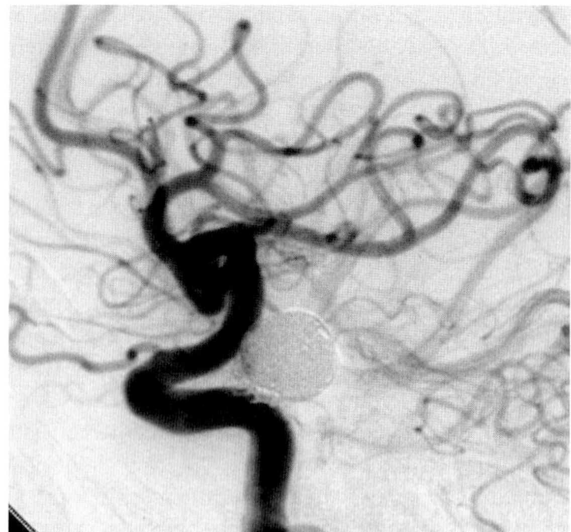
b

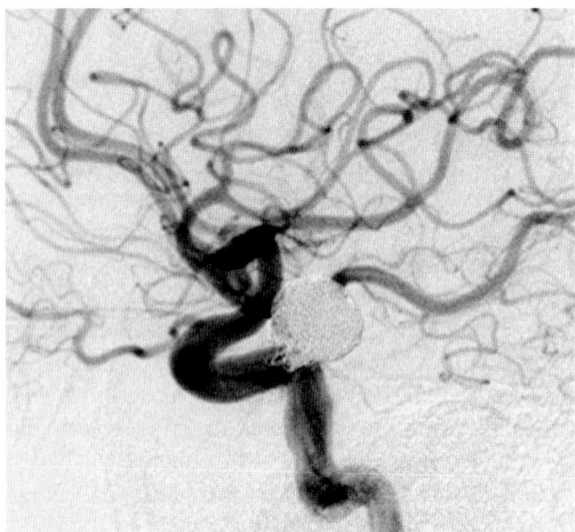
c

Fig. 5.4.10a–c. A 39-year-old male, SAH 2 years previously, second recurrent aneurysm after embolization with bare coils (**a**) after hydrogel-coil-embolization (**b**), and 6-month FU with a stable result (**c**)

tion, clot organization, and tissue integration of the coils and thereby may lead to improved aneurysm occlusion and outcome (Abrahams et al. 2000, 2001a,b; Dawson et al. 1995; Kallmes et al. 1998; Murayama et al. 1997, 2001).

5.4.7.8
Stents

The idea of using an intravascular stent followed by trans-stent placement of coils may provide another treatment option in patients with a wide-necked aneurysm in which direct surgical clipping or conventional endovascular therapy would be difficult or impossible, and in whom parent artery occlusion is not a viable option (Byrne et al. 2000; Lanzino 1999b; Horowitz et al. 2001; Lownie et al. 2000; Lylyk et al. 2001).

Stents are deployed either by balloon expansion or release of a self-expanding nitinol or steel stent from a constraining sheath. Up to now stents used for intracranial treatment, usually coronary stents (covering size ranges up to 4 mm), are balloon expandable stents bearing the risk of damaging a dysplastic aneurysm bearing segment of the artery with eventual rupture of the vessel. In addition, the large profile and relative stiffness of these stent delivery systems limit the locations that are able to be accessed and increase the risk of vessel dissection.

In summary, the balloon expandable stents were not a real treatment option. Complication rates were too high and in the majority of patients it was impossible to obtain access to the intracranial target vessel.

5.4.7.9
Neurovascular Stent

The Neuroform Stent (Boston Scientific, USA) is a new self-expanding microstent system designed specifically for intracranial vessels. It consists of three parts: the self expanding microstent, which is supplied in a 3-F delivery microcatheter, and a 2-F stabilizer. The stent comes preloaded in a 3-F delivery catheter and is currently available in diameters from 3.0 to 4.5 mm, in 0.5-mm increments, and in lengths of 15 mm and 20 mm. In our experience in a still limited number of cases the stent revealed an excellent tractability and could be easily navigated even through very tortuous vessels. We did not observe permanent parent artery occlusion nor occlusion of perforating arteries which were covered by the stent (Wanke et al. 2003). In our experience with nearly 30 implanted stents of this type the self-expandable Neuroform is an enormous improvement in treating formerly endovascularly untreatable aneurysms. Many broad-based aneurysms – most of them surgical candidates up to now – can be treated with this device.

Future developments, such as covered or coated stents lining the neck of the aneurysm would effectively exclude the aneurysm from the circulation and might theoretically present a perfect cure for selected aneurysms.

5.4.7.10
Liquid Embolic Agents

Liquid materials are commonly used for endovascular treatment of AVMs. Cyanoacrylate, the most common currently used liquid embolic material in brain AVMs, polymerises after contact with blood and becomes solid (Eskridge 1989). The use of liquid embolics for endovascular occlusion of cerebral aneurysms is still limited to a small group of patients and there is only limited experience with that technique (Macdonald et al. 1998; Tokunaga et al. 1998). An important issue of this technique is the difficulty to prevent migration of the liquid adhesive into the parent artery.

New liquid embolic agents, such as Onyx (MTI, Irvine, CA), are used in combination with protective devices, such as balloons, and/or stents. But so far we are convinced that liquids are only justified in those aneurysms than cannot be treated with any other methods because of the higher complication rate.

Onyx (MTI, Irvine, CA) is a biocompatible polymer (ethylene-vinyl alcohol copolymer, EVOH) dissolved in its organic solvent dimethyl sulfoxide (DMSO). To obtain an appropriate radiopacity micronized tantalum powder is added. When this mixture contacts a liquid agent such as blood, DMSO rapidly diffuses away from the mixture, causing in situ precipitation and solidification of the polymer. The use of Onyx and DMSO requires dedicated microcatheters to prevent material incompatibility between the solvent and the hub plastics. In their experimental study, Murayama et al. (2000) demonstrated the technical feasibility of endovascular therapy using this liquid agent and different protective devices in porcine side-wall aneurysms. Currently, mainly large or giant ICA aneurysms are treated with this technique because this approach usually allows selective occlusion of the aneurysm with preservation of the parent artery. However, clinical studies are necessary before this technique becomes clinical routine.

5.4.8
Techniques of Endovascular Therapy

Neurointerventional methods concerning aneurysm treatment are broadly classified as deconstructive or reconstructive procedures. We therefore distinguish two strategies to treat cerebral aneurysms via the endovascular approach: first, occlusion of the aneurysmal sac with embolic material preserving the parent artery, and second in otherwise untreatable aneurysms occlusion of the parent artery in order to exclude the aneurysm from the blood circulation.

Endovascular therapy for intracranial aneurysms has evolved since Serbinenko pioneered embolization of the parent artery with latex balloons in the 1970s (Serbinenko 1974a,b). Occlusion of the parent artery has become a therapeutic alternative especially in patients with giant broad-based aneurysms of the internal carotid artery which are surgically inaccessible. The basic assumption for this treatment modality is that the patient will tolerate parent vessel occlusion without ischemic complications. Although there is no general consensus about the protocol to predict patient's tolerance to permanent vessel occlusion, some authors recommend blood flow studies to decide which patient will tolerate acute balloon occlusion and who will need an extracranial-intracranial (EC-IC) bypass to avoid ischemic complications (Brunberg et al. 1994; Eckard et al. 1992; Fox et al. 1986; Linskey et al. 1994; Standard et al. 1995; Yonas et al. 1992). Complex scenarios include balloon test occlusion with SEP monitoring, SPECT imaging before, during and after test occlusion, and different degrees of hypotension during test occlusion. In our experience, a pretty simple test has a high predictive value: the compression test with injection into the contralateral ICA while the symptomatic ICA gets compressed. If the veins of the compressed side opacify not more than 1 s later than those of the injected site, anatomical preconditions for ICA occlusion are excellent. More important than the "development" of numerous test or pre-test procedures is

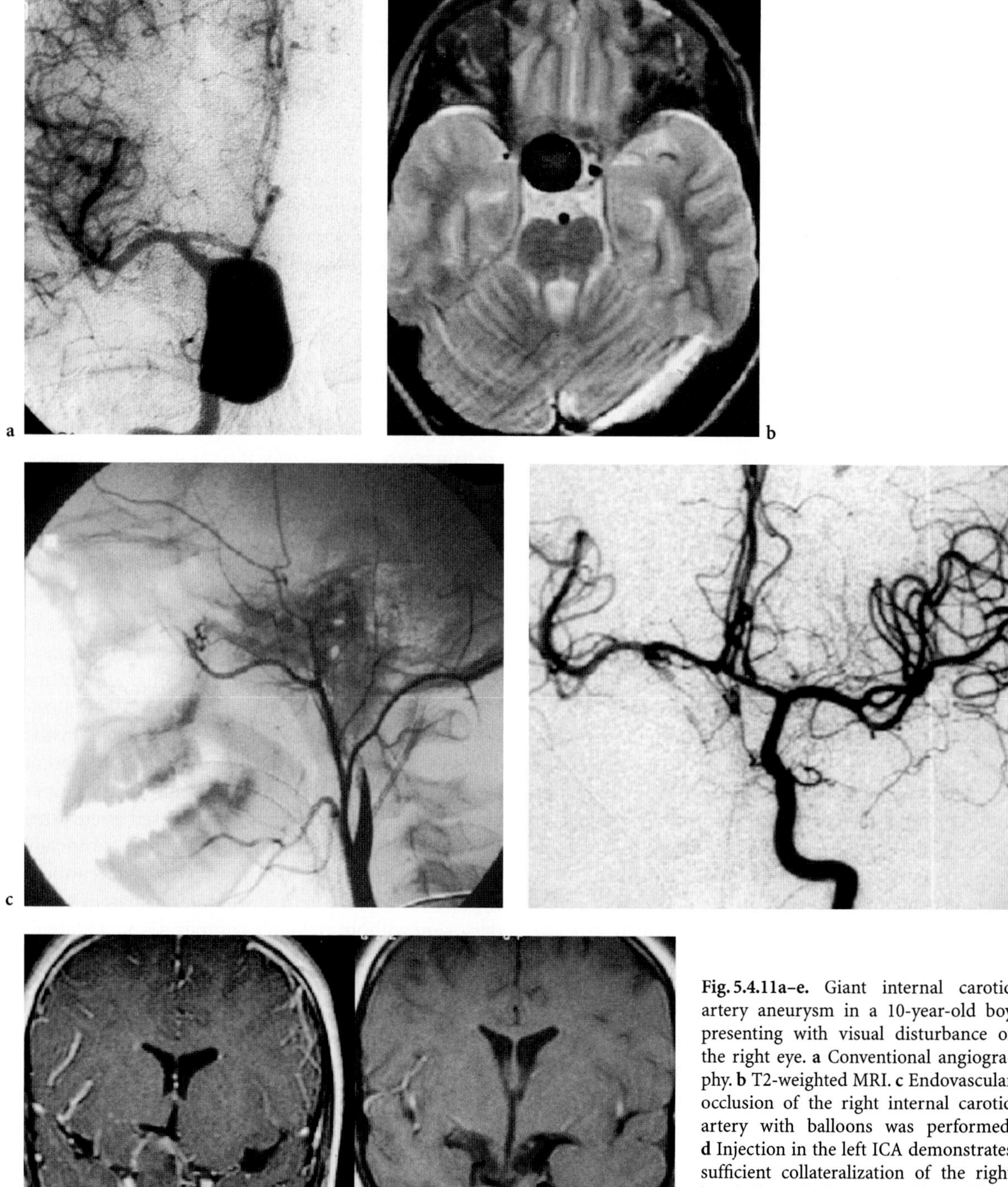

Fig. 5.4.11a–e. Giant internal carotid artery aneurysm in a 10-year-old boy presenting with visual disturbance of the right eye. **a** Conventional angiography. **b** T2-weighted MRI. **c** Endovascular occlusion of the right internal carotid artery with balloons was performed. **d** Injection in the left ICA demonstrates sufficient collateralization of the right hemisphere via the Acom. **e** T1-weighted MRI, coronal plane: before therapy and at 6-month follow-up demonstrating complete retraction of the aneurysm

probably how to take care for the patient after the procedure. Our strategy is to keep the patient recumbent and elevate his head by 30°/day. Blood pressure should be a little bit above the normal level. After the third day the patient is allowed to sit on the bed, on day 4 he can walk with assistance. In case of any problems during the first walk around, the period of laying down should be prolonged.

In experienced hands occlusion of the parent artery has proved to be safe, convenient and effective. Vessel occlusion could be done either with a detachable balloon or detachable coils positioned proximal to the aneurysm. Some authors recommend lesion trapping in order to prevent retrograde filling of the aneurysm (Berenstein et al. 1984; Debrun et al. 1981; Fox et al. 1987; Hieshima et al. 1981; Higashida et al. 1989, 1991; Kupersmith et al. 1984; Larson et al. 1995; Nelson 1998; Pasqualin et al. 1988; Serbinenko 1974a,b; Tan et al. 1986; van Rooij et al. 2000).

In order to reconstruct an aneurysm bearing vessel there exist different techniques nowadays. In the past aneurysmal sac occlusion with a detachable balloon was performed but this is now clearly obsolete. Although it is technically feasible there is no detachable balloon with different configurations which could be navigated over a microwire in order to access the aneurysm lumen in an arbitrarily manner. In addition, the relative high risk of complications – mainly due to thromboembolic events as well as aneurysm rupture during or after the procedure - with a high procedure-related mortality (reported up to 18%) as well as the fact that the balloon would not keep its configuration over time necessitated a more sophisticated endovascular technique for aneurysm embolization (Debrun et al. 1981; Higashida et al. 1989, 1990, 1991).

In the last 10 years, improvement in the development of flexible microcatheters which can navigate through cerebral vessels to lesions deep within the brain has allowed the treatment of an increasing range of intracranial aneurysms. The focus of modern endovascular therapy has shifted to the use of detachable platinum coils. In 1991, the first detachable platinum coil was introduced for treatment of cerebral aneurysms – the so-called Guglielmi detachable coil (GDC) developed by Target Therapeutics, CA, USA. Through a guiding catheter (e.g. 5 F, 6 F) a microcathether (2.3 F) is coaxially advanced into the cerebral vasculature and over a soft microwire it can be navigated into the aneurysm lumen, optimal placed in the aneurysm centre in a stable position. To ease the access into the aneurysm the microcatheter can be preshaped over steam but is also available in a preshaped configuration with different angles. Therefore, it is very important that neither the catheter nor the wire will contact the aneurysm wall too strongly in order to avoid aneurysm rupture. The interventionalist should be always aware of possible movements of the catheter while manipulating with the wire or with the coil. After gently and slowly removing the microwire the first platinum coil is delivered through the microcatheter. Pioneering in the development was that these coils are retrievable until the operator is satisfied with placement and then could be detached. The diameter of the first coil should be chosen according to the aneurysm diameter. The size of the following coils is usually the same of the first coil or smaller to densely pack the centre of the aneurysm. Introduction of coils should be continued until no more coils can be deployed into the aneurysm. The idea of this treatment is to fill the aneurysmal sack with coils and thrombus in order to exclude it from the blood circulation and thereby prevent bleeding. This technology is based on electrothrombosis and electrolytic detachment of platinum coils. Despite the extensive use of this treatment technique, the role of electrothrombosis has not been fully investigated and clarified. It is believed that the passage of electric current through the GDC induces attraction of blood constituents. This attraction may trigger a thrombotic reaction on the surface of the coil. The greater the time of current application, the more pronounced the cellular reaction and deposition of fibrin and blood cells on the surface of the GDC (Padolecchia et al. 2001).

Endosaccular embolization with platinum coils is performed in unruptured aneurysms and in patients acutely ill after subarachnoid haemorrhage. Usually and specifically in patients in the acute stage of bleeding endovascular embolization is done under general anaesthesia (GA). We recommend intubating all patients because in the case of a complication, e.g. aneurysm perforation, the patient‘s status could deteriorate suddenly and dramatically.

A standard transfemoral approach is used like in diagnostic angiography. Endovascular embolization of cerebral aneurysms could be done without GA (Qureshi et al. 2001). But in order to better manage procedure-related complications such as aneurysm perforation we recommended local anaesthesia only for those patients who clearly have an increased risk with GA.

Although there are several advantages of coil embolization over surgery, there is a disadvantage of endovascular treatment. Due to coil compaction and residual inflow in initially incompletely obliterated aneurysms there is a potential risk of recanalization with aneurysmal regrowth. In particular, the geometry of wide-necked aneurysms is less favourable for obtaining maximal coil packing (Tong et al. 2000). In cases of an unfavourable dome to neck ratio endovascular treatment can be feasible and sometimes more effective by simultaneous temporary balloon protection. Hereby, a microcatheter-mounted nondetachable balloon provides a temporary barrier across the aneurysmal neck while introducing the coils into the aneurysmal sac. Reports in the literature have offered discussions of the feasibility, efficacy, and safety of balloon-assisted coil placement in wide-necked intracranial aneurysms which was first described by J. Moret in 1997 as the "remodelling technique". The use of simultaneous temporary balloon protection may allow more dense intra-aneurysmal coil packing, especially at the neck, without parent artery compromise than did the use of Guglielmi detachable coils alone (Aletich et al. 2000; Malek et al. 2000; Mericle et al. 1997; Moret et al. 1997; Nelson and Levy 2001). Despite enormous advances in the development of flexible microcatheters, coil configurations, and embolic materials and use of remodelling technique, wide-necked aneurysms still remain a therapeutic challenge. The geometry of wide neck aneurysms sometimes makes it impossible to treat the aneurysm via the endovascular route or at least reduces the possibility of obtaining satisfactory coil packing. However, incomplete occlusion carries the risk of aneurysm recanalization, regrowth and rerupture (Byrne et al. 1999; Cognard et al. 1999). With the recent development and refinement of endovascular stents, the significant potential for these devices in the treatment of wide-necked and fusiform aneurysms has become apparent.

The technique of using an intravascular stent to create a bridging scaffold followed by endovascular placement of coils through the interstices of the stent into a wide-necked or fusiform aneurysm has been described in experimental studies (Byrne et al. 2000; Massoud et al. 1995; Szikora et al. 1994) and in humans (Higashida et al. 1997; Horowitz et al. 2001; Lanzino et al. 1999; Lownie et al. 2000; Lylyk et al. 1998, 2001; Mericle et al. 1998; Sekhon et al. 1998; Weber et al. 2000). It may provide another treatment option for patients who present with a wide-necked aneurysm in which direct surgical clipping or conventional endovascular therapy would be difficult or impossible, and in whom parent artery occlusion is not a viable option. As described before, new flexible and self expanding stents are available now and create the next shift from surgery towards endovascular therapy.

5.4.9 Anatomic Considerations for Endovascular Aneurysm Therapy

Usually, there is not only one way to treat an aneurysm. The right treatment depends on the skill and experience of the team and may differ from our recommendations. We mainly report *our* way of treating different aneurysms, but do not think that it can not be done in another way.

5.4.9.1 Internal Carotid Artery

Aneurysms of the internal carotid artery account for about 30%–40% of all intracranial aneurysms. Therefore, the ICA is the most frequent aneurysm bearing artery. In descending frequency ICA aneurysms do occur at the following sites: posterior communicating artery (52%), termination of ICA (20%), paraophthalmic segment (13%), cavernous ICA (10%), anterior choroidal artery (5%).

Due to the surgical inaccessibility the endovascular approach is the therapeutic modality of choice in proximal symptomatic aneurysms. Carotid artery occlusion is usually the therapeutic modality of choice in giant symptomatic wide-necked ICA aneurysms. This leads to subsequent thrombosis and regression of the aneurysmal sac. Ideally, ICA occlusion is performed distal and proximal to the aneurysm origin in order to prevent retrograde filling of the ICA with subsequent filling of the aneurysm (see section parent artery occlusion). However, the proximal *and* distal occlusion is more important in patients with CCF. If the passage of the aneurysm is not possible – due to elongation of the ICA itself or the giant nature of the aneurysm – proximal occlusion is usually enough and should be performed.

5.4.9.1.1 Cavernous ICA/Paraclinoid/Paraophthalmic

Aneurysms related to the carotid artery in the region of the anterior clinoid process, the so-called "paraclinoid" aneurysms are often in association with the ophthalmic artery. They may originate in the cavernous sinus and extend into the subarachnoid space, carrying the risk of subarachnoid hemorrhage, even if the origin of the aneurysm is clearly extradural.

Frequently presenting symptoms of aneurysms located within or around the cavernous sinus and the paraophthalmic region are visual deficits or cranial nerve palsies since the cavernous sinus harbours cranial

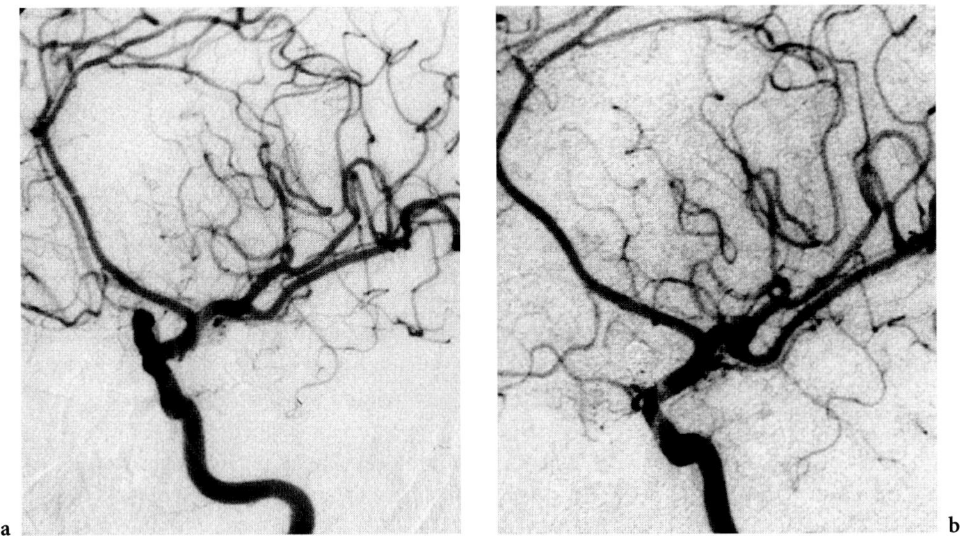

Fig. 5.4.12a,b. Before and after GDC treatment of a paraophthalmic ICA aneurysm

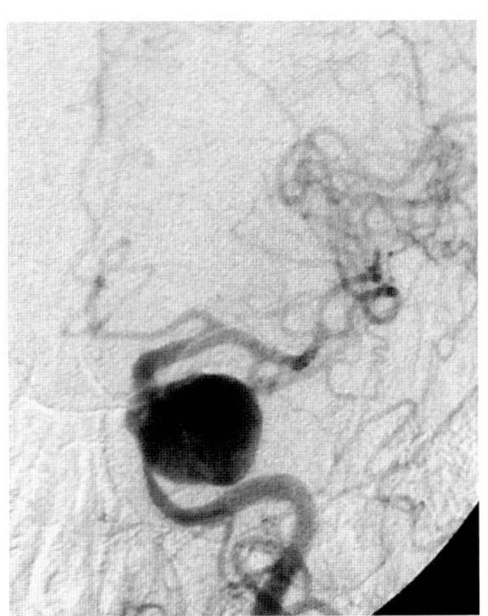

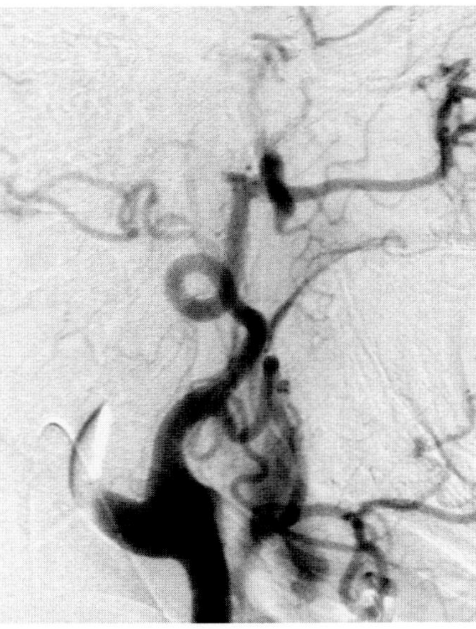

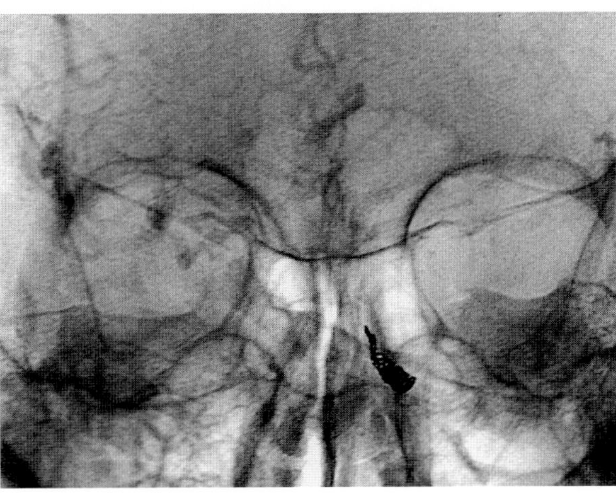

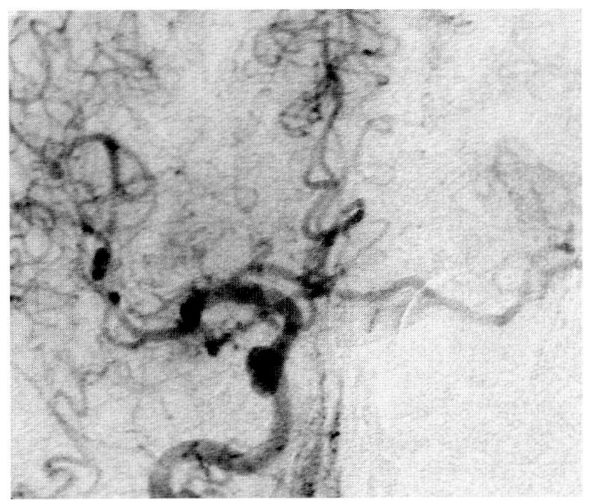

Fig. 5.4.13. a Cavernous ICA aneurysm. **b, c** After balloon test occlusion the parent artery was occluded with platinum coils. **d** Although cross filling via the Acom is flimsy the patient had no neurologic deficit after the intervention

nerves III, IV, V, and VI. Retroorbital pain due to venous congestion and visual field limitations due to compression of the optic nerve or chiasm may also occur. If aneurysms of the intracavernous portion of the carotid artery rupture they cause a carotid-cavernous fistula rather than bleeding into the subarachnoid space.

Sufficient radiologic evaluation with delineation of the extent and location of the aneurysm in relation to the subarachnoid space is extremely important to decide whether or not to treat an aneurysm in this location. For surgical planning it is important to visualize the relationship of the aneurysm to the anterior clinoid process which can be best achieved by CT angiography.

In general, treatment of this entity is controversial. Since the mortality rate from untreated cavernous aneurysms is low, treatment in asymptomatic patients should be reserved for those aneurysms extending into the subarachnoid space, because this is associated with a risk of subarachnoid hemorrhage, and those who demonstrate aneurysm enlargement (Linskey et al. 1990). Treatment in symptomatic patients should be reserved for those with progressive ophthalmoplegia or visual loss, ipsilateral facial or orbital pain, epistaxis or SAH. Treatment of these symptomatic aneurysms is aimed to eliminate mass effect and to cure symptoms. Eliminating the aneurysm also protects the patient from risk of subarachnoid hemorrhage. Treatment of choice is the endovascular approach since surgery is accompanied by significant morbidity and mortality, and those aneurysms involving the cavernous sinus are usually regarded as not surgically accessible.

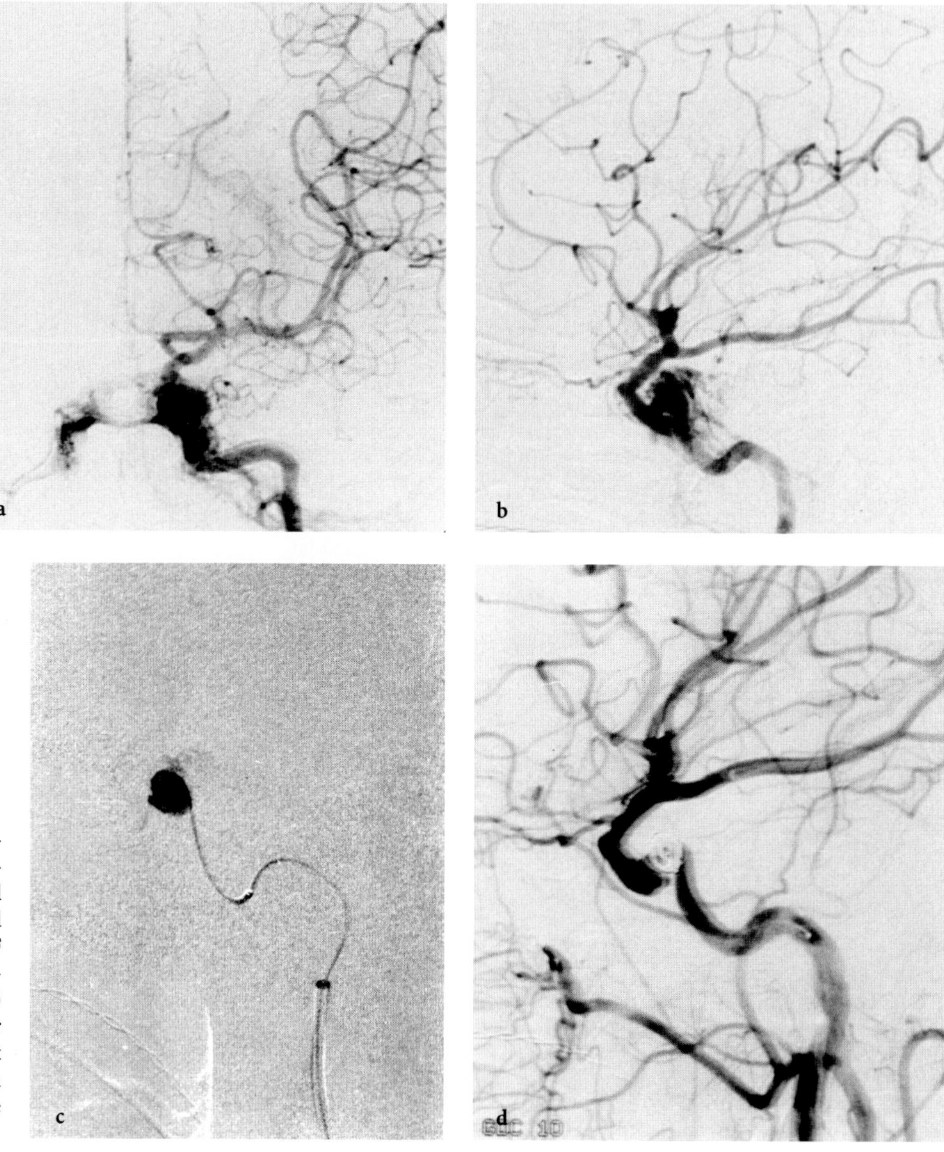

Fig. 5.4.14. a, b Conventional angiography, ap and lateral view, of the internal carotid artery: CCF due to a ruptured cavernous aneurysm (**c**) before and (**d**) after selective treatment of the aneurysm in a patient with acute ophthalmoplegia

Fig. 5.4.15a–d. Giant partially thrombosed paraophthalmic ICA aneurysm with some calcification at the ventral rim

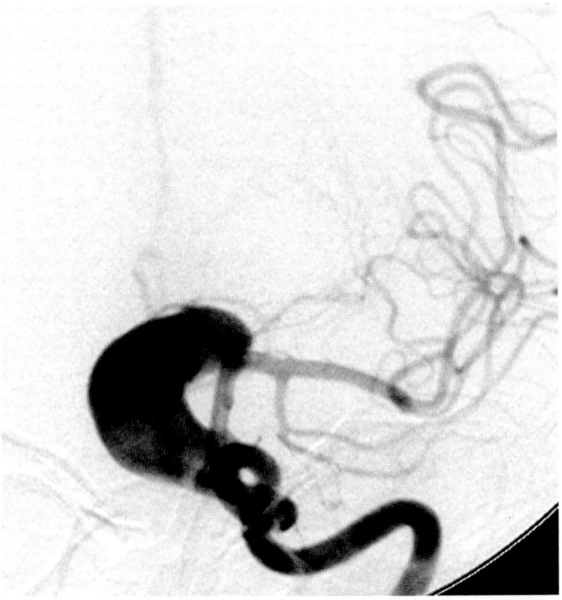

With endovascular treatment rapidly undergoing major developments, the treatment of carotid artery aneurysms have improved significantly in recent years. The primary aim is selective occlusion of the aneurysm with preservation of the parent artery. However, many aneurysms located at the paraophthalmic region have an unfavourable aneurysm geometry with a wide neck. Additionally, they may be large, partially thrombosed or calcified.

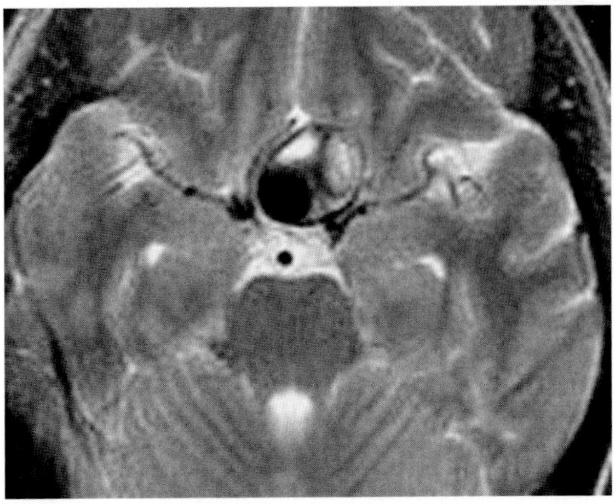

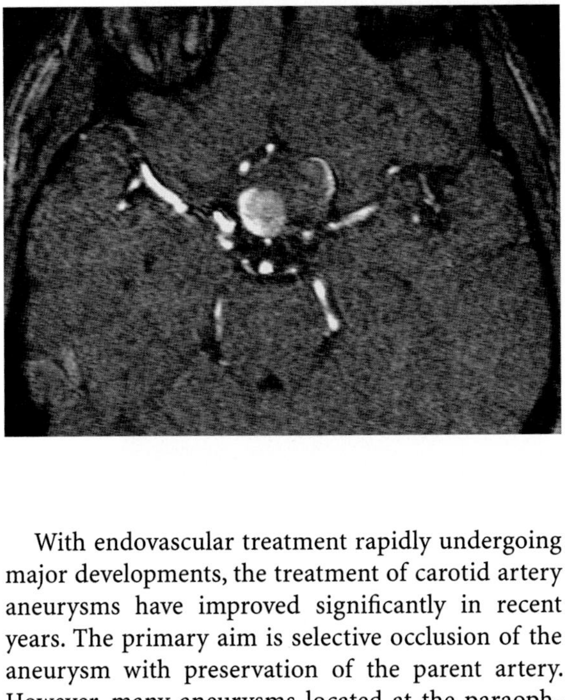

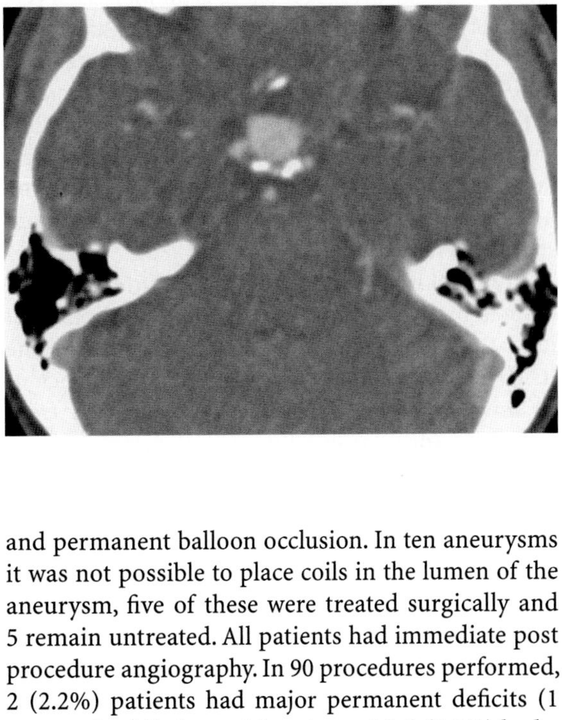

Thornton et al. reviewed 66 patients with 71 ruptured and unruptured paraclinoid aneurysms (distal to the cavernous segment of the internal carotid artery and proximal to the posterior communicating artery) treated by an endovascular approach. GDC coiling was performed in 78 aneurysms (including 45 with the remodelling technique), permanent balloon occlusion in 9, and 3 had both GDC coiling and permanent balloon occlusion. In ten aneurysms it was not possible to place coils in the lumen of the aneurysm, five of these were treated surgically and 5 remain untreated. All patients had immediate post procedure angiography. In 90 procedures performed, 2 (2.2%) patients had major permanent deficits (1 monocular blindness, 1 hemiparesis), 1 (1.1%) had a minor visual field deficit, and 2 (2.2%) patients died from major embolic events. Follow up 6 months after treatment showed more than 95% occlusion in 52/61 (85.2%) and less than 95% occlusion in 9/61 (14.8%). The authors concluded that properly selected paraclinoid aneurysms can be successfully treated by endovascular technology with a morbidity and mortality rate equal to or better than the published surgical series of similar aneurysms (Thornton et al. 2000a).

Despite these advances, occlusion of the parent artery is sometimes necessary because of the wide aneurysm neck. Balloon occlusion of the ICA is a reliable treatment for intracavernous giant aneurysms. In a series of 58 patients, Larson et al. (1995) reported a morbidity rate of 10% caused by transient cerebral ischemia, a permanent ischemic morbidity rate of 5%, and mortality rate of 5%. The authors reported a good resolution of cranial nerve deficits and visual impairment. For preocclusion work-up prior definite occlusion of the carotid artery balloon test occlusion should be performed to assess if occlusion is tolerated. In a series of 500 temporary balloon occlusions of the ICA, Mathis et al. (1995) described a complication rate of 1.6% asymptomatic, and 1.2% transient and 0.4% permanent ischemic complications. During temporary balloon occlusion, it is of crucial importance to evaluate cross-filling from the other side and simultaneous venous drainage. There is an increased risk for delayed ipsilateral ischemic deficits after ICA occlusion for treatment of aneurysms (Larson et al. 1995; Linskey et al. 1994). Ischemia associated with ICA occlusion may be secondary to thromboembolic events rather than decreased blood flow in the ICA distribution. In our opinion, prolonged heparinization for 72 h starting during treatment should therefore be performed.

Proximal ICA occlusion alone will cure the aneurysm in most cases, except those that have collateral inflow from cavernous or petrous branches of the ICA keeping the aneurysm open. The incidence of de novo aneurysm formation was reported from 1.4%–4% after carotid ligation. A direct relation between hemodynamic stress and the development of aneurysms at the anterior communicating artery has been suggested by several authors (Timperman et al. 1995). Therefore, a close long term follow-up, preferentially using non-invasive MRA to detect a possible development of an aneurysm at the Acom region should be done in these patients. In patients with bilateral aneurysms of the internal carotid artery, carotid occlusion on one side should be performed with caution since this might stress the contralateral aneurysm leading to potentially catastrophic results.

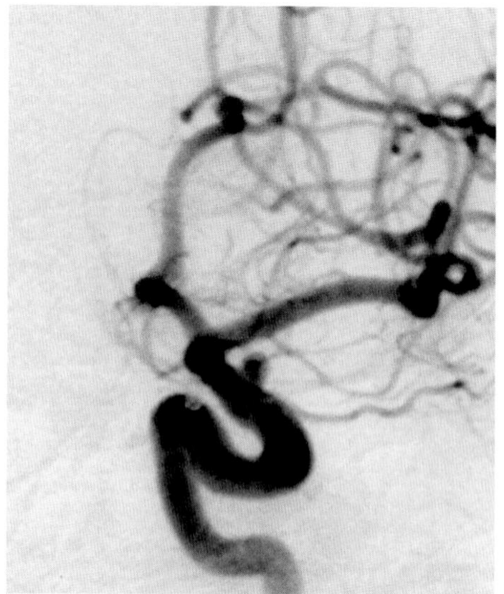

a

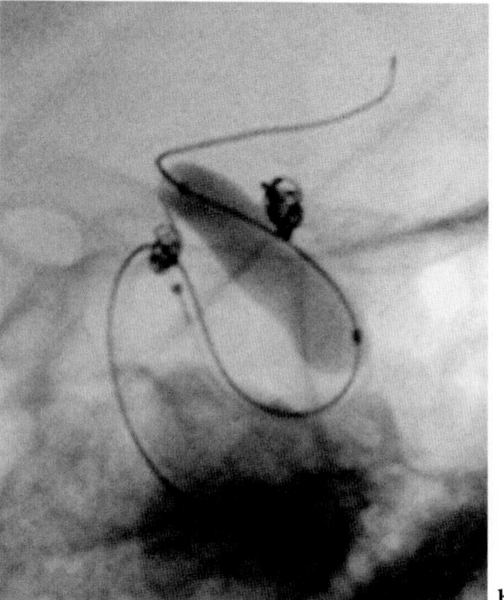

b

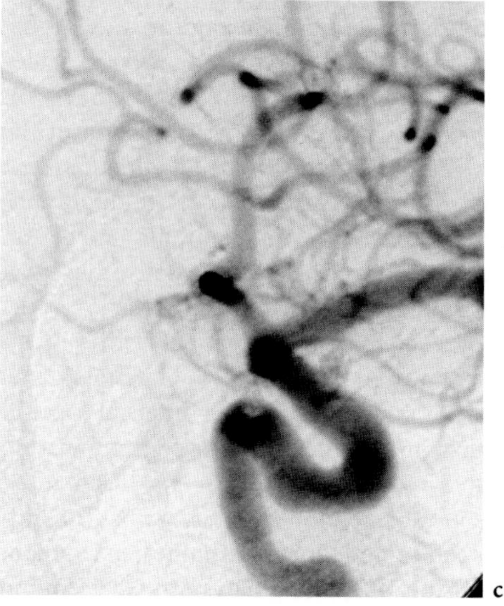

c

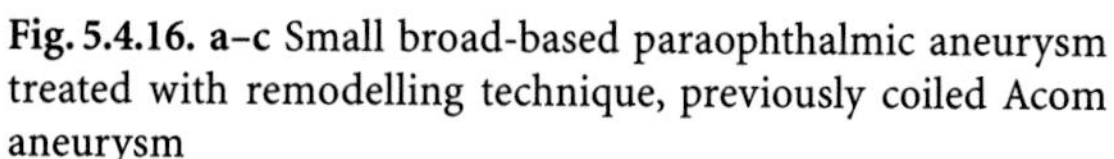

Fig. 5.4.16. a–c Small broad-based paraophthalmic aneurysm treated with remodelling technique, previously coiled Acom aneurysm

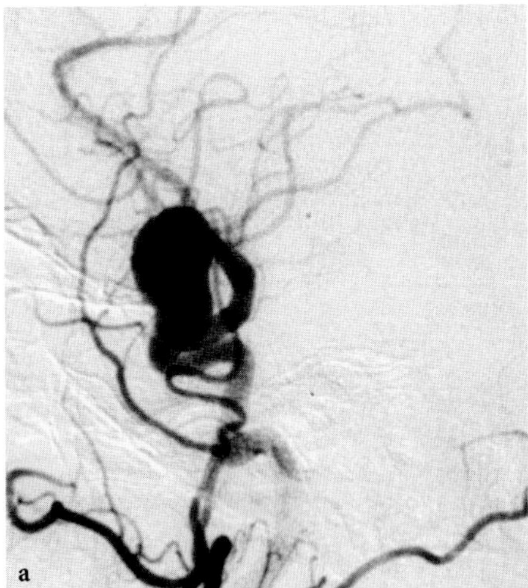

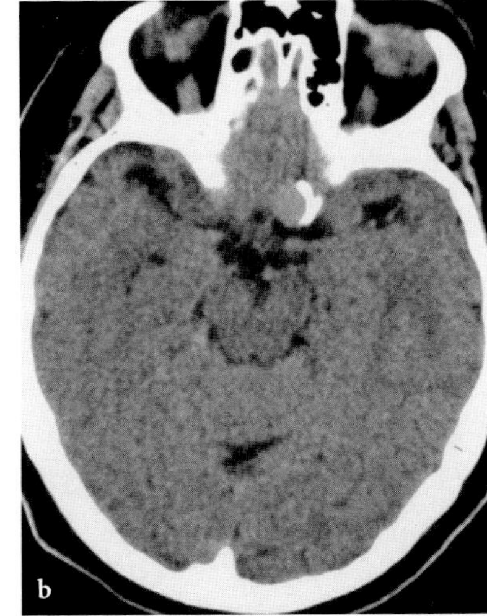

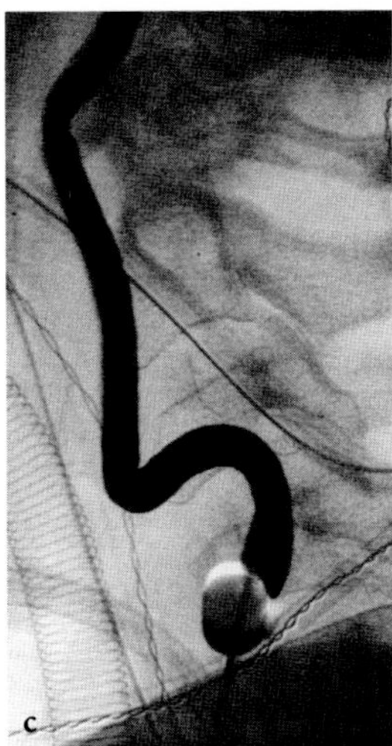

Fig. 5.4.17. a, b Large paraophthalmic broad-based ICA aneurysm extending cranially superior to the clinoid process with partial calcification. **c** "Evacuation trapping technique" during clipping was performed after transient balloon occlusion of the left internal carotid artery

5.4.9.1.2 Supraclinoid/Intracranial Carotid Bifurcation

The majority of posterior communicating artery (Pcom) aneurysms arise from the ICA at the origin of the Pcom. True Pcom aneurysms are rare and might be more difficult to catheterize. In about 30%–40% of Pcom aneurysms are associated with third nerve cranial palsy with or without subarachnoid hemorrhage (Birchall et al. 1999; Perneczky and Czech 1984). From a surgical point of view the approach to these aneurysms is not too difficult. However, many of them have a small neck and are good candidates for endovascular therapy. In our experience, those aneurysms arising from the posterior wall of the ICA might be slightly different compared to other intracranial aneurysms. They might have a higher tendency of recanalization than generally expected from a side wall aneurysm and some of them are more fragile and have a tendency not only to rupture at the dome, but also to pop out of the ICA wall. The latter situation is extremely difficult to handle and usually ends up with a parent vessel occlusion of the ICA.

Aneurysms of the intracranial carotid bifurcation usually arise at the apex of the T-shaped bifurcation and the majority of them points upward and towards the anterior perforated substance. Due to the perforating branches at this site clipping of these aneurysms is associated with a substantial risk of ischemic infarctions. The endovascular approach is usually easy from a technical point of view (like in basilar tip aneurysms). Even if these aneurysms look broad based coiling is usually possible without the aid of remodelling or stenting.

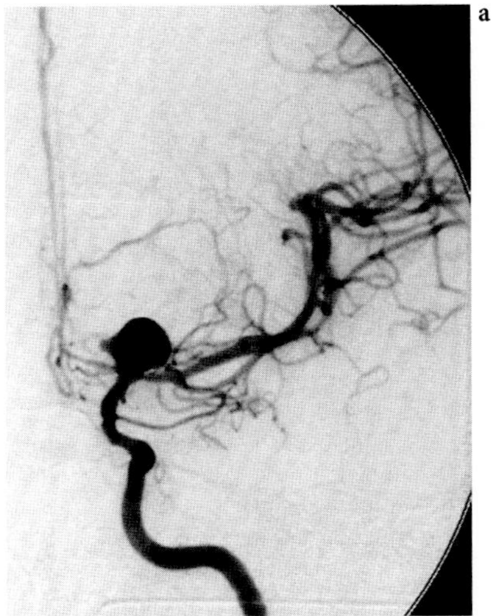

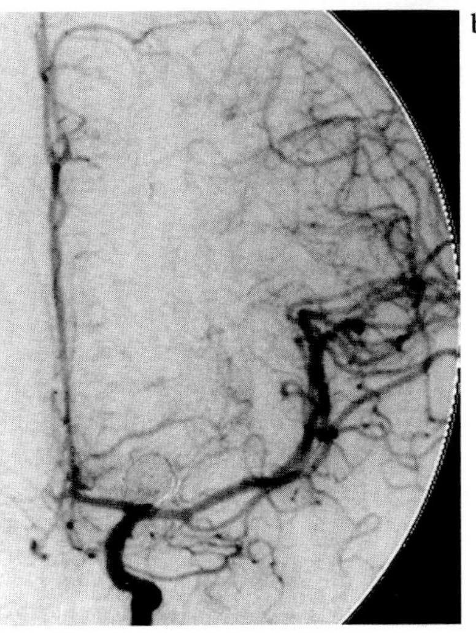

Fig. 5.4.18a,b. Conventional angiography, before and after coil treatment of a distal ICA aneurysm

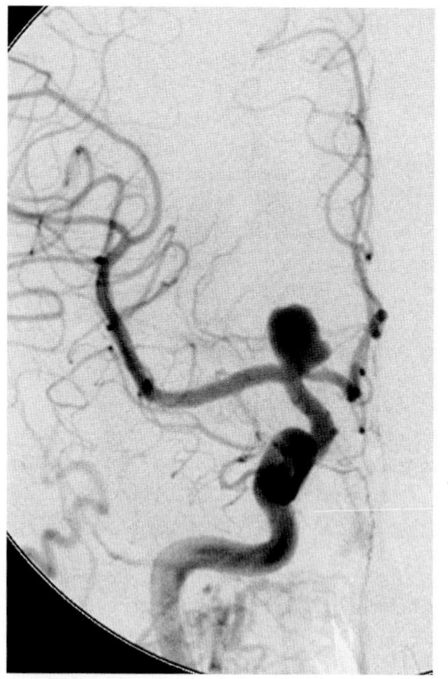

a

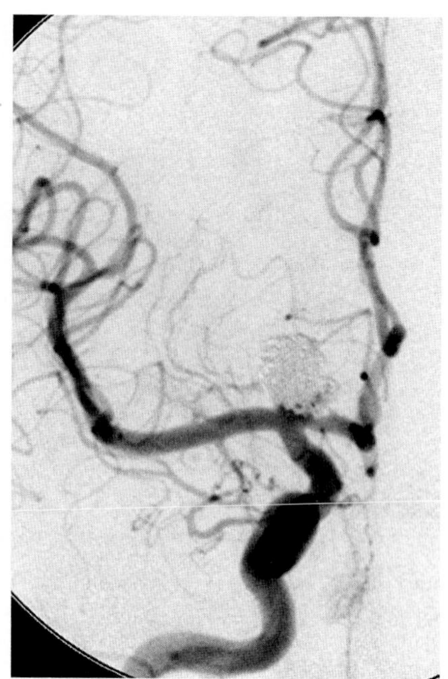

b

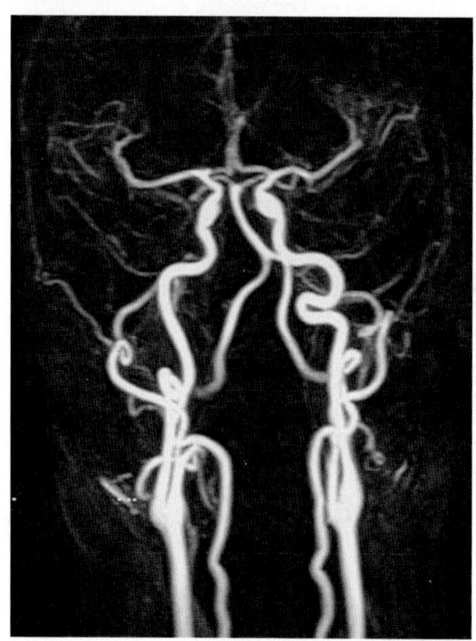

c

Fig. 5.4.19a–c. Typical intracranial carotid bifurcation aneurysm. MRA 6 month after embolization revealed stable occlusion

5.4.9.2 Anterior Cerebral Artery

5.4.9.2.1 Anterior Communicating Artery

The rupture of an aneurysm at the anterior communicating artery (Acom) is responsible for approximately 40% of subarachnoid hemorrhages (Kassell et al. 1990a,b). Treatment of these aneurysms is thus a frequent situation and of great importance. In the past, Acom aneurysms were treated nearly exclusively by surgical clipping, using either a pterional or interhemispheric approach. With the increasing use of endovascular techniques Acom aneurysms are frequently treated by coil embolization and in some institutions it is already the first-line treatment. Moret et al. (1996) reported their results on 251 berry aneurysms treated by detachable coils, of which 36 were located at the Acom and treated with GDC. There were 23 aneurysms which were completely and six were partially occluded. In three cases, no endovascular treatment was attempted because the aneurysmal neck was not clearly distinct from the adjacent, or parent vessels. In four cases, treatment failed because of atheroma of the cervical and intracranial vessels. The authors reported one permanent neurologic complication, two patients died as a result of complications of subarachnoid haemorrhage. In summary, the authors concluded that endovascular treatment using GDC is an efficient technique for treating anterior communicating artery aneurysms even in the acute phase of SAH (Moret et al. 1996). This is in accordance with our own results, demonstrating that GDC treatment of ruptured Acom aneurysms is effective and can be performed with acceptable mortality and morbidity, also during the vulnerable period of vasospasms.

Remodelling seems to be feasible for wide-necked aneurysms of the Acom (Levy 1997), but is not routine at this location. In our experience recanalization of these aneurysms is usually not a problem in downward looking aneurysms. Those aneurysms looking upward indeed have a higher tendency of recanalization even after initial complete occlusion. Follow-up is therefore of utmost importance in the latter group.

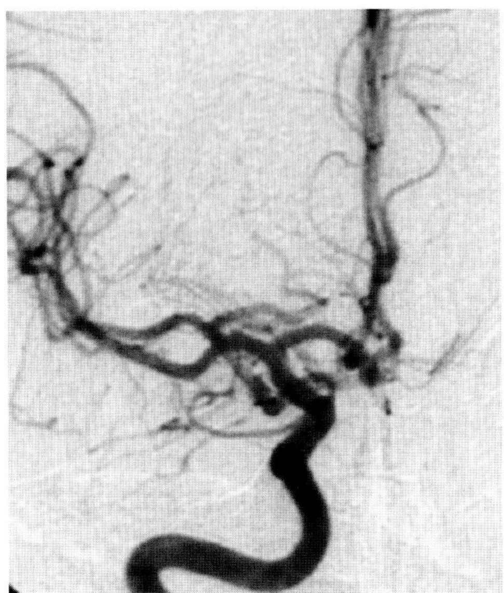
a

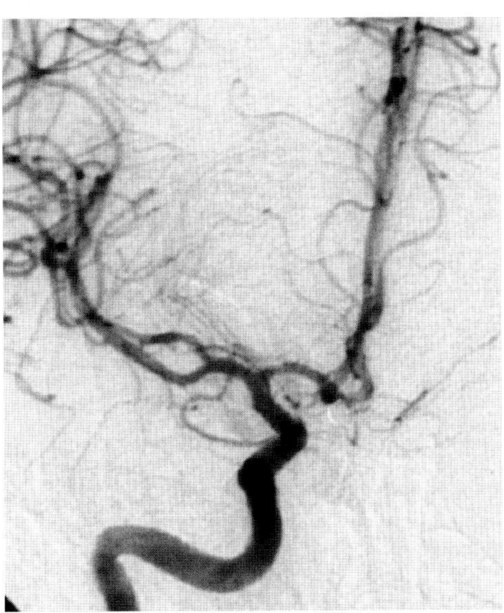
b

Fig. 5.4.20a,b. Small Acom aneurysm: (**a**) before and (**b**) after endovascular embolization

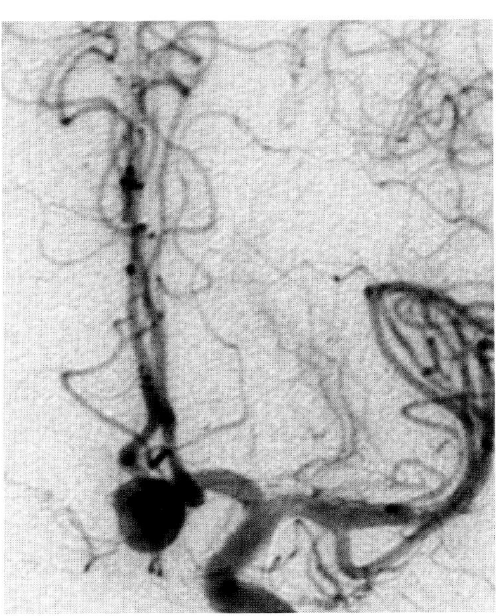
a

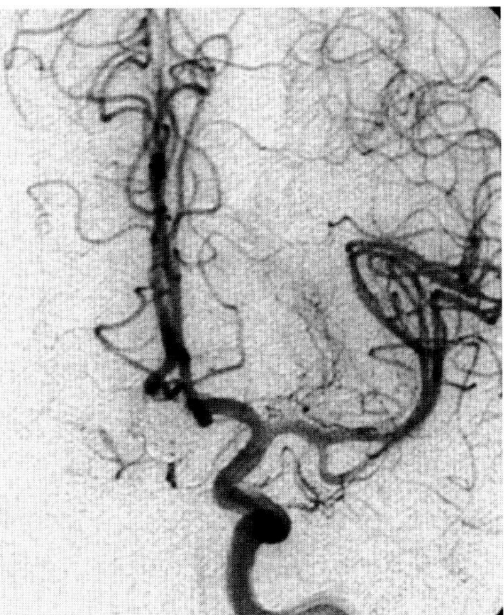
b

Fig. 5.4.21a,b. Medium sized Acom aneurysm: (**a**) before and (**b**) after endovascular treatment; the parent artery is still open

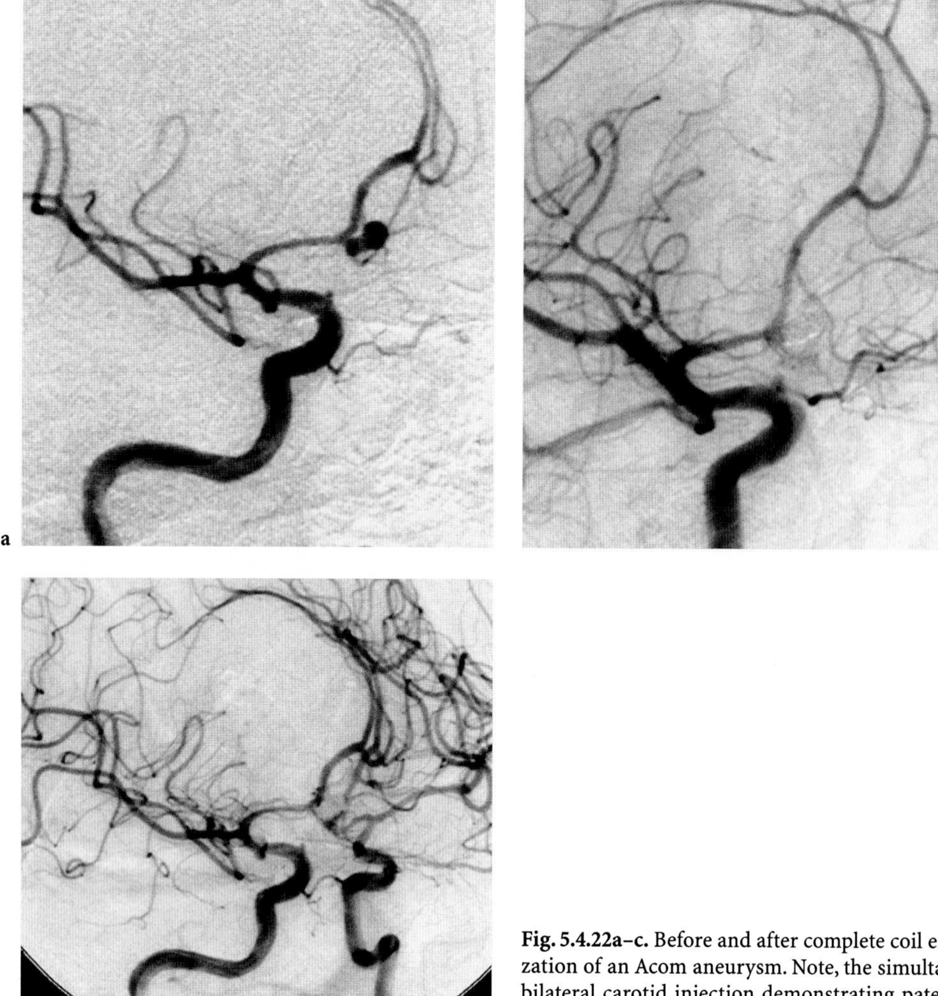

Fig. 5.4.22a–c. Before and after complete coil embolization of an Acom aneurysm. Note, the simultaneous bilateral carotid injection demonstrating patency of the Acom

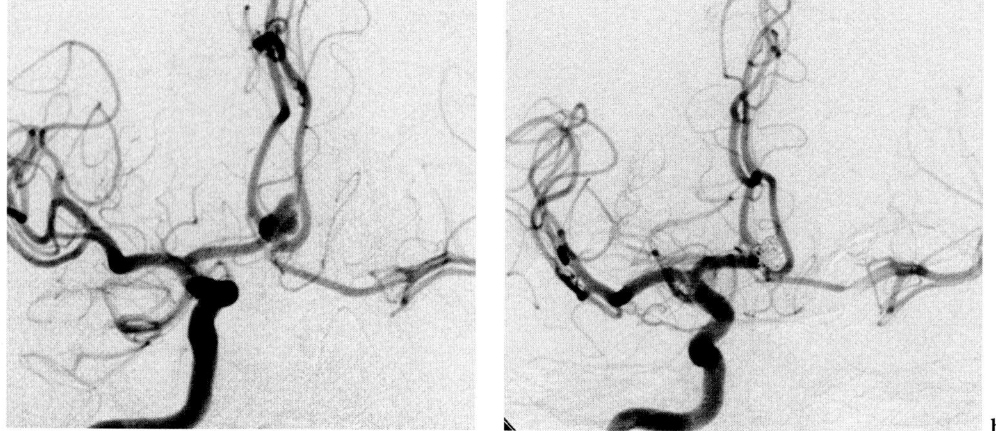

Fig. 5.4.23a,b. Before and after complete coil embolization of a multilobulated Acom aneurysm

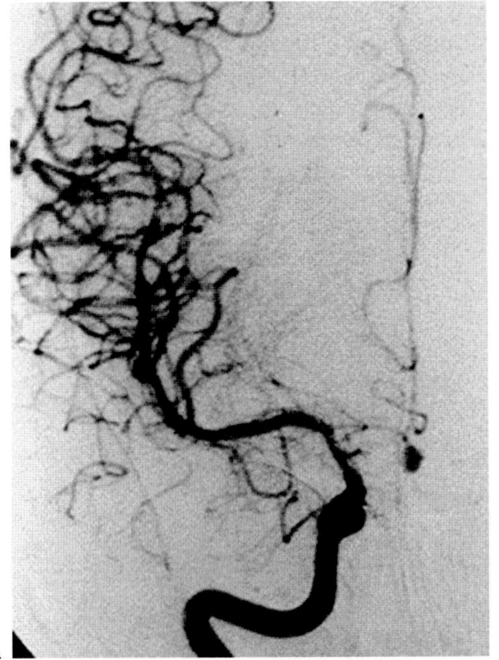

a

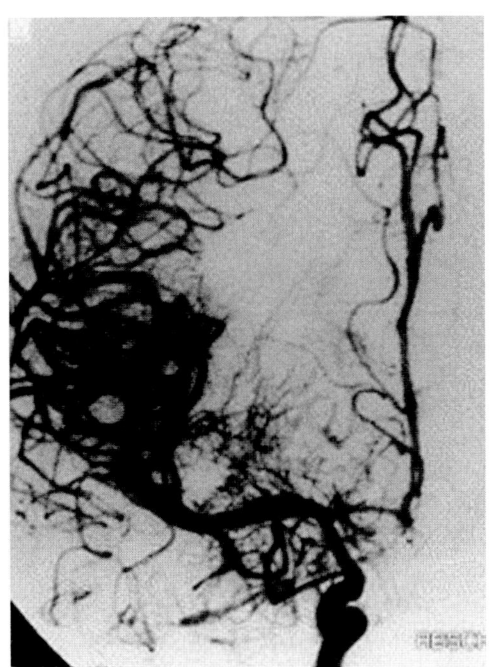

c

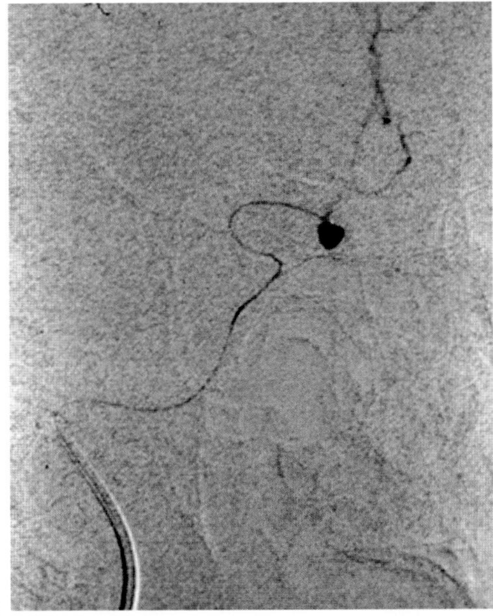

b

Fig. 5.4.24a–c. Conventional angiography before treatment revealed severe vasospasm of the ACA, despite the spasm endosaccular treatment with complete obliteration of the Acom aneurysm was performed and vasospasmolysis after treatment resulting in almost complete regression of spasm

5.4.9.2.2
Distal Anterior Cerebral Artery/Pericallosal Artery

Distal anterior cerebral artery aneurysms are rare, accounting for about 4.5% of all intracranial aneurysms (Inci et al. 1998), and usually arise at the bifurcation of the pericallosal and callosomarginal arteries. SAH due to rupture of a distal anterior cerebral artery aneurysms is frequently associated with ICH in and/or along the corpus callosum and anterior interhemispheric fissure and subsequent intraventricular hemorrhage.

Pericallosal aneurysms frequently have a broad base or absent neck associated with a small diameter of the parent vessel. In some cases the pericallosal artery arises out of the aneurysm sac. This anatomic feature is difficult for both surgery and endovascular therapy. Due to the particular anatomy of pericallosal aneurysms surgical approach is different from those of other anterior circulation aneurysms and precise neck clipping might be difficult even for an experienced surgeon. Using the frontal interhemispheric route, which is the usual approach for most surgeons, the pericallosal aneurysm neck is exposed after the fundus, which might become a delicate procedure and is frequently associated with intraoperative aneurysm rupture (Proust et al. 1997). Additionally, there might be difficulties in clip application due to the small space of the pericallosal cistern, dense adhesions between the cingulate gyri, difficulty in controlling the parent artery, and the association of vascular anomalies (Inci et al. 1998).

Proust et al. (1997) reported the results of a retrospective multicenter study in 43 patients with 50 distal anterior cerebral artery aneurysms, with only two aneurysms treated endovascularly. In their series an 11.4% incidence of thrombosis was observed on postoperative control angiography, mainly in the distal pericallosal segment or callosomarginal artery, associated with a poor outcome. The authors reported a higher tendency of rebleeding in this location. This is in accordance with the results of Sindou et al. (1988) reporting a 16% rebleeding rate in their series. But, times are changing. Recently, Menovsky et al. (2002) reported on 12 patients with pericallosal aneurysms, all treated with the endovascular method. In all 12 patients, the pericallosal aneurysm could be reached with a microcatheter and platinum coils could be deployed. There were no procedure-related complications. Initial occlusion was complete in 11 aneurysms and near complete in 1 patient. The conclusion of the authors is that coiling of ruptured pericallosal aneurysms can be considered as an alternative to surgical clipping. Increasingly improved results of endovascular therapy at different locations of the Circle of Willi are mainly based on increased skills of the interventionalist, but are also related to the continuous improvement of all parts of the material, allowing easier access to the aneurysm and denser packing with softer coils.

In our opinion, the endovascular approach in pericallosal artery aneurysms is often feasible.

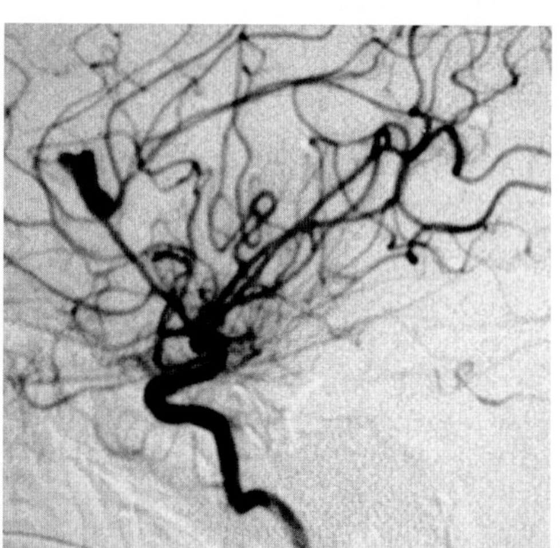

a

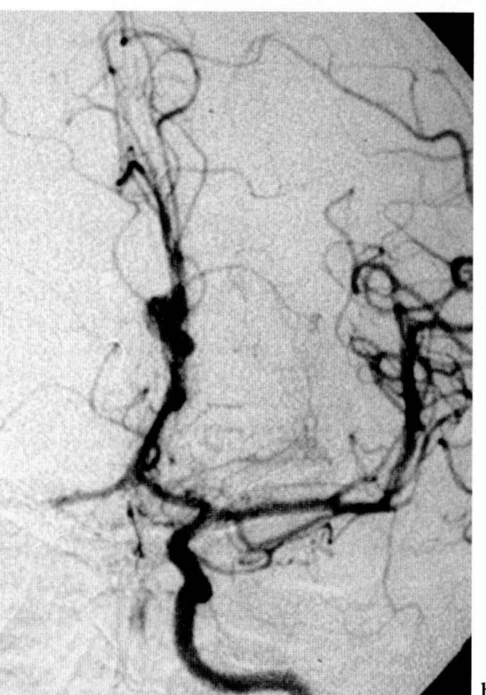

b

Fig. 5.4.25a,b. Multilobulated aneurysm of the pericallosal artery; because of an associated intraparenchymal hematoma surgery was performed

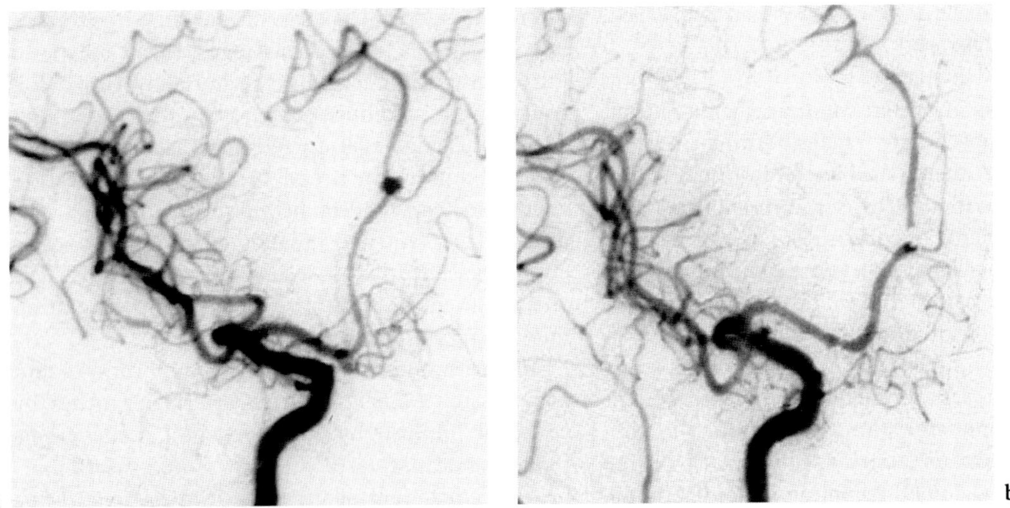

Fig. 5.4.26a,b. Before and after endovascular treatment of a small aneurysm of the pericallosal artery

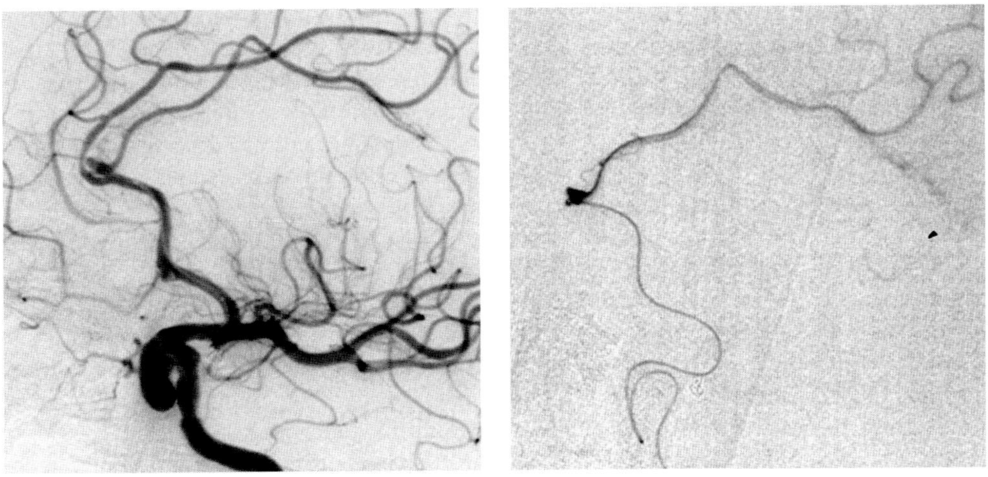

Fig. 5.4.27a–c. Before and after endovascular treatment of a small aneurysm of the pericallosal artery; aneurysmography revealed a very close relationship of the aneurysm and the callosomarginal artery

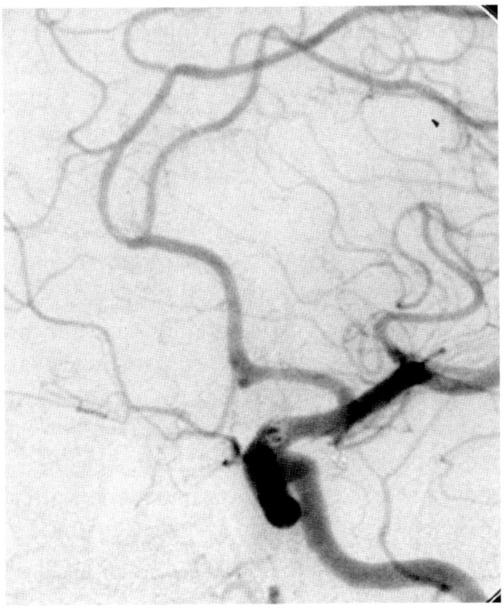

5.4.9.3
Middle Cerebral Artery

MCA aneurysms are often small and wide necked, and often incorporate neighbouring arterial branches in the aneurysm base. Additionally, they are frequently associated with multiple intracranial aneurysms ("mirror aneurysms"). Due to the local anatomy and neck configuration MCA aneurysms need particular consideration. For aneurysms with a very wide neck or difficult geometry surgery is still the therapy of choice. If a space-occupying hematoma is present, immediate evacuation of the hematoma is mandatory, in combination with clipping of the aneurysm (van Gijn and van Dongen 1982). Regli et al. (1999) recommend not to attempt coil embolization in MCA aneurysms since in their study of 35 consecutive patients harbouring 40 unruptured MCA aneurysms, only 6% could be successfully embolized with coils whereas 94% (32/34) of patients had to be clipped. The two major angioanatomic features responsible for the failure of endovascular treatment were an unfavourable dome-to-neck ratio of less than 1.5, and/or arterial branching from the aneurysm base.

Compared to other aneurysm locations, the risk of thromboembolic complications or local compression of surrounding neighbouring vessels seems to be increased. We also made the experience that endovascular treatment in this location is more often associated with complications such as thrombus formation at or near the base of the aneurysm. However, we could not confirm the results of the above mentioned study. Regarding feasibility we were able to treat almost 90% of MCA aneurysms and the clinical outcome of our consecutive series of 39 patients with 41 ruptured and unruptured aneurysms at the middle cerebral artery encountered only 2.6% with a permanent neurologic deficit due to the procedure. Although the total rate of complications including vessel occlusion, coil protrusion and groin hematoma was higher, this number of 2.6% reflects a very low procedural permanent morbidity. Therefore, we think after appropriate patient selection endovascular therapy in these aneurysms might become more applicable as it is by now. Careful evaluation of the angioarchitecture using rotational 3D angiography, superselective angiography with the microcatheter (aneurysmography), or 3D helical CT angiography might be extremely helpful in the precise visualization of the aneurysm neck, shape and the size of the aneurysm, supporting further treatment decisions and planning. MRA can provide complementary information to DSA, such as intraaneurysmal thrombus. Sometimes the endovascular attempt only with introducing the microcatheter and delivering a coil could reveal if coiling seems to be possible without an unusual high risk. In selected cases the remodelling technique in broad based MCA bifurcation aneurysms can be very helpful; in many cases it is even not necessary to inflate the balloon; it may be enough to have just a second microcatheter at the aneurysm entrance to provide coils from migration into a parent branch.

To prevent thromboembolic complications and compression of neighbouring arterial branches by coils, our "philosophy" for selected MCA aneurysms treated endovascularly is to wait longer (5–10 min) before detachment of the coils. In these aneurysms we prefer to rather underestimate the coil diameter than to choose a coil which is slightly greater than the maximum diameter of the aneurysm. In an unruptured aneurysm we administer aspirin intravenously before application of the first coil and after introducing the microcatheter into the aneurysm. If there is at least subtotal occlusion, further aneurysm thrombosis is possible and was observed in some of our patients at follow up on DSA and MRA 6 months after coil embolization.

However, Pierot et al. (1997) reported rebleeding in an only partially treated MCA aneurysm. General recommendation should imply dense packing for MCA aneurysms. In patients with loose coil packing follow up is essential like in any other locations, to see if there is growth of neck remnants or subsequent thrombosis during follow up.

When unclippable or endovascularly untreatable aneurysms involve the M1, M2, and M3 branches of the middle cerebral artery (MCA), bypass surgery can obviously be a therapeutic option in combination with parent artery occlusion (Drake and Peerless 1997; Peerless et al. 1982). However, and this again is our experience, this is the exception.

5.4.9.4
Vertebrobasilar Arteries

Aneurysms of the posterior circulation account for about 15% of all intracranial aneurysms saccular aneurysms and those of the basilar tip are the most frequent accounting for 5%–8% of all intracranial aneurysms. Ruptured aneurysms in the posterior circulation have a worse prognosis than patients with a ruptured aneurysm in another location (Schievink et al. 1995) and early rerupture occurs more often in this location.

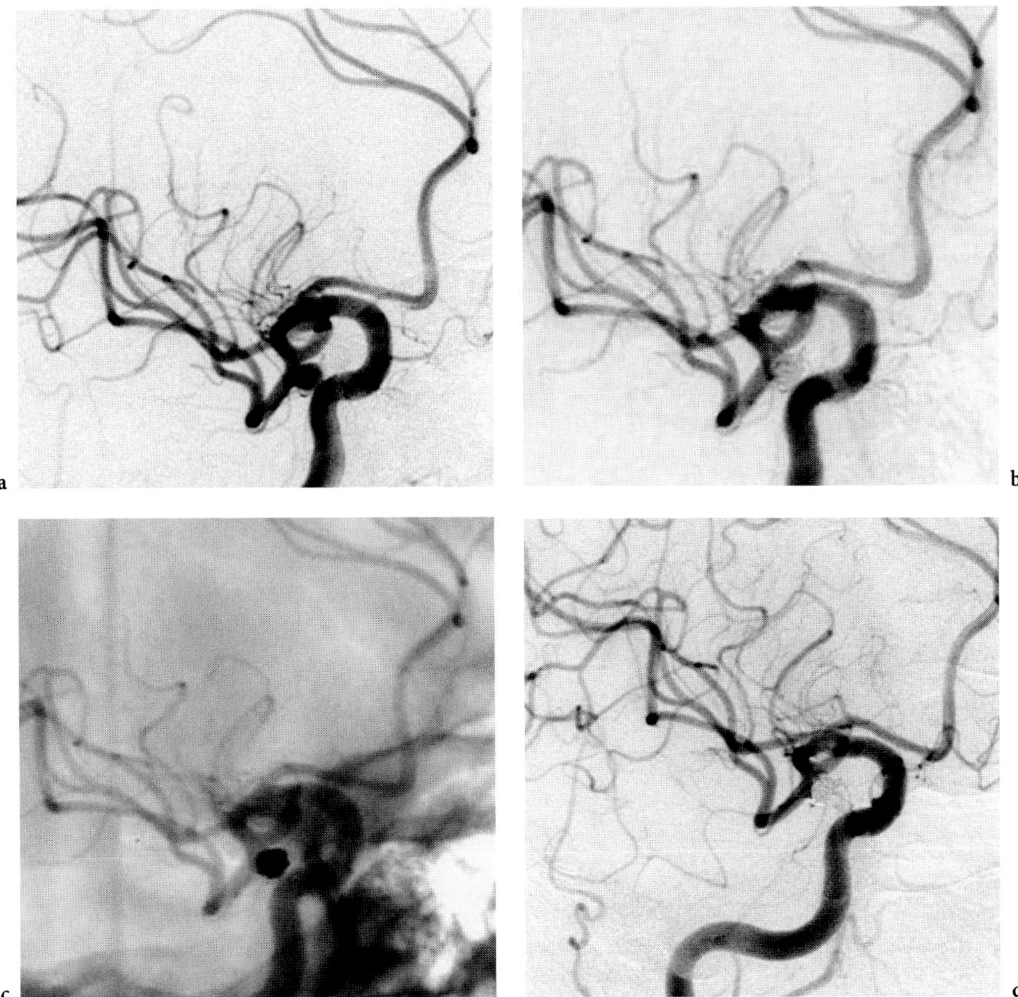

Fig. 5.4.28a–d. Small broad-based ruptured MCA bifurcation aneurysm before and after endovascular embolization with a stable occlusion after 6 months

Despite improvement in microsurgical therapy, clipping for posterior circulation aneurysms remains challenging. The main problems are the deep location, the presence of many eloquent structures around the sac and the neck as well as the restricted access to the aneurysm neck. Furthermore, SAH and cerebral edema increase the difficulties of the surgical approach much more than in any other location. Surgical complications specific for non-giant basilar bifurcation aneurysms are midbrain and/or thalamic infarctions from perforator injury or occlusion, intraoperative rupture, and frequent but nearly always transient cranial nerve paresis (Drake 1965; Horikoshi et al. 1999; Peerless et al. 1987, 1994; Rice et al. 1990). Another complication of surgery in this region is a major operative tear of the aneurysm or incomplete clipping of the aneurysm with the potential for rebleeding during closure or early in the postoperative period.

With introduction of detachable platinum coils for endovascular obliteration of cerebral aneurysms a major shift towards this method is established now specifically for aneurysms located in the posterior circulation (Bavinzski et al. 1999; Lusseveld et al. 2002; Richling et al. 1995; Tateshima et al. 2000; Vallee et al. 2003). The early recognition and acceptance that coiling is clearly better than clipping in hind brain circulation aneurysms is the reason that these aneurysms are underrepresented in the ISAT study (Molyneux et al. 2002). Almost exclusively aneurysms of the anterior circulation were involved, posterior circulation aneurysms, for which the endovascular approach is generally accepted as first-line treatment, made up only 2.7%. In most of the cases inclusion was thought to be unethical.

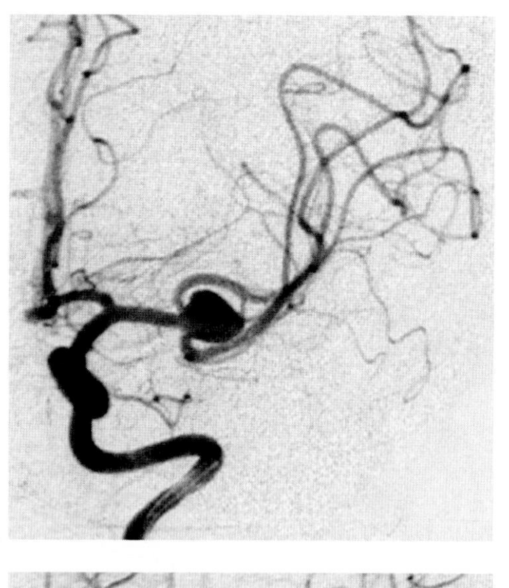
a

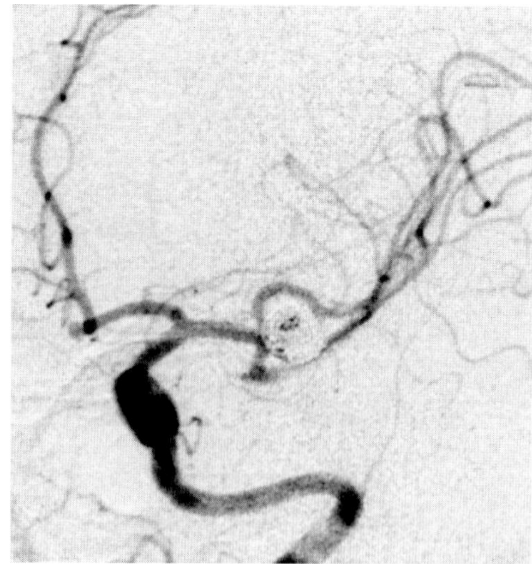
b

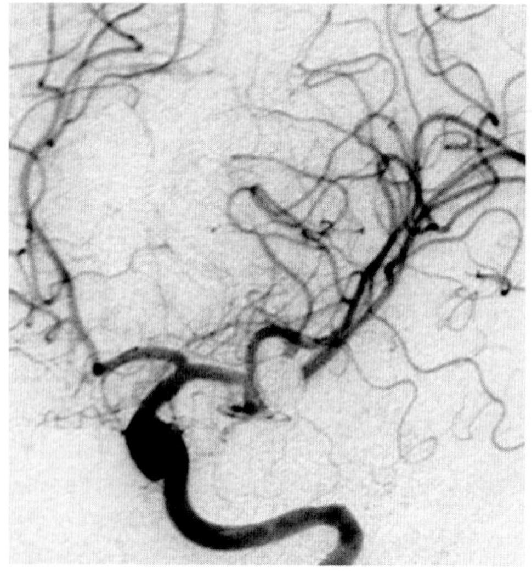
c

Fig. 5.4.29a–c. Before and after GDC treatment of a left MCA aneurysm, note the slight persistent inflow in the centre of the aneurysm **b** immediately after embolization; **c** 6-month follow-up demonstrated complete occlusion without any residual inflow

5.4.9.4.1 Tip of the Basilar Artery

Aneurysms of the basilar tip remain an extreme surgical challenge, both in terms of technical difficulties associated with the access and the significant postoperative morbidity and mortality rates reported by experienced centres following direct clipping. Clear results about morbidity and mortality rates in patients surgically clipped for an unruptured aneurysm gives the meta-analysis of Raaymakers et al. (1998). This analysis included 61 studies with a total of 2460 patients with at least 2568 unruptured aneurysms. Only 158 patients had a postoperative angiogram which revealed a residual aneurysm in 7%. Although the proportion of aneurysms in the posterior circulation of about 30% was somewhat high the study revealed a mortality and morbidity rate for non-giant aneurysms of 3% and 12.9%, respectively. The results for giant aneurysms in the same location were much worse with a morbidity and mortality of 37.9% and 9.6%, respectively.

In contrast to the surgical approach, the endovascular approach is relatively easy (unless the patient has severe arteriosclerotic disease with increased vessel elongation and stenosis). However, the access to the basilar tip plays a minor role in most cases. The main technical challenge of the endovascular procedure depends on the shape of the aneurysm and not on its location. But since the introduction of a very flexible neurostent and the development of different coil designs most of the basilar tip aneurysms are now treatable with the endovascular approach. This

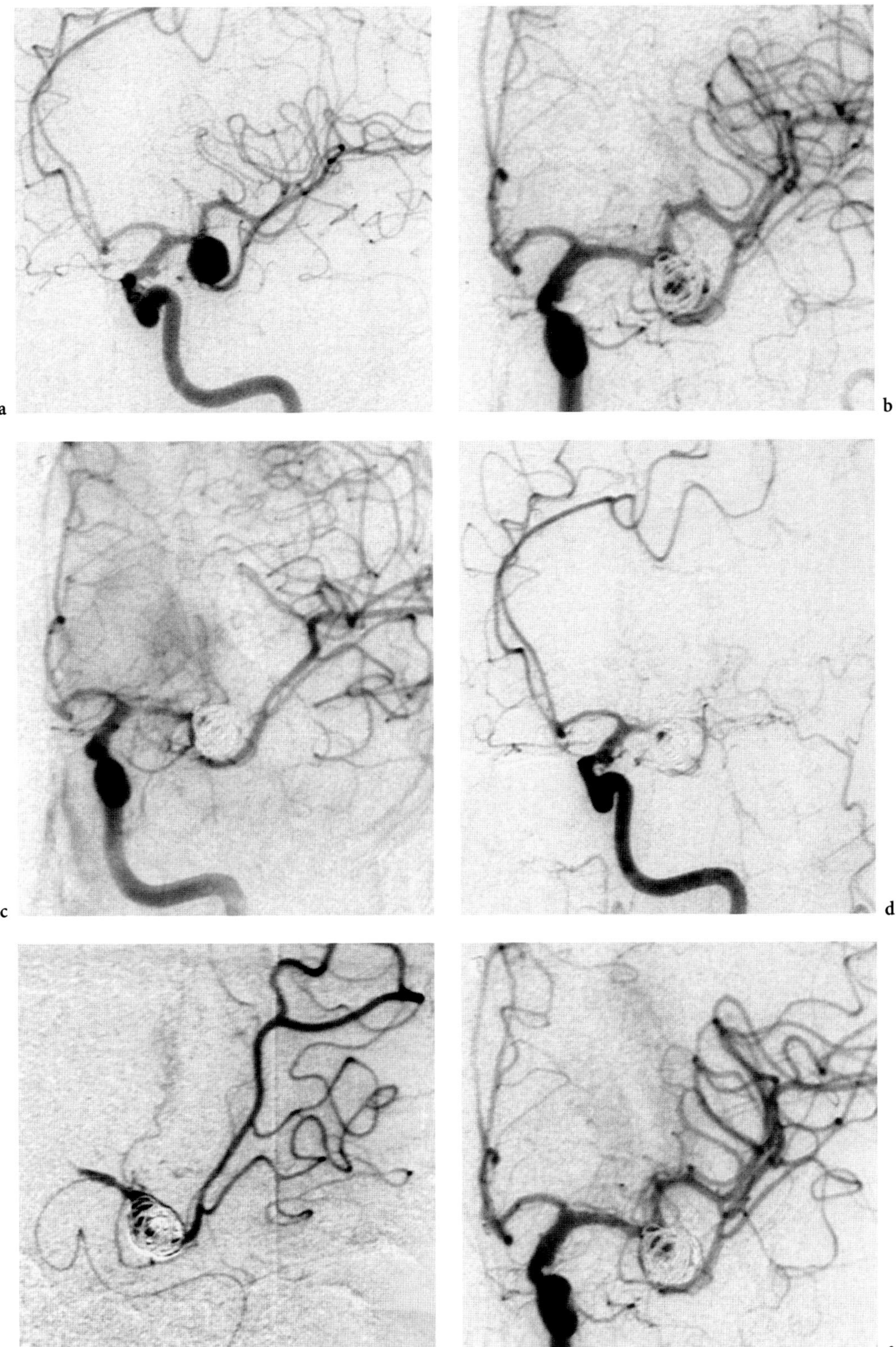

Fig. 5.4.30a–f. Angiography: before and after incomplete coil embolization of an unruptured left MCA aneurysm. Due to progressive thrombosis out of the aneurysm gradual MCA occlusion developed 4.5 h after the intervention. The vessel could be reopened by selective intraarterial thrombolysis using urokinase (1,000,000 IU). Although a small basal ganglia infarction was induced the patient had a good recovery with only mild deficits

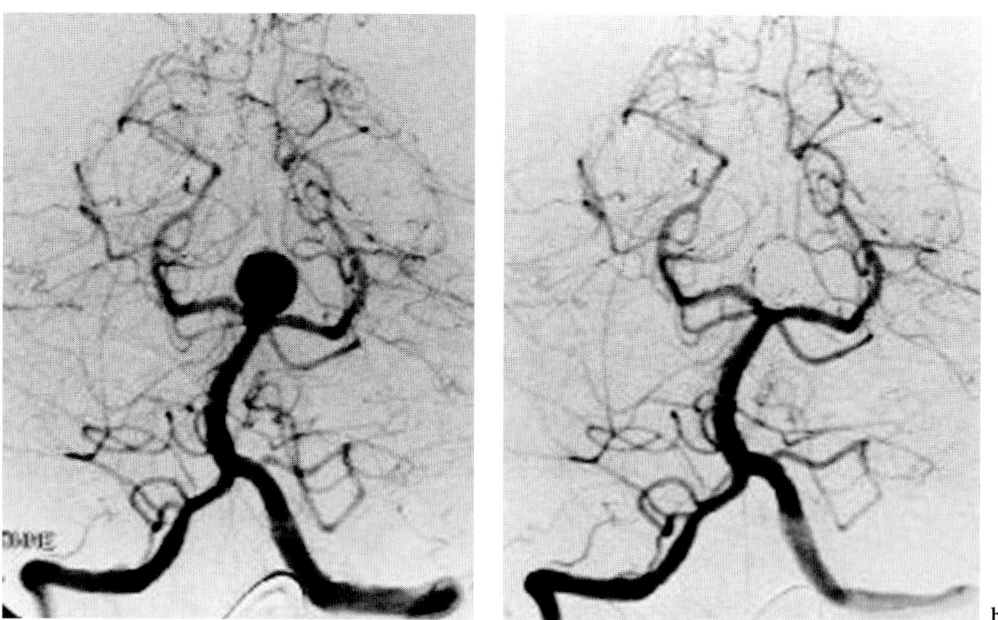

Fig. 5.4.31a,b. Before and after endovascular treatment of a non-ruptured basilar tip aneurysm

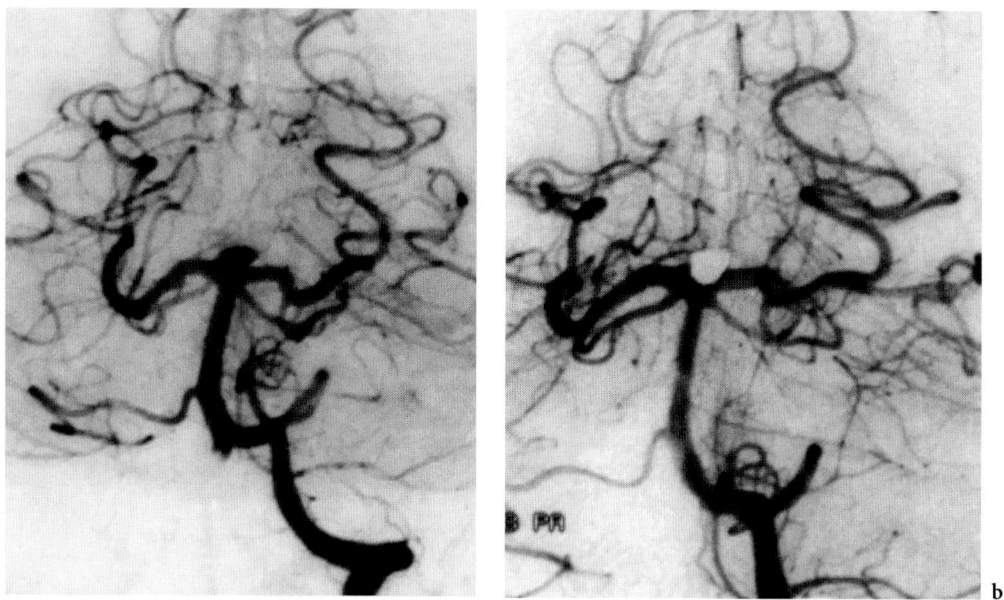

Fig. 5.4.32a,b. Before and after endovascular treatment of a broad-based ruptured basilar tip aneurysm

is also true for broad-based aneurysms which may encroach one or both P1 segments.

Bavinzski et al. (1999) treated a series of ruptured (n=34) and unruptured (n=11) basilar tip aneurysms and had a morbidity of 4.4% and a mortality of 2.2%. Even better results were obtained by the group with Tateshima (2000) who treated 73 patients with 75 basilar tip aneurysms of which 42 patients had a SAH, eight presented with symptoms due to mass effect and 23 had an incidental finding. The procedure-related morbidity was 4.1% and mortality was 1.4%.

Because most single center reports on endovascular treatment of basilar tip aneurysms revealed an

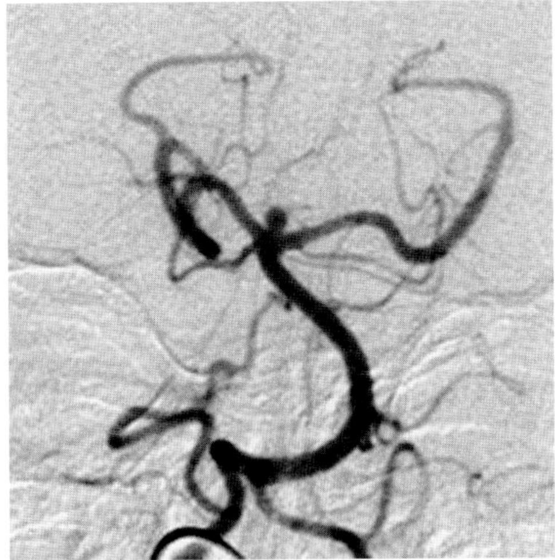

a

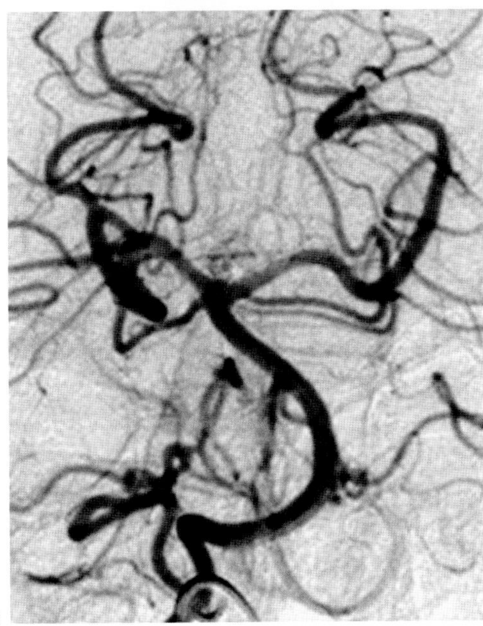

b

Fig. 5.4.33a,b. Before and after endovascular treatment of a small ruptured basilar tip aneurysm

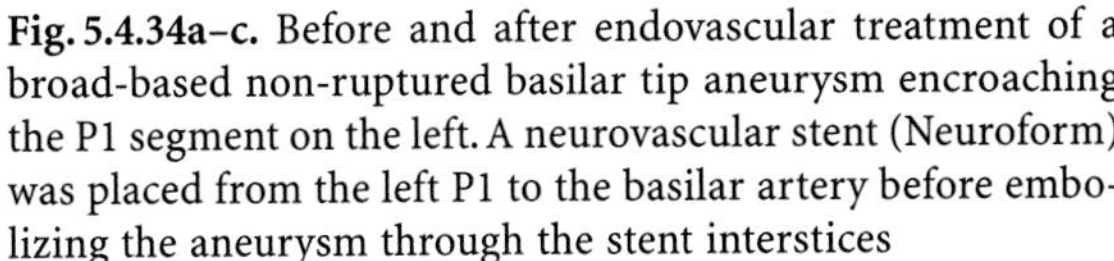

Fig. 5.4.34a–c. Before and after endovascular treatment of a broad-based non-ruptured basilar tip aneurysm encroaching the P1 segment on the left. A neurovascular stent (Neuroform) was placed from the left P1 to the basilar artery before embolizing the aneurysm through the stent interstices

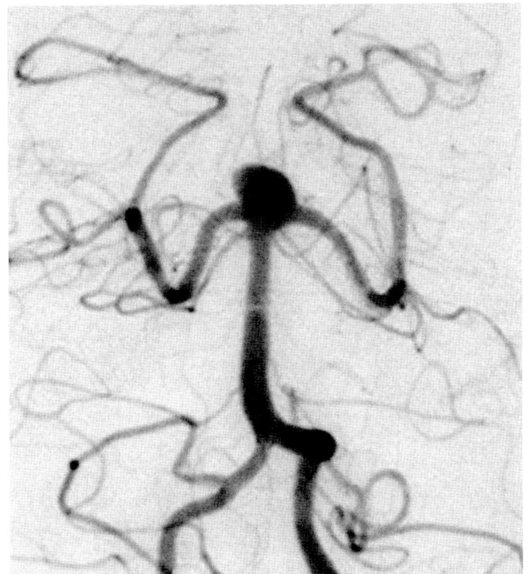

a

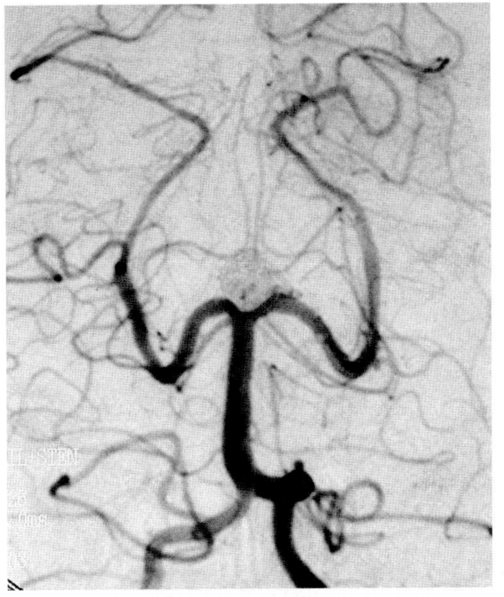

b

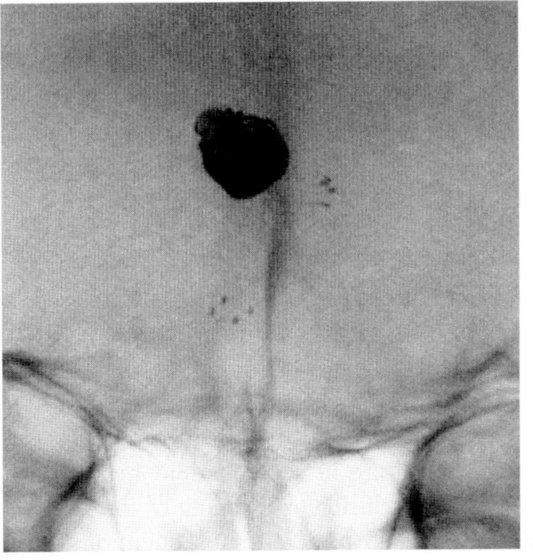

c

extremely low morbidity and mortality rate which matches our own experience we do recommend endovascular treatment as the treatment of choice in ruptured or unruptured aneurysms in this location (Bavinzski et al. 1999; Birchall et al. 2001; Pierot et al. 1996; Richling et al. 1995; Tateshima et al. 2000; Vallee et al. 2003).

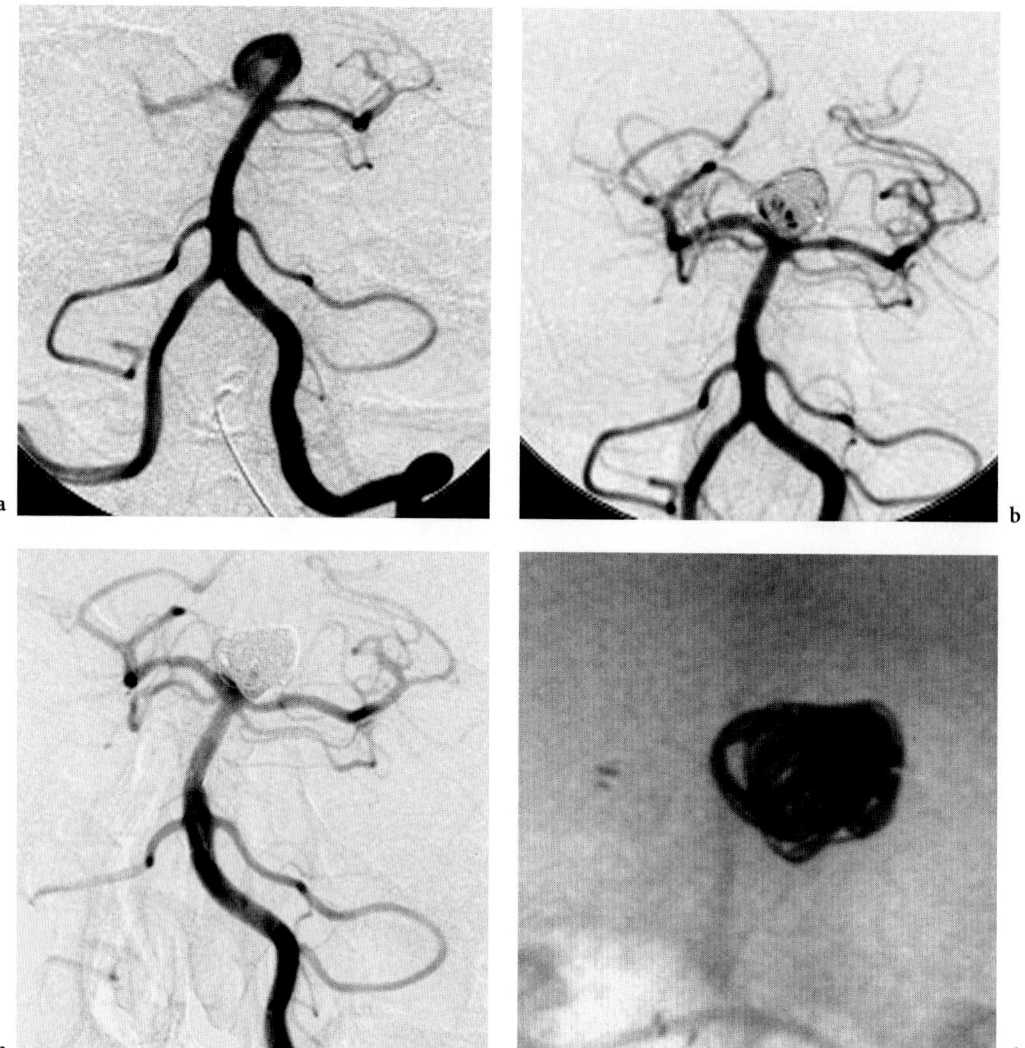

Fig. 5.4.35. a, b Before and after stent application in combination with coil treatment in a broad-based basilar tip aneurysm encroaching the P1 segment on the right side. **c** The stent was placed from the right P1 segment to the basilar artery. **d** 7-Month FU showed further obliteration of the initially subtotal occluded aneurysm

5.4.9.4.2 Vertebral Aneurysms

Aneurysms of the vertebral artery leading to SAH are located at the V4 segment. Dissecting aneurysms are more frequent in this location than non-dissecting berry aneurysms. Aneurysms are located proximal to the origin of the PICA, at the origin of the PICA (so-called PICA aneurysms) or slightly distal to the origin of the PICA.

In patients with a dissecting aneurysm of the vertebral artery resulting in subarachnoid hemorrhage, either proximal occlusion or trapping of the lesion is commonly advocated to prevent subsequent rupture. If proximal occlusion alone is performed, retrograde flow from the contralateral vertebral artery into the distal vertebral artery might be maintained. This may retard thrombosis and organization of the dissected lumen, leading to the possibility of postoperative rebleeding.

Fusiform aneurysms are usually considered due to atherosclerosis in adults. But, more common in the vertebrobasilar system, there is a subset of cerebral aneurysms with fusiform morphology, apparently unrelated to cerebral atherosclerosis or systemic connective tissue disease, thin-walled in part or whole, possibly containing thrombus (Findlay et al. 2002). These aneurysms can rupture or cause cranial nerve or brain stem compression.

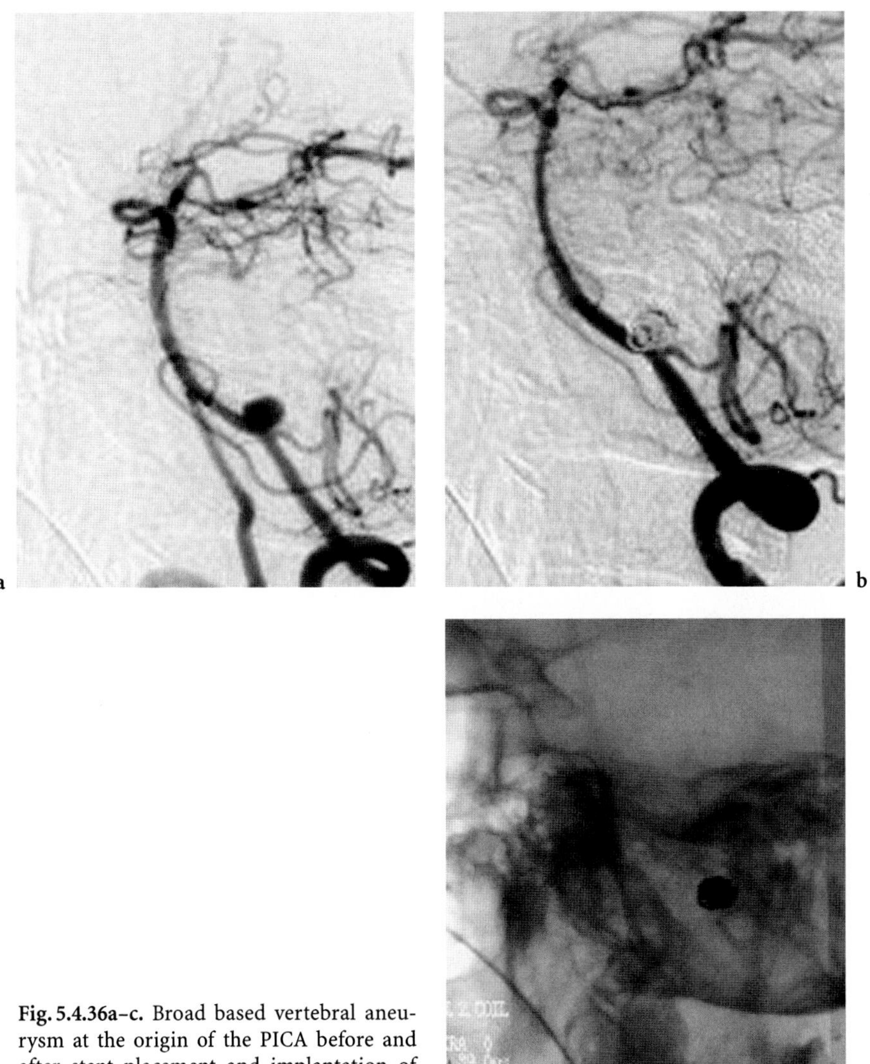

Fig. 5.4.36a–c. Broad based vertebral aneurysm at the origin of the PICA before and after stent placement and implantation of platinum coils

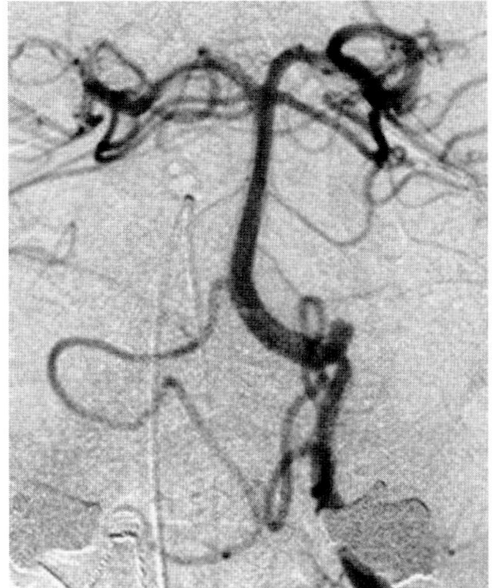

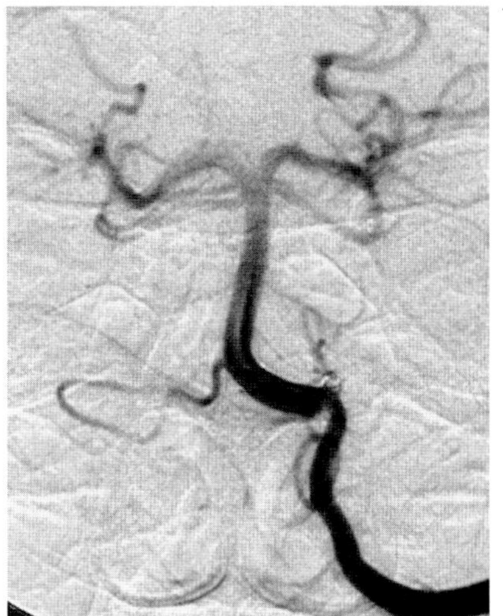

Fig. 5.4.37a,b. Small vertebral aneurysm before and after endovascular treatment

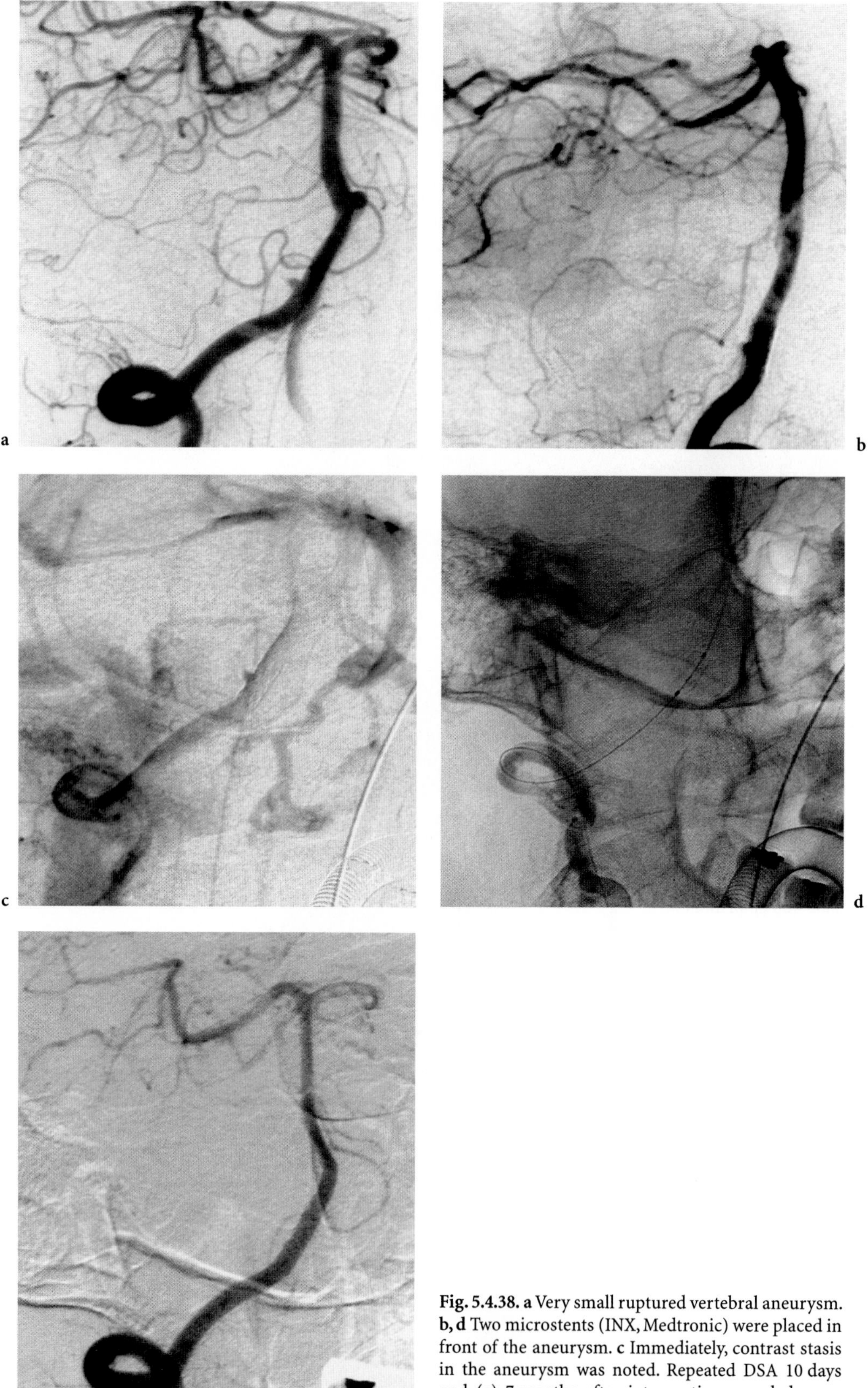

Fig. 5.4.38. **a** Very small ruptured vertebral aneurysm. **b, d** Two microstents (INX, Medtronic) were placed in front of the aneurysm. **c** Immediately, contrast stasis in the aneurysm was noted. Repeated DSA 10 days and (e) 7 months after intervention revealed complete aneurysm obliteration

5.4.9.5
Rare Locations

5.4.9.5.1
Posterior Cerebral Artery

Aneurysms of the posterior cerebral artery (PCA) are relatively rare compared with those in other locations. Extremely rare are singular berry aneurysms of the PCA. Often, this type of aneurysm is either associated with the incidence of multiple aneurysms or with other vascular disorders like arterious-venous-malformations, moyamoya disease or ipsilateral internal carotid occlusion for various reasons. Other rare causes are infectious and posttraumatic conditions. Some authors figured out that the incidence of PCA aneurysms is approximately 1% of all intracranial aneurysms (Ciceri et al. 2001; Drake 1977; Sakata et al. 1993).

Surgical treatment of these aneurysms is complex and often associated with high morbidity rates due to the close relationship to cranial nerves and the upper brain stem. A precise knowledge of the segmental anatomy of the PCA and its branches is essential when the surgical or endovascular approach to an aneurysm is planned, particularly if parent vessel occlusion is intended. In our opinion, the treatment of choice is selective endovascular obliteration of the aneurysm with preservation of the parent artery. In cases of fusiform aneurysms or wide-necked aneurysms occlusion of the parent artery might be necessary. Although no evaluation of potentially existing collaterals prior to endovascular treatment can be performed parent artery occlusion can be performed with a low incidence of visual field deficits. Nevertheless, one should be aware of the perforating arteries arising from the P1 and P2 segment supplying the brain stem and thalamus.

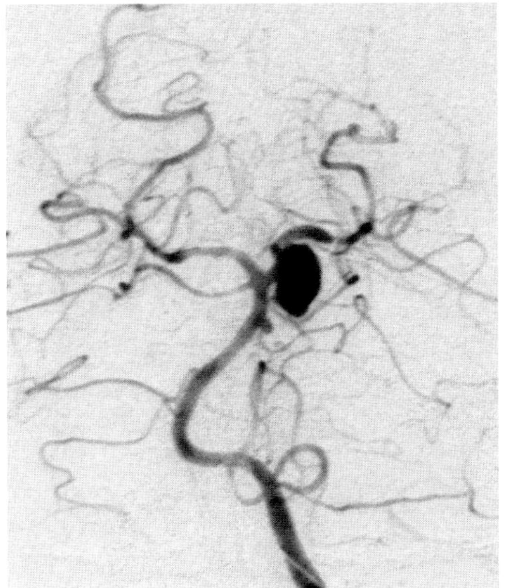

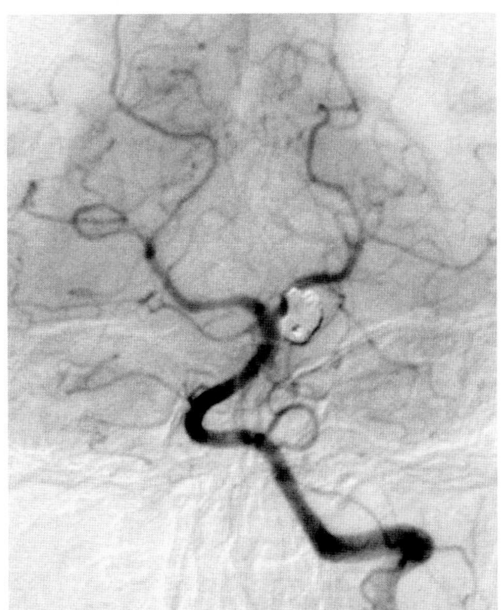

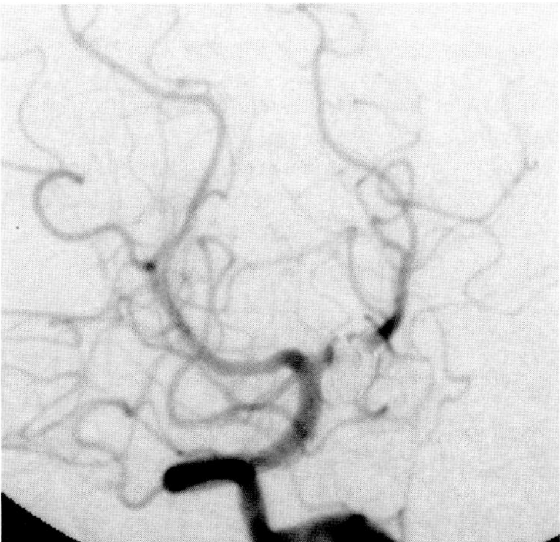

Fig. 5.4.39a–c. Before, 6 months after and 1 year after endosaccular treatment of a proximal PCA aneurysm (P1 segment), an additional small basilar stem aneurysm was not treated

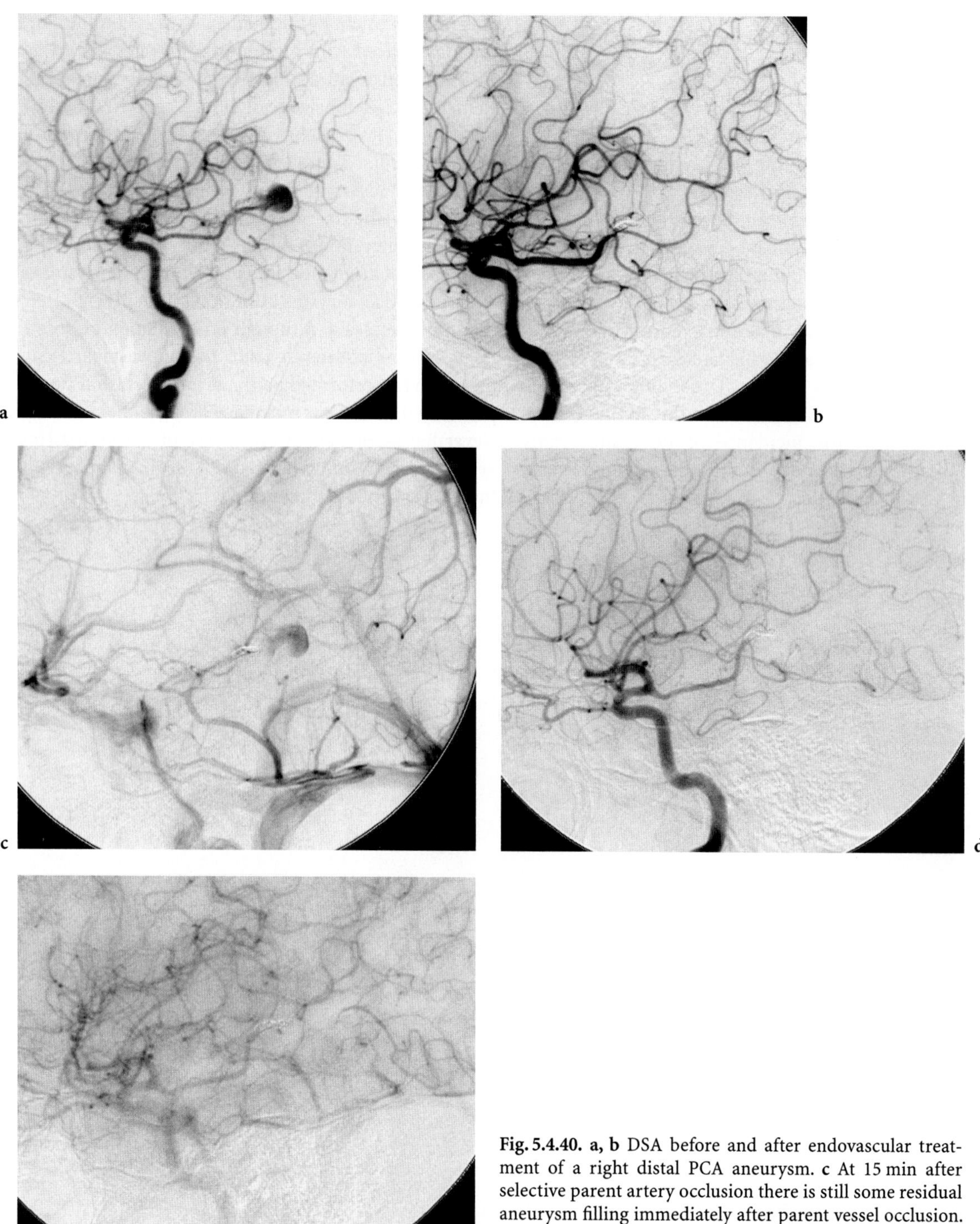

Fig. 5.4.40. a, b DSA before and after endovascular treatment of a right distal PCA aneurysm. **c** At 15 min after selective parent artery occlusion there is still some residual aneurysm filling immediately after parent vessel occlusion. Control angiography (**d, e**) 3 days after vessel occlusion demonstrated complete aneurysm occlusion

5.4.9.5.2
Posterior Inferior Cerebellar Artery

In contrast to vertebral aneurysms located at the origin of the PICA, real PICA aneurysms are located either proximally or distally at the PICA itself.

Endovascular therapy with preservation of the parent artery was thought to be very difficult in this location. Like in basilar tip aneurysms and brain stem aneurysms the access to aneurysms at the PICA is easy to perform and this is in contrast to the surgical approach. Although PICA aneurysms tend to be fusiform or at least broad based most of these aneurysms can be occluded sufficiently and often with preservation of the PICA via the endovascular route.

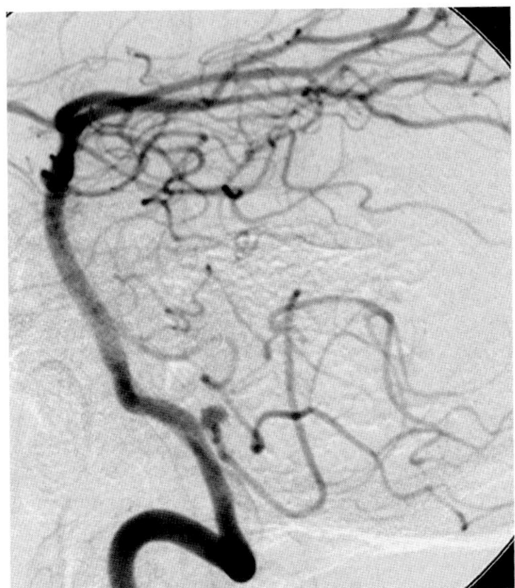

a

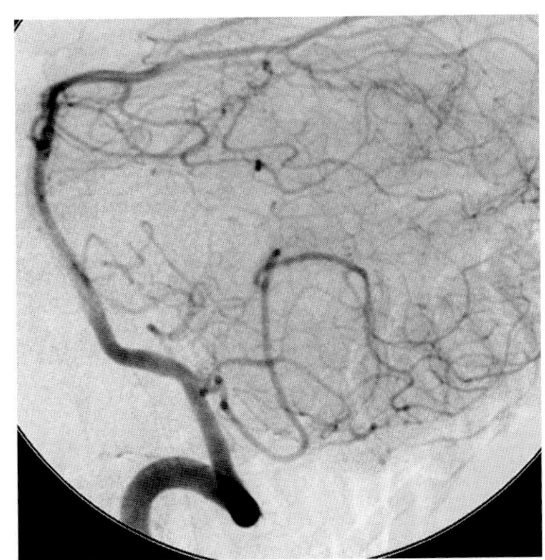

b

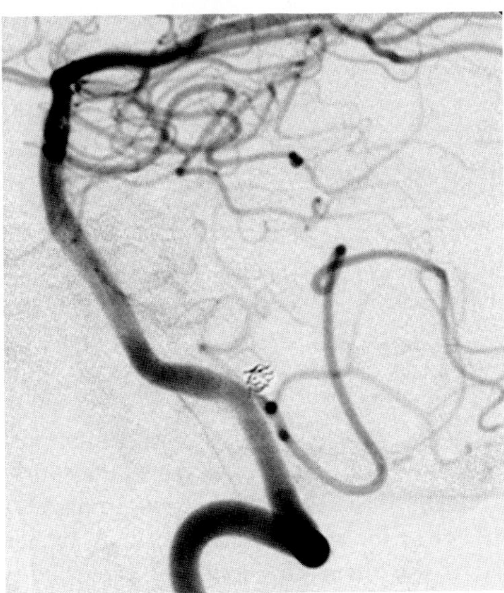

c

Fig. 5.4.41a–c. Before and after selective endosaccular treatment of a PICA aneurysm with preservation of the parent artery, 7-month FU showed a stable obliteration

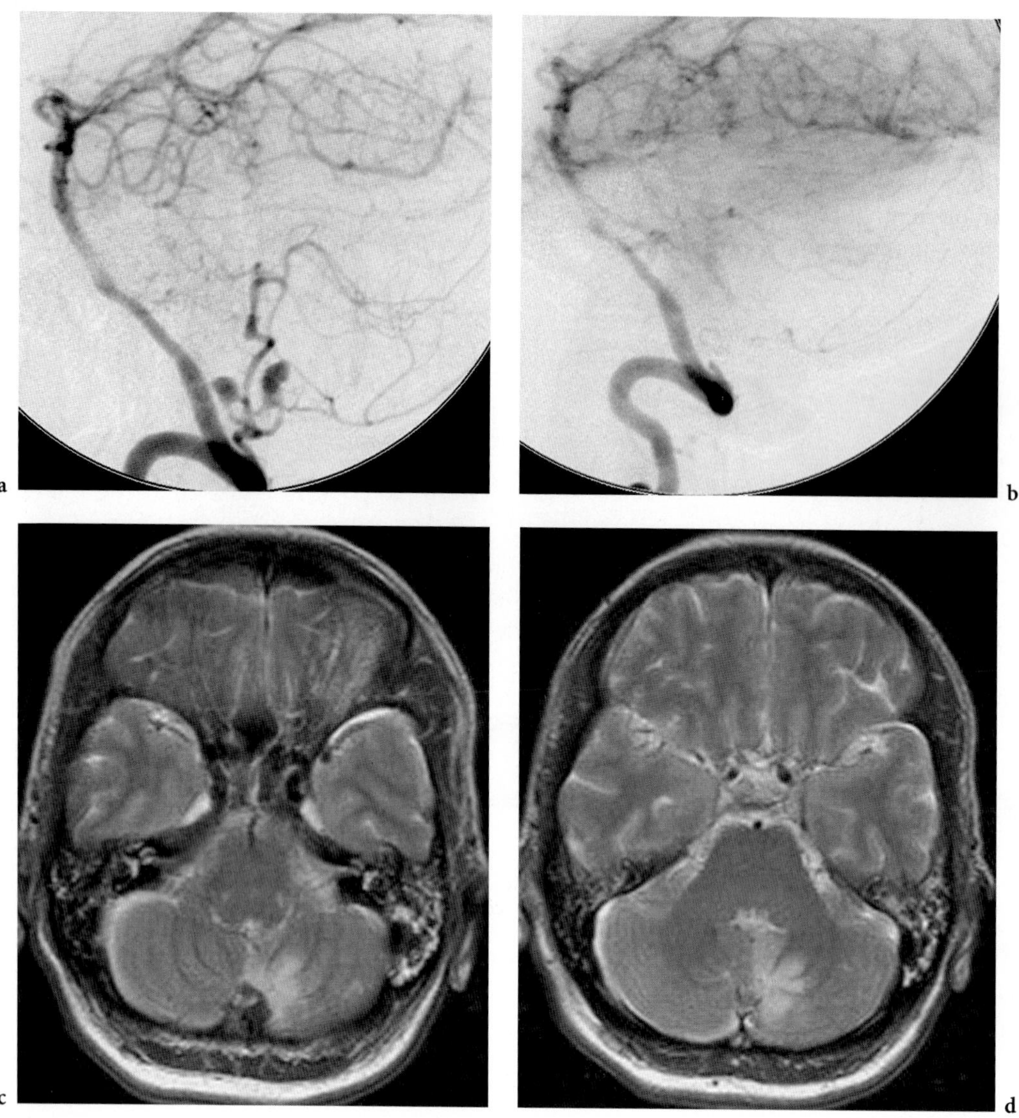

Fig. 5.4.42a–d. Before and after intended endovascular occlusion of a dysplastic PICA revealing at least four aneurysms. MRI: T2 images showed only a very small infarction in the PICA territory without causing clinical symptoms

5.4.9.5.3 Basilar Trunk Aneurysms

Saccular aneurysms of the basilar trunk are rare lesions with an incidence of less than 1% of all intracranial aneurysms. Damage to the perforating arteries is one of the major complications during surgery. Given the high risk of surgery on basilar trunk aneurysms and the simple endovascular access endovascular therapy should be first line treatment option. Van Rooij and colleagues (2003) treated a consecutive series of eight patients with this type of aneurysm, only one was non-ruptured. All patients had a good outcome except one patient who died as a consequence of the SAH. Procedure-related complications were not noted. As a consequence the authors do recommend treatment of aneurysms in this location via the endovascular route as first option. Uda et al. (2001) had the same conclusion. They treated 41 basilar trunk aneurysms and had a morbidity and mortality rate of 2.6% each. The endovascular catheterization of these lesions is relatively simple, in contrast to the complex neurosurgical approaches. Obviously, obliteration of these aneurysms decreases the possibility of unwanted occlusion of perforating arteries to the brainstem and therefore prevents brain stem infarction. In case of a broad base or a very small size a stent to bridge the neck might be necessary.

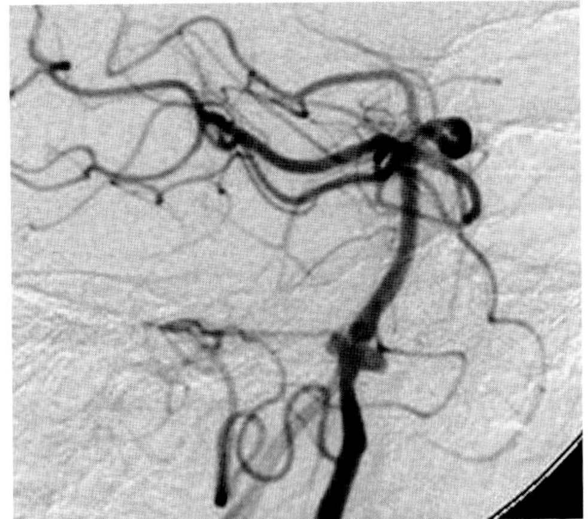
a

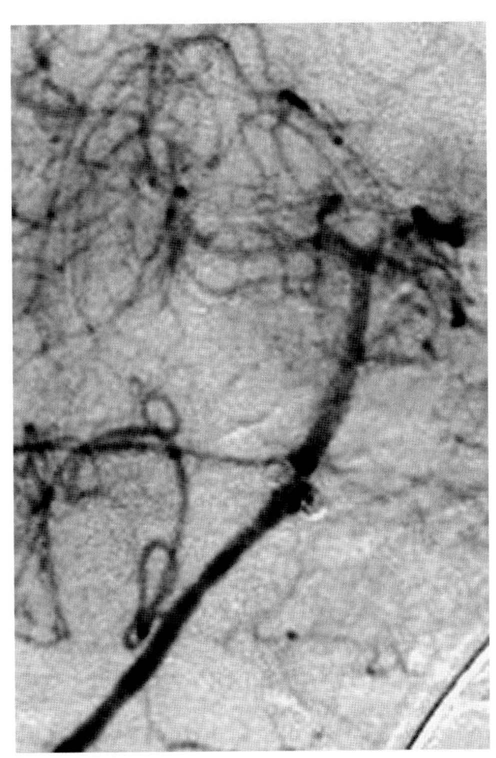
b

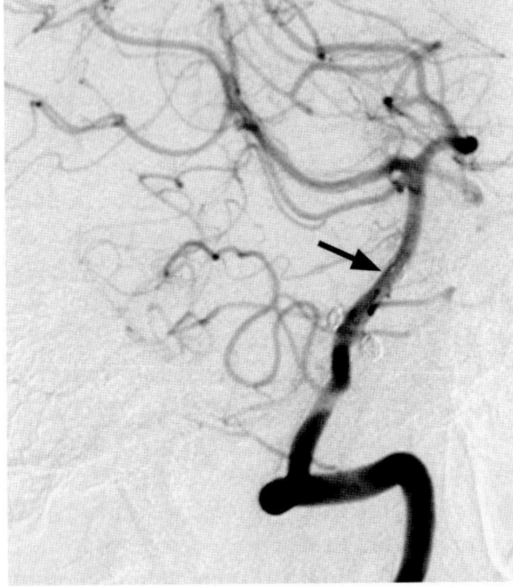
c

Fig. 5.4.43a–c. Conventional angiography: (**a, b**) before and after stent placement in combination with platinum coils to treat two small proximal located basilar stem aneurysms, (**c**) 6-month control angiography demonstrated complete obliteration of the two aneurysms, the distal markers of the stent are slightly seen (*arrow*)

a

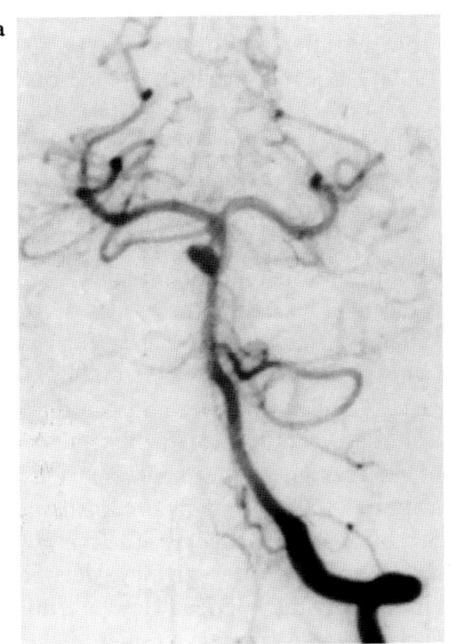

b

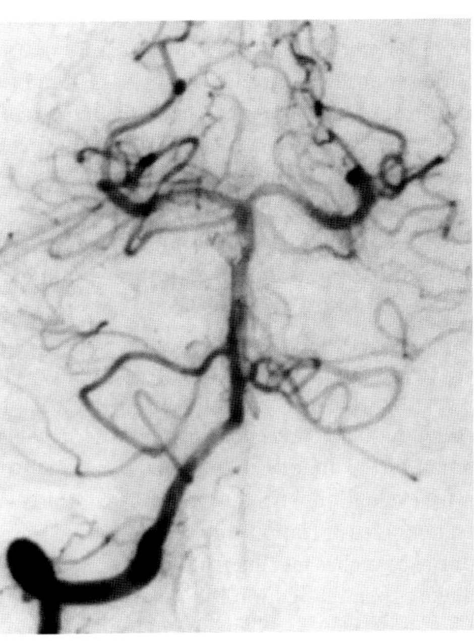

Fig. 5.4.44a,b. Conventional angiography: before and after selective obliteration of a basilar stem aneurysm located in the distal third of the vessel proximal to the origin of the superior cerebellar artery

5.4.10 Special Considerations

5.4.10.1 Giant Aneurysms

Giant aneurysms, defined as larger than 25 mm, are rare intracranial lesions with a prevalence of about 5%–8% of aneurysms. Only one fourth to one third of giant aneurysms present with subarachnoid hemorrhage. Presenting symptoms are usually due to mass effect (75%), intracerebral hemorrhage or thromboembolism. Thrombosis and stroke due to blood clot formation within the aneurysm and subsequent distant emboli, occur in 2%–5% of patients with giant aneurysms. Symptoms are related to the anatomic location, headache is also a frequent symptom. Typically, giant aneurysms in the anterior circulation are in vicinity of the optic pathway, associated with symptoms related to vision. Sixty percent of giant aneurysms occur at the internal carotid artery. The most common site is the cavernous part of the internal carotid artery. Approximately 40% have calcifications in their walls that usually make clipping difficult. These calcifications can easily be identified on CT, which should be part of the diagnostic work-up in all these giant aneurysms. An additional 10% occur at the anterior communicating artery region, 10% are located at the middle cerebral artery. Some 15% of giant aneurysms occur at the top of the basilar artery, and approximately 5% arise from the vertebral artery.

Giant aneurysms are frequently (at least 60%) associated with either partial, or less common complete thrombosis. Recanalization of a completely thrombosed giant aneurysm has been also reported (Lee et al. 1999).

Symptomatic giant aneurysms usually have a grim natural history and poor prognosis.

There are several different strategies available to manage giant aneurysms. This is mainly due to the fact that no single technique is perfect in dealing with all giant aneurysms. Treatment options for giant lesions include surgical clipping, endovascular embolization, and combined approaches. Indirect surgical techniques include proximal occlusion and trapping of the aneurysm. Trapping and proximal ligation are usually definitive treatments provided that the patient‘s collateral circulation can tolerate major vessel occlusion. Depending on the location of the aneurysm, patients should have pre-operative evaluation with temporary balloon occlusion to test tolerance of trapping or proximal ligation. Major arterial branches leaving from the aneurysm dome can make proximal ligation the only therapeutic option. In some patients inadequate collateral circulation mandates the inclusion of an arterial bypass procedure in the therapeutic approach. This is specifically true for patients with giant aneurysms at the MCA bifurcation or the intracranial ICA.

There seems to be a correlation between size and incidence of complications during surgery for unruptured intracranial aneurysms. Aneurysms larger than 2.5 cm (giant aneurysm) in diameter have a 20-fold risk of significant surgical morbidity or poor outcome during surgical treatment. However, giant aneurysms are also not real good candidates for endovascular therapy, since they carry a high risk of recanalization and regrowth, due to the size of aneurysm, nature of coils and continuous flow-related stress on the aneurysm. Pre-existing thrombus within the aneurysm and coil migration into the thrombus may additionally facilitate coil compaction. Up to now it is totally unclear, whether combined techniques with stents and coils might overcome this problem of recanalization.

Endovascular techniques also include parent vessel occlusion using balloons or coils. Proximal balloon occlusion is a useful and often used technique for giant internal carotid artery aneurysms. There are several advantages of intravascular balloon treatment over other treatment modalities. If an extradural aneurysm is excluded from circulation by placing the balloon across or proximal to the aneurysm neck, there is a very low probability of aneurysm filling by collateral circulation. The anatomical dead space is decreased, reducing the incidence of emboli potentially associated with ICA thrombosis. Additionally, there is thrombosis and shrinkage of the aneurysm and decrease of pulsatility. The mass effect is also gradually decreasing.

Unfortunately, transient worsening of mass effect can happen shortly after endovascular therapy (Hecht et al. 1991). There may be also a late increase in mass effect as reported by Blanc et al. (2001) after parent vessel occlusion of the internal carotid artery for a giant supraclinoid aneurysm in a 47-year-old woman, who became hemiparetic and dysphasic 8 days after treatment. It has been shown experimentally that a thrombosed aneurysm may swell up to 15%, specifically if located at the basilar tip. In experimental aneurysms extensive neovascularity was observed within the first week after coil embolization. Increased capillary permeability of these neovessels within the evolving thrombus likely promotes transient enlargement of the aneurysm cavity. Steroid medication (100 mg methylprednisolone three times a day) prior and up to 5 days after therapy might be indicated, and may prevent these delayed complications in an individual patient. However, this is not an evidence-based therapeutic regimen.

5.4.10.1.1 Results of Endovascular Therapy in Giant Aneurysms

Different endovascular techniques may serve as an adjunct to surgery and may further improve therapy of giant aneurysms. In general, therapy of giant aneurysms should be tailored to each patient and always arise from the combined therapeutic plan of neurosurgeons and neurointerventionalists using a multimodality approach to minimize morbidity and mortality. However, as mentioned above: parent vessel occlusion – if tolerated by the patient – is by far the most effective type of treatment. Surgery alone has an extensive risk, endovascular therapy alone has a lower procedural risk but recanalization is a frequent observation during follow-up.

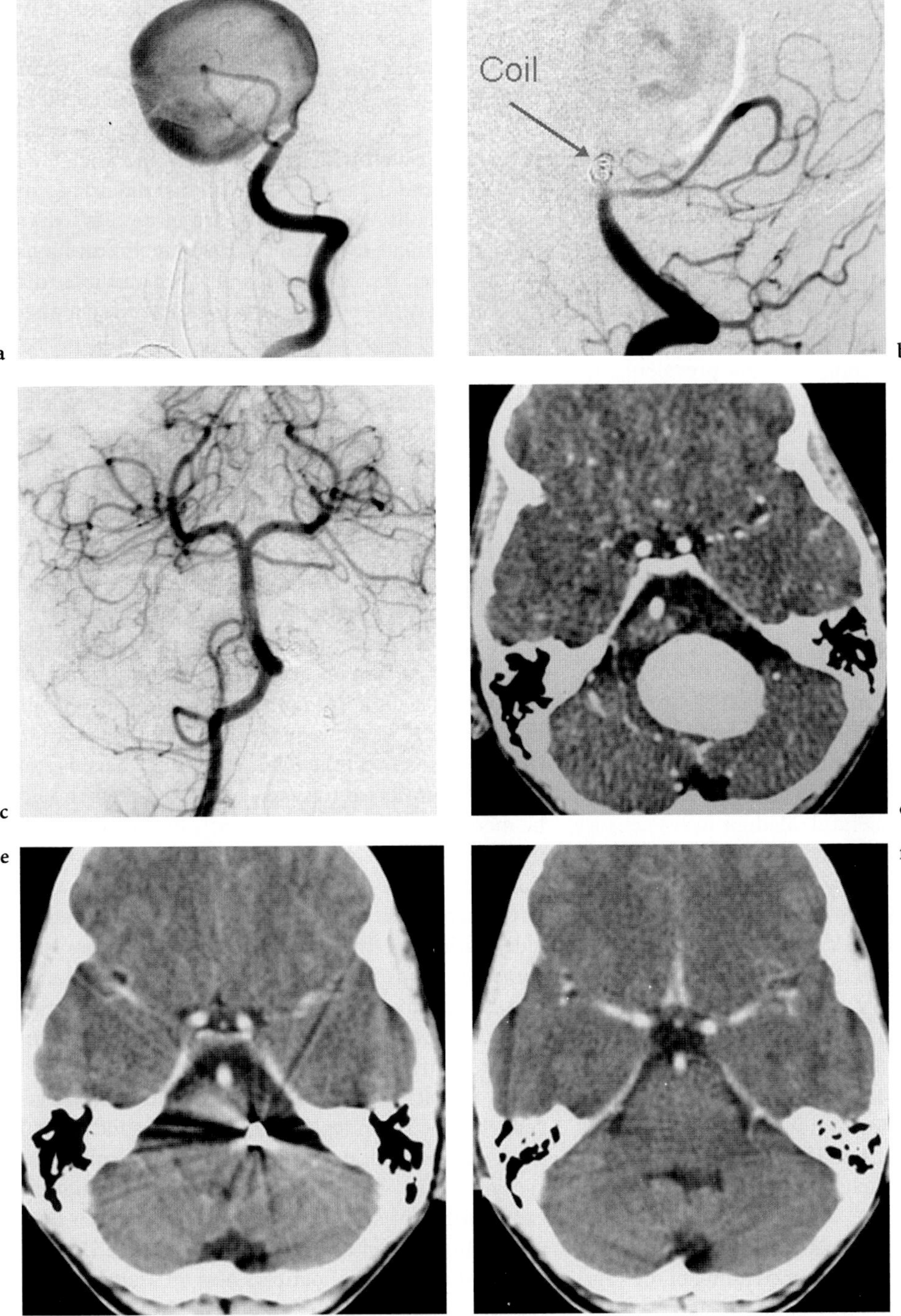

Fig. 5.4.45. **a** PA view. Giant vertebral artery aneurysm in a 9-year-old boy presenting with dizziness, vomiting and nausea. **b** Lateral view. Endovascular occlusion of the left vertebral artery was performed distal to the PICA using one GDC-Vortx-Coil. **c** Injection into the contralateral vertebral artery revealed no retrograde filling of the aneurysm. CT: (**d**) before and (**e, f**) 6 months after vessel occlusion demonstrated complete retraction of the aneurysm

5.4.10.2
Pediatric Aneurysms

The incidence of cerebral aneurysms in children is low. In patients under 15 years of age, it constitutes 1%–2% of all intracranial aneurysms (Patel and Richardson 1971), in children under 5 years, 0.1%–0.05% (Locksley et al. 1966). In a large cooperative study of intracranial aneurysms and subarachnoid hemorrhage including 2627 aneurysms, in only 1.5% of patients the aneurysm ruptured before the age of 19 (Locksley et al. 1966). Analysis of previous reports indicated several distinct characteristics of this entity. There is a predominant male:female ratio approaching 2:1 to 3:1. Compared with adults a high number of these aneurysms arise in the posterior circulation (Allison et al. 1998). Aneurysms in children tend to be large, approximately 30%–45% are giant aneurysms (Patel and Richardson 1971). Ferrante et al. (1988) reported the prevalence of giant aneurysms in children to be 26.8% compared to 2% in adults, and the prevalence for large aneurysms to be 50% compared to 27% in adults. In contrast, multiple aneurysms are less common in children (3%–5%) compared to adults (20%). Presenting symptoms are rather due to the mass effect of the aneurysm than due to aneurysm rupture. Compared to adults there is an increased incidence of infectious or mycotic aneurysms in the pediatric population, frequently secondary to bacterial endocarditis (Allison et al. 1998; Lee et al. 1998). Since general anaesthesia is mostly necessary for balloon occlusion of the internal carotid artery in children and clinical monitoring during occlusion is impossible, monitoring of somatosensory evoked potentials as a simple and reliable neurophysiological technique is very helpful. Median nerve sensory evoked potentials (SEP) may be an ideal monitoring during occlusion of aneurysms of the carotid artery territory because the ICA supplies the hand area of the somatosensory cortex. Likewise, basilar aneurysms may not be effectively monitored with SEP or brain stem auditory evoked potentials because basilar perforator occlusion may not affect either the somatosensory or auditory pathways (Friedman et al. 1987, 1991; Friedman and Grundy 1987). Again: as mentioned above, we do not perform balloon test occlusions any more, but rely more – and in the majority of patients exclusively – on the analysis of the circle of Willis.

Patients who do not tolerate the balloon test occlusion or do not have a simultaneous filling of the veins via the circle of Willis while compressing the target vessel, should undergo extracranial-intracranial bypass before parent vessel occlusion.

5.4.10.3
Aneurysms in the Elderly

Definition of the term "elderly" varies widely. Perhaps the most widely accepted definition for elderly is more than 65 years old, primarily since this is associated commonly with retirement. Incidence of SAH increases with age, from 1.5 to 2.5 per 100,000 per year in the third decade of life to 40 to 78 per 100,000 in the eighth decade of life (Phillips et al. 1980; Sacco et al. 1984). Advanced age is commonly associated with a poorer outcome after SAH (Elliott and Le Roux 1998). This might be for several reasons: older patients are more likely than younger patients to present with a poor clinical status at admission, larger amounts of SAH, and due to a diminished cerebrovascular reserve capacity a higher incidence of symptomatic vasospasm. Additionally, older patients more frequently have preexisting comorbidities, such as hypertension or atherosclerosis, which might independently have an adverse effect on outcome. Anticoagulation therapy for the treatment of atherosclerotic heart or cerebrovascular disease is also more frequent in older patients, which also increases the risk of poor outcome following aneurysmal SAH (Rinkel et al. 1997).

However, when stratifying older patients according to clinical grade, an association of advanced age and outcome is not observed (Elliott and Le Roux 1998). This is in accordance with the results of our institution. As a consequence, we think to decline treatment solely on the basis of advanced age is not justified. The decision to treat elderly patients should be made according to the patient`s overall situation, including clinical grade, overall physiologic condition and associated risk factors.

Conservative treatment of ruptured aneurysms in older patients seems to be associated with a poor outcome (Ellenbogen 1970). There is some evidence that surgically treated elderly patients do better than conservatively treated patients after aneurysm rupture. Fridikson et al. (1995) reported that two thirds of patients between 70 and 74 treated surgically returned to independent living and good mental state, whereas among 93 age-matched controls, refusion of surgery because of age, 75% suffered significant morbidity and mortality with more than 50% died within 3 months (Fridriksson et al. 1995).

In a small series of patients over 80 years old with ruptured anterior circulation aneurysms and a poor

Hunt and Hess grade of III, Hamada et al. (2001) reported a bad outcome for the conservatively treated patients, and still disappointing results for the surgically treated patients. The best results were obtained for MCA aneurysms.

Although little data is available on the results of endovascular aneurysm therapy in elderly patients, the reported results suggest this modality is promising in this age group (Rowe et al. 1996). In our opinion, endovascular therapy should be more strongly considered as first line therapy for elderly patients with SAH whenever possible. This way the aneurysms can be embolized in the acute phase with coils and preventing rebleeding (Fridriksson et al. 1995; Hamada et al. 2001).

Atherosclerotic vascular disease is more frequently in elderly patients and may be associated with more tortuous vessel anatomy. Superselective catheterizations of distal cerebral vessels might thus become technically more difficult. Atherosclerotic carotid bifurcation disease is frequently associated in patients with advanced age and might increase the risk of thromboembolic complications. In selected cases, a combined approach, first stenting of the carotid artery stenosis and subsequently coil embolization of the ruptured aneurysm might be a therapeutic option. Aneurysms at the anterior communicating artery are reported to be associated with a higher incidence of poor neuropsychologic outcome than aneurysms in other locations (Bornstein et al. 1987). In elderly patients even subtle changes in neuropsychology can have a strong influence.

5.4.10.3.1
Unruptured Aneurysms in the Elderly

Treatment decisions for unruptured aneurysms in older patients require estimation of the patient`s individual life expectancy and the risk of aneurysm rupture. Since the last results of the ISUIA study the critical size seems to be 7 mm and – beside size – location at the posterior wall of the ICA and the posterior circulation per se seem to have a higher risk of rupture.

Taylor et al. (1995) reported that only 2% of unruptured aneurysms in elderly patients rupture within 2.5 years of diagnosis. Considering these data, aggressive treatment, either surgical or endovascular do not appear to be beneficial. In any case, careful consideration should be given to the patient`s general health, coexisting morbidities, and personal and familial background before considering aneurysm therapy (Taylor et al. 1995). However, for many patients an explanation of the statistics is not the solution of the problem. If the first physician compares the – let‘s say – incidental aneurysm with a bomb in the head, quality of life usually drops dramatically and sometimes occlusion of the aneurysm is the only way to overcome the psychologic problem of the patient.

5.4.10.4
Multiple Aneurysms

The frequency of multiple aneurysms ranges from 5%–33% (Andrews and Spiegel 1979; Bigelow 1955; Inagawa 1991; McKissock et al. 1964; Mizoi et al. 1989) and seems to be higher in females than in males (Andrews and Spiegel 1979; McKissock et al. 1964). Multiple aneurysms are found in up to 34% of patients presenting with aneurysmal SAH (Rinne et al. 1994). In our patient population every third patient had two or more aneurysms.

The optimal treatment of associated – and asymptomatic aneurysms is still controversial. Treatment of multiple aneurysms should always consider location, patient‘s age, and neurological status, as well as anatomic relation to the symptomatic aneurysm. Some experts think that surgical treatment of unruptured aneurysms is not indicated. However, because of the presumed natural history of unruptured aneurysms and the progress in therapy the majority of neurosurgeons agree that associated aneurysms should be secured and that the risk of treating them is low. The symptomatic aneurysm should be treated first and the others can be treated in the same setting or alternatively later on. The localization of blood on the CT scan can help to identify the aneurysm responsible for the SAH. Nehls et al. (1985) showed that in patients presenting with multiple aneurysms and SAH the ruptured aneurysm could be correctly identified in 97.5% on the basis of clinical, CT and angiographic data. However, there is also evidence in the literature that blood distribution on CT does not enable identification of the site of the ruptured aneurysms.

Other hints may be: The larger and more irregularly shaped aneurysm is usually the one which has ruptured. If there are two aneurysms at one artery the most proximal and large aneurysm is the one that usually has ruptured.

However, little is known of the overall management outcome of multiple aneurysms. In an unselected series of 302 patients with multiple intracranial aneurysms Rinne et al. (1995) reported the management outcome one year after treatment significantly

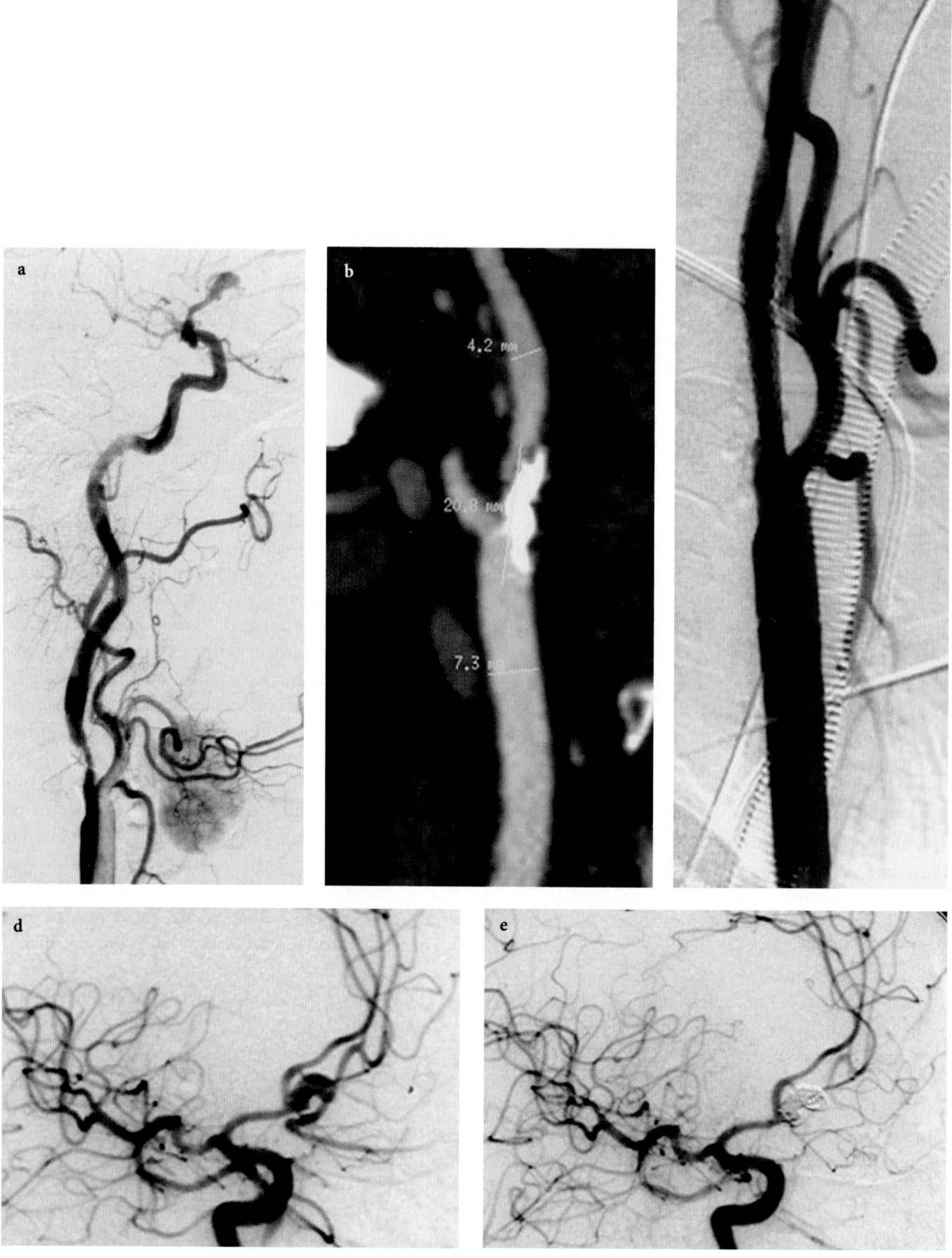

Fig. 5.4.46a–e. High-grade ICA stenosis due to atheromatous plaques in a patient with a ruptured Acom aneurysm. After stenting of the stenosis under heparin the Acom aneurysm was successfully embolized, the patient got antiplatelet therapy immediately after this two-step procedure

poorer for patients with multiple than for those with single intracranial aneurysms. The frequency of poor outcome (GCS 3–5) was most evident in patients with Hunt and Hess Grades II and III (29%), compared to patients with a single aneurysm (19%) in the same clinical grade (RINNE et al. 1995). The authors attribute their results mainly to the increased manipulation of cerebral arteries and brain tissue associated with increased delayed neurologic deficits in this patient group. This is comparable with the data by VAJDA (1992) reporting a 26% frequency of poor outcome during long-term follow-up in patients with multiple intracranial aneurysms. However, most surgical series have opposite results, with equal results in patients with multiple and single cerebral aneurysms (INAGAWA 1991; MIZOI et al. 1989; YASARGIL 1984).

A major advantage of endovascular therapy is the possibility to treat more than one aneurysm in a single procedure. Additionally, the increased manipulation of cerebral arteries and brain tissue during surgery can be avoided by the endovascular approach. There are recommendations to treat only one aneurysm of the same artery or vascular territory within a single procedure. This is not the policy in our institution. On a case-by-case selection our policy is to treat any further aneurysm during the same procedure, independent of the anatomic location, if the first symptomatic (ruptured) non-giant aneurysm was quickly treated without difficulties. This is in accordance with the results reported by SOLANDER et al. (1999) evaluating their results of GDC treatment of multiple aneurysms in single-stage procedures. The authors reported 38 consecutive patients with 101 cerebral aneurysms, 79 of which were treated with GDC, 14 neurosurgically, and eight left untreated. A total of 25 patients (66%) underwent treatment for all aneurysms within 3 days after admission. Follow up angiographic studies demonstrated unchanged or improved results in 94% of patients and an overall excellent clinical outcome in 89%. The authors conclude that endovascular GDC treatment of multiple cerebral aneurysms, regardless of their location, can be performed safely in one session. In the same way, this single-staged procedure may protect patients from rebleeding and eliminates the risk of mistakenly treating only the unruptured aneurysm (SOLANDER et al. 1999).

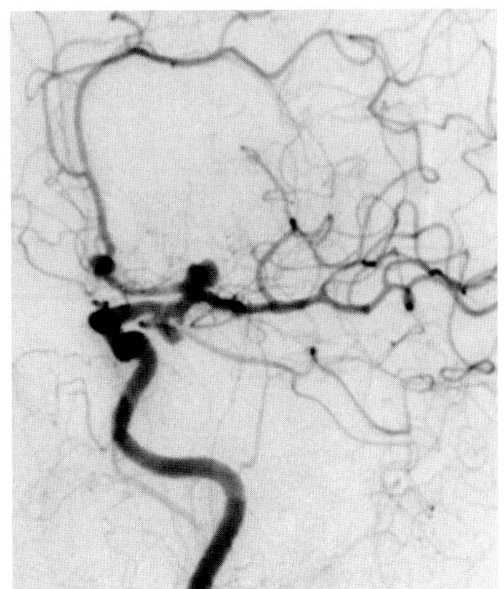
a

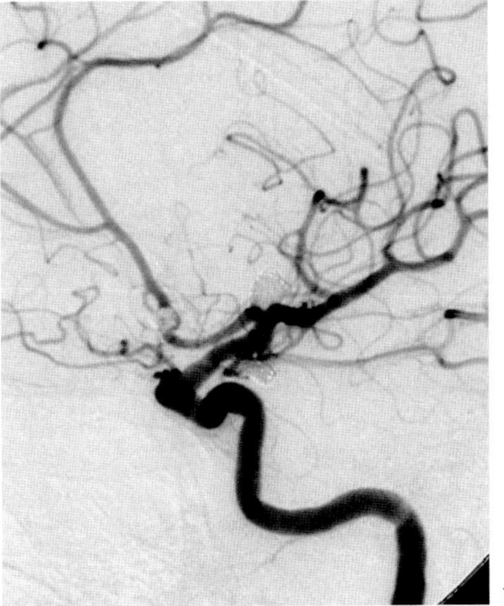
b

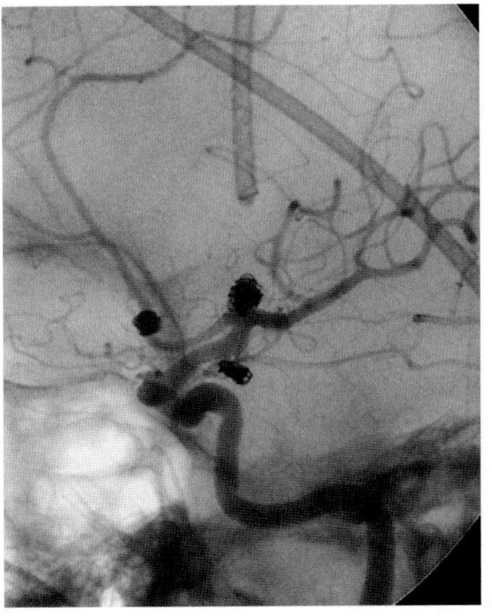
c

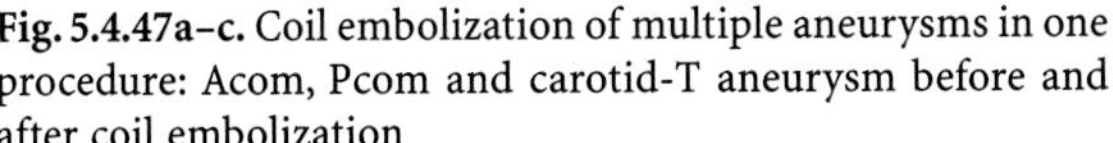

Fig. 5.4.47a–c. Coil embolization of multiple aneurysms in one procedure: Acom, Pcom and carotid-T aneurysm before and after coil embolization

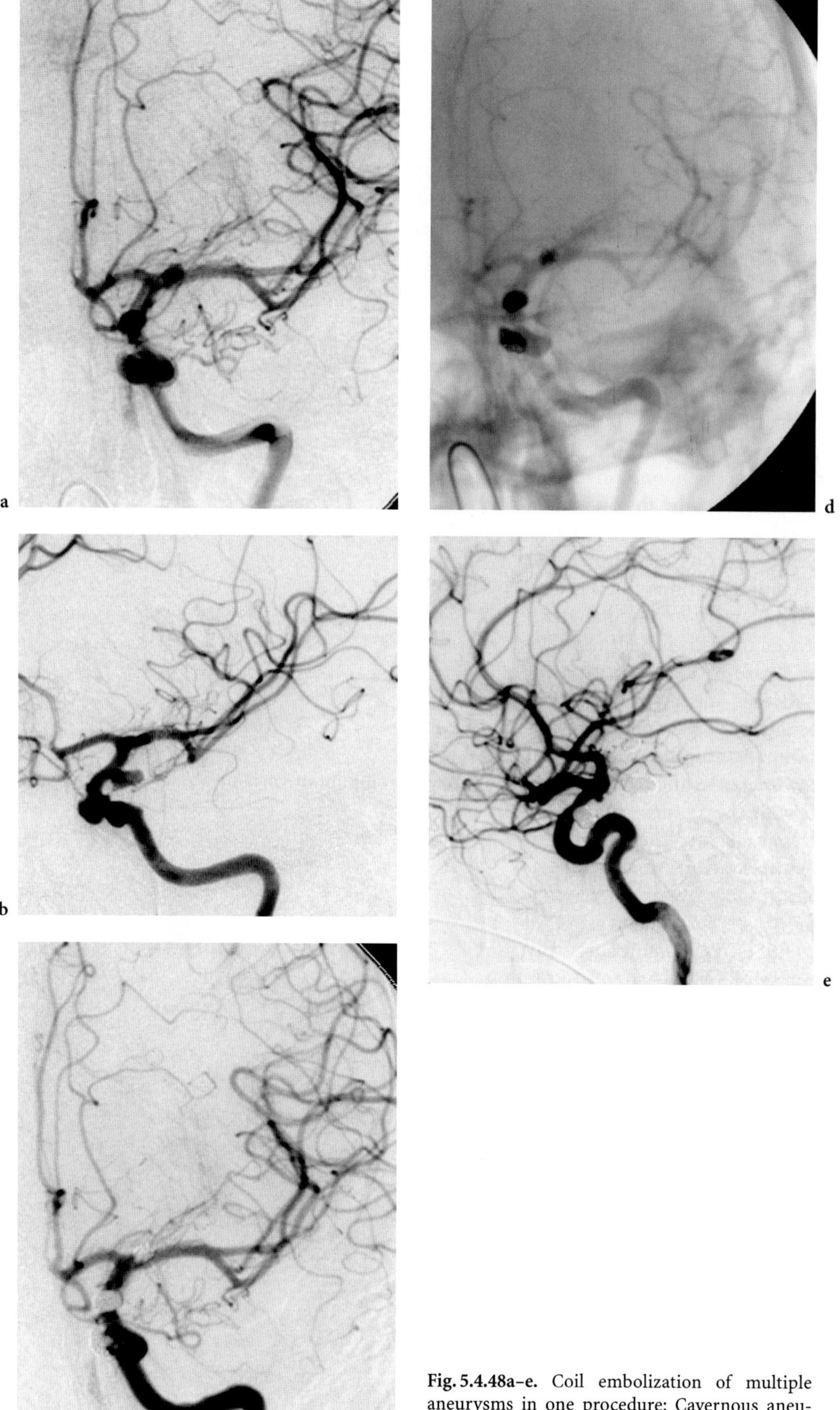

Fig. 5.4.48a–e. Coil embolization of multiple aneurysms in one procedure: Cavernous aneurysm, Pcom and carotid-T aneurysm before and after coil embolization

PIEROT et al. (1997) reported their experience of 53 patients with a total of 128 aneurysms. Endovascular treatment was performed in 67 aneurysms in 46 patients, resulting in complete occlusion in 58 aneurysms and partial occlusion in nine. Permanent neurologic complications occured in 6.5%, one patient rebled. In patients with multiple unruptured aneurysms the authors treated two aneurysms at the same time if endovascular treatment proves easy (PIEROT et al. 1997).

Because of the patients poor grade, old age, or difficult aneurysms it is not always possible to occlude all aneurysms in one setting. In the series of RINNE et al. (1995) only 58% of all patients with multiple aneurysms had all aneurysms clipped or treated endovascularly.

5.4.10.5 Incompletely Treated Aneurysms/Aneurysm Remnants

Although postoperative angiography is the only objective method for confirming the absence of any aneurysmal remnant, the widespread trend is not to perform postoperative angiography after microsurgical clipping. Since intraoperative techniques like checking exact clip location and absence of neighbouring perforators under the microscope, and needle puncture of the aneurysm are standard parts of aneurysm surgery the need of postoperative angiography may be questioned. The usefulness versus potential complications and costs have to be evaluated and its legitimacy discussed. However, we think that postoperative angiography is at least justified in all "difficult" and large aneurysms. Our institutional policy is to routinely perform postoperative angiography in all patients treated neurosurgically.

This is the only way to make completely sure that there is no remaining aneurysm or aneurysm remnant. Even opening of the aneurysm sac after clipping, a standard procedure in many neurosurgical institutions, does not exclude residual neck remnants proximal to the clip. Additionally, imperfect clip placement or delayed clip dislocation may remain unrecognized until postoperative angiography is performed.

There is another perspective that recommends postoperative angiograms in all patients: Sometimes the incomplete clipped aneurysm offers a new opportunity for the endovascular approach. A broad neck may be pretty small after incomplete clipping, a giant aneurysm may be turned into a just large one or the anatomy may have become clearer after inspection.

In up to 4% of patients postoperative angiograms reveal an expected or unexpected aneurysm residuum due to incomplete clipping (LIN et al. 1989). In a consecutive series of 305 clipped aneurysms, SINDOU et al. (1998) reported an incomplete clipping in 18 out of 305 aneurysms (5.9%), with only a neck remnant in 3.9% and neck and sac remnant in 1.9%, amenable for complementary retreatment. A recent clinical data review of six series of clipped aneurysms which were checked by early postoperative angiography, revealed that 82 aneurysms (5.2%) out of a total of 1397 patients demonstrated residual filling (THORNTON et al. 2000b).

Data on cerebral aneurysms treated by an endovascular approach also confirmed that a significant number of cases had either a residual or recurrent aneurysm. VINUELA et al. reported a multi-centre study on the results of GDC treatment for cerebral aneurysms in 403 patients. They reported an aneurysm remnant in an aneurysm-size dependent fashion: 25.6% of small aneurysms with a small neck, 52% of small aneurysms with a wide neck, 62.1% of large aneurysms and 50% of giant aneurysms demonstrated a remnant after initial treatment. During follow-up to 36 months after treatment, nine patients (2.2%) with incompletely embolized aneurysms rebled (VINUELA et al. 1997). In another review by BYRNE and coworkers (1999) 36% of cases had an aneurysm remnant of variable size after initial treatment, 14.7% of aneurysm remnants had enlarged to some degree. Giant aneurysms had a 100% recurrence rate (BYRNE et al. 1999).

The incidence of aneurysm regrowing after incomplete treatment may have been underestimated. Even a small portion of aneurysm neck has the potential to enlarge over time. Although small aneurysm remnants measuring from 1 to 2 mm may not justify retreatment, the risk of progressive enlargement to a dangerous aneurysm should be considered. Long-term angiographic – preferentially done with MR – reassessment may be valuable not to miss aneurysm enlargement (SINDOU et al. 1998).

Incomplete treatment of an aneurysm, either by clipping or endovascular, may result in recurrent hemorrhage with serious or devastating consequences (DRAKE and ALLCOCK 1973; EBINA et al. 1982; LE ROUX et al. 1998; LIN et al. 1989). The risk of rebleeding from an aneurysm remnant has not been statistically studied in a larger series of patients. One might assume that these lesions might have at least the same risk of rupture as asymptomatic aneurysms, which has been evaluated at an average of 0.5% per year (GIANNOTTA and LITOFSKY 1995;

Le Roux et al. 1998; Thielen et al. 1997). Feuerberg et al. (1987) looked at the natural history of these remnants and concluded that the rebleeding risk is between 0.38 and 0.79% per year. Lin and coworkers (1989) reported 19 patients who had an enlargement of a previously documented small aneurysm remnant after surgical clipping with 14 of these patients presenting with rebleeding.

There are some predisposing factors for postoperative aneurysm remnants such as aneurysm size and topographic peculiarities: Large or giant aneurysms are associated with a higher frequency of aneurysm remnants as well as neurosurgical difficult anatomic localizations such as carotido-ophthalmic region, which requires removal of the clinoid.

Since nowadays endovascular aneurysm therapy is an important part in the management of SAH, comparison of surgical and endovascular methods regarding completeness of obliteration is of major importance. The reported results with coil embolization are very variable according to the series, techniques used and aneurysmal size. In Raymond and Roy's (1997) series a neck remnant was present in 37%. The study by Vinuela et al. (1997) in 403 patients clearly demonstrated that the completeness of aneurysm occlusion is strongly dependent on aneurysm size. In small aneurysms the complete occlusion rate was 70.8%, whereas in large or giant aneurysms it was in the range of 50%. Using the "remodeling technique" for wide-necked aneurysms Moret et al. (1997) reported aneurysm remnants in 17% of the cases and incomplete occlusion in only 6%.

This leads to the further question concerning the management of the aneurysm remnant or residual neck: again surgical, or endovascular, or no therapy? Feuerberg and colleagues (1987) found that the incidence of rehemorrhage of an aneurysm remnant is 3.7%, and the risk of rupture is up to 0.8% per year, warranting retreatment of the residual aneurysm at least in young patients. However, Feuerberg et al. (1987) reported that up to 50% of neurosurgeons believe that a second surgical approach would not improve the situation. Perioperative scarring, the frequent need to remove the primary surgical clip, increased incidence of intraoperative rupture all add to the increased risk of such a repeat operation (Boet et al. 2001). In any case, this remains a difficult field and a complex group of patients. However, we recommend performing postoperative angiography in all patients after clipping and considering the endovascular route for those patients with aneurysm remnants. For coiled patients it is even more important to have follow-up imaging at least for 3 years.

5.4.10.6 Combined Therapies

Neurosurgery and interventional neuroradiology are not competitive therapies, but the complementary nature of techniques offers the best chance to reduce treatment morbidity and improve long-term outcome in difficult aneurysms. The primary modality of treatment, the anatomy and configuration of the aneurysm, the radiologist's and the neurosurgeon's opinion and the ease or difficulty of the retreatment procedure using either method and the risks involved with each, all have to be considered in the decision making process. However, since ISAT, the endovascular modality should clearly be the first choice, if – and this should be borne very much in mind – the endovascular expertise is available.

For complex aneurysms a combined approach of endovascular and surgical treatment may use the strength of both methods in a synergistic way. There are different management paradigms of such a combined philosophy available:

- Clipping after partial endovascular occlusion
- Coiling after partial surgical clipping
- Temporary balloon occlusion during clipping (see Fig. 5.4.17)
- Superselective angiography prior to aneurysm surgery

5.4.10.6.1 Clipping After Partial Endovascular Occlusion

GDC treatment does not exclude subsequent surgical clipping. Graves et al. (1995) reported two patients in whom surgical clipping of incompletely embolized aneurysms was performed without significant problems (Graves et al. 1995). However, in some cases clipping after coiling might be difficult, often requiring prolonged temporary vessel occlusion. Additionally, opening of the aneurysm for coil extraction might become necessary for final clip placement (Asgari et al. 2002; Batjer and Samson 1992; Solomon et al. 1996).

The primary goal of endovascular aneurysm therapy is to completely obliterate the aneurysm. However, for acutely ruptured and complex aneurysms in poor grade patients a therapeutic alternative might be a combined sequential approach: first to treat the aneurysm by partial coil embolization without the demand of achieving complete aneurysm obliteration. This way one might achieve a temporary protection against early rebleeding, give the patient the chance for clinical recovery and offer the final and definite occlusion later on.

5.4.10.6.2
Coiling After Partial Surgical Clipping

There have been several reports on completion of aneurysm occlusion by endovascular technique after partial clipping (FORSTING et al. 1996; FRASER et al. 1994). In this setting, the reduced neck size after incomplete clipping may represent a technical advantage for endovascular therapy. Wide-neck aneurysms might thereby be transformed into small-neck aneurysms. For complex aneurysms which cannot be treated by either modality alone, this staged procedure of initial partial clipping with narrowing of the aneurysm neck and subsequent endovascular aneurysm obliteration may be considered as therapy.

Entering the aneurysm with the microcatheter might sometimes represent a problem, which can be overcome in most cases by appropriate shaping of the wire and microcatheter. However, there will remain some patients in whom the partially clipped aneurysm neck may be too small to allow the microcatheter to enter the sac or too wide to retain the coils.

5.4.10.6.3
Coiling After Coiling

Surgery of a partially coiled or recanalized aneurysm can be difficult and some authors consider it to be associated with increased risk and higher morbidity (HOROWITZ et al. 1999). If at all possible, our recommendation is, if anatomy is favourable, to retreat all previously coiled, but recurrent aneurysms by a second endovascular approach. If the remnant or recurrent aneurysm is of a reasonable size the 2nd endovascular attempt is possible in the majority of patients. The decision to treat (or not to treat) is sometimes more difficult than the treatment itself. Is it really necessary to retreat a previously unruptured aneurysm with a 3-mm remnant? Probably not, if this remnant is stable during follow-up. The situation is different if a previously ruptured aneurysm reveals a growing remnant over 6–12 months. But you can probably imagine, that there is a number of patients just in between both extremes.

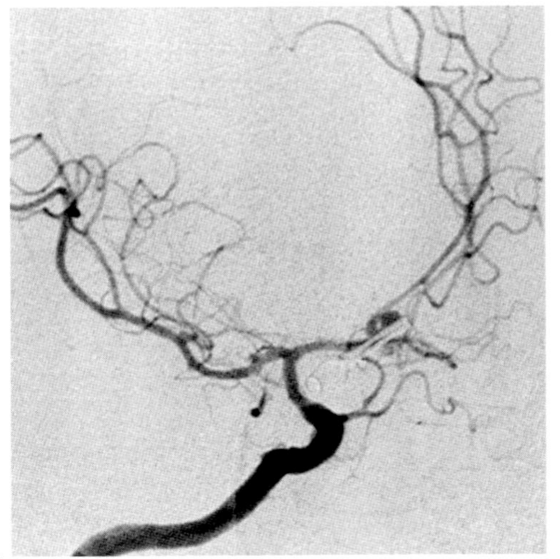
a

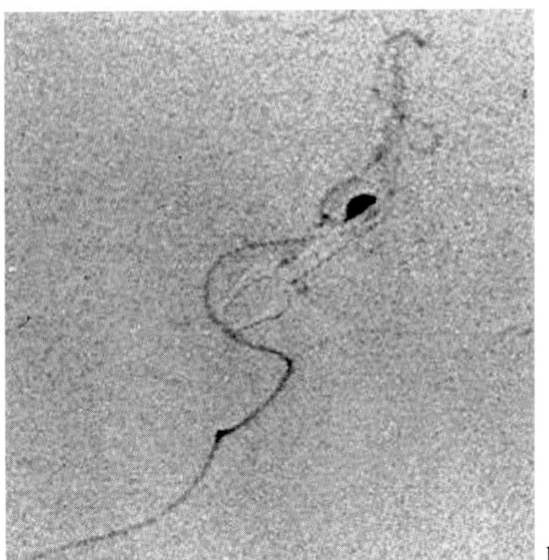
b

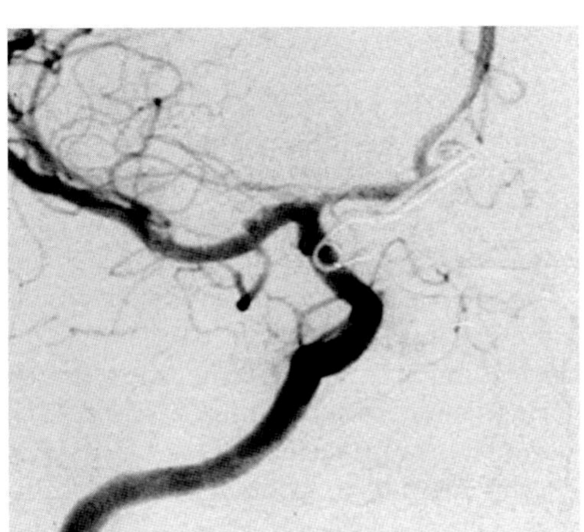
c

Fig. 5.4.49a–c. Coiling after clipping. Endovascular treatment of a small Acom aneurysm remnant after incomplete clipping.

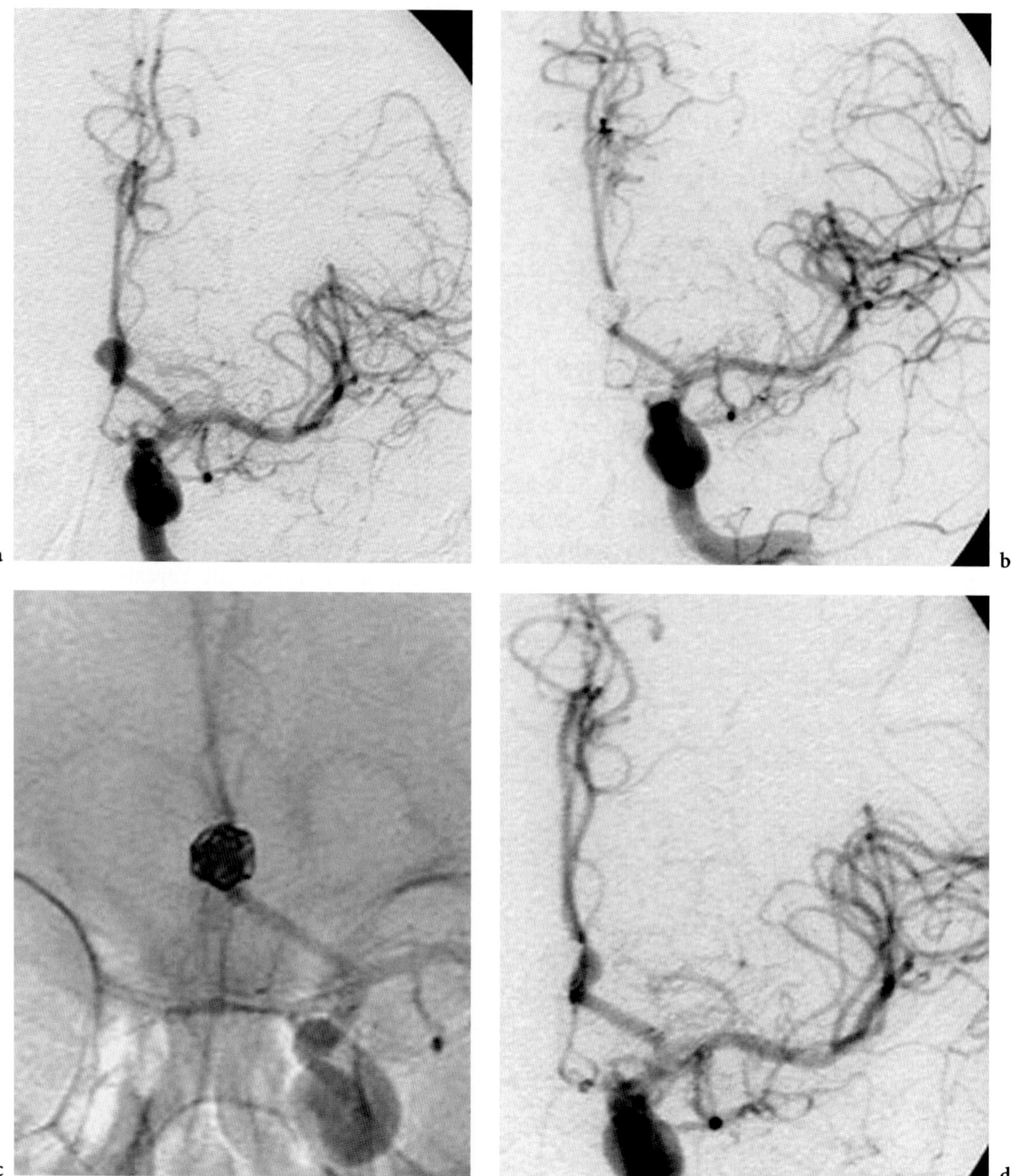

5.4.10.7 Complications of Endovascular Therapy

Endovascular treatment is potentially associated with procedural complications induced by the treatment itself. Mainly, there are two categories of complications: thromboembolic events and aneurysm rupture.

Ischemic complications are either due to a thrombosis of the aneurysm bearing arterial segment or due to an embolus either into the aneurysm bearing artery or into another artery.

Thrombosis of the parent artery probably develops at the interface of the platinum coils due to aggregation of platelets. This complication is observed more often in broad based aneurysms, e.g. in giant aneurysms of the ICA. On the other hand, an embolus generates most often in the guiding catheter system. Since this complication can occur away from the aneurysm, it is important to perform control angiograms during the intervention using a large field of view to cover all relevant vessels.

Procedural morbidity of endovascular treatment ranges between 3.7% and about 10%, mortal-

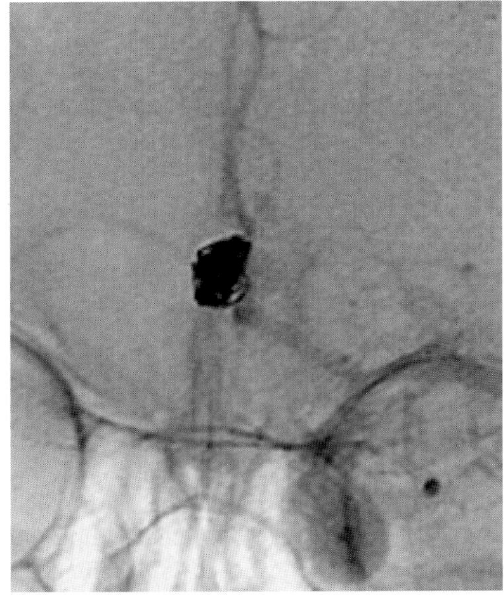
e

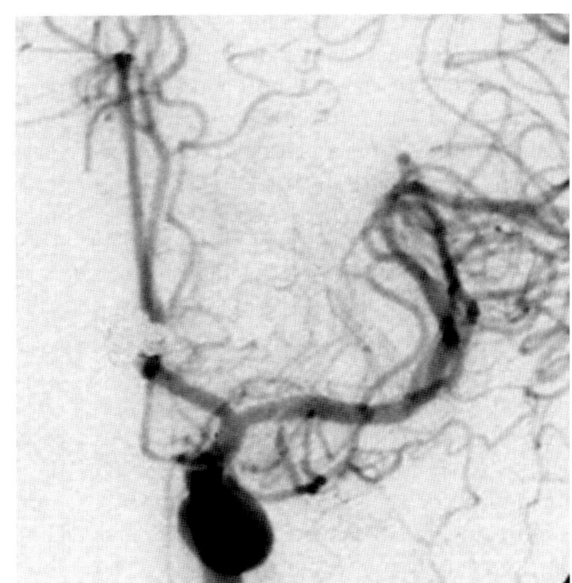
f

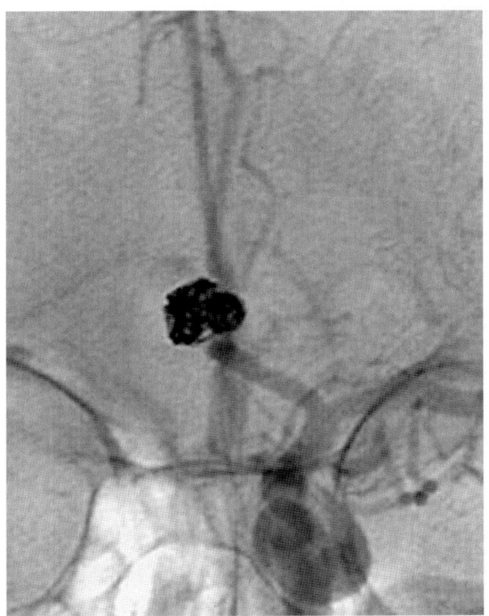
g

Fig. 5.4.50a–g. Retreatment after coil compaction („coiling after coiling"). Before and after endovascular treatment of an Acom aneurysm with complete obliteration, 6-month follow-up demonstrated partial aneurysm recanalization due to coil compaction. Retreatment was successfully performed

ity between 0% and 2.1%. These numbers are well evaluated in patients with unruptured aneurysm to exclude complications due to the SAH itself (Cognard et al. 1997; Johnston et al. 2000; Qureshi et al. 2000; Wanke et al. 2002). Johnston et al. (2000) reported about a very high number (10%) of cranial nerve palsies after endovascular therapy. This can only be explained by the large number of giant aneurysms treated with coils resulting in compression of a cranial nerve by the coil mass (Johnston et al. 2000). However, thromboembolic complications do not necessarily lead to neurologic deterioration of the patient. Qureshi et al. (2000) had 8.2% thromboembolic events during coiling which resulted in neurological deterioration in only 5.4% of the patients.

While analysing data about complications of endovascular therapy aneurysm localization plays an important role. It turns out that treating an aneurysms at the site of the MCA bifurcation is associated with a higher complication rate than treating an aneurysm at another location (7% versus 3% for Acom aneurysms (Cognard et al. 1997). Probably the complex anatomy of the MCA bifurcation might be the reason for this circumstance.

To reduce the risk of thromboembolic events, most of the neurointerventional centres anticoagulate the patient periprocedurally. Thereby, most of the groups at least double the ACT to 250–300 s. Postprocedural heparinization reduces the incidence of thromboembolic events from 9.3% to 5.9% (Qureshi et al. 2000) and is usually maintained for another 24–48 h after intervention. Although no scientific data exist about antiplatelet therapy and prevention of thromboembolic events during or after endovascular treatment, administration of low dose aspirin might (e.g. 100 mg per day) reduce symptomatic ischemic events.

If, beside this regimen, clotting occurs, elevation of blood pressure (mean arterial blood pressure 90-100mmHg), reassurance of efficient heparinization and "wait and see" for a couple of minutes is the first step. If control angiogram shows growing thrombus or no improvement occurs within 10 min and if no retrograde collateralization of the occluded vessel is visible, administration of a GPIIb/IIIa antagonist, e. g. abciximab, might be necessary. Administration should be performed in bolus fractions of 2 mg, either intra-arterial – however, this is an off-label use – or intravenously, up to 10 mg and if diminishing of the thrombus is noted, low-dose abciximab infusion should be continued. GPIIb/IIIa antagonists may induce thrombocytopenia that is probably attributed to an immunological phenomena, therefore, platelets should be monitored.

If the thrombus does not resolve local intra-arterial lysis might be necessary. In unruptured aneurysms, fibrinolytic agents are an obvious option. In ruptured aneurysms, fibrinolytic agents should be used with extreme caution because rebleeding might end in a catastrophic situation even if the aneurysm is completely occluded on DSA.

Aneurysm rupture is another complication which can occur during the intervention. Aneurysm rupture has continued to be one of the most feared complications of endovascular aneurysm therapy. Although any interventional neuroradiologist treating acutely ruptured aneurysms may be confronted with this complication, only few data regarding frequency, causes, management and outcome of such ruptures during endovascular treatment are available (Halbach et al. 1991; McDougall et al. 1998; Ricolfi et al. 1998). However, aneurysmal rupture during endovascular treatment could represent a devastating complication. There are many possible mechanisms of aneurysm rupture during treatment: rupture can occur coincidentally during diagnostic angiography or endovascular treatment. Increased blood pressure during injection of contrast may contribute to rerupture of an acutely ruptured aneurysm (Saitoh et al. 1995). Aneurysm rupture might also be due to perforation with the guidewire or microcatheter, or might occur during coil placement. Clinical sequelae may be variable, ranging from slight leakage of contrast into the subarachnoid space to massive SAH or intraparenchymal hematoma with severe intracranial hypertension.

Embolization of the aneurysm can be continued in most cases, and the majority of patients with treatment-related SAH survive without serious sequelae and with a better outcome than anticipated (Doerfler et al. 2001). In our experience the degree of vasospasms – these can occur immediately – is the most important predictor of patient's outcome: immediate severe vasospasms correlate with a bad clinical outcome. Anyway, it is extremely helpful in this situation to have the external CSF drainage in place before endovascular therapy starts.

5.4.10.8
Monitoring and Therapy of Vasospasm

Transcranial Doppler sonography (TCD) is a useful non-invasive monitoring tool in SAH patients. The detection of vasospasm is possible with transcranial Doppler, by means of increased blood flow velocity from arterial narrowing in the middle cerebral artery and the posterior circulation. However, there is uncertainty about the diagnostic specificity of TCD. Only velocities above 120–200 cm/s are highly predictive for the diagnosis of vasospasm (Vora et al. 1999). Compared to angiography, the sensitivity and specificity of TCD is good for the middle cerebral artery. For all other arteries there is a lack of evidence of accuracy or of usefulness of TCD. Additionally, TCD cannot distinguish symptomatic from asymptomatic vasospasm. The crucial point for the patient is to be in the hand's of an excellent ICU physician, preferentially a neurosurgeon or a neurologist. Both are familiar with acute or slow onset of neurological deficits and it is the clinical history that leads to an endovascular approach for vasospasm.

Quantification of cerebral tissue perfusion and earlier detection of ischemic injury would be nice to have in order to guide therapy in SAH patients with vasospasm. New imaging techniques, such as perfusion (PWI)- and diffusion (DWI)-weighted magnetic resonance imaging might enable very early identification of ischemic areas (Minematsu et al. 1992; Moseley et al. 1990; Warach et al. 1992). PWI is a non-invasive method often used to demonstrate the perfusion reduction in focal ischemia in animal

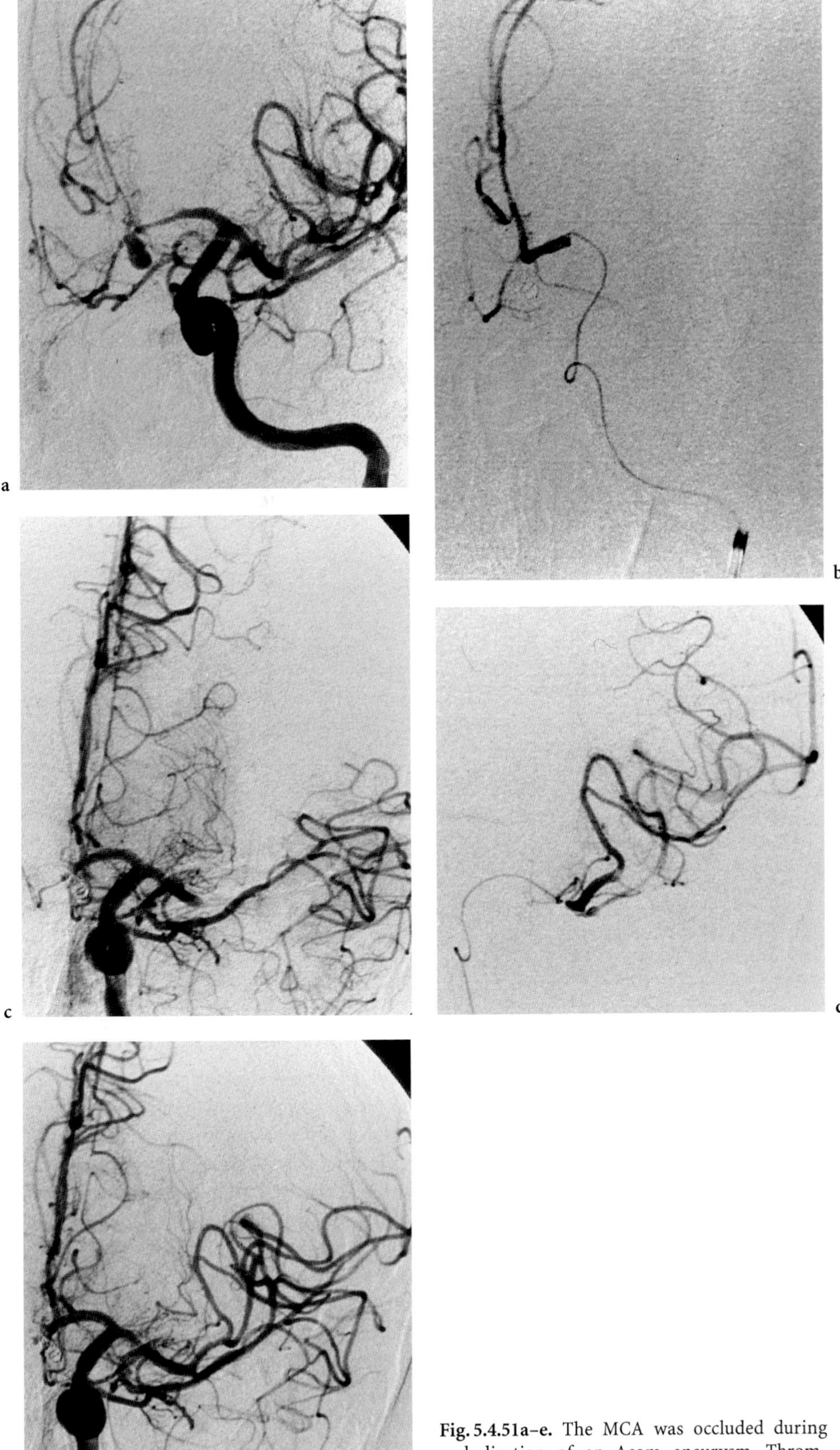

Fig. 5.4.51a–e. The MCA was occluded during embolization of an Acom aneurysm. Thrombolysis was performed using 10 mg rt-PA

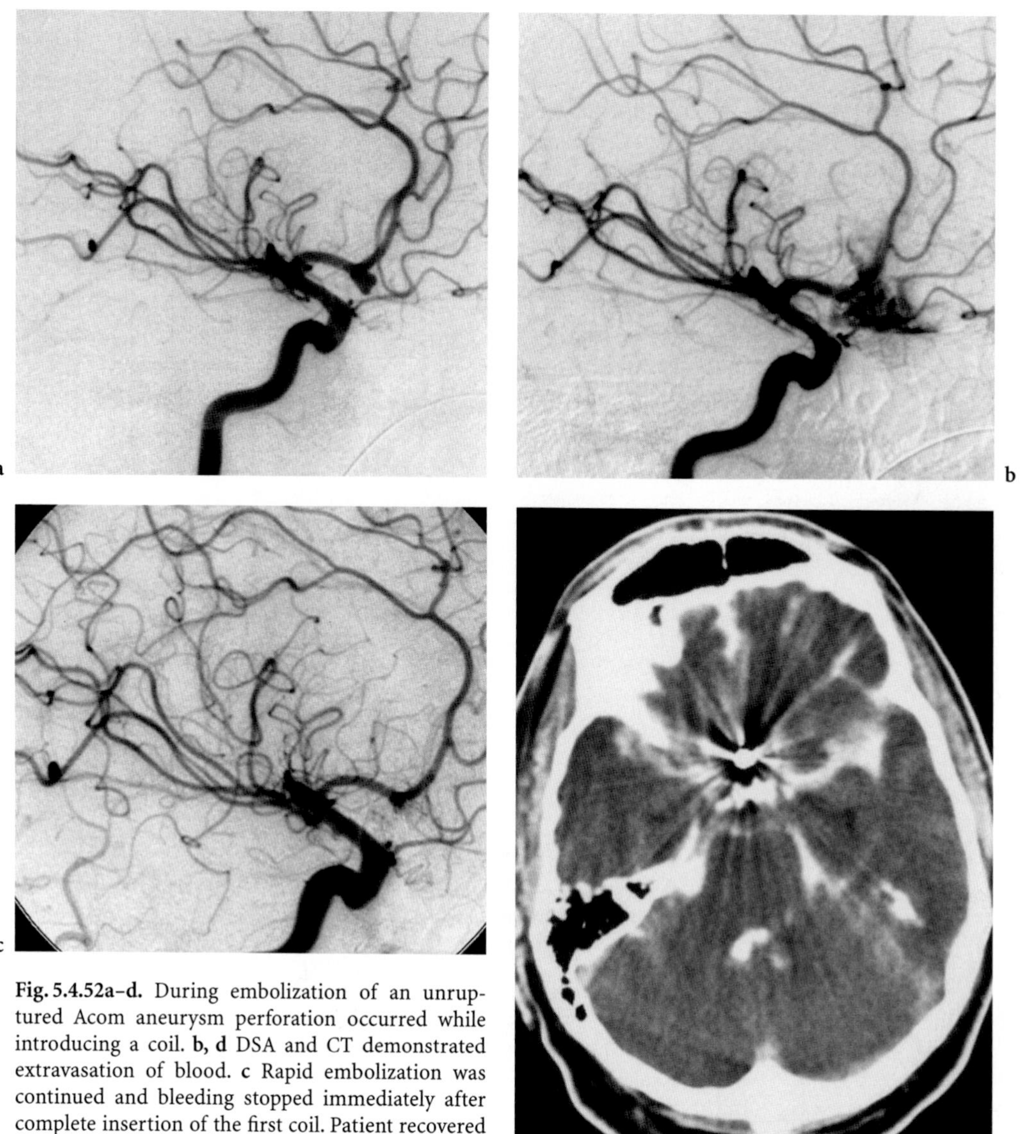

Fig. 5.4.52a–d. During embolization of an unruptured Acom aneurysm perforation occurred while introducing a coil. **b, d** DSA and CT demonstrated extravasation of blood. **c** Rapid embolization was continued and bleeding stopped immediately after complete insertion of the first coil. Patient recovered without clinical sequelae

studies and stroke patients (de Crespigny et al. 1993; Moseley et al. 1990). DWI provides potentially unique information on the viability of brain tissue and has been shown to be sensitive to early cerebral ischemia (Dardzinski et al. 1993; Moseley et al. 1990; Reith et al. 1995).

Since DWI is extremely sensitive to ischemic lesions it can be used to non-invasively assess the safety and efficacy of endovascular aneurysm therapy. DWI might be of particular help in those patients in whom clinical examination is difficult (Biondi et al. 2000).

Shimoda et al. (2001) used serial magnetic resonance imaging to prospectively investigate the incidence of infarction caused by vasospasm with or without a delayed ischemic neurological deficit in 125 patients with subarachnoid hemorrhage. The authors defined an infarct from vasospasm as a new lesion not present on the initial MRI within 3 days after SAH and therefore not attributable to primary brain damage or surgical complications. A new infarct on MRI was evident in 34% (43 patients), whereas 4% (five patients) showed no new lesion but had a delayed ischemic neurological deficit. However, 29 patients (23%) showed a new asymptomatic infarct but no delayed ischemic neurological deficit (Shimoda et al. 2001).

Vasospasms secondary to subarachnoid hemorrhage are responsible for severe ischemic complications. Condette-Auliac and colleagues (2001) studied asymptomatic vasospasms in seven patients with aneurysmal SAH to assess whether DWI provides predictive markers of silent ischemic lesions and/or progression toward symptomatic ischemia. Additionally, three patients with symptomatic vasospasm, and four patients with SAH but without vasospasm were studied at regular intervals by DWI, and their apparent diffusion coefficients (ADCs) were calculated. All patients with vasospasm including those without symptoms presented abnormalities on DWI with a reduction of the ADC prevalently in the white matter. No such abnormalities were observed in patients without vasospasm. Correlation of abnormalities on DWI with parenchymal involvement in asymptomatic patients would be of considerable clinical significance. Larger studies might be able to determine whether the ADC has a reversibility threshold, because this would facilitate patient management (Condette-Auliac et al. 2001).

Monitoring of patients with vasospasm after SAH using a combination of serial PWI and DWI might yield insight into the hemodynamics and temporal evolution of vasospasms and delayed cerebral ischemia (Rordorf et al. 1999). DWI and PWI might thereby improve our pathophysiologic understanding of the mechanisms underlying the evolution of vasospasm and delayed cerebral ischemia. Rordorf and colleagues (1999) tried to identify early ischemic injury with combined diffusion-weighted and perfusion-weighted MRI in patients with vasospasm after SAH. In patients with symptomatic vasospasm the authors found small, sometimes multiple, ischemic lesions on DWI encircled by a large area of decreased cerebral blood flow and increased mean transit time. MR images were normal in asymptomatic patients with angiographic vasospasm and patients with a normal angiogram and no clinical signs of vasospasm. This combined technique could become a useful tool in the clinical management of patients with SAH (Rordorf et al. 1999). However, at the moment the application of these techniques in SAH patients is a matter of research and not clinical routine.

Cerebral vasospasm continues to be the leading cause of morbidity and mortality following aneurysmal subarachnoid hemorrhage. Roughly 40% of patients with aneurysmal SAH develop angiographically visible vasospasm, about 20% have neurologic signs of vasospasm and 10% present with vasospasm related infarction. If vasospasm is present at the time of patient administration and before treatment of the aneurysm a combined approach might be necessary in order to occlude the aneurysm and to resolve vasospasm (Wanke et al. 2000).

After treatment of the ruptured aneurysm approaches to treat aneurysmal vasospasm currently include medical treatment with Ca-antagonists, "triple-H" therapy and endovascular methods.

Nimodipine is recommended prophylactically for all patients. Several randomized trials have demonstrated that nimodipine reduces poor outcome due to vasospasm in all grades of patients. These results are summarized by Feigin et al. (2000) who analyzed eight controlled trials on efficacy of nimodipine with 1574 randomized patients.

Aggressive hypertensive, hemodilutional, hypervolemic therapy is also recommended prophylactically and is – at least – indicated for symptomatic vasospasm. Triple-H therapy is an effective modality for elevating and sustaining CBF after SAH. In combination with early and definite aneurysm occlusion as a prerequisite for this regimen, it can minimize delayed cerebral ischemia and lead to an improved overall outcome (King and Martin 1994; Origitano et al. 1990; Seifert 1997). Assessing trial quality there exist only studies with optional recommendations for this therapy. The efficacy of triple-H therapy has yet not been demonstrated in randomized clinical trials.

The same is valid for the use of the endovascular methods. The two main endovascular treatment methods are balloon angioplasty and intra-arterial infusion of spasmolytic agents. If clinical deterioration is progressive despite intravenous medical therapy, endovascular methods to treat vasospasm should be used.

Balloon angioplasty is superior to papaverine for treatment of proximal vessel vasospasm and has a more sustained effect on the vessels. Up to date there are no series documenting a *significance* of cerebral blood flow increase or improvement of delayed ischemic neurologic deficits induced by vasospasm compared to controls, but our clinical experience and single case studies suggest that balloon angioplasty does reverse vasospasms and – if performed early enough – can improve the patient's condition.

Song et al. (1997) reported in early and aggressive treatment with balloon angioplasty clinical improvement in about two-thirds of their patients suffering from neurological deficits attributable to vasospasm. In a rabbit model an increase in endothelial proliferation and decrease in the thickness of the tunica media was shown suggesting, that angioplasty damages endothelial and smooth-muscle cells. This may be the basis for the observation that vasospastic arteries do not reconstrict after angioplasty (MacDonald et al. 1995).

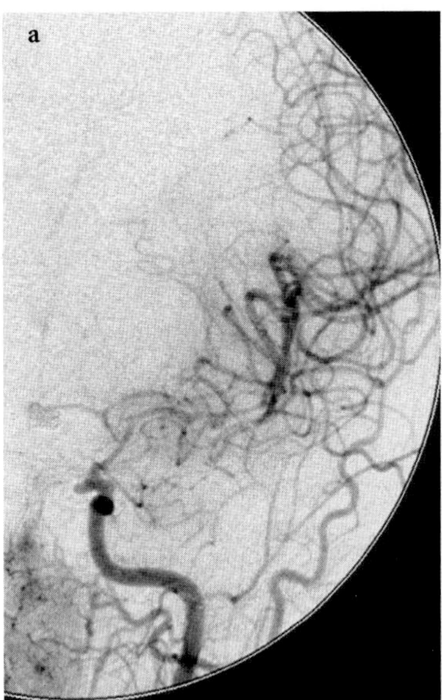

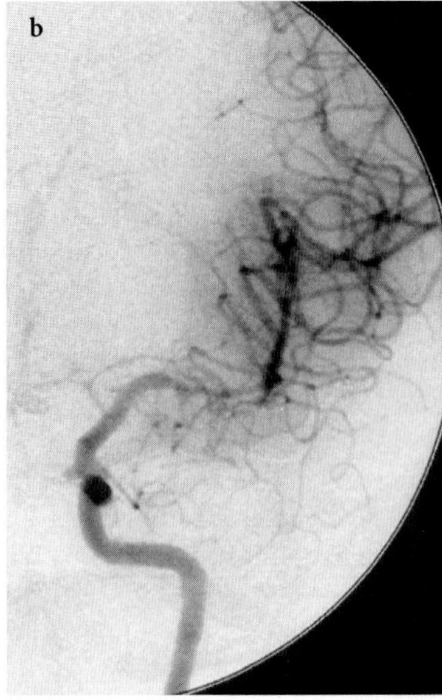

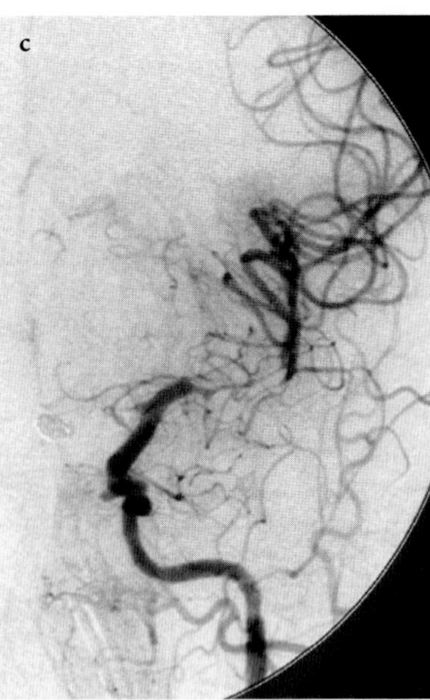

Fig. 5.4.53. **a** Severe vasospasm after rupture of an Acom aneurysm. **b** After balloon angioplasty and papaverine infusion. **c** Severe vasospasm 1 day later was noted of the previously not dilated vessels

Papaverine can be useful as an adjunct to balloon angioplasty and also for the treatment of distal vessels that are not accessible for balloon angioplasty (NEWELL et al. 1999).

Although isolated series documenting clinical successes have prompted the increased use of papaverine as a treatment for vasospasm after SAH, some authors found, as it is currently being used, the drug does not provide added benefits, compared with medical treatment of vasospasm alone but do not preclude the possibility that alterations in the timing of or indications for drug treatment might produce beneficial effects (POLIN et al. 1998).

5.4.10.9 Follow-Up and Outcome

5.4.10.9.1 Follow-Up After Endovascular Therapy

The goal of intracranial aneurysm treatment is to achieve complete aneurysm occlusion in order to avoid rebleeding. The total occlusion rate after clipping is higher than after endovascular therapy. In most of the neurosurgical centers control angiography after surgery is not performed. However, in the literature the range of incompletely clipped aneurysms range from 4% up to 17% (BYRNE et al. 1999; FEUERBERG et al. 1987; MACDONALD et al. 1993). A large series of postoperatively examined patients with a total of 837 aneurysms revealed residual aneurysms in 7.09% (SUZUKI et al. 1980).

Especially for small neck aneurysms endovascular coil embolization has become a therapeutic alternative to microneurosurgical clipping (JOHNSTON et al. 1999; KOIVISTO et al. 2000; MURAYAMA et al. 1999; RAAYMAKERS et al. 1998). However, one problem that might occur in endovascularly treated aneurysms is the relatively high number of suboptimal obliterated aneurysms with a tendency to recanalize (BYRNE et al. 1999; COGNARD et al. 1999). Therefore, careful follow-up after endovascular treatment in order to detect recurrent aneurysm is of major importance.

Up to now digital subtraction angiography (DSA) has been considered the gold standard for evaluation of residual or recurrent aneurysms. Since it is an expensive procedure and carries the risk of a permanent neurologic deficit (GRZYSKA et al. 1990; HANKEY et al. 1990) a non-invasive and more cost-effective modality would be more than nice to have. Magnetic resonance angiography (MRA) using time-of-flight (TOF) technique has an excellent spatial resolution and is – although not routinely – used for detection of both unruptured and ruptured intracranial aneurysms (BOSMANS et al. 1995; GOULIAMOS et al. 1992; HOUKIN et al. 1994; JAGER et al. 2000; RAAYMAKERS et al. 1999; ROSS et al. 1990; SEVICK et al. 1990). However, in neurosurgically clipped patients MRA is clearly not the diagnostic tool of choice to determine occlusion rate due to severe artefacts of the titanium clips (GRIEVE et al. 1999; HARTMAN et al. 1997).

However, there are still controversial studies about the value of MRA after coiling of aneurysms. Some authors report severe artefacts, others report excellent diagnostic results without producing artefacts (ANZALONE et al. 2000; DERDEYN et al. 1997; HARTMAN et al. 1997; BRUNEREAU 1999; KAHARA et al. 1999; SHELLOCK et al. 1997).

In our experience MRA is very reliable to detect recurrent aneurysms. Platinum coils do of course alter the MR signal, but not produce artefacts interfering with the evaluation of aneurysm obliteration. As always, the patient should be in a reasonable clinical condition to cooperate during the time of scanning and vasospasm and subarachnoid blood clots should not be present. The same is true if platinum coils are used in combination with a neurostent (Neuroform). Although the stent is visible on MRA source images and produces some signal loss vessel patency and aneurysm obliteration can be evaluated.

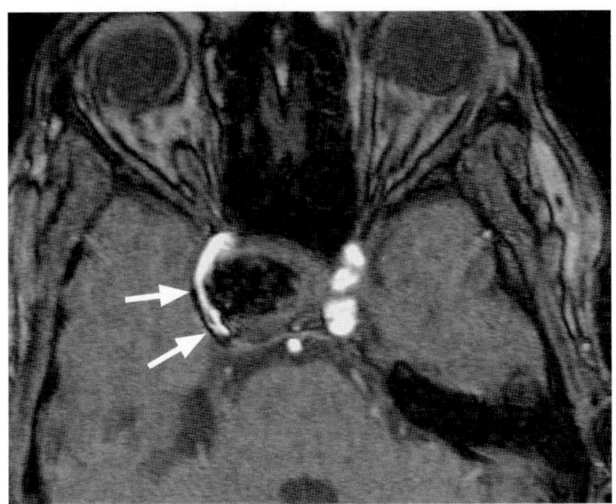
a

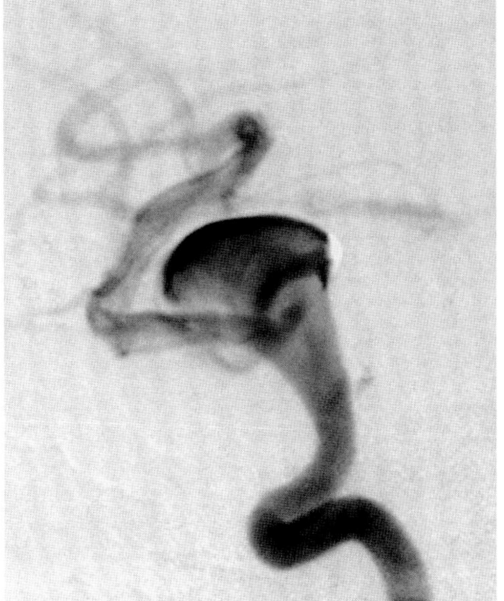
b

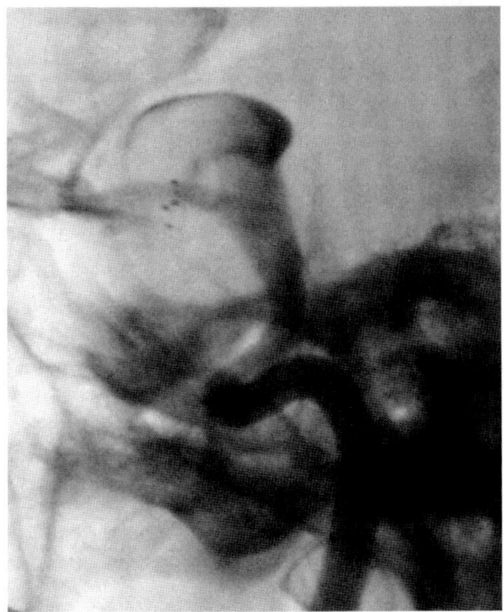
c

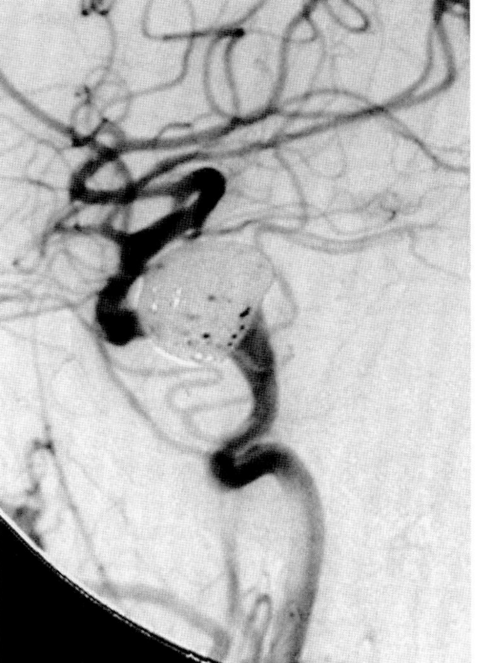
d

Fig. 5.4.54a–d. Giant broad-based ICA aneurysm: TOF axial source image demonstrating signal loss at the vessel wall at the site of the implanted stent (*arrows*). while the parent artery is patent. Although there is no flow after coiling the giant aneurysm is partially thrombosed. **b** DSA demonstrated the broad base of the aneurysm, and after (**c**) stent placement the aneurysm could be (**d**) embolized through the stent-interstices

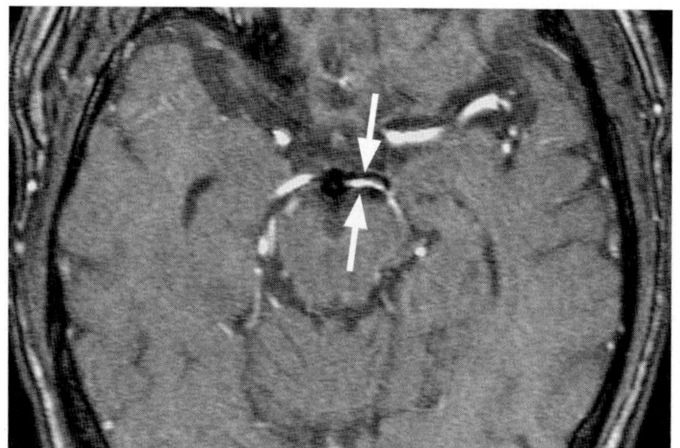

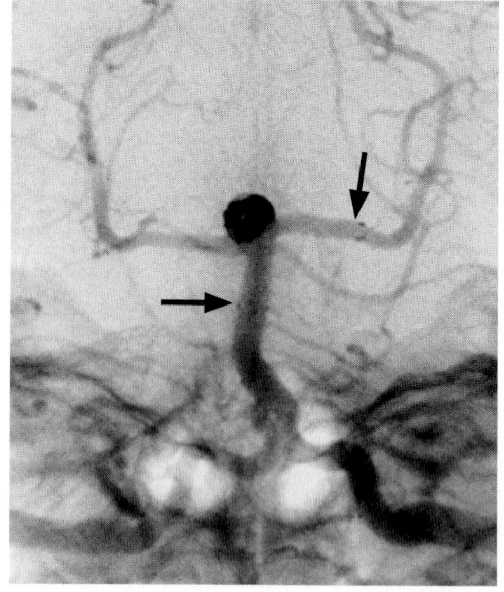

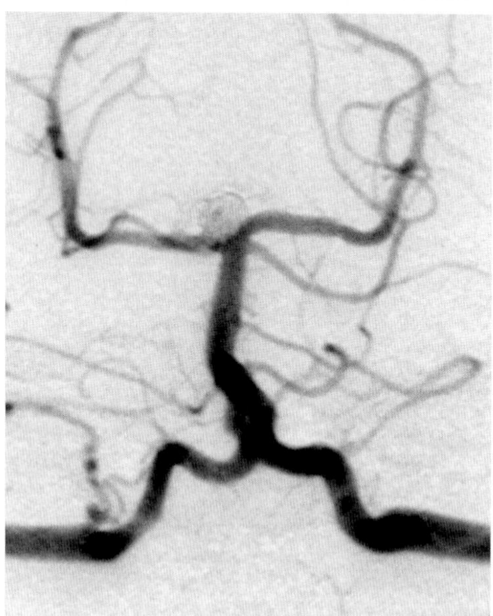

Fig. 5.4.55. **a** Broad-based basilar tip aneurysm encroaching the P1 segment. TOF axial source images revealed patency of the basilar artery as well as of the P1 segment of the left. The implanted stent is producing signal loss at the vessel wall (*arrows*). **b, c** DSA delineate the position of the proximal and distal markers of the stent (*arrows*) and complete obliteration of the aneurysm

If there is a good correlation between DSA and MRA in the first control after endovascular intervention – usually 3–6 months later – MRA seems promising as a sufficient tool for follow-up of a patient with a coiled intracranial aneurysm initially larger than 2 mm to select those who should undergo further intervention. Nevertheless, pitfalls such as aneurysm position in acquisition plane (e.g. at the basilar tip) and extraordinary vascular disease should be taken into account. To reliably evaluate aneurysmal recurrence analysis of the MRA-TOF source images is mandatory; evaluation of the 3D MIP images alone is not sufficient. However, in a series of more than 200 patients up to now we never missed an aneurysm remnant or regrowth requiring new therapy. Therefore, we consider MRA as a sufficient tool for follow-up patients after endovascular therapy of intracranial aneurysms.

5.4.10.10
Final Remarks

Aneurysm therapy has changed in recent last years. At some centers already before ISAT and in many since ISAT, endovascular therapy is the method of choice for those aneurysms that are suitable for this technique. In specialized centers, up to 70–80% of aneurysms could be treated via the endovascular approach. The remaining aneurysms are difficult and it will be a major challenge to maintain neurosurgical expertise for exactly these "non-coilable" aneurysms. However, despite all the technical improvements, occlusion of a ruptured aneurysm is often not the most difficult part of the therapy! The disease is the *subarachnoid hemorrhage* and that determines patient outcome. Instead of fighting about "who should do what" all disciplines should now focus on the remaining problems of the disease. There is still a long way ahead to overcome these difficulties.

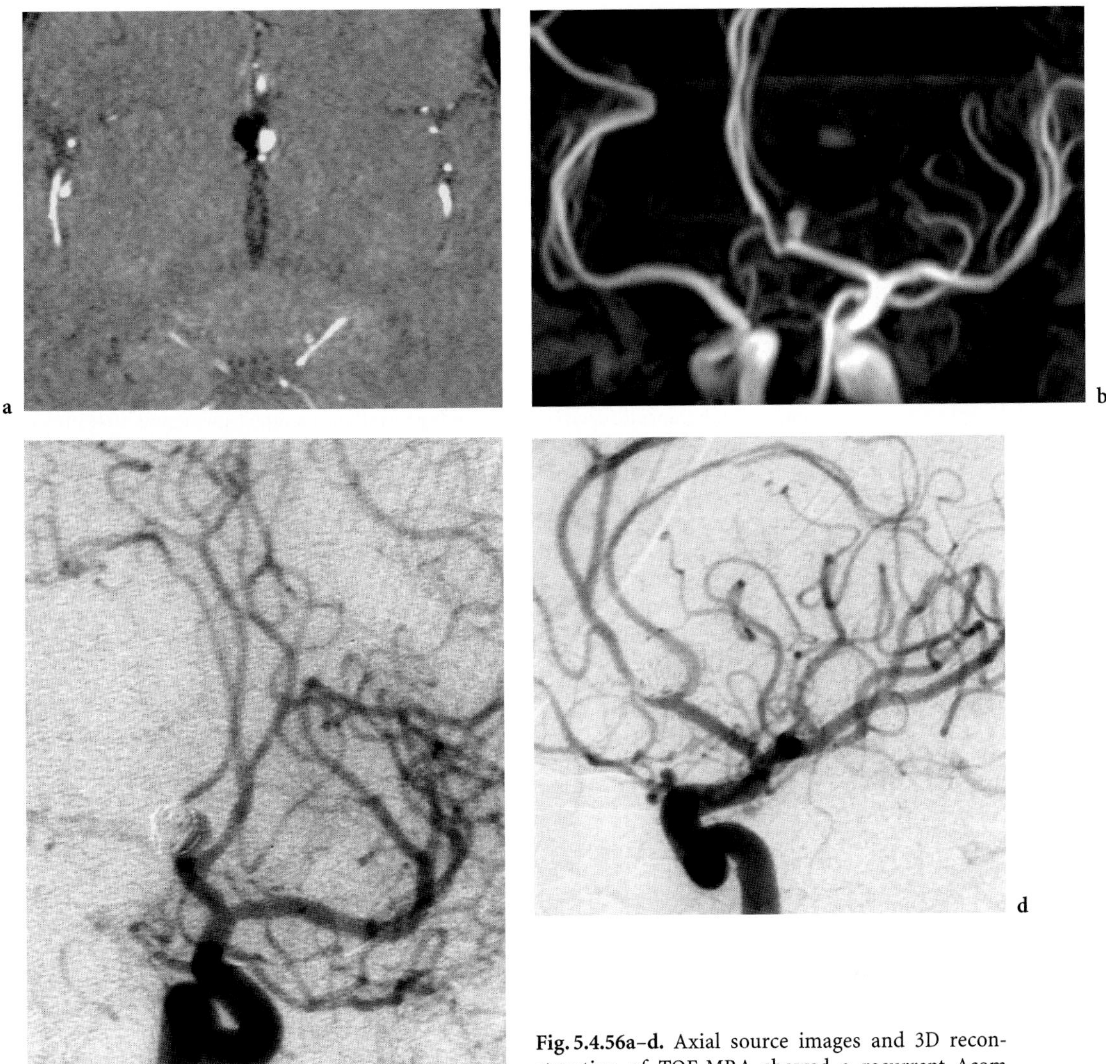

Fig. 5.4.56a–d. Axial source images and 3D reconstruction of TOF-MRA showed a recurrent Acom aneurysm which was successfully retreated

References

Abrahams JM, Diamond SL, Hurst RW, Zager EL, Grady MS (2000) Topic review: surface modifications enhancing biological activity of Guglielmi detachable coils in treating intracranial aneurysms. Surg Neurol 54:34-40; discussion 40-31

Abrahams JM, Forman MS, Grady MS, Diamond SL (2001a) Delivery of human vascular endothelial growth factor with platinum coils enhances wall thickening and coil impregnation in a rat aneurysm model. AJNR Am J Neuroradiol 22:1410-1417

Abrahams JM, Forman MS, Grady MS, Diamond SL (2001b) Biodegradable polyglycolide endovascular coils promote wall thickening and drug delivery in a rat aneurysm model. Neurosurgery 49:1187-1193; discussion 1193-1185

Adams HP Jr, Kassell NF, Torner JC, Sahs AL (1983) CT and clinical correlations in recent aneurysmal subarachnoid hemorrhage: a preliminary report of the Cooperative Aneurysm Study. Neurology 33:981-988

Adams WM, Laitt RD, Jackson A (2000) The role of MR angiography in the pretreatment assessment of intracranial aneurysms: a comparative study. AJNR Am J Neuroradiol 21:1618-1628

Aletich VA, Debrun GM, Misra M, Charbel F, Ausman JI (2000) The remodeling technique of balloon-assisted Guglielmi detachable coil placement in wide-necked aneurysms: experience at the University of Illinois at Chicago. J Neurosurg 93:388-396

Allison JW, Davis PC, Sato Y, James CA, Haque SS, Angtuaco EJ, Glasier CM (1998) Intracranial aneurysms in infants and children. Pediatr Radiol 28:223-229

Amirjamshidi A, Rahmat H, Abbassioun K (1996) Traumatic aneurysms and arteriovenous fistulas of intracranial vessels associated with penetrating head injuries occurring during war: principles and pitfalls in diagnosis and management. A survey of 31 cases and review of the literature. J Neurosurg 84:769-780

Andrews RJ, Spiegel PK (1979) Intracranial aneurysms. Age, sex, blood pressure, and multiplicity in an unselected series of patients. J Neurosurg 51:27-32

Anson JA, Lawton MT, Spetzler RF (1996) Characteristics and surgical treatment of dolichoectatic and fusiform aneurysms. J Neurosurg 84:185-193

Anxionnat R, Bracard S, Ducrocq X, Trousset Y, Launay L, Kerrien E, Braun M, Vaillant R, Scomazzoni F, Lebedinsky A, Picard L (2001) Intracranial aneurysms: clinical value of 3D digital subtraction angiography in the therapeutic decision and endovascular treatment. Radiology 218:799-808

Anzalone N, Righi C, Simionato F, Scomazzoni F, Pagani G, Calori G, Santino P, Scotti G (2000) Three-dimensional time-of-flight MR angiography in the evaluation of intracranial aneurysms treated with Guglielmi detachable coils. AJNR Am J Neuroradiol 21:746-752

Arnold H, Schwachenwald R, Nowak G, Schwachenwald D (1994) Aneurysm surgery in poor grade patients. Results, and value of external ventricular drainage. Neurol Res 16: 45-48

Asgari S, Doerfler A, Wanke I, Schoch B, Forsting M, Stolke D (2002) Complementary management of partially occluded aneurysms by using surgical or endovascular therapy. J Neurosurg 97:843-850

Atlas SW, Sheppard L, Goldberg HI, Hurst RW, Listerud J, Flamm E (1997) Intracranial aneurysms: detection and characterization with MR angiography with use of an advanced postprocessing technique in a blinded-reader study. Radiology 203:807-814

Barrow DL, Prats AR (1990) Infectious intracranial aneurysms: comparison of groups with and without endocarditis. Neurosurgery 27:562-572; discussion 572-563

Batjer HH, Samson DS (1992) Reoperation for aneurysms and vascular malformations. Clin Neurosurg 39:140-171

Bavinzski G, Killer M, Gruber A, Reinprecht A, Gross CE, Richling B (1999) Treatment of basilar artery bifurcation aneurysms by using Guglielmi detachable coils: a 6-year experience. J Neurosurg 90:843-852

Becker G, Perez J, Krone A, Demuth K, Lindner A, Hofmann E, Winkler J, Bogdahn U (1992) Transcranial color-coded real-time sonography in the evaluation of intracranial neoplasms and arteriovenous malformations. Neurosurgery 31:420-428

Benson PJ, Sung JH (1989) Cerebral aneurysms following radiotherapy for medulloblastoma. J Neurosurg 70:545-550

Berenstein A, Ransohoff J, Kupersmith M, Flamm E, Graeb D (1984) Transvascular treatment of giant aneurysms of the cavernous carotid and vertebral arteries. Functional investigation and embolization. Surg Neurol 21:3-12

Bigelow NH (1955) Multiple intracranial arterial aneurysms; an analysis of their significance. AMA Arch Neurol Psychiatry 73:76-99

Biller J, Godersky JC, Adams HP Jr (1988) Management of aneurysmal subarachnoid hemorrhage. Stroke 19:1300-1305

Biondi A, Oppenheim C, Vivas E, Casasco A, Lalam T, Sourour N, Jean LL, Dormont D, Marsault C (2000) Cerebral aneurysms treated by Guglielmi detachable coils: evaluation with diffusion-weighted MR imaging. AJNR Am J Neuroradiol 21:957-963

Birchall D, Khangure MS, McAuliffe W (1999) Resolution of third nerve paresis after endovascular management of aneurysms of the posterior communicating artery. AJNR Am J Neuroradiol 20:411-413

Birchall D, Khangure M, McAuliffe W, Apsimon H, Knuckey N (2001) Endovascular treatment of posterior circulation aneurysms. Br J Neurosurg 15:39-43

Blanc R, Weill A, Piotin M, Ross IB, Moret J (2001) Delayed stroke secondary to increasing mass effect after endovascular treatment of a giant aneurysm by parent vessel occlusion. AJNR Am J Neuroradiol 22:1841-1843

Boet R, Poon WS, Yu SC (2001) The management of residual and recurrent intracranial aneurysms after previous endovascular or surgical treatment – a report of eighteen cases. Acta Neurochir (Wien) 143:1093-1101

Bohmfalk GL, Story JL, Wissinger JP, Brown WE Jr (1978) Bacterial intracranial aneurysm. J Neurosurg 48:369-382

Bornstein RA, Weir BK, Petruk KC, Disney LB (1987) Neuropsychological function in patients after subarachnoid hemorrhage. Neurosurgery 21:651-654

Bosmans H, Wilms G, Marchal G, Demaerel P, Baert AL (1995) Characterisation of intracranial aneurysms with MR angiography. Neuroradiology 37:262-266

Brilstra EH, Hop JW, Rinkel GJ (1997) Quality of life after perimesencephalic haemorrhage. J Neurol Neurosurg Psychiatry 63:382-384

Brilstra EH, Rinkel GJ, van der Graaf Y, van Rooij WJ, Algra A (1999) Treatment of intracranial aneurysms by embolization with coils: a systematic review. Stroke 30:470-476

Brown JH, Lustrin ES, Lev MH, Ogilvy CS, Taveras JM (1999) Reduction of aneurysm clip artifacts on CT angiograms: a technical note. AJNR Am J Neuroradiol 20:694-696

Brown RD, Jr., Wiebers DO, Forbes GS (1990) Unruptured intracranial aneurysms and arteriovenous malformations: frequency of intracranial hemorrhage and relationship of lesions. J Neurosurg 73:859-863

Brunberg JA, Frey KA, Horton JA, Deveikis JP, Ross DA, Koeppe RA (1994) [15O]H2O positron emission tomography determination of cerebral blood flow during balloon test occlusion of the internal carotid artery. AJNR Am J Neuroradiol 15:725-732

Brunereau L, Cottier JP, Sonier CB, Medioni B, Bertrand P, Rouleau P, Sirinelli D, Herbreteau D (1999) Prospective evaluation of time-of-flight MR angiography in the follow-up of intracranial saccular aneurysms treated with Guglielmi detachable coils. J Comput Assist Tomogr 23:216-223

Brust JC, Dickinson PC, Hughes JE, Holtzman RN (1990) The diagnosis and treatment of cerebral mycotic aneurysms. Ann Neurol 27:238-246

Byrne JV, Sohn MJ, Molyneux AJ, Chir B (1999) Five-year experience in using coil embolization for ruptured intracranial aneurysms: outcomes and incidence of late rebleeding. J Neurosurg 90:656-663

Byrne JV, Bashiri M, Pasco A, Morris JH (2000) A novel flexible endovascular stent for use in small and tortuous vessels. Neuroradiology 42:56-61

Canhao P, Ferro JM, Pinto AN, Melo TP, Campos JG (1995) Perimesencephalic and nonperimesencephalic subarachnoid haemorrhages with negative angiograms. Acta Neurochir 132:14-19

Carey J, Numaguchi Y, Nadell J (1990) Subarachnoid hemorrhage in sickle cell disease. Childs Nerv Syst 6:47-50
Chapot R, Houdart E, Saint-Maurice JP, Aymard A, Mounayer C, Lot G, Merland JJ (2002) Endovascular treatment of cerebral mycotic aneurysms. Radiology 222:389-396
Chason J, Hindman W (1958) Berry aneurysms of the circle of Willis: results of a planned autopsy study. Neurology 8: 41-44
Church W (1869) Aneurysm of the right cerebral artery in a boy of thirteen. Trans Pathol Soc Lond 20:109
Chyatte D, Reilly J, Tilson MD (1990) Morphometric analysis of reticular and elastin fibers in the cerebral arteries of patients with intracranial aneurysms. Neurosurgery 26: 939-943
Ciceri EF, Klucznik RP, Grossman RG, Rose JE, Mawad ME (2001) Aneurysms of the posterior cerebral artery: classification and endovascular treatment. AJNR Am J Neuroradiol 22:27-34
Clare CE, Barrow DL (1992) Infectious intracranial aneurysms. Neurosurg Clin North Am 3:551-566
Cognard C, Gobin YP, Pierot L, Bailly AL, Houdart E, Casasco A, Chiras J, Merland JJ (1995) Cerebral dural arteriovenous fistulas: clinical and angiographic correlation with a revised classification of venous drainage. Radiology 194: 671-680
Cognard C, Pierot L, Boulin A, Weill A, Tovi M, Castaings L, Rey A, Moret J, Toevi M (1997) Intracranial aneurysms: endovascular treatment with mechanical detachable spirals in 60 aneurysms. Radiology 202:783-792
Cognard C, Weill A, Spelle L, Piotin M, Castaings L, Rey A, Moret J (1999) Long-term angiographic follow-up of 169 intracranial berry aneurysms occluded with detachable coils. Radiology 212:348-356
Condette-Auliac S, Bracard S, Anxionnat R, Schmitt E, Lacour JC, Braun M, Meloneto J, Cordebar A, Yin L, Picard L (2001) Vasospasm after subarachnoid hemorrhage: interest in diffusion-weighted MR imaging. Stroke 32:1818-1824
Conway JE, Hutchins GM, Tamargo RJ (1999) Marfan syndrome is not associated with intracranial aneurysms. Stroke 30:1632-1636
Conway JE, Hutchins GM, Tamargo RJ (2001) Lack of evidence for an association between neurofibromatosis type I and intracranial aneurysms: autopsy study and review of the literature. Stroke 32:2481-2485
Crompton MR (1966) The comparative pathology of cerebral aneurysms. Brain 89:789-796
Dardzinski BJ, Sotak CH, Fisher M, Hasegawa Y, Li L, Minematsu K (1993) Apparent diffusion coefficient mapping of experimental focal cerebral ischemia using diffusion-weighted echo-planar imaging. Magn Reson Med 30: 318-325
Dawson RC, Krisht AF, Barrow DL, Joseph GJ, Shengelaia GG, Bonner G (1995) Treatment of experimental aneurysms using collagen-coated microcoils. Neurosurgery 36:133-139; discussion 139-140
De Crespigny AJ, Tsuura M, Moseley ME, Kucharczyk J (1993) Perfusion and diffusion MR imaging of thromboembolic stroke. J Magn Reson Imaging 3:746-754
Debrun G, Fox A, Drake C, Peerless S, Girvin J, Ferguson G (1981) Giant unclippable aneurysms: treatment with detachable balloons. AJNR Am J Neuroradiol 2:167-173
Derdeyn CP, Graves VB, Turski PA, Masaryk AM, Strother CM (1997) MR angiography of saccular aneurysms after treatment with Guglielmi detachable coils: preliminary experience. AJNR Am J Neuroradiol 18:279-286
Derdeyn CP, Barr JD, Berenstein A, Connors JJ, Dion JE, Duckwiler GR, Higashida RT, Strother CM, Tomsick TA, Turski P (2003) The International Subarachnoid Aneurysm Trial (ISAT): a position statement from the Executive Committee of the American Society of Interventional and Therapeutic Neuroradiology and the American Society of Neuroradiology. AJNR Am J Neuroradiol 24:1404-1408
Doerfler A, Wanke I, Egelhof T, Dietrich U, Asgari S, Stolke D, Forsting M (2001) Aneurysmal rupture during embolization with Guglielmi detachable coils: causes, management, and outcome. AJNR Am J Neuroradiol 22:1825-1832
Drake CG (1965) On the surgical treatment of ruptured intracranial aneurysms. Clin Neurosurg 13:122-155
Drake CG (1977) Intracranial aneurysms. Acta Neurol Latinoam 23:43-68
Drake CG, Allcock JM (1973) Postoperative angiography and the „slipped“ clip. J Neurosurg 39:683-689
Drake CG, Peerless SJ (1997) Giant fusiform intracranial aneurysms: review of 120 patients treated surgically from 1965 to 1992. J Neurosurg 87:141-162
Ebina K, Suzuki M, Andoh A, Saitoh K, Iwabuchi T (1982) Recurrence of cerebral aneurysm after initial neck clipping. Neurosurgery 11:764-768
Eckard DA, Purdy PD, Bonte FJ (1992) Temporary balloon occlusion of the carotid artery combined with brain blood flow imaging as a test to predict tolerance prior to permanent carotid sacrifice. AJNR Am J Neuroradiol 13: 1565-1569
Ellenbogen BK (1970) Subarachnoid haemorrhage in the elderly. Gerontol Clin 12:115-120
Elliott JP, Le Roux PD (1998) Subarachnoid hemorrhage and cerebral aneurysms in the elderly. Neurosurg Clin North Am 9:587-594
Endo S, Nishijima M, Nomura H, Takaku A, Okada E (1993) A pathological study of intracranial posterior circulation dissecting aneurysms with subarachnoid hemorrhage: report of three autopsied cases and review of the literature. Neurosurgery 33:732-738
Eskridge JM (1989) Interventional neuroradiology. Radiology 172:991-1006
Fahrig R, Moreau M, Holdsworth DW (1997) Three-dimensional computed tomographic reconstruction using a C-arm mounted XRII: correction of image intensifier distortion. Med Phys 24:1097-1106
Feigin VL, Rinkel GJ, Algra A, Vermeulen M, van Gijn J (2000) Calcium antagonists for aneurysmal subarachnoid haemorrhage. Cochrane Database Syst Rev. 2002;(4):CD000277
Ferrante L, Fortuna A, Celli P, Santoro A, Fraioli B (1988) Intracranial arterial aneurysms in early childhood. Surg Neurol 29:39-56
Feuerberg I, Lindquist C, Lindqvist M, Steiner L (1987) Natural history of postoperative aneurysm rests. J Neurosurg 66: 30-34
Findlay JM, Kassell NF, Weir BK, Haley EC Jr., Kongable G, Germanson T, Truskowski L, Alves WM, Holness RO, Knuckey NW, et al. (1995) A randomized trial of intraoperative, intracisternal tissue plasminogen activator for the prevention of vasospasm. Neurosurgery 37:168–76; discussion 177–8
Findlay JM, Hao C, Emery D (2002) Non-atherosclerotic fusiform cerebral aneurysms. Can J Neurol Sci 29:41-48

Fisher CM, Kistler JP, Davis JM (1980) Relation of cerebral vasospasm to subarachnoid hemorrhage visualized by computerized tomographic scanning. Neurosurgery 6:1-9

Forsting M, Albert FK, Jansen O, von Kummer R, Aschoff A, Kunze S, Sartor K (1996) Coil placement after clipping: endovascular treatment of incompletely clipped cerebral aneurysms. Report of two cases. J Neurosurg 85:966-969

Fox AJ, Pelz DM, Vinuela F, Barnett HJ, Peerless SJ (1986) Results of the international extracranial/intracranial bypass study. Implications for neuroradiologists. Acta Radiol Suppl 369:77-78

Fox AJ, Vinuela F, Pelz DM, Peerless SJ, Ferguson GG, Drake CG, Debrun G (1987) Use of detachable balloons for proximal artery occlusion in the treatment of unclippable cerebral aneurysms. J Neurosurg 66:40-46

Fraser KW, Halbach VV, Teitelbaum GP, Smith TP, Higashida RT, Dowd CF, Wilson CB, Hieshima GB (1994) Endovascular platinum coil embolization of incompletely surgically clipped cerebral aneurysms. Surg Neurol 41:4-8

Fridriksson SM, Hillman J, Saveland H, Brandt L (1995) Intracranial aneurysm surgery in the 8th and 9th decades of life: impact on population-based management outcome. Neurosurgery 37:627-631; discussion 631-622

Friedman WA, Grundy BL (1987) Monitoring of sensory evoked potentials is highly reliable and helpful in the operating room. J Clin Monit 3:38-44

Friedman WA, Kaplan BL, Day AL, Sypert GW, Curran MT (1987) Evoked potential monitoring during aneurysm operation: observations after fifty cases. Neurosurgery 20: 678-687

Friedman WA, Chadwick GM, Verhoeven FJ, Mahla M, Day AL (1991) Monitoring of somatosensory evoked potentials during surgery for middle cerebral artery aneurysms. Neurosurgery 29:83-88

Fujii Y, Takeuchi S, Sasaki O, Minakawa T, Koike T, Tanaka R (1996) Ultra-early rebleeding in spontaneous subarachnoid hemorrhage. J Neurosurg 84:35-42

Furuya K, Sasaki T, Yoshimoto Y, Okada Y, Fujimaki T, Kirino T (1995) Histologically verified cerebral aneurysm formation secondary to embolism from cardiac myxoma. Case report. J Neurosurg 83:170-173

Gailloud P, Fasel JH, Muster M, de Tribolet N, Rufenacht DA (1997) A case in favor of aneurysmographic studies: a perforating artery originating from the dome of a basilar tip aneurysm. AJNR Am J Neuroradiol 18:1691-1694

Gallagher JP (1963) Obliteration of intracranial aneurysms by pilojection. JAMA 183:231-236

Gallagher JP (1964) Pilojection for Intracranial Aneurysms. Report of progress. J Neurosurg 21:129-134

Gallagher JP, Baiz T (1964) Pilojection for Carotid Aneurysm in the Cavernous Sinus. JAMA 188:1156-1158

Giannotta SL, Litofsky NS (1995) Reoperative management of intracranial aneurysms. J Neurosurg 83:387-393

Gobin YP, Vinuela F, Gurian JH, Guglielmi G, Duckwiler GR, Massoud TF, Martin NA (1996) Treatment of large and giant fusiform intracranial aneurysms with Guglielmi detachable coils. J Neurosurg 84:55-62

Gonner F, Lovblad KO, Heid O, Remonda L, Guzman R, Barth A, Schroth G (2002) Magnetic resonance angiography with ultrashort echo times reduces the artefact of aneurysm clips. Neuroradiology 44:755-758

Gouliamos A, Gotsis E, Vlahos L, Samara C, Kapsalaki E, Rologis D, Kapsalakis Z, Papavasiliou C (1992) Magnetic resonance angiography compared to intra-arterial digital subtraction angiography in patients with subarachnoid haemorrhage. Neuroradiology 35:46-49

Graves VB, Strother CM, Duff TA, Perl J 2nd (1995) Early treatment of ruptured aneurysms with Guglielmi detachable coils: effect on subsequent bleeding. Neurosurgery 37: 640-647; discussion 647-648

Grieve JP, Stacey R, Moore E, Kitchen ND, Jager HR (1999) Artefact on MRA following aneurysm clipping: an in vitro study and prospective comparison with conventional angiography. Neuroradiology 41:680-686

Griewing B, Motsch L, Piek J, Schminke U, Brassel F, Kessler C (1998) Transcranial power mode Doppler duplex sonography of intracranial aneurysms. J Neuroimaging 8:155-158

Grosset DG, Straiton J, du Trevou M, Bullock R (1992) Prediction of symptomatic vasospasm after subarachnoid hemorrhage by rapidly increasing transcranial Doppler velocity and cerebral blood flow changes. Stroke 23:674-679

Grote E, Hassler W (1988) The critical first minutes after subarachnoid hemorrhage. Neurosurgery 22:654-661

Grzyska U, Freitag J, Zeumer H (1990) Selective cerebral intraarterial DSA. Complication rate and control of risk factors. Neuroradiology 32:296-299

Guglielmi G, Vinuela F, Sepetka I, Macellari V (1991a) Electrothrombosis of saccular aneurysms via endovascular approach, part 1. Electrochemical basis, technique, and experimental results. J Neurosurg 75:1-7

Guglielmi G, Vinuela F, Dion J, Duckwiler G (1991b) Electrothrombosis of saccular aneurysms via endovascular approach, part 2. Preliminary clinical experience. J Neurosurg 75:8-14

Guglielmi G, Vinuela F, Duckwiler G, Dion J, Lylyk P, Berenstein A, Strother C, Graves V, Halbach V, Nichols D et al (1992) Endovascular treatment of posterior circulation aneurysms by electrothrombosis using electrically detachable coils. J Neurosurg 77:515-524

Hademenos GJ, Massoud TF, Turjman F, Sayre JW (1998) Anatomical and morphological factors correlating with rupture of intracranial aneurysms in patients referred for endovascular treatment. Neuroradiology 40:755-760

Halbach VV, Higashida RT, Dowd CF, Barnwell SL, Hieshima GB (1991) Management of vascular perforations that occur during neurointerventional procedures. AJNR Am J Neuroradiol 12:319-327

Haley EC Jr, Kassell NF, Apperson-Hansen C, Maile MH, Alves WM (1997) A randomized, double-blind, vehicle-controlled trial of tirilazad mesylate in patients with aneurysmal subarachnoid hemorrhage: a cooperative study in North America. J Neurosurg 86:467-474

Hamada J, Morioka M, Miura M, Fujioka S, Marubayashi T, Ushio Y (2001) Management outcome for ruptured anterior circulation aneurysms with a Hunt and Hess clinical grade of III in patients in the 9th decade of life. Surg Neurol 56:294-300

Hankey GJ, Warlow CP, Sellar RJ (1990) Cerebral angiographic risk in mild cerebrovascular disease. Stroke 21:209-222

Hartman J, Nguyen T, Larsen D, Teitelbaum GP (1997) MR artifacts, heat production, and ferromagnetism of Guglielmi detachable coils. AJNR Am J Neuroradiol 18:497-501

Hauerberg J, Andersen BB, Eskesen V, Rosenorn J, Schmidt K (1991) Importance of the recognition of a warning leak as a sign of a ruptured intracranial aneurysm. Acta Neurol Scand 83:61-64

Hecht ST, Horton JA, Yonas H (1991) Growth of a thrombosed giant vertebral artery aneurysm after parent artery occlusion. AJNR Am J Neuroradiol 12:449-451

Heiserman JE, Dean BL, Hodak JA, Flom RA, Bird CR, Drayer BP, Fram EK (1994) Neurologic complications of cerebral angiography. AJNR Am J Neuroradiol 15:1401-1407; discussion 1408-1411

Heiskanen O (1989) Ruptured intracranial arterial aneurysms of children and adolescents. Surgical and total management results. Childs Nerv Syst 5:66-70

Hieshima GB, Grinnell VS, Mehringer CM (1981) A detachable balloon for therapeutic transcatheter occlusions. Radiology 138:227-228

Higashida RT, Halbach VV, Cahan LD, Hieshima GB, Konishi Y (1989) Detachable balloon embolization therapy of posterior circulation intracranial aneurysms. J Neurosurg 71: 512-519

Higashida RT, Halbach VV, Barnwell SL, Dowd C, Dormandy B, Bell J, Hieshima GB (1990) Treatment of intracranial aneurysms with preservation of the parent vessel: results of percutaneous balloon embolization in 84 patients. AJNR Am J Neuroradiol 11:633-640

Higashida RT, Halbach VV, Dowd CF, Barnwell SL, Hieshima GB (1991) Intracranial aneurysms: interventional neurovascular treatment with detachable balloons–results in 215 cases. Radiology 178:663-670

Higashida RT, Smith W, Gress D, Urwin R, Dowd CF, Balousek PA, Halbach VV (1997) Intravascular stent and endovascular coil placement for a ruptured fusiform aneurysm of the basilar artery. Case report and review of the literature. J Neurosurg 87:944-949

Hijdra A, Vermeulen M, van Gijn J, van Crevel H (1987) Rerupture of intracranial aneurysms: a clinicoanatomic study. J Neurosurg 67:29-33

Hijdra A, Brouwers PJ, Vermeulen M, van Gijn J (1990) Grading the amount of blood on computed tomograms after subarachnoid hemorrhage. Stroke 21:1156-1161

Hoh BL, Rabinov JD, Pryor JC, Carter BS, Barker FG 2nd (2003) In-hospital morbidity and mortality after endovascular treatment of unruptured intracranial aneurysms in the United States, 1996-2000: effect of hospital and physician volume. AJNR Am J Neuroradiol 24:1409-1420

Holmes B, Harbaugh RE (1993) Traumatic intracranial aneurysms: a contemporary review. J Trauma 35:855-860

Hop JW, Rinkel GJ, Algra A, van Gijn J (1999) Initial loss of consciousness and risk of delayed cerebral ischemia after aneurysmal subarachnoid hemorrhage. Stroke 30: 2268-2271

Horikoshi T, Nukui H, Yagishita T, Nishigaya K, Fukasawa I, Sasaki H (1999) Oculomotor nerve palsy after surgery for upper basilar artery aneurysms. Neurosurgery 44:705-710; discussion 710-701

Horowitz M, Purdy P, Kopitnik T, Dutton K, Samson D (1999) Aneurysm retreatment after Guglielmi detachable coil and nondetachable coil embolization: report of nine cases and review of the literature. Neurosurgery 44:712-719; discussion 719-720

Horowitz MB, Levy EI, Koebbe CJ, Jungreis CC (2001) Transluminal stent-assisted coil embolization of a vertebral confluence aneurysm: technique report. Surg Neurol 55:291-296

Houkin K, Aoki T, Takahashi A, Abe H, Koiwa M, Kashiwaba T (1994) Magnetic resonance angiography (MRA) of ruptured cerebral aneurysm. Acta Neurochir 128:132-136

Housepian E, Pool J (1958) A systematic analysis of intracranial aneurysms from the autopsy file of the Presbyterian Hospital, 1914 to 1956. J Neuropathol Exp Neurol 17: 409-423

Hughes RL (1992) Identification and treatment of cerebral aneurysms after sentinel headache. Neurology 42:1118-1119

Inagawa T (1991) Surgical treatment of multiple intracranial aneurysms. Acta Neurochir 108:22-29

Inagawa T, Hirano A (1990) Autopsy study of unruptured incidental intracranial aneurysms. Surg Neurol 34:361-365

Inagawa T, Hada H, Katoh Y (1992) Unruptured intracranial aneurysms in elderly patients. Surg Neurol 38:364-370

Inci S, Erbengi A, Ozgen T (1998) Aneurysms of the distal anterior cerebral artery: report of 14 cases and a review of the literature. Surg Neurol 50:130-139; discussion 139-140

Jager HR, Mansmann U, Hausmann O, Partzsch U, Moseley IF, Taylor WJ (2000) MRA versus digital subtraction angiography in acute subarachnoid haemorrhage: a blinded multireader study of prospectively recruited patients. Neuroradiology 42:313-326

Jarus-Dziedzic K, Zub W, Wronski J, Juniewicz H, Kasper E (2000) The relationship between cerebral blood flow velocities and the amount of blood clots in computed tomography after subarachnoid haemorrhage. Acta Neurochir 142:309-318

Johnston SC, Dudley RA, Gress DR, Ono L (1999a) Surgical and endovascular treatment of unruptured cerebral aneurysms at university hospitals. Neurology 52:1799-1805

Johnston SC, Gress DR, Kahn JG (1999b) Which unruptured cerebral aneurysms should be treated? A cost-utility analysis. Neurology 52:1806-1815

Johnston SC, Wilson CB, Halbach VV, Higashida RT, Dowd CF, McDermott MW, Applebury CB, Farley TL, Gress DR (2000) Endovascular and surgical treatment of unruptured cerebral aneurysms: comparison of risks. Ann Neurol 48: 11-19

Juvela S, Poussa K, Porras M (2001) Factors affecting formation and growth of intracranial aneurysms: a long-term follow-up study. Stroke 32:485-491

Kahara VJ, Seppanen SK, Ryymin PS, Mattila P, Kuurne T, Laasonen EM (1999) MR angiography with three-dimensional time-of-flight and targeted maximum-intensity-projection reconstructions in the follow-up of intracranial aneurysms embolized with Guglielmi detachable coils. AJNR Am J Neuroradiol 20:1470-1475

Kallmes DF, Fujiwara NH (2002) New expandable hydrogel-platinum coil hybrid device for aneurysm embolization. AJNR Am J Neuroradiol 23:1580-1588

Kallmes DF, Williams AD, Cloft HJ, Lopes MB, Hankins GR, Helm GA (1998) Platinum coil-mediated implantation of growth factor-secreting endovascular tissue grafts: an in vivo study. Radiology 207:519-523

Kandel EI (1980) Complete excision of arteriovenous malformations of the cervical cord. Surg Neurol 13:135-139

Kassell NF, Torner JC (1983) Size of intracranial aneurysms. Neurosurgery 12:291-297

Kassell NF, Torner JC, Haley EC Jr, Jane JA, Adams HP, Kongable GL (1990a) The International Cooperative Study on the Timing of Aneurysm Surgery, part 1. Overall management results. J Neurosurg 73:18-36

Kassell NF, Torner JC, Jane JA, Haley EC Jr, Adams HP (1990b) The International Cooperative Study on the Timing of

Aneurysm Surgery, part 2. Surgical results. J Neurosurg 73:37-47

Kerr R, Molyneux A (2003) Results from the ISAT study, 16-19 Febr 2003, Phoenix, AZ

King WA, Martin NA (1994) Critical care of patients with subarachnoid hemorrhage. Neurosurg Clin North Am 5: 767-787

Klucznik RP, Carrier DA, Pyka R, Haid RW (1993) Placement of a ferromagnetic intracerebral aneurysm clip in a magnetic field with a fatal outcome. Radiology 187:855-856

Koivisto T, Vanninen R, Hurskainen H, Saari T, Hernesniemi J, Vapalahti M (2000) Outcomes of early endovascular versus surgical treatment of ruptured cerebral aneurysms. A prospective randomized study. Stroke 31:2369-2377

Kojima M, Nagasawa S, Lee YE, Takeichi Y, Tsuda E, Mabuchi N (1998) Asymptomatic familial cerebral aneurysms. Neurosurgery 43:776-781

Korogi Y, Takahashi M, Mabuchi N, Nakagawa T, Fujiwara S, Horikawa Y, Miki H, O'Uchi T, Shiga H, Shiokawa Y, Watabe T, Furuse M (1996) Intracranial aneurysms: diagnostic accuracy of MR angiography with evaluation of maximum intensity projection and source images. Radiology 199: 199-207

Korogi Y, Takahashi M, Katada K, Ogura Y, Hasuo K, Ochi M, Utsunomiya H, Abe T, Imakita S (1999) Intracranial aneurysms: detection with three-dimensional CT angiography with volume rendering - comparison with conventional angiographic and surgical findings. Radiology 211:497-506

Kupersmith MJ, Berenstein A, Choi IS, Ransohoff J, Flamm ES (1984) Percutaneous transvascular treatment of giant carotid aneurysms: neuro- ophthalmologic findings. Neurology 34:328-335

Landtblom AM, Fridriksson S, Boivie J, Hillman J, Johansson G, Johansson I (2002) Sudden onset headache: a prospective study of features, incidence and causes. Cephalalgia 22:354-360

Lanzino G, Kassell NF (1999) Double-blind, randomized, vehicle-controlled study of high-dose tirilazad mesylate in women with aneurysmal subarachnoid hemorrhage, part II. A cooperative study in North America. J Neurosurg 90: 1018-1024

Lanzino G, Kassell NF, Dorsch NW, Pasqualin A, Brandt L, Schmiedek P, Truskowski LL, Alves WM (1999a) Double-blind, randomized, vehicle-controlled study of high-dose tirilazad mesylate in women with aneurysmal subarachnoid hemorrhage, part I. A cooperative study in Europe, Australia, New Zealand, and South Africa. J Neurosurg 90: 1011-1017

Lanzino G, Wakhloo AK, Fessler RD, Hartney ML, Guterman LR, Hopkins LN (1999b) Efficacy and current limitations of intravascular stents for intracranial internal carotid, vertebral, and basilar artery aneurysms. J Neurosurg 91: 538-546

Larson JJ, Tew JM Jr, Tomsick TA, van Loveren HR (1995) Treatment of aneurysms of the internal carotid artery by intravascular balloon occlusion: long-term follow-up of 58 patients. Neurosurgery 36:26-30; discussion 30

Lau AH, Takeshita M, Ishii N (1991) Mycotic (Aspergillus) arteritis resulting in fatal subarachnoid hemorrhage: a case report. Angiology 42:251-255

Leblanc R (1996) Familial cerebral aneurysms. A bias for women. Stroke 27:1050-1054

Lee EK, Hecht ST, Lie JT (1998) Multiple intracranial and systemic aneurysms associated with infantile- onset arterial fibromuscular dysplasia. Neurology 50:828-829

Lee KC, Joo JY, Lee KS, Shin YS (1999) Recanalization of completely thrombosed giant aneurysm: case report. Surg Neurol 51:94-98

Le Roux PD, Winn HR (1998) Management of the ruptured aneurysm. Neurosurg Clin North Am 9:525-540

Le Roux PD, Elliott JP, Eskridge JM, Cohen W, Winn HR (1998) Risks and benefits of diagnostic angiography after aneurysm surgery: a retrospective analysis of 597 studies. Neurosurgery 42:1248-1254; discussion 1254-1245

Levine SR, Brust JC, Futrell N, Ho KL, Blake D, Millikan CH, Brass LM, Fayad P, Schultz LR, Selwa JF et al (1990) Cerebrovascular complications of the use of the „crack" form of alkaloidal cocaine. N Engl J Med 323:699-704

Levine SR, Brust JC, Futrell N, Brass LM, Blake D, Fayad P, Schultz LR, Millikan CH, Ho KL, Welch KM (1991) A comparative study of the cerebrovascular complications of cocaine: alkaloidal versus hydrochloride - a review. Neurology 41:1173-1177

Levy DI (1997) Embolization of wide-necked anterior communicating artery aneurysm: technical note. Neurosurgery 41:979-982

Liang EY, Chan M, Hsiang JH, Walkden SB, Poon WS, Lam WW, Metreweli C (1995) Detection and assessment of intracranial aneurysms: value of CT angiography with shaded-surface display. AJR Am J Roentgenol 165:1497-1502

Lin T, Fox AJ, Drake CG (1989) Regrowth of aneurysm sacs from residual neck following aneurysm clipping. J Neurosurg 70:556-560

Linn FH, Rinkel GJ, Algra A, van Gijn J (1998) Headache characteristics in subarachnoid haemorrhage and benign thunderclap headache. J Neurol Neurosurg Psychiatry 65: 791-793

Linskey ME, Sekhar LN, Hirsch WL Jr, Yonas H, Horton JA (1990) Aneurysms of the intracavernous carotid artery: natural history and indications for treatment. Neurosurgery 26:933-937; discussion 937-938

Linskey ME, Jungreis CA, Yonas H, Hirsch WL Jr, Sekhar LN, Horton JA, Janosky JE (1994) Stroke risk after abrupt internal carotid artery sacrifice: accuracy of preoperative assessment with balloon test occlusion and stable xenon- enhanced CT. AJNR Am J Neuroradiol 15:829-843

Locksley HB, Sahs AL, Knowler L (1966) Report on the cooperative study of intracranial aneurysms and subarachnoid hemorrhage. Section II. General survey of cases in the central registry and characteristics of the sample population. J Neurosurg 24:922-932

Longstreth WT Jr, Koepsell TD, Yerby MS, van Belle G (1985) Risk factors for subarachnoid hemorrhage. Stroke 16: 377-385

Lownie SP, Pelz DM, Fox AJ (2000) Endovascular therapy of a large vertebral artery aneurysm using stent and coils. Can J Neurol Sci 27:162-165

Lozano AM, Leblanc R (1987) Familial intracranial aneurysms. J Neurosurg 66:522-528

Luginbuhl M, Remonda L (1999) Interventional neuroradiology. Recent developments and anaesthesiologic aspects. Minerva Anestesiol 65:445-454

Lussenhop AJ, Spence WT (1960) Artificial embolization of cerebral arteries. Report of use in a case of arteriovenous malformation. JAMA 12; 172:1153–1155

Lusseveld E, Brilstra EH, Nijssen PC, van Rooij WJ, Sluzewski M, Tulleken CA, Wijnalda D, Schellens RL, van der Graaf Y, Rinkel GJ (2002) Endovascular coiling versus neurosurgical clipping in patients with a ruptured basilar tip aneurysm. J Neurol Neurosurg Psychiatry 73:591-593

Lylyk P, Ceratto R, Hurvitz D, Basso A (1998) Treatment of a vertebral dissecting aneurysm with stents and coils: technical case report. Neurosurgery 43:385-388

Lylyk P, Cohen JE, Ceratto R, Ferrario A, Miranda C (2001) Combined endovascular treatment of dissecting vertebral artery aneurysms by using stents and coils. J Neurosurg 94:427-432

MacDonald A, Mendelow AD (1988) Xanthochromia revisited: a re-evaluation of lumbar puncture and CT scanning in the diagnosis of subarachnoid haemorrhage. J Neurol Neurosurg Psychiatry 51:342-344

Macdonald RL, Wallace MC, Kestle JR (1993) Role of angiography following aneurysm surgery. J Neurosurg 79:826-832

Macdonald RL, Wallace MC, Montanera WJ, Glen JA (1995) Pathological effects of angioplasty on vasospastic carotid arteries in a rabbit model. J Neurosurg 83:111-117

Macdonald RL, Mojtahedi S, Johns L, Kowalczuk A (1998) Randomized comparison of Guglielmi detachable coils and cellulose acetate polymer for treatment of aneurysms in dogs. Stroke 29:478-485; discussion 485-476

Malek AM, Halbach VV, Phatouros CC, Lempert TE, Meyers PM, Dowd CF, Higashida RT (2000) Balloon-assist technique for endovascular coil embolization of geometrically difficult intracranial aneurysms. Neurosurgery 46:1397-1406; discussion 1406-1397

Massoud TF, Turjman F, Ji C, Vinuela F, Guglielmi G, Gobin YP, Duckwiler GR (1995) Endovascular treatment of fusiform aneurysms with stents and coils: technical feasibility in a swine model. AJNR Am J Neuroradiol 16:1953-1963

Mathis JM, Barr JD, Jungreis CA, Yonas H, Sekhar LN, Vincent D, Pentheny SL, Horton JA (1995) Temporary balloon test occlusion of the internal carotid artery: experience in 500 cases. AJNR Am J Neuroradiol 16:749-754

Mattle H, Kohler S, Huber P, Rohner M, Steinsiepe KF (1989) Anticoagulation-related intracranial extracerebral haemorrhage. J Neurol Neurosurg Psychiatry 52:829-837

Mawad ME, Klucznik RP (1995) Giant serpentine aneurysms: radiographic features and endovascular treatment. AJNR Am J Neuroradiol 16:1053-1060

Mayfrank L, Hutter BO, Kohorst Y, Kreitschmann-Andermahr I, Rohde V, Thron A, Gilsbach JM (2001) Influence of intraventricular hemorrhage on outcome after rupture of intracranial aneurysm. Neurosurg Rev 24:185-191

McCormick WF, Acosta-Rua GJ (1970) The size of intracranial saccular aneurysms. An autopsy study. J Neurosurg 33:422-427

McDougall CG, Halbach VV, Dowd CF, Higashida RT, Larsen DW, Hieshima GB (1998) Causes and management of aneurysmal hemorrhage occurring during embolization with Guglielmi detachable coils. J Neurosurg 89:87-92

McKissock W, Richardson A, Walsh L, Owen E (1964) Multiple intracranial aneurysms. Lancet 15:623-626

Menovsky T, van Rooij WJ, Sluzewski M, Wijnalda D (2002) Coiling of ruptured pericallosal artery aneurysms. Neurosurgery 50:11–14; discussion 14–15

Mericle RA, Wakhloo AK, Rodriguez R, Guterman LR, Hopkins LN (1997) Temporary balloon protection as an adjunct to endosaccular coiling of wide-necked cerebral aneurysms: technical note. Neurosurgery 41:975-978

Mericle RA, Lanzino G, Wakhloo AK, Guterman LR, Hopkins LN (1998) Stenting and secondary coiling of intracranial internal carotid artery aneurysm: technical case report. Neurosurgery 43:1229-1234

Minematsu K, Li L, Fisher M, Sotak CH, Davis MA, Fiandaca MS (1992) Diffusion-weighted magnetic resonance imaging: rapid and quantitative detection of focal brain ischemia. Neurology 42:235-240

Mizoi K, Suzuki J, Yoshimoto T (1989) Surgical treatment of multiple aneurysms. Review of experience with 372 cases. Acta Neurochir (Wien) 96:8-14

Mizoi K, Yoshimoto T, Nagamine Y, Kayama T, Koshu K (1995) How to treat incidental cerebral aneurysms: a review of 139 consecutive cases. Surg Neurol 44:114-120; discussion 120-111

Mohsenipour I, Ortler M, Twerdy K, Schmutzhard E, Attlmayr G, Aichner F (1994) Isolated aneurysm of a spinal radicular artery presenting as spinal subarachnoid haemorrhage. J Neurol Neurosurg Psychiatry 57:767-768

Molyneux A, Kerr R, Stratton I, Sandercock P, Clarke M, Shrimpton J, Holman R (2002) International Subarachnoid Aneurysm Trial (ISAT) of neurosurgical clipping versus endovascular coiling in 2143 patients with ruptured intracranial aneurysms: a randomised trial. Lancet 360:1267-1274

Moret J, Pierot L, Boulin A, Castaings L, Rey A (1996) Endovascular treatment of anterior communicating artery aneurysms using Guglielmi detachable coils. Neuroradiology 38:800-805

Moret J, Cognard C, Weill A, Castaings L, Rey A (1997) Reconstruction technic in the treatment of wide-neck intracranial aneurysms. Long-term angiographic and clinical results. Apropos of 56 cases. J Neuroradiol 24:30-44

Moseley ME, Mintorovitch J, Cohen Y, Asgari HS, Derugin N, Norman D, Kucharczyk J (1990) Early detection of ischemic injury: comparison of spectroscopy, diffusion-, T2-, and magnetic susceptibility-weighted MRI in cats. Acta Neurochir (Wien) [Suppl] 51:207-209

Murayama Y, Vinuela F, Suzuki Y, Do HM, Massoud TF, Guglielmi G, Ji C, Iwaki M, Kusakabe M, Kamio M, Abe T (1997) Ion implantation and protein coating of detachable coils for endovascular treatment of cerebral aneurysms: concepts and preliminary results in swine models. Neurosurgery 40:1233-1243; discussion 1243-1234

Murayama Y, Vinuela F, Duckwiler GR, Gobin YP, Guglielmi G (1999) Embolization of incidental cerebral aneurysms by using the Guglielmi detachable coil system. J Neurosurg 90:207-214

Murayama Y, Vinuela F, Tateshima S, Vinuela F Jr, Akiba Y (2000) Endovascular treatment of experimental aneurysms by use of a combination of liquid embolic agents and protective devices. AJNR Am J Neuroradiol 21:1726-1735

Murayama Y, Vinuela F, Tateshima S, Song JK, Gonzalez NR, Wallace MP (2001) Bioabsorbable polymeric material coils for embolization of intracranial aneurysms: a preliminary experimental study. J Neurosurg 94:454-463

Nakahara I, Taki W, Kikuchi H, Sakai N, Isaka F, Oowaki H, Kondo A, Iwasaki K, Nishi S (1999) Endovascular treatment of aneurysms on the feeding arteries of intracranial arteriovenous malformations. Neuroradiology 41:60-66

Nanda A, Vannemreddy PS, Polin RS, Willis BK (2000) Intracranial aneurysms and cocaine abuse: analysis of prognostic indicators. Neurosurgery 46:1063-1067; discussion 1067-1069

Nehls DG, Flom RA, Carter LP, Spetzler RF (1985) Multiple intracranial aneurysms: determining the site of rupture. J Neurosurg 63:342-348

Nelson PK (1998) Neurointerventional management of intracranial aneurysms. Neurosurg Clin North Am 9:879-895

Nelson PK, Levy DI (2001) Balloon-assisted coil embolization of wide-necked aneurysms of the internal carotid artery: medium-term angiographic and clinical follow-up in 22 patients. AJNR Am J Neuroradiol 22:19-26

Newell DW, Elliott JP, Eskridge JM, Winn HR (1999) Endovascular therapy for aneurysmal vasospasm. Crit Care Clin 15:685-699, v

Noguchi K, Ogawa T, Inugami A, Toyoshima H, Sugawara S, Hatazawa J, Fujita H, Shimosegawa E, Kanno I, Okudera T et al (1995) Acute subarachnoid hemorrhage: MR imaging with fluid-attenuated inversion recovery pulse sequences. Radiology 196:773-777

Nornes H (1973) The role of intracranial pressure in the arrest of hemorrhage in patients with ruptured intracranial aneurysm. J Neurosurg 39:226-234

Nowak G, Schwachenwald R, Arnold H (1994) Early management in poor grade aneurysm patients. Acta Neurochir (Wien) 126:33-37

Okahara M, Kiyosue H, Yamashita M, Nagatomi H, Hata H, Saginoya T, Sagara Y, Mori H (2002) Diagnostic accuracy of magnetic resonance angiography for cerebral aneurysms in correlation with 3D-digital subtraction angiographic images: a study of 133 aneurysms. Stroke 33:1803–8

Okamoto K, Horisawa R, Kawamura T, Asai A, Ogino M, Takagi T, Ohno Y (2003) Family history and risk of subarachnoid hemorrhage: a case-control study in Nagoya, Japan. Stroke 34:422-426

Origitano TC, Wascher TM, Reichman OH, Anderson DE (1990) Sustained increased cerebral blood flow with prophylactic hypertensive hypervolemic hemodilution («triple-H» therapy) after subarachnoid hemorrhage. Neurosurgery 27:729-739; discussion 739-740

Ostergaard JR (1991) Headache as a warning symptom of impending aneurysmal subarachnoid haemorrhage. Cephalalgia 11:53-55

Padolecchia R, Guglielmi G, Puglioli M, Castagna M, Nardini V, Collavoli P, Guidetti G, Dazzi M, Zucchi V, Narducci P (2001) Role of electrothrombosis in aneurysm treatment with Guglielmi detachable coils: an in vitro scanning electron microscopic study. AJNR Am J Neuoradiol 22: 1757-1760

Pasqualin A, Battaglia R, Scienza R, Da Pian R (1988) Italian cooperative study on giant intracranial aneurysms: 3. Modalities of treatment. Acta Neurochir (Wien) [Suppl] 42:60-64

Patel AN, Richardson AE (1971) Ruptured intracranial aneurysms in the first two decades of life. A study of 58 patients. J Neurosurg 35:571-576

Peerless SJ, Ferguson GG, Drake CG (1982) Extracranial-intracranial (EC/IC) bypass in the treatment of giant intracranial aneurysms. Neurosurg Rev 5:77-81

Peerless SJ, Nemoto S, Drake CG (1987) Acute surgery for ruptured posterior circulation aneurysms. Adv Tech Stand Neurosurg 15:115-129

Peerless SJ, Hernesniemi JA, Gutman FB, Drake CG (1994) Early surgery for ruptured vertebrobasilar aneurysms. J Neurosurg 80:643-649

Perneczky A, Czech T (1984) Prognosis of oculomotor palsy following subarachnoid hemorrhage due to aneurysms of the posterior communicating artery. Zentralbl Neurochir 45:189-195

Phillips LH 2nd, Whisnant JP, O'Fallon WM, Sundt TM Jr (1980) The unchanging pattern of subarachnoid hemorrhage in a community. Neurology 30:1034-1040

Phuong LK, Link M, Wijdicks E (2002) Management of intracranial infectious aneurysms: a series of 16 cases. Neurosurgery 51:1145-1151; discussion 1151-1142

Pierot L, Boulin A, Castaings L, Rey A, Moret J (1996) Selective occlusion of basilar artery aneurysms using controlled detachable coils: report of 35 cases. Neurosurgery 38:948-953; discussion 953-944

Pierot L, Boulin A, Castaings L, Rey A, Moret J (1997) The endovascular approach in the management of patients with multiple intracranial aneurysms. Neuroradiology 39:361-366

Polin RS, Hansen CA, German P, Chadduck JB, Kassell NF (1998) Intra-arterially administered papaverine for the treatment of symptomatic cerebral vasospasm. Neurosurgery 42:1256-1264; discussion 1264-1257

Proust F, Toussaint P, Hannequin D, Rabenenoina C, Le Gars D, Freger P (1997) Outcome in 43 patients with distal anterior cerebral artery aneurysms. Stroke 28:2405-2409

Qureshi AI, Mohammad Y, Yahia AM, Luft AR, Sharma M, Tamargo RJ, Frankel MR (2000a) Ischemic events associated with unruptured intracranial aneurysms: multicenter clinical study and review of the literature. Neurosurgery 46: 282-289; discussion 289-290

Qureshi AI, Luft AR, Sharma M, Guterman LR, Hopkins LN (2000b) Prevention and treatment of thromboembolic and ischemic complications associated with endovascular procedures, part II. Clinical aspects and recommendations. Neurosurgery 46:1360-1375; discussion 1375-1366

Qureshi AI, Suri MF, Khan J, Kim SH, Fessler RD, Ringer AJ, Guterman LR, Hopkins LN (2001) Endovascular treatment of intracranial aneurysms by using Guglielmi detachable coils in awake patients: safety and feasibility. J Neurosurg 94:880-885

Raaymakers T (1999) Aneurysms in relatives of patients with subarachnoid hemorrhage: frequency and risk factors. MARS study group. Magnetic Resonance Angiography in relatives of patients with subarachnoid hemorrhage. Neurology 53:982-988

Raaymakers T (2000) Functional outcome and quality of life after angiography and operation for unruptured intracranial aneurysms. On behalf of the MARS Study Group. J Neurol Neurosurg Psychiatry 68:571-576

Raaymakers T, Rinkel G, Limburg M, Algra A (1998a) Mortality and morbidity of surgery for unruptured intracranial aneurysms. Stroke 29:1531-1538

Raaymakers TW, Rinkel GJ, Ramos LM (1998b) Initial and follow-up screening for aneurysms in families with familial subarachnoid hemorrhage. Neurology 51:1125-1130

Raaymakers TW, Buys PC, Verbeeten B Jr, Ramos LM, Witkamp TD, Hulsmans FJ, Mali WP, Algra A, Bonsel GJ, Bossuyt PM, Vonk CM, Buskens E, Limburg M, van Gijn J, Gorissen A, Greebe P, Albrecht KW, Tulleken CA, Rinkel GJ (1999) MR angiography as a screening tool for intracranial aneurysms: feasibility, test characteristics, and interobserver agreement. AJR Am J Roentgenol 173:1469-1475

Raymond J, Roy D (1997) Safety and efficacy of endovascular treatment of acutely ruptured aneurysms. Neurosurgery 41:1235-1245; discussion 1245-1236

Regli L, Uske A, de Tribolet N (1999) Endovascular coil placement compared with surgical clipping for the treatment of unruptured middle cerebral artery aneurysms: a consecutive series. J Neurosurg 90:1025-1030

Reith W, Hasegawa Y, Latour LL, Dardzinski BJ, Sotak CH, Fisher M (1995) Multislice diffusion mapping for 3-D evolution of cerebral ischemia in a rat stroke model. Neurology 45:172-177

Rice BJ, Peerless SJ, Drake CG (1990) Surgical treatment of unruptured aneurysms of the posterior circulation. J Neurosurg 73:165-173

Richling B, Gruber A, Bavinzski G, Killer M (1995) GDC-system embolization for brain aneurysms – location and follow-up. Acta Neurochir 134:177-183

Ricolfi F, Le Guerinel C, Blustajn J, Combes C, Brugieres P, Melon E, Gaston A (1998) Rupture during treatment of recently ruptured aneurysms with Guglielmi electrodetachable coils. AJNR Am J Neuroradiol 19:1653-1658

Rinkel GJ, Wijdicks EF, Hasan D, Kienstra GE, Franke CL, Hageman LM, Vermeulen M, van Gijn J (1991) Outcome in patients with subarachnoid haemorrhage and negative angiography according to pattern of haemorrhage on computed tomography. Lancet 338:964-968

Rinkel GJ, Prins NE, Algra A (1997) Outcome of aneurysmal subarachnoid hemorrhage in patients on anticoagulant treatment. Stroke 28:6-9

Rinkel GJ, Djibuti M, Algra A, van Gijn J (1998) Prevalence and risk of rupture of intracranial aneurysms: a systematic review. Stroke 29:251-256

Rinne J, Hernesniemi J, Puranen M, Saari T (1994) Multiple intracranial aneurysms in a defined population: prospective angiographic and clinical study. Neurosurgery 35:803-808

Rinne J, Hernesniemi J, Niskanen M, Vapalahti M (1995) Management outcome for multiple intracranial aneurysms. Neurosurgery 36:31-37; discussion 37-38

Ronkainen A, Hernesniemi J, Puranen M, Niemitukia L, Vanninen R, Ryynanen M, Kuivaniemi H, Tromp G (1997) Familial intracranial aneurysms. Lancet 349:380-384

Roos YB, Hasan D, Vermeulen M (1995) Outcome in patients with large intraventricular haemorrhages: a volumetric study. J Neurol Neurosurg Psychiatry 58:622-624

Roos YB, de Haan RJ, Beenen LF, Groen RJ, Albrecht KW, Vermeulen M (2000) Complications and outcome in patients with aneurysmal subarachnoid haemorrhage: a prospective hospital based cohort study in the Netherlands. J Neurol Neurosurg Psychiatry 68:337-341

Rordorf G, Koroshetz WJ, Copen WA, Gonzalez G, Yamada K, Schaefer PW, Schwamm LH, Ogilvy CS, Sorensen AG (1999) Diffusion- and perfusion-weighted imaging in vasospasm after subarachnoid hemorrhage. Stroke 30:599-605

Ross JS, Masaryk TJ, Modic MT, Ruggieri PM, Haacke EM, Selman WR (1990) Intracranial aneurysms: evaluation by MR angiography. AJNR Am J Neuroradiol 11:449-455

Rowe JG, Molyneux AJ, Byrne JV, Renowden S, Aziz TZ (1996) Endovascular treatment of intracranial aneurysms: a minimally invasive approach with advantages for elderly patients. Age Ageing 25:372-376

Rumboldt Z, Kalousek M, Castillo M (2003) Hyperacute subarachnoid hemorrhage on T2-weighted MR images. AJNR Am J Neuroradiol 24:472-475

Sacco RL, Wolf PA, Bharucha NE, Meeks SL, Kannel WB, Charette LJ, McNamara PM, Palmer EP, D'Agostino R (1984) Subarachnoid and intracerebral hemorrhage: natural history, prognosis, and precursive factors in the Framingham Study. Neurology 34:847-854

Saitoh H, Hayakawa K, Nishimura K, Okuno Y, Teraura T, Yumitori K, Okumura A (1995) Rerupture of cerebral aneurysms during angiography. AJNR Am J Neuroradiol 16:539-542

Sakata S, Fujii K, Matsushima T, Fujiwara S, Fukui M, Matsubara T, Nagatomi H, Kuromatsu C, Kamikaseda K (1993) Aneurysm of the posterior cerebral artery: report of eleven cases – surgical approaches and procedures. Neurosurgery 32:163-167; discussion 167-168

Sasaki O, Ogawa H, Koike T, Koizumi T, Tanaka R (1991) A clinicopathological study of dissecting aneurysms of the intracranial vertebral artery. J Neurosurg 75:874-882

Schievink WI (1997) Genetics of intracranial aneurysms. Neurosurgery 40:651-662; discussion 662-653

Schievink WI (2001) Spontaneous dissection of the carotid and vertebral arteries. N Engl J Med 344:898-906

Schievink WI, Wijdicks EF, Piepgras DG, Chu CP, O'Fallon WM, Whisnant JP (1995) The poor prognosis of ruptured intracranial aneurysms of the posterior circulation. J Neurosurg 82:791-795

Schievink WI, Parisi JE, Piepgras DG (1997) Familial intracranial aneurysms: an autopsy study. Neurosurgery 41:1247-1251; discussion 1251-1242

Schwartz RB, Tice HM, Hooten SM, Hsu L, Stieg PE (1994) Evaluation of cerebral aneurysms with helical CT: correlation with conventional angiography and MR angiography. Radiology 192:717-722

Schwartz TH, Solomon RA (1996) Perimesencephalic nonaneurysmal subarachnoid hemorrhage: review of the literature. Neurosurgery 39:433-440; discussion 440

Seifert V (1997) Neurosurgical therapy of subarachnoid hemorrhage. Wien Med Wochenschr 147:152-158

Sekhon LH, Morgan MK, Sorby W, Grinnell V (1998) Combined endovascular stent implantation and endosaccular coil placement for the treatment of a wide-necked vertebral artery aneurysm: technical case report. Neurosurgery 43: 380-383; discussion 384

Serbinenko FA (1974a) Balloon occlusion of saccular aneurysms of the cerebral arteries. Vopr Neirokhir. 1974 Jul-Aug; (4):8-15

Serbinenko FA (1974b) Balloon catheterization and occlusion of major cerebral vessels. J Neurosurg 41:125-145

Sethi H, Moore A, Dervin J, Clifton A, MacSweeney JE (2000) Hydrocephalus: comparison of clipping and embolization in aneurysm treatment. J Neurosurg 92:991-994

Sevick RJ, Tsuruda JS, Schmalbrock P (1990) Three-dimensional time-of-flight MR angiography in the evaluation of cerebral aneurysms. J Comput Assist Tomogr 14:874-881

Shellock FG, Detrick MS, Brant-Zawadski MN (1997) MR compatibility of Guglielmi detachable coils. Radiology 203:568-570

Shimoda M, Takeuchi M, Tominaga J, Oda S, Kumasaka A, Tsugane R (2001) Asymptomatic versus symptomatic infarcts from vasospasm in patients with subarachnoid hemorrhage: serial magnetic resonance imaging. Neurosurgery 49:1341-1348; discussion 1348-1350

Sindou M, Pelissou-Guyotat I, Mertens P, Keravel Y, Athayde AA (1988) Pericallosal aneurysms. Surg Neurol 30:434-440

Sindou M, Acevedo JC, Turjman F (1998) Aneurysmal remnants

after microsurgical clipping: classification and results from a prospective angiographic study (in a consecutive series of 305 operated intracranial aneurysms). Acta Neurochir (Wien) 140:1153-1159

Solander S, Ulhoa A, Vinuela F, Duckwiler GR, Gobin YP, Martin NA, Frazee JG, Guglielmi G (1999) Endovascular treatment of multiple intracranial aneurysms by using Guglielmi detachable coils. J Neurosurg 90:857-864

Solomon RA, Mayer SA, Tarmey JJ (1996) Relationship between the volume of craniotomies for cerebral aneurysm performed at New York state hospitals and in-hospital mortality. Stroke 27:13-17

Song JK, Elliott JP, Eskridge JM (1997) Neuroradiologic diagnosis and treatment of vasospasm. Neuroimaging Clin North Am 7:819-835

Standard SC, Ahuja A, Guterman LR, Chavis TD, Gibbons KJ, Barth AP, Hopkins LN (1995) Balloon test occlusion of the internal carotid artery with hypotensive challenge. AJNR Am J Neuroradiol 16:1453-1458

Stapf C, Mohr JP, Pile-Spellman J, Sciacca RR, Hartmann A, Schumacher HC, Mast H (2002) Concurrent arterial aneurysms in brain arteriovenous malformations with haemorrhagic presentation. J Neurol Neurosurg Psychiatry 73:294-298

Stehbens WE (1989) Etiology of intracranial berry aneurysms. J Neurosurg 70:823-831

Steinberg GK, Guppy KH, Adler JR, Silverberg GD (1992) Stereotactic, angiography-guided clipping of a distal, mycotic intracranial aneurysm using the Cosman-Roberts-Wells system: technical note. Neurosurgery 30:408-411

Suzuki J, Komatsu S, Sato T, Sakurai Y (1980) Correlation between CT findings and subsequent development of cerebral infarction due to vasospasm in subarachnoid haemorrhage. Acta Neurochir (Wien) 55:63-70

Suzuki J, Kwak R, Katakura R (1980) Review of incompletely occluded surgically treated cerebral aneurysms. Surg Neurol 13:306-310

Szikora I, Guterman LR, Wells KM, Hopkins LN (1994) Combined use of stents and coils to treat experimental wide-necked carotid aneurysms: preliminary results. AJNR Am J Neuroradiol 15:1091-1102

Tan WS, Jafar JJ, Abejo R, Spigos DG, Crowell RM, Capek V (1986) Regional cerebral blood flow assessment prior to balloon detachment in the treatment of intracranial giant aneurysms. Acta Radiol [Suppl] 369:116-119

Tateshima S, Murayama Y, Gobin YP, Duckwiler GR, Guglielmi G, Vinuela F (2000) Endovascular treatment of basilar tip aneurysms using Guglielmi detachable coils: anatomic and clinical outcomes in 73 patients from a single institution. Neurosurgery 47:1332-1339; discussion 1339-1342

Taylor CL, Yuan Z, Selman WR, Ratcheson RA, Rimm AA (1995) Cerebral arterial aneurysm formation and rupture in 20,767 elderly patients: hypertension and other risk factors. J Neurosurg 83:812-819

Teunissen LL, Rinkel GJ, Algra A, van Gijn J (1996) Risk factors for subarachnoid hemorrhage: a systematic review. Stroke 27:544-549

Thielen KR, Nichols DA, Fulgham JR, Piepgras DG (1997) Endovascular treatment of cerebral aneurysms following incomplete clipping. J Neurosurg 87:184-189

Thompson RC, Steinberg GK, Levy RP, Marks MP (1998) The management of patients with arteriovenous malformations and associated intracranial aneurysms. Neurosurgery 43:202-211; discussion 211-202

Thornton J, Aletich VA, Debrun GM, Alazzaz A, Misra M, Charbel F, Ausman JI (2000a) Endovascular treatment of paraclinoid aneurysms. Surg Neurol 54:288-299

Thornton J, Bashir Q, Aletich VA, Debrun GM, Ausman JI, Charbel FT (2000b) What percentage of surgically clipped intracranial aneurysms have residual necks? Neurosurgery 46:1294-1298; discussion 1298-1300

Timperman PE, Tomsick TA, Tew JM Jr, van Loveren HR (1995) Aneurysm formation after carotid occlusion. AJNR Am J Neuroradiol 16:329-331

Tokunaga K, Kinugasa K, Mandai S, Handa A, Hirotsune N, Ohmoto T (1998) Partial thrombosis of canine carotid bifurcation aneurysms with cellulose acetate polymer. Neurosurgery 42:1135-1142; discussion 1142-1134

Tong FC, Cloft HJ, Dion JE (2000) Endovascular treatment of intracranial aneurysms with Guglielmi detachable coils: emphasis on new techniques. J Clin Neurosci 7:244-253

Torner JC, Kassell NF, Wallace RB, Adams HP Jr (1981) Preoperative prognostic factors for rebleeding and survival in aneurysm patients receiving antifibrinolytic therapy: report of the Cooperative Aneurysm Study. Neurosurgery 9:506-513

Turjman F, Massoud TF, Vinuela F, Sayre JW, Guglielmi G, Duckwiler G (1994) Aneurysms related to cerebral arteriovenous malformations: superselective angiographic assessment in 58 patients. AJNR Am J Neuroradiol 15:1601-1605

Uda K, Murayama Y, Gobin YP, Duckwiler GR, Vinuela F (2001) Endovascular treatment of basilar artery trunk aneurysms with Guglielmi detachable coils: clinical experience with 41 aneurysms in 39 patients. J Neurosurg 95:624-632

Vajda J (1992) Multiple intracranial aneurysms: a high risk condition. Acta Neurochir (Wien) 118:59-75

Vallee JN, Aymard A, Vicaut E, Reis M, Merland JJ (2003) Endovascular treatment of basilar tip aneurysms with Guglielmi detachable coils: predictors of immediate and long-term results with multivariate analysis 6-year experience. Radiology 226:867-879

Van der Wee N, Rinkel GJ, Hasan D, van Gijn J (1995) Detection of subarachnoid haemorrhage on early CT: is lumbar puncture still needed after a negative scan? J Neurol Neurosurg Psychiatry 58:357-359

Van Gijn J, van Dongen KJ (1982) The time course of aneurysmal haemorrhage on computed tomograms. Neuroradiology 23:153-156

Van Rooij WJ, Sluzewski M, Metz NH, Nijssen PC, Wijnalda D, Rinkel GJ, Tulleken CA (2000) Carotid balloon occlusion for large and giant aneurysms: evaluation of a new test occlusion protocol. Neurosurgery 47:116-121; discussion 122

Van Rooij WJ, Sluzewski M, Menovsky T, Wijnalda D (2003) Coiling of saccular basilar trunk aneurysms. Neuroradiology 45:19-21

Vermeulen M, van Gijn J, Hijdra A, van Crevel H (1984) Causes of acute deterioration in patients with a ruptured intracranial aneurysm. A prospective study with serial CT scanning. J Neurosurg 60:935-939

Vermeulen M, Hasan D, Blijenberg BG, Hijdra A, van Gijn J (1989) Xanthochromia after subarachnoid haemorrhage needs no revisitation. J Neurol Neurosurg Psychiatry 52: 826-828

Vieco PT, Shuman WP, Alsofrom GF, Gross CE (1995) Detection of circle of Willis aneurysms in patients with acute subarachnoid hemorrhage: a comparison of CT angiography and digital subtraction angiography. AJR Am J Roentgenol 165:425-430

Vieco PT, Morin EE 3rd, Gross CE (1996) CT angiography in the examination of patients with aneurysm clips. AJNR Am J Neuroradiol 17:455-457

Vinuela F, Duckwiler G, Mawad M (1997) Guglielmi detachable coil embolization of acute intracranial aneurysm: perioperative anatomical and clinical outcome in 403 patients. J Neurosurg 86:475-482

Vora YY, Suarez-Almazor M, Steinke DE, Martin ML, Findlay JM (1999) Role of transcranial Doppler monitoring in the diagnosis of cerebral vasospasm after subarachnoid hemorrhage. Neurosurgery 44:1237-1247; discussion 1247-1238

Wanke I, Dorfler A, Dietrich U, Aalders T, Forsting M (2000) Combined endovascular therapy of ruptured aneurysms and cerebral vasospasm. Neuroradiology 42:926-929

Wanke I, Doerfler A, Dietrich U, Egelhof T, Schoch B, Stolke D, Forsting M (2002) Endovascular treatment of unruptured intracranial aneurysms. AJNR Am J Neuroradiol 23: 756-761

Wanke I, Doerfler A, Schoch B, Stolke D, Forsting M (2003) Treatment of wide-necked intracranial aneurysms with a self-expanding stent system: initial clinical experience. AJNR Am J Neuroradiol 24:1192-1199

Warach S, Chien D, Li W, Ronthal M, Edelman RR (1992) Fast magnetic resonance diffusion-weighted imaging of acute human stroke. Neurology 42:1717-1723

Wardlaw J, White P (2000) The detection and management of unruptured intracranial aneurysms. Brain 123:205-221

Wardlaw JM, Cannon JC (1996) Color transcranial „power“ Doppler ultrasound of intracranial aneurysms. J Neurosurg 84:459-461

Wardlaw JM, White PM (2000) The detection and management of unruptured intracranial aneurysms. Brain 123:205-221

Weaver JP, Fisher M (1994) Subarachnoid hemorrhage: an update of pathogenesis, diagnosis and management. J Neurol Sci 125:119-131

Weber W, Henkes H, Kuhne D (2000) Stent implantation into the basilar artery for supporting endovascular aneurysm treatment. Nervenarzt 71:843-848

Weber W, Yousry TA, Felber SR, Henkes H, Nahser HC, Roer N, Kuhne D (2001) Noninvasive follow-up of GDC-treated saccular aneurysms by MR angiography. Eur Radiol 11: 1792-1797

Weir B, MacDonald N, Mielke B (1978) Intracranial vascular complications of choriocarcinoma. Neurosurgery 2:138-142

Weir BK, Kongable GL, Kassell NF, Schultz JR, Truskowski LL, Sigrest A (1998) Cigarette smoking as a cause of aneurysmal subarachnoid hemorrhage and risk for vasospasm: a report of the Cooperative Aneurysm Study. J Neurosurg 89:405-411

White PM, Wardlaw JM, Easton V (2000) Can noninvasive imaging accurately depict intracranial aneurysms? A systematic review. Radiology 217:361-370

White PM, Wardlaw JM, Teasdale E, Sloss S, Cannon J, Easton V (2001) Power transcranial Doppler ultrasound in the detection of intracranial aneurysms. Stroke 32:1291-1297

Wiebers D (1998) Unruptured intracranial aneurysms – risk of rupture and risks of surgical intervention. The international study of unruptured intracranial aneurysms investigators. New Engl J Med 339:1725-1733

Wiebers D, Whisnant JP, O'Fallon WM (1981) The natural history of unruptured intracranial aneurysms. N Engl J Med 304:696-698

Wiebers D, Torner J, Meissner I (1992) Impact of unruptured intracranial aneurysms on public health in the United States. Stroke 23:1416-1419

Wiebers D, Whisnant JP, Huston J 3rd, Meissner I, Brown RD Jr, Piepgras DG, Forbes GS, Thielen K, Nichols D, O'Fallon WM, Peacock J, Jaeger L, Kassell NF, Kongable-Beckman GL, Torner JC (2003) Unruptured intracranial aneurysms: natural history, clinical outcome, and risks of surgical and endovascular treatment. Lancet 362:103-110

Wiesmann M, Mayer TE, Yousry I, Medele R, Hamann GF, Bruckmann H (2002) Detection of hyperacute subarachnoid hemorrhage of the brain by using magnetic resonance imaging. J Neurosurg 96:684-689

Winn HR, Richardson AE, Jane JA (1977) The long-term prognosis in untreated cerebral aneurysms I. The incidence of late hemorrhage in cerebral aneurysm: a 10-year evaluation of 364 patients. Ann Neurol 1:358-370

Winn HR, Almaani WS, Berga SL, Jane JA, Richardson AE (1983) The long-term outcome in patients with multiple aneurysms. Incidence of late hemorrhage and implications for treatment of incidental aneurysms. J Neurosurg 59:642-651

Wintermark M, Uske A, Chalaron M, Regli L, Maeder P, Meuli R, Schnyder P, Binaghi S (2003) Multislice computerized tomography angiography in the evaluation of intracranial aneurysms: a comparison with intraarterial digital subtraction angiography. J Neurosurg 98:828-836

Yalamanchili K, Rosenwasser RH, Thomas JE, Liebman K, McMorrow C, Gannon P (1998) Frequency of cerebral vasospasm in patients treated with endovascular occlusion of intracranial aneurysms. AJNR Am J Neuroradiol 19:553-558

Yamaura A, Ono J, Hirai S (2000) Clinical picture of intracranial non-traumatic dissecting aneurysm. Neuropathology 20:85-90

Yasargil MG (1984) Multiple aneurysms in microneurosurgery, vol 1. Thieme, Stuttgart, pp 305-328

Yasui N, Suzuki A, Nishimura H, Suzuki K, Abe T (1997) Long-term follow-up study of unruptured intracranial aneurysms. Neurosurgery 40:1155-1159; discussion 1159-1160

Yonas H, Linskey M, Johnson DW, Horton JA, Janecka IP, Witt JP, Jungreis C, Hirsch WL, Sekhar LN (1992) Internal carotid balloon test occlusion does require quantitative CBF. AJNR Am J Neuroradiol 13:1147-1152

Yong-Zhong G, van Alphen HA (1990) Pathogenesis and histopathology of saccular aneurysms: review of the literature. Neurol Res 12:249-255

Subject Index

List of Contributors

CHRISTOPHE COGNARD, MD
Service de Neuroradiologie
Diagnostique et Therapeutique
Hôpital Purpan
Centre Hospitalier Universitaire
Place du Docteur-Baylac
31059 Toulouse Cedex
France

ARND DÖRFLER, MD
Institute of Diagnostic and Interventional Radiology
Department of Neuroradiology
University of Essen
Hufelandstrasse 55
45122 Essen
Germany

MICHAEL FORSTING, MD, PhD
Professor of Neuroradiology
Institute of Diagnostic and Interventional Radiology
Department of Neuroradiology
University of Essen
Hufelandstrasse 55
45122 Essen
Germany

WILHELM KÜKER, MD
Department of Neuroradiology
University of Tübingen
Hoppe-Seyler-Strasse 3
72076 Tübingen
Germany

LAURENT PIEROT, MD
Service de Radiologie
Hôpital Maison-Blanche
45 rue Cognacq-Jay
51092 Reims Cedex
France

LAURENT SPELLE, MD
Département de Neuroradiologie interventionelle
et fonctionelle
Fondation A. de Rothschild
25–29 Rue Manin
75940 Paris Cedex
France

ISTVÁN SZIKORA, MD
Professor of Neuroradiology
Nagybányai ut 86/b
1025 Budapest
Hungary

ISABEL WANKE, MD
Institute of Diagnostic and Interventional Radiology
Department of Neuroradiology
University of Essen
Hufelandstrasse 55
45122 Essen
Germany

List of Co[illegible]

MEDICAL RADIOLOGY Diagnostic Imaging and Radiation Oncology

Titles in the series already published

DIAGNOSTIC IMAGING

Innovations in Diagnostic Imaging
Edited by J. H. Anderson

Radiology of the Upper Urinary Tract
Edited by E. K. Lang

The Thymus - Diagnostic Imaging, Functions, and Pathologic Anatomy
Edited by E. Walter, E. Willich, and W. R. Webb

Interventional Neuroradiology
Edited by A. Valavanis

Radiology of the Pancreas
Edited by A. L. Baert, co-edited by G. Delorme

Radiology of the Lower Urinary Tract
Edited by E. K. Lang

Magnetic Resonance Angiography
Edited by I. P. Arlart, G. M. Bongartz, and G. Marchal

Contrast-Enhanced MRI of the Breast
S. Heywang-Köbrunner and R. Beck

Spiral CT of the Chest
Edited by M. Rémy-Jardin and J. Rémy

Radiological Diagnosis of Breast Diseases
Edited by M. Friedrich and E.A. Sickles

Radiology of the Trauma
Edited by M. Heller and A. Fink

Biliary Tract Radiology
Edited by P. Rossi

Radiological Imaging of Sports Injuries
Edited by C. Masciocchi

Modern Imaging of the Alimentary Tube
Edited by A. R. Margulis

Diagnosis and Therapy of Spinal Tumors
Edited by P. R. Algra, J. Valk, and J. J. Heimans

Interventional Magnetic Resonance Imaging
Edited by J.F. Debatin and G. Adam

Abdominal and Pelvic MRI
Edited by A. Heuck and M. Reiser

Orthopedic Imaging
Techniques and Applications
Edited by A. M. Davies and H. Pettersson

Radiology of the Female Pelvic Organs
Edited by E. K.Lang

Magnetic Resonance of the Heart and Great Vessels
Clinical Applications
Edited by J. Bogaert, A.J. Duerinckx, and F. E. Rademakers

Modern Head and Neck Imaging
Edited by S. K. Mukherji and J. A. Castelijns

Radiological Imaging of Endocrine Diseases
Edited by J. N. Bruneton in collaboration with B. Padovani and M.-Y. Mourou

Trends in Contrast Media
Edited by H. S. Thomsen, R. N. Muller, and R. F. Mattrey

Functional MRI
Edited by C. T. W. Moonen and P. A. Bandettini

Radiology of the Pancreas
2nd Revised Edition
Edited by A. L. Baert
Co-edited by G. Delorme and L. Van Hoe

Emergency Pediatric Radiology
Edited by H. Carty

Spiral CT of the Abdomen
Edited by F. Terrier, M. Grossholz,and C. D. Becker

Liver Malignancies
Diagnostic and Interventional Radiology
Edited by C. Bartolozzi and R. Lencioni

Medical Imaging of the Spleen
Edited by A. M. De Schepper and F. Vanhoenacker

Radiology of Peripheral Vascular Diseases
Edited by E. Zeitler

Diagnostic Nuclear Medicine
Edited by C. Schiepers

Radiology of Blunt Trauma of the Chest
P. Schnyder and M. Wintermark

Portal Hypertension
Diagnostic Imaging-Guided Therapy
Edited by P. Rossi
Co-edited by P. Ricci and L. Broglia

Recent Advances in Diagnostic Neuroradiology
Edited by Ph. Demaerel

Virtual Endoscopy and Related 3D Techniques
Edited by P. Rogalla, J. Terwisscha Van Scheltinga, and B. Hamm

Multislice CT
Edited by M. F. Reiser, M. Takahashi, M. Modic, and R. Bruening

Pediatric Uroradiology
Edited by R. Fotter

Transfontanellar Doppler Imaging in Neonates
A. Couture and C. Veyrac

Radiology of AIDS
A Practical Approach
Edited by J.W.A.J. Reeders and P.C. Goodman

CT of the Peritoneum
Armando Rossi and Giorgio Rossi

Magnetic Resonance Angiography
2nd Revised Edition
Edited by I. P. Arlart, G. M. Bongratz,and G. Marchal

Pediatric Chest Imaging
Edited by Javier Lucaya and Janet L. Strife

Applications of Sonography in Head and Neck Pathology
Edited by J. N. Bruneton in collaboration with C. Raffaelli and O. Dassonville

Imaging of the Larynx
Edited by R. Hermans

3D Image Processing
Techniques and Clinical Applications
Edited by D. Caramella and C. Bartolozzi

Imaging of Orbital and Visual Pathway Pathology
Edited by W. S. Müller-Forell

Pediatric ENT Radiology
Edited by S. J. King and A. E. Boothroyd

Radiological Imaging of the Small Intestine
Edited by N. C. Gourtsoyiannis

Imaging of the Knee
Techniques and Applications
Edited by A. M. Davies and V. N. Cassar-Pullicino

Perinatal Imaging
From Ultrasound to MR Imaging
Edited by Fred E. Avni

Radiological Imaging of the Neonatal Chest
Edited by V. Donoghue

Diagnostic and Interventional Radiology in Liver Transplantation
Edited by E. Bücheler, V. Nicolas, C. E. Broelsch, X. Rogiers, and G. Krupski

Radiology of Osteoporosis
Edited by S. Grampp

Imaging Pelvic Floor Disorders
Edited by C. I. Bartram and J. O. L. DeLancey
Associate Editors: S. Halligan, F. M. Kelvin, and J. Stoker

Imaging of the Pancreas
Cystic and Rare Tumors
Edited by C. Procassi and A. J. Megibow

High Resolution Sonography of the Peripheral Nervous System
Edited by S. Peer and G. Bodner

Imaging of the Foot and Ankle
Techniques and Applications
Edited by A. M. Davies, R. W. Whitehouse, and J. P. R. Jenkins

Radiology Imaging of the Ureter
Edited by F. Joffre, Ph. Otal, and M. Soulie

Imaging of the Shoulder
Techniques and Applications
Edited by A. M. Davies and J. Hodler

Radiology of the Petrous Bone
Edited by M. Lemmerling and S. S. Kollias

Interventional Radiology in Cancer
Edited by A. Adam, R. F. Dondelinger, and P. R. Mueller

Duplex and Color Doppler Imaging of the Venous System
Edited by G. H. Mostbeck

Multidetector-Row CT of the Thorax
Edited by U. J. Schoepf

Functional Imaging of the Chest
Edited by H.-U. Kauczor

Radiology of the Pharynx and the Esophagus
Edited by O. Ekberg

Radiological Imaging in Hematological Malignancies
Edited by A. Guermazi

Imaging and Intervention in Abdominal Trauma
Edited by R. F. Dondelinger

Multislice CT
2nd Revised Edition
Edited by M. F. Reiser, M. Takahashi, M. Modic, and C. R. Becker

Intracranial Vascular Malformations and Aneurysms
From Diagnostic Work-Up to Endovascular Therapy
Edited by M. Forsting

Radiology and Imaging of the Colon
Edited by A. H. Chapman

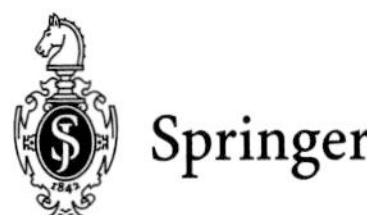

Medical Radiology Diagnostic Imaging and Radiation Oncology

Titles in the series already published

Radiation Oncology

Lung Cancer
Edited by C.W. Scarantino

Innovations in Radiation Oncology
Edited by H. R. Withers and L. J. Peters

Radiation Therapy of Head and Neck Cancer
Edited by G. E. Laramore

Gastrointestinal Cancer – Radiation Therapy
Edited by R.R. Dobelbower, Jr.

Radiation Exposure and Occupational Risks
Edited by E. Scherer, C. Streffer, and K.-R. Trott

Radiation Therapy of Benign Diseases
A Clinical Guide
S. E. Order and S. S. Donaldson

Interventional Radiation Therapy Techniques – Brachytherapy
Edited by R. Sauer

Radiopathology of Organs and Tissues
Edited by E. Scherer, C. Streffer, and K.-R. Trott

Concomitant Continuous Infusion Chemotherapy and Radiation
Edited by M. Rotman and C. J. Rosenthal

Intraoperative Radiotherapy – Clinical Experiences and Results
Edited by F. A. Calvo, M. Santos, and L.W. Brady

Radiotherapy of Intraocular and Orbital Tumors
Edited by W. E. Alberti and R. H. Sagerman

Interstitial and Intracavitary Thermoradiotherapy
Edited by M. H. Seegenschmiedt and R. Sauer

Non-Disseminated Breast Cancer
Controversial Issues in Management
Edited by G. H. Fletcher and S.H. Levitt

Current Topics in Clinical Radiobiology of Tumors
Edited by H.-P. Beck-Bornholdt

Practical Approaches to Cancer Invasion and Metastases
A Compendium of Radiation Oncologists' Responses to 40 Histories
Edited by A. R. Kagan with the Assistance of R. J. Steckel

Radiation Therapy in Pediatric Oncology
Edited by J. R. Cassady

Radiation Therapy Physics
Edited by A. R. Smith

Late Sequelae in Oncology
Edited by J. Dunst and R. Sauer

Mediastinal Tumors. Update 1995
Edited by D. E. Wood and C. R. Thomas, Jr.

Thermoradiotherapy and Thermochemotherapy
Volume 1:
Biology, Physiology, and Physics
Volume 2:
Clinical Applications
Edited by M.H. Seegenschmiedt, P. Fessenden, and C.C. Vernon

Carcinoma of the Prostate
Innovations in Management
Edited by Z. Petrovich, L. Baert, and L.W. Brady

Radiation Oncology of Gynecological Cancers
Edited by H.W. Vahrson

Carcinoma of the Bladder
Innovations in Management
Edited by Z. Petrovich, L. Baert, and L.W. Brady

Blood Perfusion and Micro-environment of Human Tumors
Implications for Clinical Radiooncology
Edited by M. Molls and P. Vaupel

Radiation Therapy of Benign Diseases
A Clinical Guide
2nd Revised Edition
S. E. Order and S. S. Donaldson

Carcinoma of the Kidney and Testis, and Rare Urologic Malignancies
Innovations in Management
Edited by Z. Petrovich, L. Baert, and L.W. Brady

Progress and Perspectives in the Treatment of Lung Cancer
Edited by P. Van Houtte, J. Klastersky, and P. Rocmans

Combined Modality Therapy of Central Nervous System Tumors
Edited by Z. Petrovich, L. W. Brady, M. L. Apuzzo, and M. Bamberg

Age-Related Macular Degeneration
Current Treatment Concepts
Edited by W. A. Alberti, G. Richard, and R. H. Sagerman

Radiotherapy of Intraocular and Orbital Tumors
2nd Revised Edition
Edited by R. H. Sagerman, and W. E. Alberti

Biological Modification of Radiation Response
Edited by C. Nieder, L. Milas, and K. K. Ang

Palliative Radiation Oncology
R. G. Parker. N. A. Janjan, and M. T. Selch

Clinical Target Volumes in Conformal and Intensity Modulated Radiation Therapy
A Clinical Guide to Cancer Treatment
Edited by V. Grégoire, P. Scalliet, and K. K. Ang

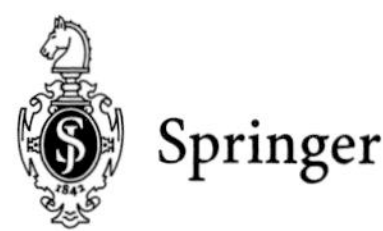

Springer

Printing and Binding: Stürtz AG, Würzburg